Imperial College London
240769168X

AF616039

Pulmonary Vascular Disorders

Progress in Respiratory Research

Vol. 41

Series Editor

Chris T. Bolliger Cape Town

Pulmonary Vascular Disorders

Volume Editors

Marc Humbert Clamart

Rogerio Souza Sao Paulo

Gérald Simonneau Clamart

82 figures, 21 in color, 45 tables, 2012

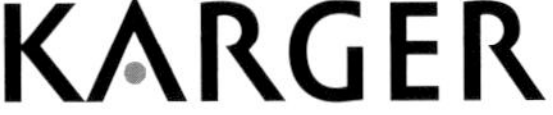

Basel · Freiburg · Paris · London · New York · New Delhi · Bangkok · Beijing · Tokyo · Kuala Lumpur · Singapore · Sydney

Marc Humbert, MD, PhD
Service de Pneumologie et Réanimation Respiratoire
Centre National de Référence de l'Hypertension Artérielle
Pulmonaire Sévère
Inserm U999
Hôpital Antoine Béclère
Asssitance Publique Hôpitaux de Paris
Université Paris-Sud 11
157, rue de la Porte de Trivaux
F-92140 Clamart
France

Rogerio Souza, MD, PhD
Pulmonary Circulation Unit
Pulmonary Department
Heart Institute
University of Sao Paulo Medical School
Av. Dr. Eneas de Carvalho Aguiar, 44
Sao Paulo 05403–000
Brazil

Gérald Simonneau, MD
Service de Pneumologie et Réanimation Respiratoire
Centre National de Référence de l'Hypertension Artérielle
Pulmonaire Sévère
Inserm U999
Hôpital Antoine Béclère
Asssitance Publique Hôpitaux de Paris
Université Paris-Sud 11
157, rue de la Porte de Trivaux
F-92140 Clamart
France

Library of Congress Cataloging-in-Publication Data

Pulmonary vascular disorders / volume editors, Marc Humbert, Rogerio Souza,
Gérald Simonneau.
p. ; cm. -- (Progress in respiratory research, ISSN 1422-2140 ; v.
41)
Includes bibliographical references and indexes.
ISBN 978-3-8055-9914-6 (hard cover : alk. paper) -- ISBN 978-3-8055-9915-3
(e-ISBN)
I. Humbert, Marc, 1963- II. Souza, Rogerio. III. Simonneau, Gérald. IV.
Series: Progress in respiratory research, v. 41. 1422-2140
[DNLM: 1. Hypertension, Pulmonary. 2. Vascular Diseases. W1 PR681DM
v.41 2012 / WG 340]

616.2'4--dc23

2012002107

Bibliographic Indices. This publication is listed in bibliographic services, including Current Contents®.

Drug Dosage. The authors and the publisher have exerted every effort to ensure that drug selection and dosage set forth in this text are in accord with current recommendations and practice at the time of publication. However, in view of ongoing research, changes in government regulations, and the constant flow of information relating to drug therapy and drug reactions, the reader is urged to check the package insert for each drug for any change in indications and dosage and for added warnings and precautions. This is particularly important when the recommended agent is a new and/or infrequently employed drug.

www.karger.com
Printed in Germany on acid-free and non-aging paper (ISO 9706) by Bosch-Druck GmbH, Ergolding
ISSN 1422–2140
e-ISSN 1662–3932
ISBN 978–3–8055–9914–6
e-ISBN 978–3–8055–9915–3

Contents

Foreword **VII**
Preface **VIII**

Chapter 1 **Updated Clinical Classification of Pulmonary Hypertension** **1**
Montani, D.; Simonneau, G. (Clamart)

Chapter 2 **Pathology of Pulmonary Arterial Hypertension** **14**
Dorfmüller, P. (Le Plessis Robinson)

Chapter 3 **Invasive Rest and Exercise Hemodynamics in the Modern Management of Pulmonary Vascular Disease: An Expanding Role in the Future** **23**
Whyte, K.F. (Auckland); Hervé, P. (Le Plessis-Robinson); Hoette, S.; Chemla, D. (Clamart)

Chapter 4 **Exercise Testing in Pulmonary Arterial Hypertension** **37**
Provencher, S.; Mainguy, V. (Québec, Qué.)

Chapter 5 **Noninvasive Exploration of the Pulmonary Circulation and the Right Heart** **48**
Vonk Noordegraaf, A. (Amsterdam); Peacock, A. (Glasgow); Naeije, R. (Brussels)

Chapter 6 **Biomarkers in Pulmonary Arterial Hypertension** **59**
Souza, R.; Hoette, S.; Dias, B.; Jardim, C. (Sao Paulo)

Chapter 7 **Genetics of Pulmonary Arterial Hypertension and the Concept of Heritable Pulmonary Arterial Hypertension** **65**
Girerd, B.; Montani, D.; Yaici, A. (Clamart); Eyries, M.; Coulet, F.; Soubrier, F. (Paris); Humbert, M. (Clamart)

Chapter 8 **Drug- and Toxin-Induced Pulmonary Arterial Hypertension** **76**
Price, L.; Bouillon, K.; Wort, S.J. (London); Humbert, M. (Clamart)

Chapter 9 **Idiopathic Pulmonary Arterial Hypertension and Its Prognosis in the Modern Management Era in Developed and Developing Countries** **85**
Jiang, X. (Shanghai); Humbert, M. (Clamart); Jing, Z.-C. (Shanghai)

Chapter 10 **Pulmonary Arterial Hypertension Complicating Connective Tissue Disorders** **94**
Le Pavec, J. (Clamart); Hassoun, P.M. (Baltimore, Md.)

Chapter 11 **Pulmonary Arterial Hypertension and HIV and Other Viral Infections** **105**
Degano, B.; Valmary, S. (Besançon); Sitbon, O.; Humbert, M. (Clamart)

Chapter 12 **Portopulmonary Hypertension and Hepatopulmonary Syndrome** **113**
Savale, L.; Hervé, P.; Sitbon, O. (Clamart)

Chapter 13 **Pulmonary Hypertension in Congenital Heart Diseases** **122**
Tissot, C.; Beghetti, M. (Geneva)

Chapter 14 **Pulmonary Hypertension in Sickle Cell Disease** **137**
Parent, F.; Savale, L. (Clamart); Maitre, B. (Créteil); Simonneau, G. (Clamart)

Chapter 15 **Schistosomiasis and Pulmonary Hypertension** **143**
Fernandes, C.J.C.; Jardim, C.; Hovnanian, A.; Hoette, S.; Morinaga, L.K.; Souza, R. (Sao Paulo)

Chapter 16 **Pulmonary Veno-Occlusive Disease** **149**
Montani, D.; Huertas, A.; Dorfmüller, P.; Humbert, M. (Clamart)

Chapter 17 **Pulmonary Hypertension and Left Heart Disease** **161**
Adir, Y. (Haifa); Galiè, N. (Bologna)

Chapter 18 **Pulmonary Hypertension in Chronic Obstructive Pulmonary Disease** **169**
Weitzenblum, E. (Strasbourg); Chaouat, A. (Nancy); Canuet, M.; Ducoloné, A.; Kessler, R. (Strasbourg)

Chapter 19 **Pulmonary Hypertension Complicating Interstitial and Granulomatous Lung Diseases** **178**
Nunes, H.; Uzunhan, Y.; Gille, T. (Bobigny); Dauriat, G. (Paris); Brauner, M.; Kambouchner, M.; Valeyre, D. (Bobigny)

Chapter 20 **High-Altitude Pulmonary Hypertension** **199**
Di, R.-M.; Jing, Z.-C. (Shanghai)

Chapter 21 **Acute Pulmonary Venous Thromboembolic Disease** **207**
Sanchez, O.; Meyer, G. (Paris)

Chapter 22 **Anticoagulation for Venous Thromboembolism in the Modern Management Era** **218**
Le Gal, G.; Leroyer, C.; Mottier, D. (Brest)

Chapter 23 **Chronic Thromboembolic Pulmonary Hypertension** **226**
Lang, I.M. (Vienna); Jais, X. (Clamart)

Chapter 24 **Medical Treatment of Pulmonary Arterial Hypertension** **237**
O'Callaghan, D.S. (Clamart); Gaine, S.P. (Dublin)

Chapter 25 **Lung Transplantation and Role for Novel Extracorporeal Support in Pulmonary Hypertension** **246**
Hoeper, M.M. (Hannover)

Chapter 26 **Atrial Septostomy** **254**
Vachiéry, J.-L. (Brussels)

Chapter 27 **Pulmonary Vascular Disorders in Hereditary Hemorrhagic Telangiectasia** **262**
Cottin, V.; Khouatra, C.; Dupuis-Girod, S.; Cordier, J.-F. (Lyon)

Chapter 28 **Future Perspectives in Pulmonary Arterial Hypertension** **276**
Rubin, L.J. (La Jolla, Calif.)

Author Index **280**

Subject Index **281**

Foreword

The aim of *Progress in Respiratory Research*, the so-called blue series, has always been to cover a broad range of topics in respiratory medicine. When looking for a topic for the next volume to follow the most recent one on *Antituberculosis Chemotherapy* (vol. 40), I realized that we never had an entire book dedicated to pulmonary vascular disorders during my tenure as series editor. I actually had to go back all the way to 1990, i.e. 22 years ago, to find the last such volume entitled: *Pulmonary Blood Vessels in Lung Disease*. While paging through it, I was stunned to realize how much progress has been made during the last two decades. On the therapeutic side for primary pulmonary hypertension, the only options that were discussed back then were the use of warfarin and a first hint at calcium channel blockers, which probably would have to have been administered in high doses. It was thus clear to me that we urgently needed a state-of-the-art update in that field.

To ask Marc Humbert to become a volume editor was an easy choice, and to my delight he not only accepted the task but also brought along two other eminent specialists, Rogerio Souza and Gérald Simonneau, as volume co-editors. As usual for *Progress in Respiratory Research*, the 'who's who' were invited from all over the world to contribute chapters to the current book and cover the entire range of pulmonary vascular disorders. Careful attention was paid to have the latest scientific findings reported.

The result is an outstanding stand-alone volume which – as the volume editors mention in the following Preface – should appeal to health care providers interested in the field, ranging from nurses to top specialists in the field.

I hope that you as the reader will enjoy the read, and would like to express my gratitude to the volume editors and chapter authors, as well as the editorial team at Karger Publishers, in particular Linda Haas and Stefan Sessler, who helped us all to have this book out in time.

C.T. Bolliger, Cape Town

Preface

World health is generally improving with fewer people dying from infectious diseases, and therefore chronic diseases are more prevalent. In that context, the burden of chronic respiratory diseases is increasing and conditions such as asthma and chronic obstructive pulmonary diseases are clear public health priorities worldwide. Pulmonary vascular diseases and their consequences on right heart function also contribute markedly to the global burden of chronic pulmonary diseases.

Pulmonary hypertension has previously been called an orphan disease, that is, a condition which affects few individuals and is overlooked by the medical profession and pharmaceutical companies. Although undoubtedly rare, the concept that pulmonary hypertension is overlooked cannot be considered to be the case today. Indeed, there have been a number of important discoveries in recent years that have significantly improved our understanding of the disease, helped guide patient management, and laid foundations for future research. Since the middle of the twentieth century, amazing achievements have been made in the field from the development of right heart catheterization techniques to the first description of 'primary' pulmonary hypertension and the progress achieved as a result of the National Institute of Health Registry and the World Pulmonary Hypertension conferences which have taken place only four times: in 1973 (Geneva, Switzerland), 1998 (Evian, France), 2003 (Venice, Italy), and 2008 (Dana Point, California, USA). The more recent set of European guidelines have been jointly published by the European Society of Cardiology and the European Respiratory Society and endorsed by the International Society for Heart and Lung Transplantation. These guidelines give a robust hemodynamic definition of pulmonary hypertension as an increase in mean pulmonary arterial pressure ≥25 mm Hg at rest, as assessed by right heart catheterization. These guidelines also provide a very clear classification of the five major clinical subcategories of pulmonary hypertension. Of these, pulmonary arterial hypertension and chronic thromboembolic pulmonary hypertension have seen the most rapid advancements in terms of knowledge and treatment options in the past decades.

By contrast, pulmonary venous thromboembolic disease is one of the most frequent diseases encountered in clinical practice, and diagnostic and treatment options have been revolutionized by large studies allowing robust recommendations in terms of diagnosis, prevention, and treatment. Only a small minority of patients with acute pulmonary embolism (sometimes subclinical) will develop chronic thromboembolic disease, a major cause of pulmonary hypertension which can be cured by pulmonary endarterectomy, an outstanding but difficult surgical procedure developed in a few expert centers.

We have come a long way since 1973 when the World Health Organization sponsored the first international meeting on a mysterious condition named 'primary pulmonary hypertension', spurned by the interest created by the sudden increase in patients who had used the anorexigen aminorex fumarate. It remains widely believed that pulmonary hypertension is a rare disease. Although true for idiopathic pulmonary arterial hypertension, a condition affecting less than 15 individuals per million inhabitants in Europe, the true burden of pulmonary hypertension is currently unknown and largely underestimated. In the developing world, highly prevalent diseases such as schistosomiasis in Brazil are associated with an increased risk of pulmonary hypertension. In addition, patients with

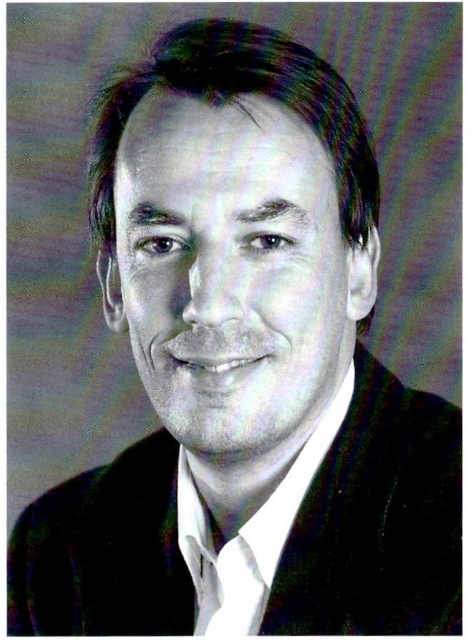

Marc Humbert

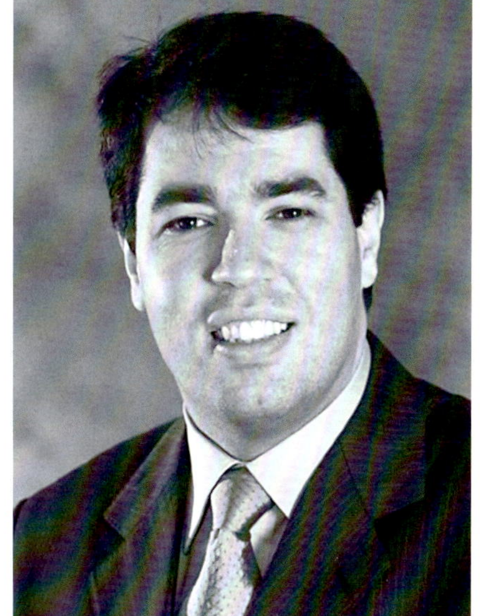

Rogerio Souza

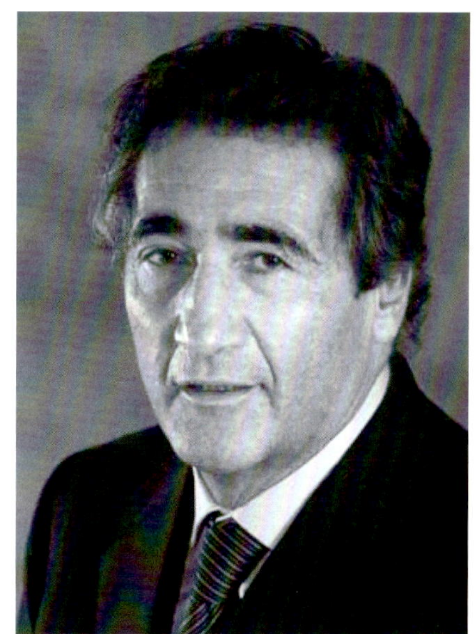

Gérald Simonneau

sickle cell disease, human immunodeficiency virus infection, liver cirrhosis, autoimmune diseases, and congenital heart diseases are at risk for pulmonary hypertension. Moreover, hypoxia is a major worldwide risk factor for pulmonary hypertension. The predominant causes of hypoxia are inadequate oxygenation of arterial blood as a result of either lung disease, impaired control of breathing, or residence at high altitude. Indeed, more than 140 million individuals live above 2,500 m worldwide, including more than 80 million in Asia and 35 million in South America.

Altogether, the burden of pulmonary vascular diseases is certainly underestimated worldwide and requires much attention from the medical community. Better characterization and management of the subjects displaying pulmonary vascular conditions is of major importance in order to improve patients' outcomes. We hope that this book will be helpful to nurses, medical trainees, and medical doctors from various fields (cardiology, internal medicine, intensive care medicine, pneumology, thoracic surgery, rheumatology, etc.) who witness the burden of pulmonary vascular diseases in their daily practice.

Marc Humbert, Clamart
Rogerio Souza, Sao Paulo
Gérald Simonneau, Clamart

Chapter 1

Humbert M, Souza R, Simonneau G (eds): Pulmonary Vascular Disorders.
Prog Respir Res. Basel, Karger, 2012, vol 41, pp 1–13

Updated Clinical Classification of Pulmonary Hypertension

David Montani[a–c] · Gérald Simonneau[a–c]

[a]Université Paris-Sud, Faculté de Médecine, Kremlin- Bicêtre; [b]AP-HP, Centre National de Référence de l'Hypertension Pulmonaire Sévère, Service de Pneumologie et Réanimation Respiratoire, Hôpital Antoine Béclère, Clamart; [c]INSERM U999, Hypertension Artérielle Pulmonaire: Physiopathologie et Innovation Thérapeutique, LabEx LERMIT, Centre Chirurgical, Marie-Lannelongue, Le Plessis-Robinson, France

Abstract

The fourth World Symposium on Pulmonary Hypertension and the conjoint ERS/ESC guidelines revise previous classifications of pulmonary hypertension (PH) in order to accurately reflect information published over the past 5 years. PH has been defined as an increase in mean pulmonary arterial pressure (mPAP) ≥25 mm Hg at rest as assessed by right heart catheterization. No definition for PH on exercise was considered. PH was defined as precapillary when pulmonary capillary wedge pressure was ≤15 mm Hg associated with a normal or reduced cardiac output. In Group 1 (PAH), the term familial PAH has been replaced by heritable PAH, including sporadic idiopathic PAH with germline mutations and familial cases. Pulmonary veno-occlusive disease and pulmonary capillary hemangiomatosis have been individualized and designated as clinical Group 1'. Group 2 'pulmonary hypertension due to left heart diseases' has been divided into three subgroups: systolic dysfunction, diastolic dysfunction, and valvular disease. Group 3 includes only chronic thromboembolic pulmonary hypertension without any distinction of proximal or distal forms.

The classification of pulmonary hypertension (PH) has gone through a series of changes since the first classification proposed in 1973 which designated only two categories, primary PH or secondary PH, depending on the presence or absence of identifiable causes or risk factors [1, 2]. During the second World Symposium on Pulmonary Arterial Hypertension held in France in 1998, a new classification was proposed which attempted to create categories of PH that shared similar pathogenesis, clinical features, and therapeutic options [3]. This classification defined homogenous groups of patients in order to conduct clinical trials and obtain approval for specific pulmonary arterial hypertension (PAH) therapies. In 2003, the 3rd World Symposium on Pulmonary Arterial Hypertension (Venice, Italy) proposed only minor changes, except for the introduction of the terms of idiopathic PAH, familial PAH, and/or associated PAH (table 1) defining three groups sharing broadly similar physiopathology and response to therapy. The other prominent change was to move pulmonary veno-occlusive disease (PVOD) and pulmonary capillary hemangiomatosis (PCH) from separate categories into a single subcategory of PAH. These two entities have many similarities with idiopathic PAH, including clinical presentation, hemodynamic characteristics, and risk factors, which justified placing them together in Group 1 (table 1).

In 2008, the 4th World Symposium on Pulmonary Hypertension held in Dana Point (Calif., USA) and the consensus of an international group of experts revised previous classifications in order to accurately reflect information published over the previous 5 years, as well as to clarify some areas that were unclear. The current Dana Point classification is presented in table 2.

Group 1: Pulmonary Arterial Hypertension

The nomenclature of the subgroups and associated conditions has evolved since the first classification, and additional modifications were added in this revised classification.

Group 1.1/1.2: Idiopathic and Heritable Pulmonary Arterial Hypertension

Idiopathic PAH corresponds to sporadic disease in which there is neither a family history of PAH nor an identified risk factor. When PAH occurs in a familial context, germline mutations in the bone morphogenetic protein receptor 2 *(BMPR2)* gene, a member of the transforming growth

Table 1. Venice clinical classification of PH (2003)

1.	PAH
1.1.	Idiopathic PAH
1.2.	Familial PAH
1.3.	Associated with PAH:
1.3.1.	Collagen vascular disease
1.3.2.	Congenital systemic-to-pulmonary shunts
1.3.3.	Portal hypertension
1.3.4.	HIV infection
1.3.5.	Drugs and toxins
1.3.6.	Other (thyroid disorders, glycogen storage disease, Gaucher's disease, hereditary hemorrhagic telangiectasia, hemoglobinopathies, myeloproliferative disorders, splenectomy)
1.4.	Associated with significant venous or capillary involvement
1.4.1.	PVOD
1.4.2.	PCH
1.5.	Persistent PH of the newborn
2.	PH with left heart disease
2.1.	Left-sided atrial or ventricular heart disease
2.2.	Left-sided valvular heart disease
3.	PH associated with lung diseases and/or hypoxemia
3.1.	Chronic obstructive pulmonary disease
3.2.	Interstitial lung disease
3.3.	Sleep-disordered breathing
3.4.	Alveolar hypoventilation disorders
3.5.	Chronic exposure to high altitude
3.6.	Developmental abnormalities
4.	PH due to chronic thrombotic and/or embolic disease
4.1.	Thromboembolic obstruction of proximal pulmonary arteries
4.2.	Thromboembolic obstruction of distal pulmonary arteries
4.3.	Nonthrombotic pulmonary embolism (tumor, parasites, foreign material)
5.	Miscellaneous

Sarcoidosis, histiocytosis X, lymphangiomatosis, compression of pulmonary vessels (adenopathy, tumor, fibrosing mediastinitis)

Table 2. Updated clinical classification of PH (Dana Point, 2008)

1.	PAH
1.1	Idiopathic
1.2	**Heritable**
1.2.1	***BMPR2***
1.2.2	***ALK1, endoglin*** **(with or without hereditary hemorrhagic telangiectasia)**
1.2.3	**Unknown**
1.3	Drug- and toxin-induced
1.4	Associated with
1.4.1	Connective tissue diseases
1.4.2	HIV infection
1.4.3	Portal hypertension
1.4.4	Congenital heart diseases
1.4.5	**Schistosomiasis**
1.4.6	**Chronic hemolytic anemia**
1.5	Persistent PH of the newborn
1′	**PVOD and/or PCH**
2.	PH due to left heart disease
2.1	**Systolic dysfunction**
2.2	**Diastolic dysfunction**
2.3	Valvular disease
3.	PH due to lung diseases and/or hypoxia
3.1	Chronic obstructive pulmonary disease
3.2	Interstitial lung disease
3.3	**Other pulmonary diseases with mixed restrictive and obstructive pattern**
3.4	Sleep-disordered breathing
3.5	Alveolar hypoventilation disorders
3.6	Chronic exposure to high altitude
3.7	Developmental abnormalities
4.	**CTEPH**
5.	PH with unclear multifactorial mechanisms
5.1	Hematologic disorders: myeloproliferative disorders splenectomy
5.2	Systemic disorders, sarcoidosis, pulmonary Langerhans cell histiocytosis, lymphangioleiomyomatosis, neurofibromatosis, vasculitis
5.3	Metabolic disorders: glycogen storage disease, Gaucher's disease, thyroid disorders
5.4	Other: tumoral obstruction, fibrosing mediastinitis, chronic renal failure on dialysis.

Main modifications to the previous Venice classification are set in bold.

factor-β (TGF-β) signaling family, can be detected in about 70% of cases [4, 5]. Recently, it has been suggested that PAH patients carrying a *BMPR2* mutation had more severe disease and were less likely to demonstrate vasoreactivity than idiopathic PAH patients without a *BMPR2* mutation [6–8]. More rarely, mutations in activin receptor-like kinase type 1 *(ACVRL1* or *ALK1)* or *endoglin* genes, also coding for members of the TGF-β signaling family, have been identified in patients with PAH, predominantly with coexistent hereditary hemorrhagic telangiectasia.

Table 3. Updated risk factors and associated conditions for PAH

Definite	*Possible*
Aminorex	Cocaine
Fenfluramine	Phenylpropanolamine
Dexfenfluramine	St. John's wort
Toxic rapeseed oil	Chemotherapeutic agents
Benfluorex	SSRI
Likely	*Unlikely*
Amphetamines	Oral contraceptives
L-tryptophan	Estrogen
Methamphetamines	Cigarette smoking

BMPR2 mutations have also been detected in 11–40% of apparently idiopathic cases with no family history [9, 10]. Indeed, the distinction between idiopathic and familial PAH with *BMPR2* mutations is artificial, as all patients with a *BMPR2* mutation have heritable disease. In addition, *BMPR2* mutations were identified in only 70% families with PAH. Thus, it was decided to abandon the term 'familial PAH' in favor of the term 'heritable PAH'. Heritable forms of PAH include idiopathic PAH with germline mutations (mainly *BMPR2,* but also *ACVRL1* or *endoglin*) and familial cases with or without identified mutations [11, 12]. Genetic testing should be performed as a part of a comprehensive program that includes genetic counseling and discussion of the risks, benefits, and limitations of such testing [13].

Group 1.3: Drug- and Toxin-Induced PAH

A number of risk factors for the development of PAH have been included in the previous classifications [3, 14]. In the current classification, the categorization of risk factors and the likelihood of developing PAH have been modified (table 3).

Aminorex, fenfluramine derivatives, and toxic rapeseed oil represent the only identified 'definite' risk factors for PAH [3, 14]. Souza et al. [15] recently demonstrated that this subgroup of PAH shares clinical, functional, hemodynamic, and genetic features with idiopathic PAH, suggesting that fenfluramine exposure represents a potential trigger for PAH without influencing its clinical course. The association of fenfluramine and dexfenfluramine intake with the development of PAH was confirmed by the Surveillance Of Pulmonary Hypertension In America (SOPHIA), which enrolled 1,335 subjects at tertiary PH centers in the United States between 1998 and 2001 [16]. Benfluorex is a benzoate ester that shares similar structural and pharmacologic characteristics with dexfenfluramine and fenfluramine. The active and common metabolite of each of these molecules is norfenfluramine, which itself has a chemical structure similar to that of the amphetamines. Given its pharmacological properties, benfluorex would be expected to have similar toxic effects to the fenfluramine derivatives. We recently reported an outbreak of valvular diseases and PAH associated with benfluorex use in France and the drug has now been completely withdrawn from the market. A novel finding was that St. John's wort (OR: 3.6 vs. thromboembolic PH) and over-the-counter antiobesity agents containing phenylpropanolamine (OR: 5.2 vs. thromboembolic PH) also increased the risk of developing idiopathic PAH. The SOPHIA study examined intake of a variety of nonselective monoamine reuptake inhibitors, selective serotonin reuptake inhibitors, antidepressants, and anxiolytics, and found no increased risk for developing PAH [16]. However, a case-control study of selective serotonin reuptake inhibitor use during pregnancy showed an increased risk (OR: 6.1) in the offspring of developing persistent PH of the newborn [17]. Based on this study, selective serotonin reuptake inhibitors were reclassified in the 'possible' category.

Amphetamine use represents a 'likely' risk factor, although they are frequently used in combination with fenfluramine. A recent comprehensive retrospective study suggested a strong relationship with the use of methamphetamines (inhaled, smoked, oral, or intravenous) and the occurrence of idiopathic PAH [18]. Based primarily on the results of this study, methamphetamine use is now considered a 'very likely' risk factor for the development of PAH.

Group 1.4.1: Pulmonary Arterial Hypertension Associated with Connective Tissue Diseases

PAH associated with connective tissue diseases represents an important clinical subgroup. The prevalence of PAH has been well established only for systemic sclerosis. Two recent prospective studies using echocardiography as a screening method and right heart catheterization for confirmation found a prevalence of PAH of between 7 and 12% [19, 20]. Several long-term studies suggest the outcome of patients with PAH associated with systemic sclerosis is markedly worse than that of patients with idiopathic PAH. However, PAH does not represent the only cause of PH in systemic sclerosis. Pulmonary hypertension due to lung fibrosis [21], diastolic left heart dysfunction [22], and primary cardiac involvement [23] are also frequent, emphasizing the importance of a complete evaluation with right heart catheterization to accurately classify its etiology so as to determine appropriate treatment.

In systemic lupus erythematosis [24, 25] and mixed connective tissue diseases [26, 27], the prevalence of PAH remains unknown, but likely occurs less frequently than in systemic sclerosis. In the absence of chronic lung disease, PAH has been reported infrequently in other connective tissue diseases such as Sjögren's syndrome [28], polymyositis [29], or rheumatoid arthritis [30].

Group 1.4.2: HIV Infection
PAH is a rare but well-established complication of HIV infection [31, 32]. HIV-associated PAH has clinical, hemodynamic, and histologic characteristics similar to those seen in idiopathic PAH. Epidemiologic data in the early 1990s, a time when therapy with highly active antiretroviral therapy was not yet available, indicated a prevalence of 0.5% [33]. The prevalence of HIV-associated PAH was evaluated more recently and showed a stable prevalence of 0.46% [34]. Uncontrolled studies suggest that patients with severe HIV-associated PAH could benefit from specific PAH therapies, such as bosentan or continuous intravenous epoprostenol [35, 36]. Interestingly, normalization of hemodynamics has been reported with specific PAH therapies in a substantial number of cases [37].

Group 1.4.3: Portopulmonary Hypertension
Portopulmonary hypertension (PoPH) is defined by the development of PAH associated with increased pressure in the portal circulation [38, 39]. Prospective hemodynamic studies have shown that 2–6% of patients with portal hypertension had PH [40, 41]. However, right heart catheterization is mandatory for the diagnosis of PoPH, as several mechanisms may increase pulmonary artery pressure in the setting of advanced liver disease: hyperdynamic circulatory state with high cardiac output, fluid overload, and diastolic dysfunction. Pulmonary vascular resistance (PVR) is usually normal in these cases. Pathologic changes in the small arteries appear identical to those seen in idiopathic PAH. A recent multicenter case-control study identified that female gender and autoimmune hepatitis were independent risk factors for the development of PoPH and that hepatitis C infection was associated with a decreased risk [42]. A recent, large cohort study of PoPH showed that long-term prognosis was related to the presence and severity of cirrhosis as well to cardiac function [43].

Group 1.4.4: Congenital Heart Diseases
A significant proportion of patients with congenital heart disease, in particular those with systemic-to-pulmonary shunts, will develop PAH if left untreated. Eisenmenger's syndrome is defined as congenital heart disease with an initial large systemic-to-pulmonary shunt that induces progressive pulmonary vascular disease and PAH, with resultant reversal of the shunt and central cyanosis [44, 45]. It represents the most advanced form of PAH associated with congenital heart disease. It has been reported that a large proportion of patients with congenital heart disease develop some degree of PAH [46–48]. The prevalence of PAH associated with congenital systemic-to-pulmonary shunts in Europe and North America has been estimated between 1.6 and 12.5 cases per million adults, with 25–50% of this population affected by Eisenmenger's syndrome. The histopathologic and pathobiologic changes seen in patients with PAH associated with congenital systemic-to-pulmonary shunts, in particular endothelial dysfunction, are similar to those observed in idiopathic or other associated forms of PAH. Following the Dana Point meeting, it was decided to update the pathologic and pathophysiologic classification of congenital heart disease with systemic-to-pulmonary shunts (table 4) in order to provide a more detailed description of each condition, with the result that four quite distinct phenotypes were individualized (table 5).

Group 1.4.5: Schistosomiasis
In the new classification, PH associated with schistosomiasis was included in Group 1 even though it was subcategorized in Group 4 as PH due to chronic embolic disease in the previous classification. Embolic obstruction of pulmonary arteries by schistosoma eggs was thought to be the primary mechanism responsible for the development of PH [49]. However, it has recently been demonstrated that PH associated with schistosomiasis may have similar clinical presentation and histologic findings as idiopathic PAH [50, 51]. The mechanism of PAH in patients with schistosomiasis is probably multifactorial including PoPH, a frequent complication of this disease [52], and local vascular inflammation, whereas mechanical obstruction by schistosoma eggs seems to play a minor role. More than 200 million people are infected and 4–8% will develop hepatosplenic disease. PAH associated with schistosomiasis represents a frequent form of PAH, especially in countries where the infection is endemic. Data from a recent study based on invasive hemodynamics provided evidence showing the prevalence of PAH in patients with hepatosplenic disease to be 4.6%. The prevalence of postcapillary hypertension (3.0%) was also important, reinforcing the need for invasive hemodynamics for the specific diagnosis of PAH in schistosomiasis [53].

Group 1.4.6: Chronic Hemolytic Anemia

Chronic hemolytic anemia represents a new subcategory of PAH previously subcategorized under 'other conditions' associated with PAH. There is increasing evidence that PAH is a complication of chronic hereditary and acquired hemolytic anemia, including sickle cell disease [54, 55], thalassemia [56], hereditary spherocytosis [57], stomatocytosis [58], and microangiopathic hemolytic anemia [59].

PH has been reported most frequently in patients with sickle cell disease; however, the prevalence of PAH is not yet clearly established. A large study of sickle cell disease patients, which defined PH echocardiographically by the presence of tricuspid regurgitation jet velocity (TRV) ≥2.5 m/s, found that 32% of patients had PH [55]. However, TRV ≥2.5 m/s is a low threshold to define PH and leads to a substantial number of false positive cases of PH not confirmed by right heart catheterization [19, 34, 60]. When a TRV >3.0 m/s was used, only 9% of the cohort met the criteria for PH. In this study, right heart catheterization was carried out in only 18 of 63 patients with TRV >2.5 m/s and PH defined by a mean pulmonary arterial pressure (PAP) >25 mm Hg was confirmed in 17 patients; however, pulmonary wedge pressure was elevated in some patients. A substantial proportion of sickle cell disease patients have pulmonary venous hypertension: 46% in one study of 26 patients with sickle cell disease and PH [61]. In addition, some patients present with a hyperkinetic state with moderate elevation in mean pulmonary artery pressure and normal PVR. Thus, the prevalence of PAH in sickle cell disease is undoubtedly much lower than 32%. Prospective epidemiologic studies using echocardiographic screening and direct hemodynamic confirmation with right heart catheterization in all patients with suspected PH are ongoing and will assess the precise prevalence of PAH in sickle cell disease.

The mechanism of PAH in sickle cell disease remains uncertain. Histologic lesions similar to those found in idiopathic PAH, including plexiform lesions in one case series [62]. A probable hypothesis is that chronic hemolysis results in high rates of nitric oxide consumption, and produces a state of resistance to nitric oxide bioactivity, leading to a decrease in activation of smooth muscle guanosine monophosphate, a potent vasodilator/antiproliferative mediator [63, 64].

Group 1′: Pulmonary Veno-Occlusive Disease and/or Pulmonary Capillary Hemangiomatosis

PVOD and PCH are uncommon conditions, but they are increasingly recognized as causes of PH [65]. In the Evian

Table 4. Anatomic-pathophysiologic classification of congenital systemic-to-pulmonary shunts associated with PAH (modified from Venice 2003)

1.	Type
1.1	Simple pretricuspid shunts
1.1.1	ASD
1.1.1.1	Ostium secundum
1.1.1.2	Sinus venosus
1.1.1.3	Ostium primum
1.1.2	Total or partial unobstructed anomalous pulmonary venous return
1.2	Simple posttricuspid shunts
1.2.1	VSD
1.2.2	Patent ductus arteriosus
1.3	Combined shunts
	Describe combination and define predominant defect
1.4	Complex CHD
1.4.1	Complete atrioventricular septal defect
1.4.2	Truncus arteriosus
1.4.3	Single ventricle physiology with unobstructed pulmonary blood flow
1.4.4	Transposition of the great arteries with VSD (without pulmonary stenosis) and/or patent ductus arteriosus
1.4.5	Other
2.	Dimension (specify for each defect if more than one congenital heart defect)
2.1	Hemodynamic (specify Qp/Qs)[1]
2.1.1	Restrictive (pressure gradient across the defect)
2.1.2	Nonrestrictive
2.2	Anatomic
2.2.1	Small-to-moderate (ASD ≤2.0 and VSD ≤1.0 cm)
2.2.2	Large (ASD >2.0 and VSD >1.0 cm)
3.	Direction of shunt
3.1	Predominantly systemic-to-pulmonary
3.2	Predominantly pulmonary-to-systemic
3.3	Bidirectional
4.	Associated cardiac and extracardiac abnormalities
5.	Repair status
5.1	Unoperated
5.2	Palliated (specify type of operation/s, age at surgery)
	Repaired (specify type of operation/s, age at surgery)

[1] Ratio of pulmonary (Qp) to systemic (Qs) blood flow. ASD = Atrial septal defect; VSD = ventricular septal defect.

Table 5. Clinical classification of congenital systemic-to-pulmonary shunts associated to PAH

Eisenmenger syndrome Includes all systemic-to-pulmonary shunts resulting from large defects and leading to a severe increase in PVR and a reversed (pulmonary-to-systemic) or bidirectional shunt; cyanosis, erythrocytosis, and multiple organ involvement are present.
PAH associated with systemic-to-pulmonary shunts Includes moderate-to-large defects; PVR is mildly to moderately increased, systemic-to-pulmonary shunt is still prevalent, and no cyanosis is present at rest
PAH with small defects Small defects (usually ventricular septal defects <1 cm and atrial septal defects <2 cm of effective diameter assessed by echocardiography); the clinical picture is very similar to idiopathic PAH
PAH after corrective cardiac surgery Congenital heart disease has been corrected, but PAH is still present immediately after surgery or recurs several months or years after surgery in the absence of significant postoperative residual lesions

classification, these two entities were placed in two different groups, both distinct from PAH (table 1). Similarities in pathologic features and clinical presentation suggest that these disorders may overlap [66]; thus, PVOD and PCH were included in the same subgroup of PAH. The decision to leave PVOD and PCH in the same subgroup is supported by a recent clinicopathologic study [66] analyzing specimens from 35 patients diagnosed as having either PVOD (n = 30) or PCH (n = 5). PCH was identified in 24 cases (73%) diagnosed as PVOD. Indeed, venous involvement was present in 4 of 5 cases initially diagnosed as PCH. These findings suggest that PCH may be an angioproliferative process frequently associated with PVOD.

PVOD and PCH were included in Group 1 because the two entities share a number of characteristics with idiopathic PAH. First, some histologic changes in the small pulmonary arteries (intimal fibrosis and medial hypertrophy), observed in PAH, were also found in PVOD/PCH. Second, the clinical presentations and hemodynamics of PVOD/PCH and PAH are often indistinguishable [14, 65, 67]. Third, PVOD/PCH and PAH share similar risk factors, including the scleroderma spectrum of disease [68], HIV infection [69, 70], and the use of anorexigens [65]. Lastly, familial occurrence has been reported with both PVOD and PCH, and mutations in the *BMPR2* gene have been documented in patients with PVOD [67, 71]. These findings suggest that PVOD, PCH, and PAH may represent different components of a single spectrum of disease.

Although PVOD and PCH may present similarly to idiopathic PAH, there are a number of important differences. These include the presence of crackles on examination, radiologic abnormalities on high-resolution CT of the chest (ground glass opacities, septal thickening, mediastinal adenopathy) [67, 72–74], hemosiderin-laden macrophages on bronchoalveolar lavage [75], and a lower DLCO and PaO_2 in patients with PVOD or PCH [67]. In addition, the response to medical therapy and prognosis of PVOD/PCH are quite different from PAH. A recent study compared 24 patients with histologic evidence of PVOD with or without PCH and 24 randomly selected patients with idiopathic, familial, or anorexigen-associated PAH [65]. Among the 16 PVOD patients who received PAH-specific therapy, 7 (43.8%) developed pulmonary edema. These patients were treated mainly with continuous intravenous epoprostenol, but also with oral therapies, bosentan, and calcium-channel blockers, and clinical outcomes were worse in PVOD patients than in idiopathic PAH patients.

PVOD/PCH remains a difficult disorder to categorize, as it shares characteristics with idiopathic PAH but also has a number of distinct differences. Given the current evidence, it was decided that PVOD/PCH should be a distinct category but not completely separated from PAH. As a result, PVOD and PCH are designated as 1' in the current classification.

Group 2: Pulmonary Hypertension Due to Left Heart Disease

Left-sided ventricular or valvular diseases may produce an increase of left atrial pressure, leading to a backward transmission of the pressure and a passive increase of pulmonary arterial pressure. Left heart disease probably represents the most frequent cause of PH [76]. In this situation, PVR is normal or near normal (<3.0 Wood units) and there is no gradient between mean PAP and pulmonary wedge pressure (transpulmonary gradient <12 mm Hg). In the previous classification, these entities were divided into two subgroups based on the presence or absence of valvular disease. In the recent classification, the increasing recognition of left-sided heart dysfunction with preserved ejection fraction led to changes in the subcategories of Group 2 and this group now includes three distinct etiologies: left heart systolic dysfunction, left heart diastolic dysfunction, and left heart valvular disease. In some patients with left heart disease, the elevation of PAP is out of proportion to that expected from the elevation of left arterial pressure (transpulmonary gradient >12 mm Hg), and PVR is increased to >3.0 Wood units (19–35% of patients) [76]. Some patients with left heart valvular disease or even left heart dysfunction can develop severe PH of the same magnitude as that seen in PAH [77–79]. The elevation of PAP and PVR may be due to either the increase of pulmonary artery vasomotor tone and/or pulmonary vascular remodeling [80, 81]. No studies using medications approved for PAH have been performed in this patient population, and the efficacy and safety of PAH medications remain unknown.

Group 3: Pulmonary Hypertension due to Lung Diseases and/or Hypoxia

In this group, the predominant cause of PH is alveolar hypoxia as a result of either chronic lung disease, impaired control of breathing, or residence at high altitude; however, the precise prevalence of PH in all these conditions remains largely unknown. In the revised classification, the heading has been modified to reinforce the link with the development of PH. A category of lung disease characterized by a mixed obstructive and restrictive pattern was added, including chronic bronchiectasis, cystic fibrosis, and the recently described syndrome of combined pulmonary fibrosis and emphysema in which the prevalence of PH is almost 50% [82, 83]. In PAH associated with parenchymal lung disease, the increase of PAP is usually modest (mean PAP <35 mm Hg) [84]. Interestingly, in some patients, the increase of PAP is out of proportion and may be >35 mm Hg [85]. In a retrospective study of 998 patients with chronic obstructive pulmonary disease who underwent right heart catheterization, only 1% had severe PH [86]. These patients with more severe PH were characterized by mild-to-moderate airway obstruction, severe hypoxemia, hypocapnia, and a very low diffusing capacity for carbon monoxide. Large randomized controlled studies of specific PAH therapies are not available for PH 'out of proportion' associated with parenchyma lung disease.

Group 4: Chronic Thromboembolic Pulmonary Hypertension

In the Venice classification, Group 4 was heterogeneous including obstruction of pulmonary arterial vessels by thromboemboli, tumors, or foreign bodies. However, depending on the origin of the obstruction, the clinical and radiologic findings are different, and management is unique to each etiology. Even if the incidence of chronic thromboembolic pulmonary hypertension (CTEPH) is uncertain, CTEPH represents a frequent cause of PH and occurs in up to 4% of patients after an acute pulmonary embolism [87, 88]. In contrast, other etiologies of 'obstructive PH' are very rare. Therefore, in the new classification, only CTEPH was included in Group 4. In the previous classification, CTEPH was divided into two subgroups: proximal CTEPH and distal CTEPH, depending on the feasibility of performing pulmonary thromboendarterectomy. Currently, there is no consensus about the definitions of proximal and distal CTEPH and the decision of surgery may vary depending on individual centers [89]. Thus, in the new classification, it was decided to maintain in Group 4 only a single category of CTEPH without distinction between proximal and distal forms. However, patients with suspected or confirmed CTEPH need to be referred to a center with expertise in the management of CTEPH in order to consider the feasibility of performing surgery, which depends on the location of the obstruction, the correlation between hemodynamic findings and the degree of mechanical obstruction assessed by angiography, comorbidities, the willingness of the patient, and the experience of the surgeon [90, 91]. Patients who are not candidates for surgery may benefit from PAH-specific medical therapy [27, 92]; however, further evaluation of these therapies in randomized control trials are needed [93].

Group 5: Pulmonary Hypertension with Unclear or Multifactorial Etiologies

Group 5.1: Hematologic Disorders
PH has been reported in chronic myeloproliferative disorders including polycythemia vera, essential thrombocythemia, and chronic myeloid leukemia [94, 95]. Several mechanisms may be implicated in PH associated with

chronic myeloproliferative disorders, including high cardiac output, asplenia, direct obstruction of pulmonary arteries by circulating megakaryocytes [96], CTEPH [97], PoPH, and congestive heart failure. Splenectomy as a result of trauma or as a treatment for hematologic disorders may increase the risk of developing PH [98]. CTEPH [95, 99] and several cases of PAH [95, 100] with medial hypertrophy, intimal fibrosis, and plexiform lesions in the pulmonary vasculature have been reported in association with splenectomy.

Group 5.2: Systemic Disorders

The second subgroup includes systemic disorders, including sarcoidosis, pulmonary Langerhans cell histiocytosis, lymphangioleiomyomatosis, neurofibromatosis, and vasculitis.

Sarcoidosis is a common systemic granulomatous disease of unknown origin. PH is an increasingly recognized complication of sarcoidosis [101], with a reported prevalence of 1–28% [101–103]. PH is often attributed to the destruction of the capillary bed by the fibrotic process and/or to the resultant chronic hypoxemia [104]. However, the severity of PH may be out of proportion with the degree of parenchymal lung disease and blood gas abnormalities, suggesting that other mechanisms may be contributing to the development of PH [102]. In this setting, such mechanisms include extrinsic compression of large pulmonary arteries by lymph node enlargement and granulomatous infiltration of the pulmonary vasculature, especially the pulmonary veins, which sometimes mimic PVOD [105]. More rarely, sarcoidosis with hepatic involvement can be associated with PoPH.

Pulmonary Langerhans cell histiocytosis is an uncommon cause of infiltrative and destructive lung disease. Severe PH is a common feature in patients with end-stage disease [106], and PH in these patients is usually related to chronic hypoxemia and/or abnormal pulmonary mechanics. However, in some patients, especially those with more severe elevation of PAP, PH is unrelated to lung parenchymal injury. Histopathologic examination has shown severe diffuse pulmonary vasculopathy involving predominantly intralobular pulmonary veins and, to a lesser extent, muscular pulmonary arteries [107].

Lymphangioleiomyomatosis is a rare multisystem disorder predominantly affecting women and is characterized by cystic lung destruction, lymphatic abnormalities, and abdominal tumors. PH is relatively uncommon in patients with lymphangioleiomyomatosis [108, 109]. Chronic hypoxemia and pulmonary capillary destruction caused by cystic lung lesions probably represent the predominant causes of PH.

Neurofibromatosis type 1, also known as von Recklinghausen's disease, is an autosomal dominant disease that can be recognized by its characteristic 'café au lait' skin lesions and cutaneous fibromas. The disease is occasionally complicated by systemic vasculopathy. Several cases of PH have recently been reported in the setting of von Recklinghausen's disease [110–113]. The mechanism of PH is unclear and lung fibrosis and CTEPH may play a role in the development of PH. In rare cases, histologic examination found both arteries and veins narrowed by medial and/or intimal hypertrophy and fibrosis [113, 114].

Lastly, some rare cases of PH have been observed in anti-neutrophil cytoplasmic antibodies-associated vasculitis with clinical presentation similar to PAH; however, histologic data are not available [115].

Group 5.3: Metabolic Disorders

PH has been reported in a few cases of type Ia glycogen storage disease, a rare autosomal recessive disorder caused by a deficiency of glucose-6-phosphatase [116–118]. The mechanisms of PH are uncertain, but portacaval shunts, atrial septal defects, severe restrictive pulmonary function defects, and thrombosis are thought to play a role. In one case, autopsy findings revealed the presence of plexiform lesions [119].

Gaucher's disease is a rare disorder characterized by a deficiency of lysosomal B-glucosidase, which results in an accumulation of glucocerebroside in reticuloendothelial cells. In a study of 134 patients with Gaucher's disease who were systematically screened by echocardiography, PH was not uncommon [120]. In this setting, several potential mechanisms for PH have been suggested, including interstitial lung disease, chronic hypoxemia, capillary plugging by Gaucher cells, and splenectomy [120, 121]. One case of histologic findings similar to idiopathic PAH has been reported [122].

The association between thyroid diseases and PH has been reported in a number of studies [123, 124]. In a recent prospective study using echocardiographic evaluation, more than 40% of patients with thyroid diseases had PH [125]. One case of PVOD confirmed by histology has been observed in a patient with a Hashimoto's thyroiditis [126]. Interestingly, a recent prospective study of 63 consecutive adult patients with PAH found a prevalence of autoimmune thyroid disease, including both hypothyroidism and hyperthyroidism, in 49%, suggesting that these conditions may share a common immunogenetic susceptibility [127].

Group 5.4: Miscellaneous Conditions
The last subgroup includes a number of miscellaneous conditions, including tumoral obstruction, fibrosing mediastinitis, and chronic renal failure on dialysis.

A progressive obstruction of proximal pulmonary arteries leading to PH may be observed in tumor obstruction when a tumor grows into the central pulmonary arteries with additional thrombosis. Such cases are due principally to pulmonary artery sarcomas, which occur rarely but are usually rapidly fatal [128, 129]. The differential diagnosis with CTEPH can be difficult and CT or MRI angiography may be useful to differentiate an obstruction from a tumor or thrombotic material [128, 130, 131]. Occlusion of the microvasculature by metastatic tumor emboli represents another rare cause of rapidly progressive PH [132]. The initial laboratory evaluation shows hypoxemia, often severe, with a clear lung field [133]. CT scanning does not show proximal thrombi, but often shows thickening of septa. In contrast, the V/Q lung scan is generally abnormal with multiple subsegmental perfusion defects. Pulmonary microvascular cytology sampling through a pulmonary artery catheter in the wedge position is an important diagnostic tool [133]. The majority of reported cases occur in association with breast, lung, or gastric carcinoma.

Fibrosing mediastinitis may be associated with severe PH due to compression of both pulmonary arteries and veins [134, 135]. V/Q scan, CT, and pulmonary angiography are useful for an accurate diagnosis; however, findings can mimic proximal thrombotic obstruction. The predominant etiologies are histoplasmosis [135], other fungal organisms, tuberculosis [136], and sarcoidosis.

Lastly, PH has been reported in patients with end-stage renal disease maintained on long-term hemodialysis. Based on echocardiographic studies, the prevalence of PH in this patient population is estimated to be as high as 40% [137]. There are several potential explanations for the development of PH in these patients. PAP may be increased by high cardiac output (resulting from the arteriovenous access and anemia) as well as fluid overload. In addition, diastolic and systolic left heart dysfunctions are also frequent in this setting [137, 138]. Furthermore, hormonal and metabolic derangement associated with end-stage renal disease might lead to dysfunction of normal pulmonary vascular tone.

Conclusion

In this updated classification of PH, recent findings were incorporated to clarify areas of ambiguity. The major modifications adopted principally concern Group 1 of PAH in order to define a more homogeneous group. This subgroup introduces the term of 'heritable PAH' for patients with a family history or idiopathic PAH patients with germline mutations (e.g. *BMPR2, ACVRL1* or *endoglin*). In the new classification, schistosomiasis and chronic hemolytic anemia appear as separate entities in the subgroup of PAH associated with identified conditions. Finally, it was decided to place PVOD and PCH in a separate group, distinct from but very close to Group 1 (now called Group 1').

References

1 Hatano S, Strasser T: Primary Pulmonary Hypertension. Report on a WHO Meeting. October 15–17, 1973. Geneva, WHO, 1975.

2 Wagenvoort CA, Wagenvoort N: Primary pulmonary hypertension: a pathological study of the lung vessels in 156 clinically diagnosed cases. Circulation 1970;42:1163–1184.

3 Fishman AP: Clinical classification of pulmonary hypertension. Clin Chest Med 2001;22:385–391, vii.

4 Cogan JD, Pauciulo MW, Batchman AP, Prince MA, Robbins IM, Hedges LK, Stanton KC, Wheeler LA, Phillips JA 3rd, Loyd JE, Nichols WC: High frequency of BMPR2 exonic deletions/duplications in familial pulmonary arterial hypertension. Am J Respir Crit Care Med 2006;174:590–598.

5 Aldred MA, Vijayakrishnan J, James V, Soubrier F, Gomez-Sanchez MA, Martensson G, Galie N, Manes A, Corris P, Simonneau G, Humbert M, Morrell NW, Trembath RC: BMPR2 gene rearrangements account for a significant proportion of mutations in familial and idiopathic pulmonary arterial hypertension. Hum Mutat 2006;27:212–213.

6 Sztrymf B, Coulet F, Girerd B, Yaici A, Jais X, Sitbon O, Montani D, Souza R, Simonneau G, Soubrier F, Humbert M: Clinical outcomes of pulmonary arterial hypertension in carriers of BMPR2 mutation. Am J Respir Crit Care Med 2008;177:1377–1383.

7 Elliott CG, Glissmeyer EW, Havlena GT, Carlquist J, McKinney JT, Rich S, McGoon MD, Scholand MB, Kim M, Jensen RL, Schmidt JW, Ward K: Relationship of BMPR2 mutations to vasoreactivity in pulmonary arterial hypertension. Circulation 2006;113:2509–2515.

8 Rosenzweig EB, Morse JH, Knowles JA, Chada KK, Khan AM, Roberts KE, McElroy JJ, Juskiw NK, Mallory NC, Rich S, Diamond B, Barst RJ: Clinical implications of determining BMPR2 mutation status in a large cohort of children and adults with pulmonary arterial hypertension. J Heart Lung Transplant 2008;27:668–674.

9 Machado RD, Aldred MA, James V, Harrison RE, Patel B, Schwalbe EC, Gruenig E, Janssen B, Koehler R, Seeger W, Eickelberg O, Olschewski H, Elliott CG, Glissmeyer E, Carlquist J, Kim M, Torbicki A, Fijalkowska A, Szewczyk G, Parma J, Abramowicz MJ, Galie N, Morisaki H, Kyotani S, Nakanishi N, Morisaki T, Humbert M, Simonneau G, Sitbon O, Soubrier F, Coulet F, Morrell NW, Trembath RC: Mutations of the TGF-beta type II receptor BMPR2 in pulmonary arterial hypertension. Hum Mutat 2006;27:121–132.

10 Thomson JR, Machado RD, Pauciulo MW, Morgan NV, Humbert M, Elliott GC, Ward K, Yacoub M, Mikhail G, Rogers P, Newman J, Wheeler L, Higenbottam T, Gibbs JSR, Egan J, Crozier A, Peacock A, Allcock R, Corris P, Loyd JE, Trembath RC, Nichols WC: Sporadic primary pulmonary hypertension is associated with germline mutations of the gene encoding BMPR-II, a receptor member of the TGF-β family. J Med Genet 2000;37:741–745.
11 Chaouat A, Coulet F, Favre C, Simonneau G, Weitzenblum E, Soubrier F, Humbert M: Endoglin germline mutation in a patient with hereditary haemorrhagic telangiectasia and dexfenfluramine associated pulmonary arterial hypertension. Thorax 2004;59:446–448.
12 Trembath RC, Thomson JR, Machado RD, Morgan NV, Atkinson C, Winship I, Simonneau G, Galie N, Loyd JE, Humbert M, Nichols WC, Morrell NW, Berg J, Manes A, McGaughran J, Pauciulo M, Wheeler L: Clinical and molecular genetic features of pulmonary hypertension in patients with hereditary hemorrhagic telangiectasia. N Engl J Med 2001;345:325–334.
13 McGoon M, Gutterman D, Steen V, Barst R, McCrory DC, Fortin TA, Loyd JE: Screening, early detection, and diagnosis of pulmonary arterial hypertension: ACCP evidence-based clinical practice guidelines. Chest 2004;126:14S–34S.
14 Simonneau G, Galie N, Rubin LJ, Langleben D, Seeger W, Domenighetti G, Gibbs S, Lebrec D, Speich R, Beghetti M, Rich S, Fishman A: Clinical classification of pulmonary hypertension. J Am Coll Cardiol 2004;43:5S–12S.
15 Souza R, Humbert M, Sztrymf B, Jais X, Yaici A, Le Pavec J, Parent F, Herve P, Soubrier F, Sitbon O, Simonneau G: Pulmonary arterial hypertension associated with fenfluramine exposure: report of 109 cases. Eur Respir J 2008;31:343–348.
16 Walker AM, Langleben D, Korelitz JJ, Rich S, Rubin LJ, Strom BL, Gonin R, Keast S, Badesch D, Barst RJ, Bourge RC, Channick R, Frost A, Gaine S, McGoon M, McLaughlin V, Murali S, Oudiz RJ, Robbins IM, Tapson V, Abenhaim L, Constantine G: Temporal trends and drug exposures in pulmonary hypertension: an American experience. Am Heart J 2006;152:521–526.
17 Chambers CD, Hernandez-Diaz S, Van Marter LJ, Werler MM, Louik C, Jones KL, Mitchell AA: Selective serotonin-reuptake inhibitors and risk of persistent pulmonary hypertension of the newborn. N Engl J Med 2006;354:579–587.
18 Chin KM, Channick RN, Rubin LJ: Is methamphetamine use associated with idiopathic pulmonary arterial hypertension? Chest 2006;130:1657–1663.
19 Hachulla E, Gressin V, Guillevin L, Carpentier P, Diot E, Sibilia J, Kahan A, Cabane J, Frances C, Launay D, Mouthon L, Allanore Y, Tiev KP, Clerson P, de Groote P, Humbert M: Early detection of pulmonary arterial hypertension in systemic sclerosis: a French nationwide prospective multicenter study. Arthritis Rheum 2005;52:3792–3800.
20 Mukerjee D, St George D, Coleiro B, Knight C, Denton CP, Davar J, Black CM, Coghlan JG: Prevalence and outcome in systemic sclerosis associated pulmonary arterial hypertension: application of a registry approach. Ann Rheum Dis 2003;62:1088–1093.
21 Launay D, Mouthon L, Hachulla E, Pagnoux C, de Groote P, Remy-Jardin M, Matran R, Lambert M, Queyrel V, Morell-Dubois S, Guillevin L, Hatron PY: Prevalence and characteristics of moderate to severe pulmonary hypertension in systemic sclerosis with and without interstitial lung disease. J Rheumatol 2007;34:1005–1011.
22 de Groote P, Gressin V, Hachulla E, Carpentier P, Guillevin L, Kahan A, Cabane J, Frances C, Lamblin N, Diot E, Patat F, Sibilia J, Petit H, Cracowski JL, Clerson P, Humbert M: Evaluation of cardiac abnormalities by Doppler echocardiography in a large nationwide multicentric cohort of patients with systemic sclerosis. Ann Rheum Dis 2008;67:31–36.
23 Meune C, Avouac J, Wahbi K, Cabanes L, Wipff J, Mouthon L, Guillevin L, Kahan A, Allanore Y: Cardiac involvement in systemic sclerosis assessed by tissue-doppler echocardiography during routine care: a controlled study of 100 consecutive patients. Arthritis Rheum 2008;58:1803–1809.
24 Tanaka E, Harigai M, Tanaka M, Kawaguchi Y, Hara M, Kamatani N: Pulmonary hypertension in systemic lupus erythematosus: evaluation of clinical characteristics and response to immunosuppressive treatment. J Rheumatol 2002;29:282–287.
25 Asherson RA, Higenbottam TW, Dinh Xuan AT, Khamashta MA, Hughes GR: Pulmonary hypertension in a lupus clinic: experience with twenty-four patients. J Rheumatol 1990;17:1292–1298.
26 Burdt MA, Hoffman RW, Deutscher SL, Wang GS, Johnson JC, Sharp GC: Long-term outcome in mixed connective tissue disease: longitudinal clinical and serologic findings. Arthritis Rheum 1999;42:899–909.
27 Jais X, Launay D, Yaici A, Le Pavec J, Tcherakian C, Sitbon O, Simonneau G, Humbert M: Immunosuppressive therapy in lupus- and mixed connective tissue disease-associated pulmonary arterial hypertension: a retrospective analysis of twenty-three cases. Arthritis Rheum 2008;58:521–531.
28 Launay D, Hachulla E, Hatron PY, Jais X, Simonneau G, Humbert M: Pulmonary arterial hypertension: a rare complication of primary Sjogren syndrome: report of 9 new cases and review of the literature. Medicine (Baltimore) 2007;86:299–315.
29 Bunch TW, Tancredi RG, Lie JT: Pulmonary hypertension in polymyositis. Chest 1981;79:105–107.
30 Dawson JK, Goodson NG, Graham DR, Lynch MP: Raised pulmonary artery pressures measured with Doppler echocardiography in rheumatoid arthritis patients. Rheumatology (Oxford) 2000;39:1320–1325.
31 Kim KK, Factor SM: Membranoproliferative glomerulonephritis and plexogenic pulmonary arteriopathy in a homosexual man with acquired immunodeficiency syndrome. Hum Pathol 1987;18:1293–1296.
32 Mehta NJ, Khan IA, Mehta RN, Sepkowitz DA: HIV-Related pulmonary hypertension: analytic review of 131 cases. Chest 2000;118:1133–1141.
33 Opravil M, Pechere M, Speich R, Joller-Jemelka HI, Jenni R, Russi EW, Hirschel B, Luthy R: HIV-associated primary pulmonary hypertension. A case control study. Swiss HIV Cohort Study. Am J Respir Crit Care Med 1997;155:990–995.
34 Sitbon O, Lascoux-Combe C, Delfraissy JF, Yeni PG, Raffi F, De Zuttere D, Gressin V, Clerson P, Sereni D, Simonneau G: Prevalence of HIV-related pulmonary arterial hypertension in the current antiretroviral therapy era. Am J Respir Crit Care Med 2008;177:108–113.
35 Nunes H, Humbert M, Sitbon O, Morse JH, Deng Z, Knowles JA, Le Gall C, Parent F, Garcia G, Herve P, Barst RJ, Simonneau G: Prognostic factors for survival in human immunodeficiency virus-associated pulmonary arterial hypertension. Am J Respir Crit Care Med 2003;167:1433–1439.
36 Sitbon O, Gressin V, Speich R, Macdonald PS, Opravil M, Cooper DA, Fourme T, Humbert M, Delfraissy JF, Simonneau G: Bosentan for the treatment of human immunodeficiency virus-associated pulmonary arterial hypertension. Am J Respir Crit Care Med 2004;170:1212–1217.
37 Degano B, Yaïci A, Le Pavec J, Savale L, Jaïs X, Camara B, Humbert M, Simonneau G, Sitbon O: Long-term effects of bosentan in patients with HIV-associated pulmonary arterial hypertension. Eur Respir J 2009;33:92–98.
38 Herve P, Lebrec D, Brenot F, Simonneau G, Humbert M, Sitbon O, Duroux P: Pulmonary vascular disorders in portal hypertension. Eur Respir J 1998;11:1153–1166.
39 Rodriguez-Roisin R, Krowka MJ, Herve P, Fallon MB, ERS Task Force Pulmonary-Hepatic Vascular Disorders Scientific Committee ERS Task Force PHD Scientific Committee: Pulmonary-hepatic vascular disorders (PHD). Eur Respir J 2004;24:861–880.
40 Hadengue A, Benhayoun MK, Lebrec D, Benhamou JP: Pulmonary hypertension complicating portal hypertension: prevalence and relation to splanchnic hemodynamics. Gastroenterology 1991;100:520–528.
41 Krowka MJ, Swanson KL, Frantz RP, McGoon MD, Wiesner RH: Portopulmonary hypertension: results from a 10-year screening algorithm. Hepatology 2006;44:1502–1510.
42 Kawut SM, Krowka MJ, Trotter JF, Roberts KE, Benza RL, Badesch DB, Taichman DB, Horn EM, Zacks S, Kaplowitz N, Brown RS Jr, Fallon MB: Clinical risk factors for portopulmonary hypertension. Hepatology 2008;48:196–203.
43 Le Pavec J, Souza R, Herve P, Lebrec D, Savale L, Tcherakian C, Jais X, Yaici A, Humbert M, Simonneau G, Sitbon O: Portopulmonary hypertension: survival and prognostic factors. Am J Respir Crit Care Med 2008;178:637–643.

44 Eisenmenger V: Die angeborene Defecte der Kammersheidewand das Herzen. Z Klin Med 1897;132:131.
45 Wood P: The Eisenmenger syndrome or pulmonary hypertension with reversed central shunt. I. Br Med J 1958;2:701–709.
46 Daliento L, Somerville J, Presbitero P, Menti L, Brach-Prever S, Rizzoli G, Stone S: Eisenmenger syndrome. Factors relating to deterioration and death. Eur Heart J 1998;19:1845–1855.
47 Besterman E: Atrial septal defect with pulmonary hypertension. Br Heart J 1961;23:587–598.
48 Hoffman JI, Rudolph AM: The natural history of ventricular septal defects in infancy. Am J Cardiol 1965;16:634–653.
49 Mazzei JA, Mazzei: A tribute: Abel Ayerza and pulmonary hypertension. Eur Respir Rev 2011;20:220–221.
50 Lapa MS, Ferreira EV, Jardim C, Martins Bdo C, Arakaki JS, Souza R: Clinical characteristics of pulmonary hypertension patients in two reference centers in the city of Sao Paulo (in Portuguese). Rev Assoc Med Bras 2006;52:139–143.
51 Chaves E: The pathology of the arterial pulmonary vasculature in Manson's schistosomiasis. Dis Chest 1966;50:72–77.
52 de Cleva R, Herman P, Pugliese V, Zilberstein B, Saad WA, Rodrigues JJ, Laudanna AA: Prevalence of pulmonary hypertension in patients with hepatosplenic Mansonic schistosomiasis – prospective study. Hepatogastroenterology 2003;50:2028–2030.
53 Lapa M, Dias B, Jardim C, Fernandes CJ, Dourado PM, Figueiredo M, Farias A, Tsutsui J, Terra-Filho M, Humbert M, Souza R: Cardiopulmonary manifestations of hepatosplenic schistosomiasis. Circulation 2009;119:1518–1523.
54 Castro O, Hoque M, Brown BD: Pulmonary hypertension in sickle cell disease: cardiac catheterization results and survival. Blood 2003;101:1257–1261.
55 Gladwin MT, Sachdev V, Jison ML, Shizukuda Y, Plehn JF, Minter K, Brown B, Coles WA, Nichols JS, Ernst I, Hunter LA, Blackwelder WC, Schechter AN, Rodgers GP, Castro O, Ognibene FP: Pulmonary hypertension as a risk factor for death in patients with sickle cell disease. N Engl J Med 2004;350:886–895.
56 Aessopos A, Stamatelos G, Skoumas V, Vassilopoulos G, Mantzourani M, Loukopoulos D: Pulmonary hypertension and right heart failure in patients with beta-thalassemia intermedia. Chest 1995;107:50–53.
57 Smedema JP, Louw VJ: Pulmonary arterial hypertension after splenectomy for hereditary spherocytosis. Cardiovasc J Afr 2007;18:84–89.
58 Jais X, Till SJ, Cynober T, Ioos V, Garcia G, Tchernia G, Dartevelle P, Simonneau G, Delaunay J, Humbert M: An extreme consequence of splenectomy in dehydrated hereditary stomatocytosis: gradual thrombo-embolic pulmonary hypertension and lung-heart transplantation. Hemoglobin 2003;27:139–147.
59 Stuard ID, Heusinkveld RS, Moss AJ: Microangiopathic hemolytic anemia and thrombocytopenia in primary pulmonary hypertension. N Engl J Med 1972;287:869–870.
60 Parent F, Egels S, Stzrymf B, Girot R, Dreiss F, Galacteros F, Simonneau G: Haemodynamic characteristics of patients with sickle cell disease and suspected pulmonary hypertension on the basis of a tricuspid regurgitation jet velocity >2.5 m/s on Doppler echocardiography (abstract). Eur Respir J 2006;28:544s.
61 Anthi A, Machado RF, Jison ML, Taveira-Dasilva AM, Rubin LJ, Hunter L, Hunter CJ, Coles W, Nichols J, Avila NA, Sachdev V, Chen CC, Gladwin MT: Hemodynamic and functional assessment of patients with sickle cell disease and pulmonary hypertension. Am J Respir Crit Care Med 2007;175:1272–1279.
62 Haque AK, Gokhale S, Rampy BA, Adegboyega P, Duarte A, Saldana MJ: Pulmonary hypertension in sickle cell hemoglobinopathy: a clinicopathologic study of 20 cases. Hum Pathol 2002;33:1037–1043.
63 Reiter CD, Wang X, Tanus-Santos JE, Hogg N, Cannon RO 3rd, Schechter AN, Gladwin MT: Cell-free hemoglobin limits nitric oxide bioavailability in sickle-cell disease. Nat Med 2002;8:1383–1389.
64 Gladwin MT, Lancaster JR Jr, Freeman BA, Schechter AN: Nitric oxide's reactions with hemoglobin: a view through the SNO-storm. Nat Med 2003;9:496–500.
65 Montani D, Achouh L, Dorfmuller P, Le Pavec J, Sztrymf B, Tcherakian C, Rabiller A, Haque R, Sitbon O, Jais X, Dartevelle P, Maitre S, Capron F, Musset D, Simonneau G, Humbert M: Pulmonary veno-occlusive disease: clinical, functional, radiologic, and hemodynamic characteristics and outcome of 24 cases confirmed by histology. Medicine (Baltimore) 2008;87:220–233.
66 Lantuejoul S, Sheppard MN, Corrin B, Burke MM, Nicholson AG: Pulmonary veno-occlusive disease and pulmonary capillary hemangiomatosis: a clinicopathologic study of 35 cases. Am J Surg Pathol 2006;30:850–857.
67 Montani D, Price LC, Dorfmuller P, Achouh L, Jais X, Yaici A, Sitbon O, Musset D, Simonneau G, Humbert M: Pulmonary veno-occlusive disease. Eur Respir J 2009;33:189–200.
68 Dorfmuller P, Humbert M, Perros F, Sanchez O, Simonneau G, Muller KM, Capron F: Fibrous remodeling of the pulmonary venous system in pulmonary arterial hypertension associated with connective tissue diseases. Hum Pathol 2007;38:893–902.
69 Escamilla R, Hermant C, Berjaud J, Mazerolles C, Daussy X: Pulmonary veno-occlusive disease in a HIV-infected intravenous drug abuser. Eur Respir J 1995;8:1982–1984.
70 Ruchelli ED, Nojadera G, Rutstein RM, Rudy B: Pulmonary veno-occlusive disease. Another vascular disorder associated with human immunodeficiency virus infection? Arch Pathol Lab Med 1994;118:664–666.
71 Runo JR, Vnencak-Jones CL, Prince M, Loyd JE, Wheeler L, Robbins IM, Lane KB, Newman JH, Johnson J, Nichols WC, Phillips JA 3rd: Pulmonary veno-occlusive disease caused by an inherited mutation in bone morphogenetic protein receptor II. Am J Respir Crit Care Med 2003;167:889–894.
72 Resten A, Maitre S, Humbert M, Rabiller A, Sitbon O, Capron F, Simonneau G, Musset D: Pulmonary hypertension: CT of the chest in pulmonary venoocclusive disease. AJR Am J Roentgenol 2004;183:65–70.
73 Holcomb BW Jr, Loyd JE, Ely EW, Johnson J, Robbins IM: Pulmonary veno-occlusive disease: a case series and new observations. Chest 2000;118:1671–1679.
74 Dufour B, Maitre S, Humbert M, Capron F, Simonneau G, Musset D: High-resolution CT of the chest in four patients with pulmonary capillary hemangiomatosis or pulmonary venoocclusive disease. AJR Am J Roentgenol 1998;171:1321–1324.
75 Rabiller A, Jais X, Hamid A, Resten A, Parent F, Haque R, Capron F, Sitbon O, Simonneau G, Humbert M: Occult alveolar haemorrhage in pulmonary veno-occlusive disease. Eur Respir J 2006;27:108–113.
76 Oudiz RJ: Pulmonary hypertension associated with left-sided heart disease. Clin Chest Med 2007;28:233–241.
77 Abramson SV, Burke JF, Kelly JJ Jr, Kitchen JG 3rd, Dougherty MJ, Yih DF, McGeehin FC 3rd, Shuck JW, Phiambolis TP: Pulmonary hypertension predicts mortality and morbidity in patients with dilated cardiomyopathy. Ann Intern Med 1992;116:888–895.
78 Zener JC, Hancock EW, Shumway NE, Harrison DC: Regression of extreme pulmonary hypertension after mitral valve surgery. Am J Cardiol 1972;30:820–826.
79 Braunwald E, Braunwald NS, Ross J Jr, Morrow AG: Effects of mitral-valve replacement on the pulmonary vascular dynamics of patients with pulmonary hypertension. N Engl J Med 1965;273:509–514.
80 Delgado JF, Conde E, Sanchez V, Lopez-Rios F, Gomez-Sanchez MA, Escribano P, Sotelo T, Gomez de la Camara A, Cortina J, de la Calzada CS: Pulmonary vascular remodeling in pulmonary hypertension due to chronic heart failure. Eur J Heart Fail 2005;7:1011–1016.
81 Moraes DL, Colucci WS, Givertz MM: Secondary pulmonary hypertension in chronic heart failure: the role of the endothelium in pathophysiology and management. Circulation 2000;102:1718–1723.
82 Fraser KL, Tullis DE, Sasson Z, Hyland RH, Thornley KS, Hanly PJ: Pulmonary hypertension and cardiac function in adult cystic fibrosis: role of hypoxemia. Chest 1999;115:1321–1328.
83 Cottin V, Nunes H, Brillet PY, Delaval P, Devouassoux G, Tillie-Leblond I, Israel-Biet D, Court-Fortune I, Valeyre D, Cordier JF: Combined pulmonary fibrosis and emphysema: a distinct underrecognised entity. Eur Respir J 2005;26:586–593.

84 Weitzenblum E, Hirth C, Ducolone A, Mirhom R, Rasaholinjanahary J, Ehrhart M: Prognostic value of pulmonary artery pressure in chronic obstructive pulmonary disease. Thorax 1981;36:752–758.
85 Thabut G, Dauriat G, Stern JB, Logeart D, Levy A, Marrash-Chahla R, Mal H: Pulmonary hemodynamics in advanced COPD candidates for lung volume reduction surgery or lung transplantation. Chest 2005;127:1531–1536.
86 Chaouat A, Bugnet AS, Kadaoui N, Schott R, Enache I, Ducolone A, Ehrhart M, Kessler R, Weitzenblum E: Severe pulmonary hypertension and chronic obstructive pulmonary disease. Am J Respir Crit Care Med 2005;172:189–194.
87 Tapson VF, Humbert M: Incidence and prevalence of chronic thromboembolic pulmonary hypertension: from acute to chronic pulmonary embolism. Proc Am Thorac Soc 2006;3:564–567.
88 Pengo V, Lensing AW, Prins MH, Marchiori A, Davidson BL, Tiozzo F, Albanese P, Biasiolo A, Pegoraro C, Iliceto S, Prandoni P: Incidence of chronic thromboembolic pulmonary hypertension after pulmonary embolism. N Engl J Med 2004;350:2257–2264.
89 Kim NH: Assessment of operability in chronic thromboembolic pulmonary hypertension. Proc Am Thorac Soc 2006;3:584–588.
90 Dartevelle P, Fadel E, Mussot S, Chapelier A, Herve P, de Perrot M, Cerrina J, Ladurie FL, Lehouerou D, Humbert M, Sitbon O, Simonneau G: Chronic thromboembolic pulmonary hypertension. Eur Respir J 2004;23:637–648.
91 Jamieson SW, Kapelanski DP, Sakakibara N, Manecke GR, Thistlethwaite PA, Kerr KM, Channick RN, Fedullo PF, Auger WR: Pulmonary endarterectomy: experience and lessons learned in 1,500 cases. Ann Thorac Surg 2003;76:1457–1462, discussion 62–64.
92 Suntharalingam J, Treacy CM, Doughty NJ, Goldsmith K, Soon E, Toshner MR, Sheares KK, Hughes R, Morrell NW, Pepke-Zaba J: Long-term use of sildenafil in inoperable chronic thromboembolic pulmonary hypertension. Chest 2008;134:229–236.
93 Rubin LJ, Hoeper MM, Klepetko W, Galie N, Lang IM, Simonneau G: Current and future management of chronic thromboembolic pulmonary hypertension: from diagnosis to treatment responses. Proc Am Thorac Soc 2006;3:601–607.
94 Dingli D, Utz JP, Krowka MJ, Oberg AL, Tefferi A: Unexplained pulmonary hypertension in chronic myeloproliferative disorders. Chest 2001;120:801–808.
95 Guilpain P, Montani D, Damaj G, Achouh L, Lefrère F, Marfaing-Koka A, Dartevelle P, Simonneau G, Humbert M, Hermine O: Pulmonary hypertension associated with myeloproliferative disorders: a retrospective study of ten cases. Respiration 2008;76:295–302.
96 Marvin KS, Spellberg RD: Pulmonary hypertension secondary to thrombocytosis in a patient with myeloid metaplasia. Chest 1993;103:642–644.
97 Nand S, Orfei E: Pulmonary hypertension in polycythemia vera. Am J Hematol 1994;47:242–244.
98 Peacock AJ: Pulmonary hypertension after splenectomy: a consequence of loss of the splenic filter or is there something more? Thorax 2005;60:983–984.
99 Jais X, Ioos V, Jardim C, Sitbon O, Parent F, Hamid A, Fadel E, Dartevelle P, Simonneau G, Humbert M: Splenectomy and chronic thromboembolic pulmonary hypertension. Thorax 2005;60:1031–1034.
100 Hoeper MM, Niedermeyer J, Hoffmeyer F, Flemming P, Fabel H: Pulmonary hypertension after splenectomy? Ann Intern Med 1999;130:506–509.
101 Gluskowski J, Hawrylkiewicz I, Zych D, Wojtczak A, Zielinski J: Pulmonary haemodynamics at rest and during exercise in patients with sarcoidosis. Respiration 1984;46:26–32.
102 Handa T, Nagai S, Miki S, Fushimi Y, Ohta K, Mishima M, Izumi T: Incidence of pulmonary hypertension and its clinical relevance in patients with sarcoidosis. Chest 2006;129:1246–1252.
103 Shorr AF, Helman DL, Davies DB, Nathan SD: Pulmonary hypertension in advanced sarcoidosis: epidemiology and clinical characteristics. Eur Respir J 2005;25:783–788.
104 Bourbonnais JM, Samavati L: Clinical predictors of pulmonary hypertension in sarcoidosis. Eur Respir J 2008;32:296–302.
105 Nunes H, Humbert M, Capron F, Brauner M, Sitbon O, Battesti JP, Simonneau G, Valeyre D: Pulmonary hypertension associated with sarcoidosis: mechanisms, haemodynamics and prognosis. Thorax 2006;61:68–74.
106 Dauriat G, Mal H, Thabut G, Mornex JF, Bertocchi M, Tronc F, Leroy-Ladurie F, Dartevelle P, Reynaud-Gaubert M, Thomas P, Pison C, Blin D, Stern M, Bonnette P, Dromer C, Velly JF, Brugiere O, Leseche G, Fournier M: Lung transplantation for pulmonary Langerhans' cell histiocytosis: a multicenter analysis. Transplantation 2006;81:746–750.
107 Fartoukh M, Humbert M, Capron F, Maitre S, Parent F, Le Gall C, Sitbon O, Herve P, Duroux P, Simonneau G: Severe pulmonary hypertension in histiocytosis X. Am J Respir Crit Care Med 2000;161:216–223.
108 Taveira-DaSilva AM, Hathaway OM, Sachdev V, Shizukuda Y, Birdsall CW, Moss J: Pulmonary artery pressure in lymphangioleiomyomatosis: an echocardiographic study. Chest 2007;132:1573–1578.
109 Harari S, Simonneau G, De Juli E, Brenot F, Cerrina J, Colombo P, Gronda E, Micallef E, Parent F, Dartevelle P: Prognostic value of pulmonary hypertension in patients with chronic interstitial lung disease referred for lung or heart-lung transplantation. J Heart Lung Transplant 1997;16:460–463.
110 Simeoni S, Puccetti A, Chilosi M, Tinazzi E, Prati D, Corrocher R, Lunardi C: Type 1 neurofibromatosis complicated by pulmonary artery hypertension: a case report. J Med Invest 2007;54:354–358.
111 Engel PJ, Baughman RP, Menon SG, Kereiakes DJ, Taylor L, Scott M: Pulmonary hypertension in neurofibromatosis. Am J Cardiol 2007;99:1177–1178.
112 Aoki Y, Kodama M, Mezaki T, Ogawa R, Sato M, Okabe M, Aizawa Y: von Recklinghausen disease complicated by pulmonary hypertension. Chest 2001;119:1606–1608.
113 Samuels N, Berkman N, Milgalter E, Bar-Ziv J, Amir G, Kramer MR: Pulmonary hypertension secondary to neurofibromatosis: intimal fibrosis versus thromboembolism. Thorax 1999;54:858–859.
114 Stewart DR, Cogan JD, Kramer MR, Miller WT Jr, Christiansen LE, Pauciulo MW, Messiaen LM, Tu GS, Thompson WH, Pyeritz RE, Ryu JH, Nichols WC, Kodama M, Meyrick BO, Ross DJ: Is pulmonary arterial hypertension in neurofibromatosis type 1 secondary to a plexogenic arteriopathy? Chest 2007;132:798–808.
115 Launay D, Souza R, Guillevin L, Hachulla E, Pouchot J, Simonneau G, Humbert M: Pulmonary arterial hypertension in ANCA-associated vasculitis. Sarcoidosis Vasc Diffuse Lung Dis 2006;23:223–228.
116 Hamaoka K, Nakagawa M, Furukawa N, Sawada T: Pulmonary hypertension in type I glycogen storage disease. Pediatr Cardiol 1990;11:54–56.
117 Inoue S, Nakamura T, Hasegawa K, Tadaoka S, Samukawa M, Nezuo S, Sawayama T, Higashi Y, Shirabe T: Pulmonary hypertension due to glycogen storage disease type II (Pompe's disease): a case report (in Japanese). J Cardiol 1989;19:323–332.
118 Humbert M, Labrune P, Sitbon O, Le Gall C, Callebert J, Herve P, Samuel D, Machado R, Trembath R, Drouet L, Launay JM, Simonneau G: Pulmonary arterial hypertension and type-I glycogen-storage disease: the serotonin hypothesis. Eur Respir J 2002;20:59–65.
119 Pizzo CJ: Type I glycogen storage disease with focal nodular hyperplasia of the liver and vasoconstrictive pulmonary hypertension. Pediatrics 1980;65:341–343.
120 Elstein D, Klutstein MW, Lahad A, Abrahamov A, Hadas-Halpern I, Zimran A: Echocardiographic assessment of pulmonary hypertension in Gaucher's disease. Lancet 1998;351:1544–1546.
121 Lee R, Yousem S: The frequency and type of lung involvement in patients with Gaucher's disease (abstract). Lab Invest 1998;58:54 A.
122 Theise ND, Ursell PC: Pulmonary hypertension and Gaucher's disease: logical association or mere coincidence? Am J Pediatr Hematol Oncol 1990;12:74–76.
123 Li JH, Safford RE, Aduen JF, Heckman MG, Crook JE, Burger CD: Pulmonary hypertension and thyroid disease. Chest 2007;132:793–797.

124 Ferris A, Jacobs T, Widlitz A, Barst RJ, Morse JH: Pulmonary arterial hypertension and thyroid disease. Chest 2001;119:1980–1981.
125 Merce J, Ferras S, Oltra C, Sanz E, Vendrell J, Simon I, Camprubi M, Bardaji A, Ridao C: Cardiovascular abnormalities in hyperthyroidism: a prospective Doppler echocardiographic study. Am J Med 2005;118:126–131.
126 Kokturk N, Demir N, Demircan S, Memis L, Kurul C, Akyurek N, Turktas H: Pulmonary veno-occlusive disease in a patient with a history of Hashimoto's thyroiditis. Indian J Chest Dis Allied Sci 2005;47:289–292.
127 Chu JW, Kao PN, Faul JL, Doyle RL: High prevalence of autoimmune thyroid disease in pulmonary arterial hypertension. Chest 2002;122:1668–1673.
128 Mayer E, Kriegsmann J, Gaumann A, Kauczor HU, Dahm M, Hake U, Schmid FX, Oelert H: Surgical treatment of pulmonary artery sarcoma. J Thorac Cardiovasc Surg 2001;121:77–82.
129 Anderson MB, Kriett JM, Kapelanski DP, Tarazi R, Jamieson SW: Primary pulmonary artery sarcoma: a report of six cases. Ann Thorac Surg 1995;59:1487–1490.
130 Kim HK, Choi YS, Kim K, Shim YM, Sung K, Lee YT, Park PW, Kim J: Surgical treatment for pulmonary artery sarcoma. Eur J Cardiothorac Surg 2008;33:712–716.
131 Ishiguro T, Kasahara K, Matsumoto I, Waseda R, Minato H, Kimura H, Katayama N, Yasui M, Ohta Y, Fujimura M: Primary pulmonary artery sarcoma detected with a pulmonary infarction. Intern Med 2007;46:601–604.
132 Roberts KE, Hamele-Bena D, Saqi A, Stein CA, Cole RP: Pulmonary tumor embolism: a review of the literature. Am J Med 2003;115:228–232.
133 Dot JM, Sztrymf B, Yaici A, Dorfmuller P, Capron F, Parent F, Jais X, Sitbon O, Simonneau G, Humbert M: Pulmonary arterial hypertension due to tumor emboli (in French). Rev Mal Respir 2007;24:359–366.
134 Davis AM, Pierson RN, Loyd JE: Mediastinal fibrosis. Semin Respir Infect 2001;16:119–130.
135 Loyd JE, Tillman BF, Atkinson JB, Des Prez RM: Mediastinal fibrosis complicating histoplasmosis. Medicine (Baltimore) 1988;67:295–310.
136 Goodwin RA, Nickell JA, Des Prez RM: Mediastinal fibrosis complicating healed primary histoplasmosis and tuberculosis. Medicine (Baltimore) 1972;51:227–246.
137 Yigla M, Nakhoul F, Sabag A, Tov N, Gorevich B, Abassi Z, Reisner SA: Pulmonary hypertension in patients with end-stage renal disease. Chest 2003;123:1577–1582.
138 Nakhoul F, Yigla M, Gilman R, Reisner SA, Abassi Z: The pathogenesis of pulmonary hypertension in haemodialysis patients via arterio-venous access. Nephrol Dial Transplant 2005;20:1686–1692.

David Montani, MD, PhD
Centre de Référence de l'Hypertension Pulmonaire Sévère, Service de Pneumologie
Hôpital Antoine-Béclère, Assistance Publique – Hôpitaux de Paris, Université Paris-Sud 11
157 rue de la Porte de Trivaux
FR–92140 Clamart (France)
Tel. +33 1 45 37 47 72, E-Mail david.montani@abc.aphp.fr

Chapter 2

Humbert M, Souza R, Simonneau G (eds): Pulmonary Vascular Disorders.
Prog Respir Res. Basel, Karger, 2012, vol 41, pp 14–22

Pathology of Pulmonary Arterial Hypertension

Peter Dorfmüller

Service d'Anatomie et de Cytologie Pathologiques, Hôpital Marie Lannelongue and INSERM U999 'Hypertension Artérielle Pulmonaire: Physiopathologie et Innovation Thérapeutique', Le Plessis Robinson, France

Abstract

Vascular lesions found in lungs of patients with pulmonary hypertension are probably responsible for the increase of pulmonary arterial pressures and share some peculiarities that appear characteristic. The fibrotic and proliferative lesions mainly concern small lung vessels; precapillary lesions are typically located in muscular arteries <500 μm diameter and arterioles in patients with pulmonary arterial hypertension (PAH), while septal veins and preseptal venules are involved in patients with postcapillary pulmonary veno-occlusive disease (PVOD)/pulmonary capillary hemangiomatosis (PCH). During the World Symposium at Dana Point, California, in 2008, PVOD/PCH was assigned to a novel, distinctive category of pulmonary venous hypertension (Group 1') due to important differences in clinical management. However, many similarities between those two conditions can be observed, and conditions with mixed (arterial and venous) involvement may be encountered, a fact that is taken into consideration by this 'soft' prime separation.

The Correlate of Pulmonary Arterial Hypertension in Histopathology – A View from a Different Standpoint

Pathological anatomy, or pathology, is first of all a descriptive discipline. It necessitates a primary 'starting point', an initial rigid and objective observation, which will initiate a cascade of suppositions, deductions, and consequently a directional (influenced) analysis of the diseased sample. Although the pathological report appears as additional and, in most cases, terminal information to other clinical data, it actually represents far more: as the morphological observation is dissociated from the patient and its acute symptoms [pulmonary arterial hypertension (PAH) samples are mostly collected during transplantation or autopsy], it may be a possibility to countercheck the disease from the 'other side', i.e. from the inside. This of course will not always produce concordance with the clinical image, but sometimes contradiction, or morphological diversity, that cannot be translated directly into the clinical language/symptoms. The descriptive approach to diseased pulmonary arteries and the histological phenotyping in PAH is based on the different vascular compartments affected and the different cell types involved in their pathological anatomy. Sadly enough, we lack longitudinal temporal information of histological changes: in most cases, observations and hypotheses are based on transversal time points of different subjects. And as stated above, most PAH cases are diagnosed initially on clinical grounds, while histological confirmation is often achieved preterminally via analysis of lung explants or autopsy samples. In the actual diagnostic setting, lung biopsy is contraindicated for the vast majority of patients suffering from PAH and consequently the morphological correlate will be a late one: a 'photo-finish' for all PAH patients a few weeks before total right heart failure. This final picture of the complete workings of the disease probably fails to underline important levels of disease evolution. Many research groups from the international PAH community still invest a lot of time and energy into the constitution of animal models mimicking PAH; the possibility to look into a 4-dimensional vascular time tube and to influence different compartments at different moments of the disease process makes it clear why it is worth the trouble.

Vascular Lesions in Pulmonary Arterial Hypertension

Vascular lesions found in the lungs of patients suffering from PAH are most likely responsible for the increase of pulmonary arterial pressure and share some peculiarities that appear characteristic, but should not be regarded as specific or even pathognomonic. The fibrotic and proliferative lesions mainly concern small lung vessels; precapillary lesions are typically located in muscular arteries with diameters less than 500 μm diameter and arterioles in patients with PAH, while septal veins (running within the lobular septa) and preseptal venules are involved in patients with postcapillary pulmonary veno-occlusive disease (PVOD)/pulmonary capillary hemangiomatosis (PCH). Although clinical differentiation between these entities is not always simple, and although PVOD has been considered until recently as a subgroup of PAH, in 2008, during the World Symposium at Dana Point, California, PVOD/PCH was assigned to a novel category of pulmonary venous hypertension (Group 1') [1]. However, contrary to what the dichotomy of 'arterial' and 'venous' implies in this nomenclature, many similarities between these two conditions can be observed, a fact that is taken into consideration by this 'soft' prime separation. Hence, both conditions will be revisited in this chapter.

Arterial Lesions

Typical arterial lesions in lungs of patients with PAH do not involve the larger pulmonary arteries of the elastic type; intimal and medial lesions on this level may be found in patients with chronically increased pulmonary arterial pressures, but mainly correspond to nonobstructing atherosclerotic lesions as are typically found in the systemic vasculature [2]. Obliterating PAH lesions are found in pre- and intra-acinar arteries with a muscular medial layer. Different vessel wall compartments may contribute to the thickening of the arterial wall, and hence various histological patterns may occur (presented below).

Medial Hypertrophy

This abnormality of the vessel wall can be observed in all subgroups of PAH and may be encountered in other forms of pulmonary hypertension (PH), e.g. Group 2 or 3 (PH owing to left heart disease, and PH owing to lung diseases and/or hypoxia). The lesion corresponds to a proliferation of smooth muscle cells within the tunica media. The histological criterion of medial hypertrophy (which corresponds more precisely to hypertrophy and hyperplasia, i.e. increase in volume and number of smooth muscle cells, respectively) is fulfilled when the diameter of a single medial layer, delineated by its internal and external elastic lamina, exceeds 10% of the artery's cross-sectional diameter (fig. 1a, b). Isolated hypertrophy of the medial layer may be considered as an early and even reversible event, as has been shown for PH due to hypoxia at high altitude [3]. Also, as recently stated by Sakao et al. [4], new therapeutic concepts that appear to work in experimental PH, e.g. the tyrosine-kinase receptor-inhibitor imatinib, solely reduce the pulmonary arterial/arteriolar muscularization, an observation which underlines the reversibility of muscular remodeling. In a recent study and review of the literature, Penazola and Arias-Stella [5] noted that healthy natives of high-altitude regions over 3,500 m above sea level have PH, right ventricular hypertrophy, and an increased amount of smooth muscle cells in the distal pulmonary arterial branches. Clinical and histological findings from 30 healthy high-altitude natives and 30 sea-level natives revealed that the main factor responsible for PH in healthy highlanders is the increased amount of smooth muscle cells in the distal pulmonary arteries and arterioles. Vasoconstriction is a secondary factor in this setting because the administration of oxygen decreases the pulmonary arterial pressure only by 15–20%. The adaptive increase in cardiac and smooth muscle cell mass reverses after a prolonged residence at sea level. In PAH, medial hypertrophy is commonly associated with the remodeling of other vascular compartments, which is discussed below.

Intimal Fibrosis

Fibrotic lesions of the intimal layer are frequent in PAH-diseased lungs. The intima may be thickened by proliferation and recruitment of fibroblasts, myofibroblasts, and other connective tissue cells, and consequently by the interstitial deposition of collagen. In a purely descriptive approach, this thickening may be uniform and concentric, or focally predominating and eccentric (fig. 1c, d). Both forms can lead to a complete occlusion of the artery. The gain in intimal cellularity is generally understood as a reaction of the inner arterial layer to a luminal stimulus, e.g. chronic pressure and shear stress or as a scarring process after primary endothelial damage [6]. In many cases, adventitial fibrosis is associated with intimal changes, but remains difficult to evaluate due to the lack of a clear anatomical delimitation. Eccentric intimal thickening is frequently observed in cases with thrombotic events and probably represents residues of wall-adherent, organized thrombi. Thrombotic lesions, or so-called in situ thrombosis, are a frequent pattern in different PAH subgroups and PVOD: organization and recanalization of totally occluding thrombotic material may lead to bizarre fibrotic multichannel lesions (so-called 'colander-

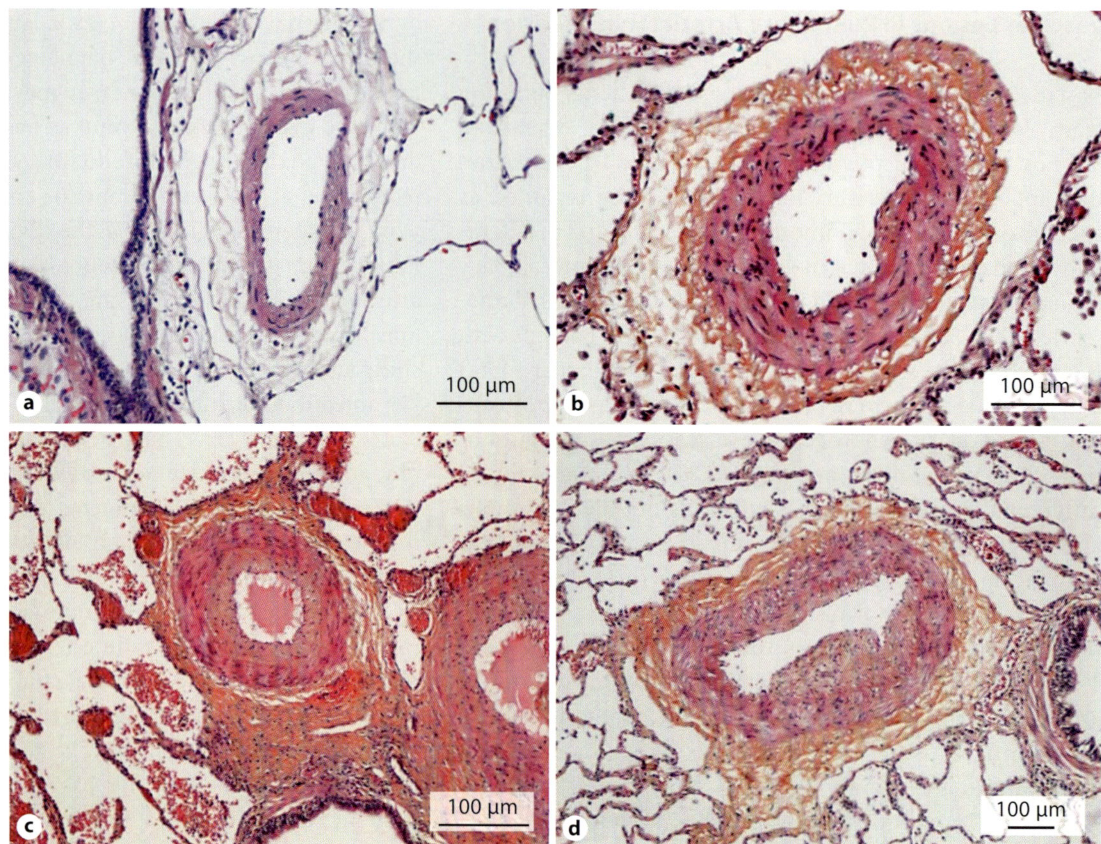

Fig. 1. Histology of lung samples from a control and from patients suffering from idiopathic PAH. **a** Pulmonary artery with adjacent bronchiole from a control (undiseased lung parenchyma at distance from a pulmonary carcinoma). The medial layer is slender, there is no intimal thickening. HE-staining (hematoxylin-eosin), magnification ×100. **b** Medial hypertrophy and moderate adventitial fibrosis in a muscular artery. The intima is not significantly remodeled. HES-staining (hematoxylin-eosin-saffron), magnification ×100. **c** Two branches of a pulmonary artery and their adjacent bronchiole (below). The intima (of the centered artery) displays concentric nonlaminar fibrosis (inner, orange-colored layer), the media is hypertrophic (outer, fuchsia-colored layer). HES-staining, magnification ×100. **d** Pulmonary artery displaying eccentric intimal fibrosis forming a cushion-like protrusion into the lumen. Again, adventitial fibrosis is present. HES-staining, magnification ×40.

like' lesions) which can easily be confounded with proliferative complex lesions (see below).

Concentric Laminar Intimal Fibrosis

This morphologically conspicuous phenotype of intimal fibrosis is also known as an 'onion skin' or 'onion bulb' lesion. Numerous concentrically arranged fibrotic layers occlude the arterial lumen of small (diameter: 100–200 µm) arteries (fig. 2a). The scar-like, cell-lacking morphology of this lesion may be found in lungs of patients suffering from different forms of PAH, including PAH associated with connective tissue disease (CTD) [7]. Nevertheless, the observation that intimal thickening proximal to plexiform lesions in supernumerary arteries usually displays a concentric laminar phenotype seems to closely associate these two lesions. Immunohistochemical analysis reveals fibroblasts, myofibroblasts, and smooth muscle cells.

Complex Lesions

Complex pulmonary arterial lesions comprise three different patterns, which are commonly observed in close topographic association. Most often, they have been interpreted as a 3-dimensional continuum, but despite several descriptive studies based on 3-dimensional imaging techniques remain a poorly understood construct, at least in its pathophysiology. To date, it is not clear if this very special and in global lung vascular pathology infrequent anomaly is the (or a) reason for increased vascular resistance or simply

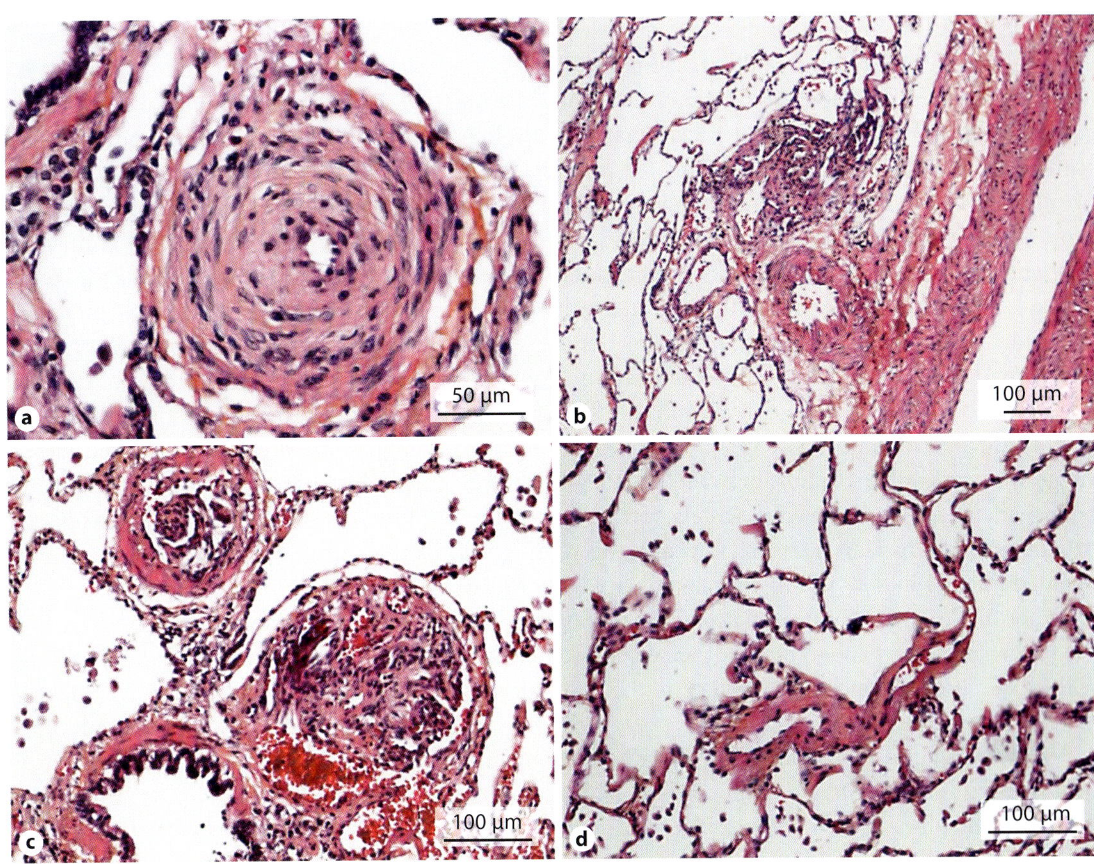

Fig. 2. Histology of lung samples from patients suffering from idiopathic PAH. **a** Small pulmonary artery with concentric laminar fibrosis: note the onion skin-like layers. HES-staining, magnification ×200. **b** Complex lesion occurring within a supernumerary artery branching of a larger pulmonary artery. Sinusoidal, endothelial-lined channels fill out the former lumen of the small vessel. HES-staining, magnification ×40. **c** Another complex lesion: the plexiform remodeling occupies the entire lumen, displaying a 'glomeruloid' appearance. The rest of the lumen seems to feed into dilated vessels below (dilation lesion). HES-staining, magnification ×100. **d** Muscularized arteriole with thickened walls, feeding into the capillary network. HES-staining, magnification ×100.

a secondary reaction, a failed attempt to decrease PH. The three histological patterns are the following:

(1) The plexiform lesion probably represents the most illustrious form of vascular lesions in PAH: for a long time it was considered as a pathognomonic pattern of idiopathic PAH (formerly known as primary PH) [8]. Since then, this presumption has been revised, as plexiform lesions have been shown to occur in other PAH subgroups like congenital heart disease-associated PAH or portopulmonary hypertension. The peculiar lesion affects various vascular compartments: a focal intimal thickening of small pulmonary arteries, preferably beyond branching points, is followed by an exuberant endothelial cell proliferation, leading to the formation of capillary-like, sinusoidal channels on a smooth muscle cell and collagen-rich matrix within the native arterial lumen and resulting in obstruction (fig. 2b, c) [9]. This glomerular-like arterial zone appears to feed into dilated, vein-like congestive vessels, which are perceivable at low magnification and may be helpful as sentinel lesions when tracing plexiform lesions.

(2) The latter vein-like congestive pulmonary vessels, also known as 'dilation lesions', may predominate the histological pattern, but are most frequently associated with plexiform lesions. Pulmonary hemorrhage in PAH patients could be in part a consequence of the unstable and thin-walled vessel structure.

(3) Classical arteritis with transmural inflammation and fibrinoid necrosis, as first described by Heath and Edwards [10], may be observed, but is a rather infrequent phenomenon in PAH, possibly due to the prolonged survival

of patients and new drug therapies. Nevertheless, perivascular inflammatory infiltrates of diseased pulmonary arteries in PAH patients are commonly found. Infiltrates mainly consisting of T lymphocytes and macrophages, as well as scattered mast cells are frequently associated with plexiform or other intimal lesions. This inflammatory phenotype, in most cases, is evaluated as 'mild' to 'moderate'.

Complex lesions were first described in patients with congenital cardiac left-to-right shunts [10], and eventually in other forms of PAH, all belonging to Group 1 of the Venice and Dana Point classifications. In a publication from 1993 [11], plexiform lesions were detected in 20 of 31 patients with confirmed chronic major vessel thromboembolic PH, suggesting a possible relation between organizing thromboembolic and complex lesions, which mirrors an old theory first inspired by Harrison [12]. Recently, this finding has been confirmed in a review by Piazza and Goldhaber [13]. Another historic hypothesis explaining the pathogenesis of the glomerular-like exuberant endothelial cell proliferation within the affected pulmonary artery is the formation of arteriovenous shunts [14].

Wagenvoort and Wagenvoort [8] explained the generation of plexiform lesions in cardiac left-to-right shunting by increased blood flow eliciting reflective vasoconstriction with subsequent development of endothelial alteration. More interestingly, they speculated that vascular necrosis with arteritis might result from intense vasospasms, as seen in the systemic circulation. Here, the pathogenetic plot is that plexiform lesions develop in the focal areas of fibrinoid necrosis by active cellular reorganization and recanalization of the thrombus composed of fibrin and platelets, usually present in this setting and observed within plexiform lesions. In fact, the only animal model leading to obvious plexiform lesions was achieved by producing necrosis of pulmonary arterioles in dogs after 2 weeks of severe PH due to the creation of a shunt between the pulmonary and systemic circulations [15]. This explanation would take into consideration that elements of inflammation are consistently present in the range of plexiform and other vascular lesions in PAH [16, 17].

On the other hand, Lee et al. [18] proposed a neoplastic approach to the hardly understandable proliferation of intraluminal neovessels at the core of plexiform lesions: they found that a large proportion of the endothelial cells in this area show monoclonality, raising the question of possible tumor-like growth. These different observations of arterial wall alteration within plexiform lesions are probably connected in a temporary line. However, they could fit into a broader concept of pathogenesis first mentioned by Wagenvoort and Wagenvoort [8], but interestingly developed by Yaginuma et al. [19]. They submitted histological data from 11 patients with PH due to congenital heart disease to a computer-based 3-dimensional image reconstruction and found that plexiform lesions mostly occurred in supernumerary arteries branching off from larger pulmonary arteries, proximal to arterial lesions with intimal fibrosis and medial hypertrophy. They also gathered evidence for generation of indirect anastomoses between the postplexiform arterial segment and the bronchial arteries running along the close bronchiole, passing via arterioles and the capillary bed and thereby creating the thin-walled congestive dilation lesions. In this view, the generation of proximal complex lesions might merely be an attempt of the pulmonary vasculature to bypass the primary downstream obstruction and to ensure capillary oxygenation through overt contact with arterial blood from proximal pulmonary and bronchial arteries.

Plexiform lesions, however, are not restricted to supernumerary branching and can be observed after distal dichotomous branching of pulmonary arteries. Cool et al. [20] came to different conclusions after a computerized 3-dimensional study on 5 patients with severe PH of different causes. In their view, plexiform lesions are functionally important because blood flow is severely obstructed along the entire length of a vessel affected by a single lesion. This at least puts a working shunt concept into question. They hypothesize that the plexiform lesion could be an early vascular alteration in severe PH, independent of a component of medial smooth muscle cell hypertrophy. At a later time-point in disease evolution, the plexiform lesion could transform into an intraluminal concentric obstruction composed of endothelial cells and recruited myofibroblasts, following the path of the plexiform lesion and thus representing a fibrous scar of the latter. The close association that can be observed between concentric laminar intimal fibrosis and plexiform lesions in lungs of patients suffering from PAH makes this thought a tempting assumption. Nevertheless, a shunt hypothesis would not be contradictory if seen in the light of a failed attempt to shortcut other correlates of obstruction found in PAH, such as medial hypertrophy, muscularization of arterioles (< 80 microns in diameter) (fig. 2d), intimal nonlaminar fibrosis, and thrombotic lesions.

Vascular Inflammation

It has not yet been elucidated whether the inflammatory pattern seen in plexiform lesions and other intimal lesions is of pathogenetic importance or if it represents a pure epiphenomenon within disease evolution. The reported evidence of proinflammatory mediators, so-called chemokines, released

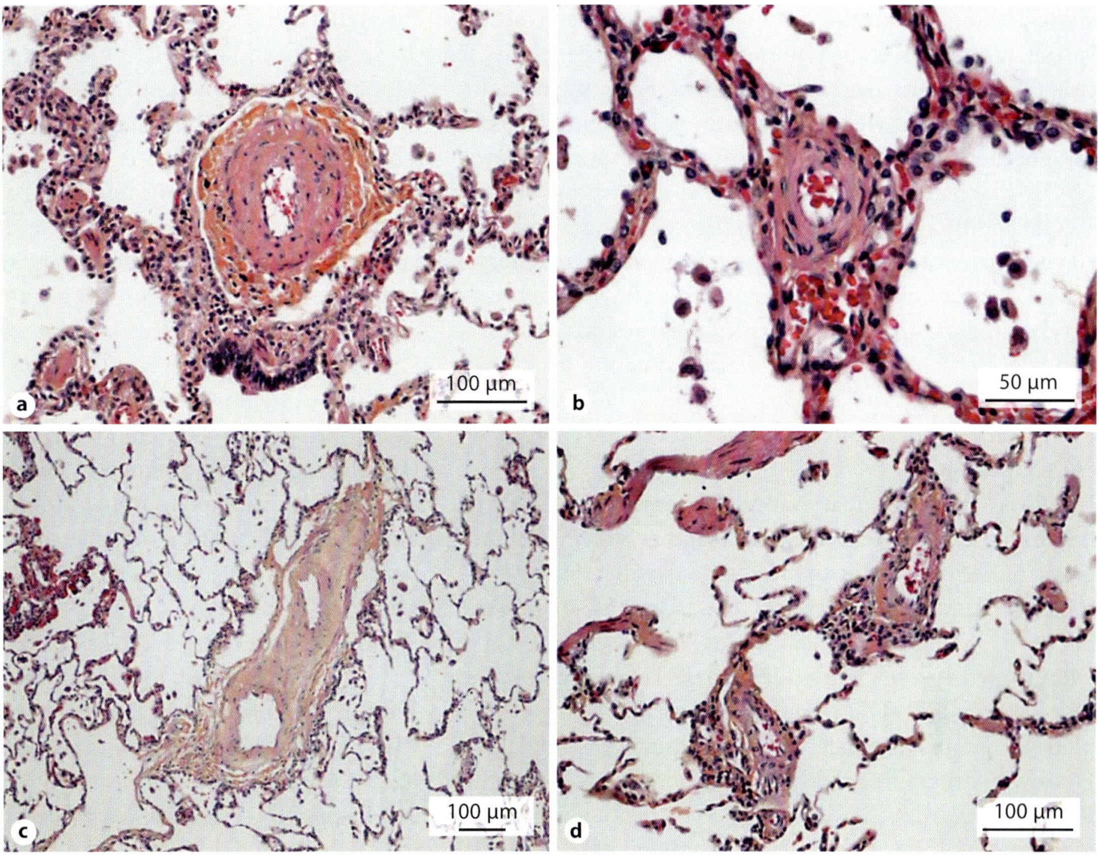

Fig. 3. Histology of lung samples from patients suffering from PVOD. **a** Most arteries are involved and show intimal thickening, sometimes with adventitial fibrosis as seen in this pulmonary artery. Note the thickened alveolar septa. HES-staining, magnification ×100. **b** Pulmonary arteriole showing typical muscularization and pericytic hyperplasia. The alveolar septa are thickened due to doubling and trebling of the alveolar capillary layers (filled with erythrocytes) in a hemangiomatosis-like fashion (see text). Note the increase of alveolar macrophages (many are siderin-laden macrophages, so-called siderophages). HES-staining, magnification ×200. **c** Septal vein with occlusive intimal fibrosis (orange-colored). HES-staining, magnification ×40. **d** Small, preseptal venules displaying intimal fibrosis. Note the numerous black dots in the periphery of the vessels corresponding to perivascular lymphocytic infiltrates. HES-staining, magnification ×100.

by altered endothelial cells of PAH lungs strongly indicates a self-supporting and self-amplifying process [21–23]. As elements of inflammation seem to be present in affected arteries of patients displaying PAH in various associated disease conditions, as well as in idiopathic PAH, the specific role of immune cells within installation and/or maintenance of obstructive lesions remains unclear. It seems unlikely that intimal proliferation and medial hypertrophy of pulmonary arteries could be the sole result of ‘scarring’ vasculitis-like lesions because lymphocytic and macrophagic infiltrates observed in the setting of PAH remain perivascular and are less abundant than in pulmonary forms of vasculitis, e.g. as seen in Wegener’s granulomatosis [24]. Nonetheless, Wagenvoort and Wagenvoort [8] discussed such a possibility 40 years ago, and it cannot be excluded that a phase of intense inflammatory activity precedes a clinically symptomatic arterial remodeling with proliferation and recruitment of smooth muscle cells, endothelial cells, and fibroblasts/myofibroblasts. In fact, the latest investigations provide evidence that chemokines with specific chemotactic activity for T lymphocytes and macrophages can increase smooth muscle proliferation [25].

Venous and Venular Lesions

During the Dana Point meeting in 2008 a consensus was reached, formally separating group 1 (PAH) of the classification of PH from the rare entities of PVOD and PCH, now categorized as the new Group 1’ (one prime): pulmonary venous hypertension. This differentiation seemed necessary because of particularities regarding therapeutic strategies and the cautious, if not restrictive, use of potent vasodilating drugs, such as intravenous epoprostenol, in the case of pulmonary venous involvement. From the pathologist's standpoint of view, this separation is comprehensible, but not ideal. In fact, some cases of PAH (Group 1) show a PVOD-like pattern (see beneath), and the vast majority of PVOD and PCH cases (Group 1') present at least mild arterial and arteriolar (fig. 3a, b). The frequent occurrence of mixed vascular involvement seems to demand a less absolutistic evaluation into pulmonary vascular lesions predominating either the arterial or the venous system.

Pulmonary Veno-Occlusive Disease/Pulmonary Capillary Hemangiomatosis

PVOD is a rare pulmonary vascular disease causing PH and has until recently been considered together with PCH a subgroup of PAH according to the Venice classification of 2003. It has an estimated prevalence of 0.1–0.2 per million persons per year [26]. Historical reports and large case studies have extrapolated a proportion of PVOD in PAH ranging from 5 to 25% [26, 27]. In PVOD as in PCH, vascular lesions predominate on the postcapillary level of pulmonary vasculature. However, lesions frequently involve both veins *and* arteries in lungs of patients with PVOD. Interestingly, a recent report has indicated that certain subgroups of PAH regarded as precapillary forms simultaneously display a PVOD-like pattern (see below). In PVOD, the observed postcapillary lesions involves septal veins and preseptal venules, and frequently consist of loose fibrous remodeling of the intima, which may totally occlude the lumen (fig. 3c, d). The involvement of preseptal venules should be considered as necessary for the histological diagnosis of PVOD; fibrous occlusion of large septal veins may be seen in many forms of pulmonary venous hypertension, including a frequently reported obstruction of large pulmonary veins following catheter ablation for cardiac atrial fibrillation [28].

While septal veins usually display a paucicellular cushion-like fibrous obstruction, intimal thickening of preseptal venules can present with a dense pattern and increased cellularity. Anti-α-actin staining may reveal involvement of smooth muscle cells and/or myofibroblasts within such venular lesions. Thrombotic occlusion of small postcapillary microvessels has also been observed, corresponding to 'colander-like' lesions, which otherwise can be seen in small pulmonary arteries. The tunica media may be muscularized in both septal veins and preseptal venules. Pleural and pulmonary lymphatic vessels are usually dilated [2]. The presence of calcium-encrusting elastic fibers in the vessel wall or the perivascular space, and inflammatory activation through a foreign body giant cell response is considered as an argument in favor of PVOD as compared to secondary venous hypertension [29]. Importantly, occult pulmonary hemorrhage regularly occurs in patients displaying PVOD. This particularity, which is certainly due to the postcapillary block, is of diagnostic interest as bronchoalveolar lavage can reveal occult hemorrhage. The degree of hemorrhage can be evaluated semiquantitatively and qualitatively using the Golde score, which assesses intra-alveolar siderin-laden macrophages by Perls' Prussian blue staining [30, 31].

In addition to an increased number of siderophages, large amounts of hemosiderin can be found in type II pneumocytes, and within the interstitial space. Moreover, postcapillary obstruction may frequently lead to capillary angiectasia and even capillary angioproliferation; in PVOD-cases, doubling and tripling of the alveolar septal capillary layers may be focally present. Lately, this histological peculiarity has raised questions concerning a possible overlap between PVOD and cases of PCH, a disease classically characterized by an aggressive patch-like angioproliferation of capillaries. Indeed, Lantuejoul et al. [32] recently reported 35 cases of PVOD and PCH with more or less a similar pattern, evoking the possibility of a same disease entity.

Historically, PCH was described by Wagenvoort et al. [33] as an aggressive capillary proliferation with patchy to nodular distribution: several rows of capillaries along alveolar walls progressed to nodules and sheets of back-to-back capillaries in advanced lesions. However, a malignant disorder which had been evoked with the term of 'angiomatous growth' seems unlikely because cytological atypia and mitoses are usually absent. An infiltration of bronchiolar structures has also been described. A possible explanation for this angiomatoid expansion might be a hemodynamically relevant postcapillary block. Occult hemorrhage or hemosiderosis, therefore, is frequently found. As in PVOD, these characteristics lead to compensatory muscularization of arterioles and medial hypertrophy in pulmonary arteries. As previously mentioned, the similarities in clinical and histological presentation suggest that PVOD and PCH are the same disease entity with either a venule-predominating or a capillary-predominating phenotype [32].

Forms of Pulmonary Hypertension with Significant Arterial and Venous Remodeling

Pulmonary Arterial Hypertension Associated with Connective Tissue Disease.

Until recently, lesions of the pulmonary arterial system, more or less similar to those occurring in idiopathic PAH, have been held responsible for PH in patients with CTD-associated PAH. In a published analysis of 8 patients suffering from CTD-associated PAH, we observed that 6 of 8 patients (75%) exhibited occlusive lesions of pulmonary veins and venules, as can typically be seen in PVOD. In contrast, only 5 of 29 non-CTD control patients with the primary diagnosis PAH displayed venous involvement [34]. Though all of the investigated CTD-associated PAH patients exhibited pulmonary arterial changes, venous and venular fibrous remodeling, when present, was more pronounced than arterial changes, concerning the quantity of affected vessels. All cases of CTD-associated PAH revealed pulmonary arterial lesions involving small muscular vessels on the pre- and intra-acinar level. The vessel wall remodeling corresponded to arterial changes found in PAH, ranging from intimal constrictive and nonconstrictive lesions to associated medial hypertrophy and adventitial thickening. In another major report on this subject, Overbeek et al. [35] analyzed lung tissue of 8 PAH patients with limited cutaneous systemic sclerosis and compared it to samples of 11 idiopathic PAH patients. They found that all systemic sclerosis PAH patients displayed arterial and venous remodeling, while venous lesions were present in only 3 of the 11 idiopathic PAH patients. It is notable that 4 systemic sclerosis PAH cases displayed a PVOD-like pattern with patchy capillary congestion and signs of occult alveolar hemorrhage.

Systemic sclerosis represents one of the leading pathological conditions associated with PH and CTD-associated PH belongs to Group 1 of the Dana Point classification. Prevalence of PAH in certain forms of CTD has been estimated to be as high as 50% [36]. In a recent cross-sectional national screening, at least 8% of scleroderma patients displayed moderate-to-severe PAH [37]. In patients with CTD, PAH is the leading cause of mortality and necessitates intensive medical treatment, which frequently proves to be both difficult and only yielding mixed results [38]. Treatment with vasodilators like continuous intravenous epoprostenol has shown improvement of exercise capacity and cardiopulmonary hemodynamics, but the response is less effective than in idiopathic PAH and survival remains poor among patients with associated CTD [39, 40]. Equally, endothelin receptor antagonists seem to show less impressive effects in systemic sclerosis patients than in other forms of PAH [41]. In addition, adverse effects of vasoactive treatment in PAH associated with CTD can occur and may lead to severe pulmonary edema [42]. Considering this background, the described findings of a PVOD-like setting in CTD-associated PAH highlight the important hemodynamic effect of postcapillary occlusion on the pulmonary vasculature. Resistance of CTD-associated PAH to common vasodilator therapies and complications such as pulmonary edema could merely be the consequence of a higher prevalence of veno-occlusive remodeling in these patients as compared to other forms of PAH.

Conclusion

Regarding the pathology of PH, it appears important to stress that the differentiation of lesions and their localization seem to influence the outcome and should have an impact on therapeutic decisions. However, a clear-cut separation of different forms of PH through recognition of a histological phenotype will always be difficult or even impossible: different etiological factors (e.g. hypoxia vs. anorexigen intake) may trigger a final common step in the cascade of pathologic events (e.g. oxidative stress and consecutive growth factor expression) and finally lead to the same morphologic pattern (e.g. medial hypertrophy). Nonetheless and as a general statement, a look at the disease from the 'other side', i.e. the pathologists' view, can be both intriguing and illuminating. An apparently rich and inexplicable variety of lesions is described and categorized without obvious clinical relevance, but then again parallels between the outcome of disease subgroups and the involvement of specific anatomical structures, such as veins and venules in CTD-associated PAH, emerge to obviousness and shed some light onto a more or less obscure pathogenesis – a beautiful and overall necessary exercise in medicine.

References

1 Simonneau G, Robbins IM, et al: Updated clinical classification of pulmonary hypertension. J Am Coll Cardiol 2009;54:S43–S54.
2 Pietra G: Pathology of Primary Pulmonary Hypertension. New York, Marcel Dekker, 1997.
3 Heath D, Williams D: High-Altitude Medicine and Pathology. London, Butterworths, 1989.
4 Sakao S, Tatsumi K, et al: Reversible or irreversible remodeling in pulmonary arterial hypertension. Am J Respir Cell Mol Biol 2010;43:629–634.
5 Penaloza D, Arias-Stella J: The heart and pulmonary circulation at high altitudes: healthy highlanders and chronic mountain sickness. Circulation 2007;115:1132–1146.
6 Voelkel NF, Tuder RM: Cellular and molecular mechanisms in the pathogenesis of severe pulmonary hypertension. Eur Respir J 1995;8: 2129–2138.

7 Cool C, Kennedy D, et al: Pathogenesis and evolution of plexiform lesions in pulmonary hypertension associated with scleroderma and human immunodeficiency virus infection. Hum Pathol 1997;28:434–442.
8 Wagenvoort C, Wagenvoort N: Primary pulmonary hypertension: a pathologic study of the lung vessels in 156 clinically diagnosed cases. Circulation 1970;42:1163–1184.
9 Tuder RM, Abman SH, et al: Development and pathology of pulmonary hypertension. J Am Coll Cardiol 2009;54(1 suppl): S3–S9.
10 Heath D, Edwards JE: The pathology of hypertensive pulmonary vascular disease; a description of six grades of structural changes in the pulmonary arteries with special reference to congenital cardiac septal defects. Circulation 1958;18(4 Part 1):533–547.
11 Moser KM, Bloor CM: Pulmonary vascular lesions occurring in patients with chronic major vessel thromboembolic pulmonary hypertension. Chest 1993;103:685–692.
12 Harrison CV: IV. The pathology of the pulmonary vessels in pulmonary hypertension. Br J Radiol 1958;31:217–226.
13 Piazza G, Goldhaber SZ: Chronic thromboembolic pulmonary hypertension. N Engl J Med 2011;364:351–360.
14 Kucsko L: Arteriovenous communications in the human lung and their functional significance (in German). Frankf Z Pathol 1953;64:54–83.
15 Saldaña ME, Harley RA, et al: Experimental extreme pulmonary hypertension and vascular disease in relation to polycythemia. Am J Pathol 1968;52:935–981.
16 Tuder R, Groves B, et al: Exuberant endothelial cell growth and elements of inflammation are present in plexiform lesions of pulmonary hypertension. Am J Pathol 1994;144:275–285.
17 Dorfmüller P, Perros F, et al: Inflammation in pulmonary arterial hypertension. Eur Respir J 2003;22:358–363.
18 Lee SD, Shroyer KR, et al: Monoclonal endothelial cell proliferation is present in primary but not secondary pulmonary hypertension. J Clin Invest 1998;101:927–934.
19 Yaginuma G, Mohri H, et al: Distribution of arterial lesions and collateral pathways in the pulmonary hypertension of congenital heart disease: a computer aided reconstruction study. Thorax 1990;45:586–590.
20 Cool CD, Stewart JS, et al: Three-dimensional reconstruction of pulmonary arteries in plexiform pulmonary hypertension using cell-specific markers. Evidence for a dynamic and heterogeneous process of pulmonary endothelial cell growth. Am J Pathol 1999;155:411–419.
21 Balabanian K, Foussat A, et al: CX(3)C chemokine fractalkine in pulmonary arterial hypertension. Am J Respir Crit Care Med 2002;165:1419–1425.
22 Dorfmüller P, Zarka V, et al: Chemokine RANTES in severe pulmonary arterial hypertension. Am J Respir Crit Care Med 2002;165:534–539.
23 Sanchez O, Marcos E, et al: Role of endothelium-derived CC chemokine ligand 2 in idiopathic pulmonary arterial hypertension. Am J Respir Crit Care Med 2007;176:1041–1047.
24 Dorfmüller P, Humbert M, et al: Pathology and aspects of pathogenesis in pulmonary arterial hypertension. Sarcoidosis Vasc Diffuse Lung Dis 2003;20:9–19.
25 Perros F, Dorfmüller P, et al: Fractalkine-induced smooth muscle cell proliferation in pulmonary hypertension. Eur Respir J 2007;29: 937–943.
26 Mandel J, Mark EJ, et al: Pulmonary veno-occlusive disease. Am J Respir Crit Care Med 2000;162:1964–1973.
27 Rich S, Dantzker DR, et al: Primary pulmonary hypertension. A national prospective study. Ann Intern Med 1987;107:216–223.
28 Di Biase L, Fahmy TS, et al: Pulmonary vein total occlusion following catheter ablation for atrial fibrillation: clinical implications after long-term follow-up. J Am Coll Cardiol 2006;48:2493–2499.
29 Pietra GG, Capron F, et al: Pathologic assessment of vasculopathies in pulmonary hypertension. J Am Coll Cardiol 2004;43(12 suppl S):25S–32S.
30 Golde DW, Drew WL, et al: Occult pulmonary haemorrhage in leukaemia. Br Med J 1975;2: 166–168.
31 Capron F: Bronchoalveolar lavage and alveolar hemorrhage (in French). Ann Pathol 1999;19:395–400.
32 Lantuéjoul S, Sheppard MN, et al: Pulmonary veno-occlusive disease and pulmonary capillary hemangiomatosis: a clinicopathologic study of 35 cases. Am J Surg Pathol 2006;30:850–857.
33 Wagenvoort CA, Beetstra A, et al: Capillary haemangiomatosis of the lungs. Histopathology 1978;2:401–406.
34 Dorfmüller P, Humbert M, et al: Fibrous remodeling of the pulmonary venous system in pulmonary arterial hypertension associated with connective tissue diseases. Hum Pathol 2007;38:893–902.
35 Overbeek MJ, Vonk MC, et al: Pulmonary arterial hypertension in limited cutaneous systemic sclerosis: a distinctive vasculopathy. Eur Respir J 2009;34:371–379.
36 Ungerer RG, Tashkin DP, et al: Prevalence and clinical correlates of pulmonary arterial hypertension in progressive systemic sclerosis. Am J Med 1983;75:65–74.
37 Hachulla E, Gressin V, et al: Early detection of pulmonary arterial hypertension in systemic sclerosis: a French nationwide prospective multicenter study. Arthritis Rheum 2005; 52:3792–3800.
38 Sanchez O, Humbert M, et al: Treatment of pulmonary hypertension secondary to connective tissue diseases. Thorax 1999;54:273–277.
39 Badesch DB, Tapson VF, et al: Continuous intravenous epoprostenol for pulmonary hypertension due to the scleroderma spectrum of disease. A randomized, controlled trial. Ann Intern Med 2000;132:425–434.
40 Ramirez A, Varga J: Pulmonary arterial hypertension in systemic sclerosis: clinical manifestations, pathophysiology, evaluation, and management. Treat Respir Med 2004;3:339–352.
41 Humbert M, Simonneau G: Drug insight: endothelin-receptor antagonists for pulmonary arterial hypertension in systemic rheumatic diseases. Nat Clin Pract Rheumatol 2005;1:93–101.
42 Humbert M, Sanchez O, et al: Short-term and long-term epoprostenol (prostacyclin) therapy in pulmonary hypertension secondary to connective tissue diseases: results of a pilot study. Eur Respir J 1999;13:1351–1356.

Peter Dorfmüller, MD, PhD
Service d'Anatomie et de Cytologie Pathologiques, Hôpital Marie Lannelongue and INSERM U999 'Hypertension Artérielle Pulmonaire: Physiopathologie et Innovation Thérapeutique'
133, Avenue de la Résistance
FR–92350 Le Plessis Robinson (France)
Tel. +33 1 40948708, E-Mail peter.dorfmuller@u-psud.fr

Chapter 3

Humbert M, Souza R, Simonneau G (eds): Pulmonary Vascular Disorders.
Prog Respir Res. Basel, Karger, 2012, vol 41, pp 23–36

Invasive Rest and Exercise Hemodynamics in the Modern Management of Pulmonary Vascular Disease: An Expanding Role in the Future

Kenneth F. Whyte[a] · Philipe Hervé[b] · Susanna Hoette[c] · Denis Chemla[c]

[a]Greenlane Respiratory Service, Auckland City Hospital, Auckland, New Zealand; [b]Department of Thoracic and Vascular Surgery, Marie Lannelongue Hospital, Le Plessis-Robinson, and [c]Service de Pneumologie, Hospital Antoine Béclère, Clamart, France

Abstract

The central role of invasive hemodynamic measurements remains incontestable despite many recent noninvasive technologies. Understanding the physiology and the limitations of our current knowledge of the pulmonary circulation during exercise and in pulmonary vascular disease is crucial in both the investigation and the management of patients. Modern invasive hemodynamic testing is a short, simple, comfortable, and safe procedure. As a result, its use will increase allowing us to better assess the pathophysiology of pulmonary vascular disease, to provide essential data on individual patient's disease state, prognosis, and potentially their response to targeted vasodilator therapies.

The last 30 years has seen a dramatic increase in both our understanding of pulmonary vascular diseases and the incidence of these diseases as our ability to screen high-risk groups and investigate symptomatic patients has expanded.

With this explosion of knowledge, the pivotal role of invasive pulmonary hemodynamic measurements has been overshadowed and their importance emphasized less. Invasive hemodynamic measurements are essential in the diagnosis and management of patients and no other investigative tool is capable of providing the breadth of clinically relevant information we obtain at right heart catheterization, which remains the 'gold standard' diagnostic procedure (table 1). In addition to describing the current 'best practice' for carrying out invasive hemodynamic investigation, this chapter outlines the hemodynamic physiology of the pulmonary circulation and discusses the impact of pulmonary vascular disease on hemodynamics at rest and during exercise.

Invasive hemodynamic data is essential for definitive diagnosis in all current guidelines [1–3] for the management of these diseases, as other investigative tools such as echocardiography have poorer diagnostic sensitivity and are not interchangeable [4, 5]. Hemodynamic variables at the first diagnostic right heart catheterization continue to be powerful predictors of prognosis even in the current era of targeted pulmonary vasodilator therapies [6–10]. Acute vasodilator responses continue to influence decisions on therapeutic interventions at the initiation of therapy and further hemodynamic data are routinely part of the data used to make decisions regarding changing or escalating therapy in individual patients.

The right ventricle (RV) and the pulmonary vasculature are an inextricably linked functional unit and right heart catheterization provides important data to assess right ventricular function.

The role of exercise hemodynamics remains controversial, and although no longer recommended as a diagnostic tool, we will discuss its role in potentially recognizing patients with abnormal pulmonary exercise responses with a high risk of developing overt pulmonary vascular disease and its role in expanding our understanding of the physiology of the pulmonary circulation and the pathophysiology of pulmonary vascular disease. Exercise hemodynamics has the potential to link our understanding of the pathobiology of the small muscular pulmonary arteries with the very variable clinical outcomes observed in clinical practice in different types of pulmonary arterial hypertension (PAH) and between individual patients within diagnostic groups.

Table 1. Clinical indications and utility of invasive hemodynamic measurements (evidence grading from Galie et al. [2])

Clinical situation	Significant variables	Clinical importance	Class of evidence	Level of evidence
Diagnosis	mPAP	essentially the diagnostic test	I	C
Prognosis	mRA, mPAP, cardiac index, mixed venous PO_2	best validated prognostic variables	I	C
Choice of therapy	response to vasodilator challenge	identifies potential responders to CCB therapy	IIa	C
Response to therapy	failure to increase cardiac index	utility, but has to be combined with other functional and clinical measurements	IIa	C
Escalation of therapy	deteriorating CI, rising PVR/mPAP or mRA	Contributes to overall clinical assessment of need for escalation	IIa	C

Physiology of the Pulmonary Circulation

With the increasing interest in pulmonary vascular disease over the last 30 years, it has become clear that our understanding of the physiology of the normal pulmonary circulation on exercise and how the RV and pulmonary circulation adapt both to increasing age and to the stress of exercise in pulmonary vascular disease are neither well described nor well understood. From the beginning, physiologists have recognized that the RV and pulmonary circulation are a linked unit, whereas in recent years there has been a tendency to consider manipulation of the pulmonary vasculature independent of the RV's response to load.

The invasive pulmonary hemodynamic pioneering work of physiologists in the middle of last century, mostly in normal younger volunteers, described the human pulmonary circulation and viewed it as a simple elastic system with low resistance and high compliance that both recruits and distends easily to the fluctuating demands of day-to-day activities and minimizes the workload of the RV. The proximal elastic arterial vessels had minimal resistance, but more distal vessels were resistance vessels. The pathologists identified that the small and precapillary pulmonary arteries were muscularized and that muscular control of pulmonary arterial tone at this level was involved in the regulation of the pulmonary circulation peripherally.

Physiologists recognized that although its control via the autonomic system is minimal, the pulmonary circulation has a complex task on exercise to maximize gas exchange and maintain V/Q close to 1 throughout the fluctuating pulmonary blood flow that occurs during a bout of physical exercise. In addition, pulmonary capillary pressure and pulsatile flow, essential for gas exchange, has to be tightly regulated to protect the fragile pulmonary capillary bed from excessive pressure and shear force injury. In health, the pulmonary circulation achieves these objectives remarkably efficiently while avoiding overloading the RV.

An additional challenge for the pulmonary circulation is to maintain a uniform time constant by balancing resistance and compliance to maximize ventilation/perfusion and gas exchange in health and disease [11].

Originally, the primary mediators of pulmonary vascular tone described were hypoxia and hormonal influences such as noradrenaline, isoprenaline, and histamine which could have both local effects, e.g. hypoxic pulmonary vasoconstriction in a segment of atelectatic lung or global as with histamine release in anaphylaxis. Over the last 25 years there has been recognition of the importance of 'local control' of pulmonary arterial blood flow, with the endothelium playing a crucial role along with a host of paracrines and cytokines. Control appears centered at the level of the precapillary small muscular pulmonary arteries which has given some insight into the mechanisms involved in the successful regulation of flow at the level of the small muscular pulmonary arteries [12]. The extent of involvement of the proximal pulmonary arteries, which are elastic arteries with very low resistance in pulmonary vascular disease, will vary from disease to disease, e.g. proximal involvement is more likely in chronic thromboembolic pulmonary hypertension (PH).

How local control of flow responds and 'fine tunes' the system during the constantly changing circulatory loads of exercise to maintain a uniform time constant for all lung segments to achieve maximal gas exchange and minimize right ventricular load remains to be elucidated. It is probable that 'passive' factors have a significant contribution with a variable rise in wedge pressure during exercise in normal subjects, leading potentially to both more recruitment and increased distension of pulmonary vessels. Therefore, it does not just limit rises in pulmonary vascular resistance (PVR), but reduces PVR despite the four- to eightfold exercise-induced increase in pulmonary blood flow in healthy adults [13].

The Hemodynamic Definition of Pulmonary Hypertension

Currently, PH is defined as a mean pulmonary arterial pressure (mPAP) at rest of ≥25 mm Hg. The normal range of mPAP is 14 ± 3.3 mm Hg (SD). As a rule normal ranges are mean ±2 SD and would include 95% of the normal population. As PAH is an orphan disease, using 21 mm Hg (mean + 2 SD) would result in more normals being diagnosed with disease (2.5% of population) than individuals with disease. At the Dana Point meeting in 2008, an upper limit of normal using 3 SD was proposed, 24 mm Hg, to decrease this high false positive rate [1]. Patients with a mPAP of 21–24 mm Hg at rest are in a borderline or gray zone, but should not be diagnosed as suffering from PAH. Some PAH centers will recommend regular monitoring to detect the development of PH in individuals in the 'gray zone', especially if they have risk factors for pulmonary vascular disease such as collagen vascular disease.

PAH or precapillary PH is defined as mPAP ≥25 mm Hg combined with a pulmonary capillary wedge pressure (PCWP) of <15 mm Hg and a PVR >3 Wood units (240 dynes•s•cm^{-5}). Postcapillary PH is defined as mPAP ≥25 mm Hg with PCWP ≥15 mm Hg. As the major determinant of PVR is precapillary resistance to flow, the PVR is usually <3 Wood units (240 dynes•cm•s^{-5}). There is a group of patients who have postcapillary PH mPAP ≥25 mm Hg and raised PCWP, but in addition the transpulmonary gradient (TPG) is >12 mm Hg and are considered to have postcapillary PH with resultant pulmonary artery remodeling raising PVR. Some authors have argued that the diastolic PAP minus PCWP gradient may define pulmonary venous hypertension more appropriately [14].

Exercise-Induced Pulmonary Hypertension

mPAP on exercise is dependent on exercise level and age, and there is very limited data across the extensive age range of patients seen at PAH centers. As a result, it is not possible to set absolute upper limits of normal mPAP on exercise to allow recognition of abnormal pulmonary hemodynamic responses to exercise due to pulmonary vascular disease. However, it is clear from case series that patients with resting mPAP in the normal range can have dramatic increases in mPAP on exercise. Frequently, such patients subsequently develop abnormal resting mPAP and are diagnosed with PAH. In those under 50 years of age, exercise mPAP rarely exceeds 30 mm Hg (mean ± SD = 19.4 ± 4.8 mm Hg) [15]. In patients over 50 years of age, the upper limit of normal for mPAP may be as high as 46 mm Hg (29.4 ± 8.4 mm Hg) on mild exercise, which is equivalent to day-to-day activities [15]. The number of normal older subjects from each decade of life who have undergone progressive supine exercise during heart catheterization is small and, thus, confidence limits are wide. We do not know the range of normal responses in terms of mPAP, PVR, RVEDP, and PCWP during progressive exercise and increasing cardiac output (CO) in order to reliably recognize abnormal pulmonary hemodynamic responses in older adults and diagnose with certainty pulmonary vascular disease.

Right Ventricular Afterload

Resistive Load: The Overt Load

Though the pulmonary circulation is a pulsatile system, the standard approach using heart catheterization in assessing RV load measures only the resistive component, i.e. PVR, and ignores pulsatility. This 'classical' approach assumes the pulmonary circulation is at a mean constant flow and pulmonary driving pressure, and measures PVR as the pressure fall across the pulmonary circulation (TPG) divided by CO. TPG is the mPAP minus left atrial pressure, measured as the pulmonary artery occlusion pressure (PAOP), which is often referred to as the PCWP, i.e. PVR = TPG/CO or PVR = (mPAP – PAOP)/CO.

This can be rewritten as mPAP = (CO × PVR) + PAOP, emphasizing that when PVR and CO are constant, a rise in downstream pressure increases mPAP, e.g. as in left heart disease.

PVR in this model is governed by Poiseuille's law and, thus, the radius to the fourth power is the major determinant of resistance. This ignores the fact that Poiseuille's law is specific to constant flow in a series of rigid tubes applied to newtonian fluids. The major site of resistance in the normal pulmonary circulation is the small muscular pulmonary arteries, and PVR is determined by their tone and distensibility. In humans, the influence of pleural pressure and perivascular alveoli surrounding peripheral vessels is currently unclear [14].

Exactly which downstream pressure is being measured when a Swan-Ganz balloon is inflated in a small pulmonary artery is open to discussion [16]. Unlike the systemic circulation, the pulmonary circulation is surrounded by varying pressure during respiration which can further complicate determining downstream pressure. Theoretically, when a subject is supine, all pulmonary vessels are in West zone 3, i.e. pulmonary venous pressure exceeds alveolar pressure throughout the respiratory cycle. This assumption does not hold true for patients with obstructive lung disease when end-expiratory pressure may be positive, resulting in alveolar pressure exceeding pulmonary capillary pressure and pulmonary vessels will narrow or collapse changing resistance and flow within each respiratory cycle. In this situation alveolar pressure replaces left atrial pressure in the above equation for some lung units. It has been proposed that a waterfall model better describes the pulmonary circulation rather than a simple resistance model [17, 18] (fig. 1).

These concepts are important as changes in downstream pressure can alter mPAP when CO is constant, thus altering PVR even though there has been no dilatation or constriction of the pulmonary vascular bed [19, 20]. This has led some authors to argue that PVR is a meaningless measurement which should be abandoned [21] – a suggestion that should be rejected [19, 22]. However, an understanding of the factors that influence PVR, other than changes in pulmonary arterial vascular tone, is essential for any individual interpreting hemodynamic studies [14].

Impedance: The Hidden Load

It is crucial to be aware of the impedance of the pulmonary circulation and its components which are the opposition to the pulsatile component, compliance, and inertance, and account for approximately one third of the hydraulic power of right ventricular afterload in healthy individuals [23].

The classical model physiologists apply to pulsatile systems is a Windkessel model based on the electrical current theory with a resistive component and capacitance (= compliance) in parallel (fig. 2) [24]. In health, even at rest, the literature is limited on the contributions of these components to RV workload, reflecting the challenges in making such measurements both in health and disease requiring high-fidelity catheters to analyze wave reflection, measure interventricular dependence, and using MRI scanning to generate pressure volume loops for the RV. Simpler approaches with standard catheters and simultaneous echocardiography have yet to gain widespread acceptance [25].

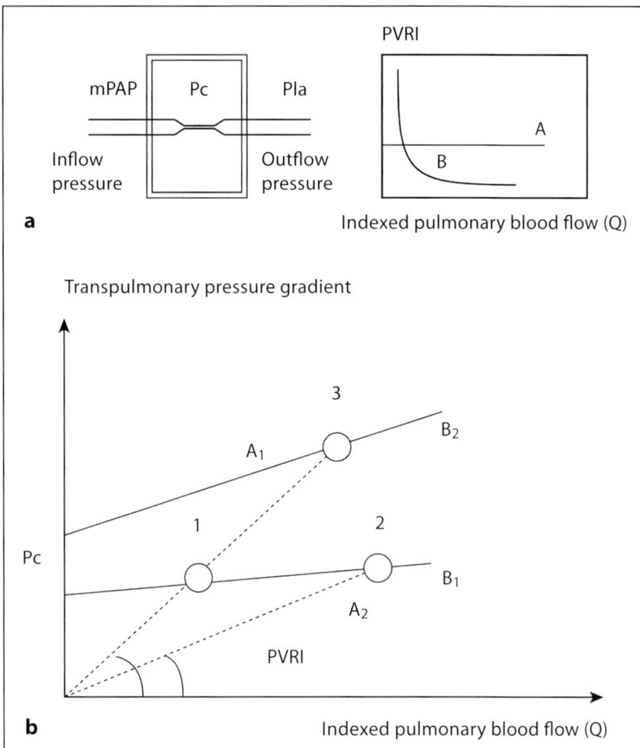

Fig. 1. a Starling resistor model to explain the concept of closing pressure within the circulatory system. Flow (Q) is determined by the gradient between inflow pressure (mPAP) and an outflow pressure which is either closing pressure (Pc) or left atrial pressure (Pla). When left atrial pressure is greater than Pc, then PVRI is constant at all levels of blood flow decreases (line B), e.g. reflecting derecruitment and less distension (adapted from Naeije [19] with permission from the publisher). **b** Dotted lines (A_1 and A_2) both assume left atrial pressure is the downstream pressure and the line passes through the origin. If with a change in pulmonary blood flow a patient moves from point 1 (on line A_1) to point 2 (on line A_2), then the slope (slope = PVRI) of the dotted line changes and apparent vasodilation has occurred; however if the 'true' downstream closing pressure is higher (Pc on the y-axis) than left atrial pressure (e.g. Starling resistor effect occurs due to alveolar pressure), then point 1 and point 2 are on the same line (solid line B_1) and the PVRI (= the slope) is actually unchanged. If a patient moves from point 1 to point 3 and we assume the downstream pressure goes through the origin (dotted line A_2), then there is no apparent change in PVRI as the slope is unchanged; however if downstream pressure is higher than zero, then the slope has changed and PVRI has increased (adapted from Chemla et al. [14] with permission from the publisher).

The initial impedance load is the energy required in stretching pulmonary vessels during early systole, characteristic impedance. Later in systole, there is a load due to wave reflection [26]. In the diseased pulmonary circulation, wave reflection is enhanced and anticipated, and the pattern of alteration has been shown to differ between diseases, e.g. in proximal chronic embolic disease the pattern is different

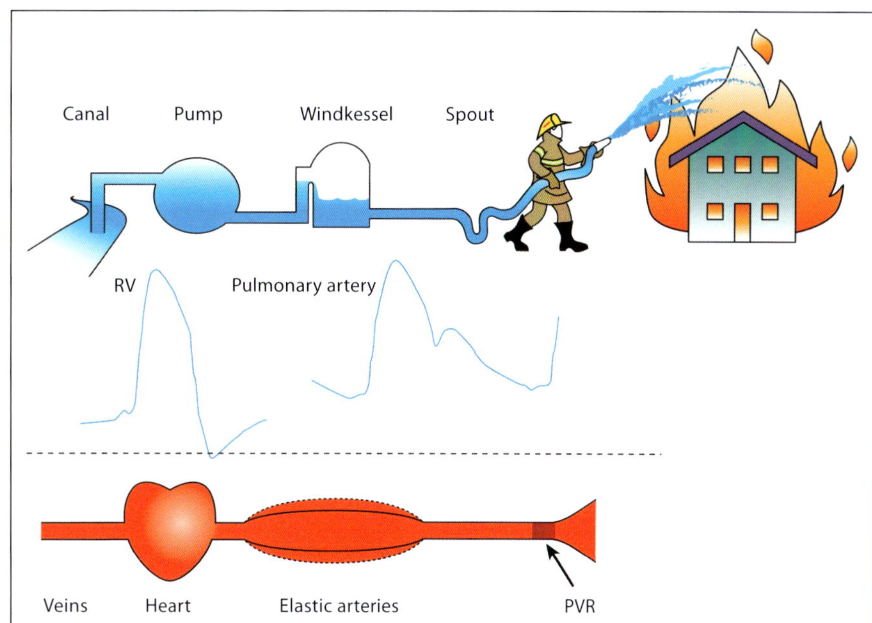

Fig. 2. Comparison of the circulation with a fire engine, with the veins as the source of water pumped by the RV into the air.

compared to PAH [26]. In addition, impedance is frequency dependent, and as the frequency, i.e. heart rate, changes with exercise, impedance will be altered not just by changes in CO, but also frequency.

It should be noted that models of the pulmonary circulation based on distensibility (compliance) and hematocrit (inertance) fit data derived from the human pulmonary circulation better than 'resistive' models [27].

Right Ventricle Adaption to Increased Load

In recent years, attention has increasingly been focused on right ventricular function both at the physiological and cellular level and the mechanisms involved in the RV's adaption to increased load and the factors that may influence decompensation of the RV [28, 29].

A further area of importance, at least in the diseased pulmonary circulation, is interventricular dependence with the prolonged contraction of the RV, after the left ventricle (LV) begins to relax, due to increased afterload, and interventricular septal bulging into the LV in diastole altering LV mechanics and lowering CO, venous return, and potentially coronary artery filling.

In the face of an increased afterload, the first response of the compliant RV is to increase end-diastolic volume (preload) using the Frank-Starling mechanism to maintain CO. The increased volume leads to increased RV wall stress (Laplace's law), which is offset to an extent by the resultant RV hypertrophy. RV hypertrophy is very variable and rarely as pronounced in idiopathic PAH as the RV hypertrophy noted in congenital heart disease where the load is a mixture of volume and pressure overload. Eventually, RV load exceeds capacity and the RV decompensates (fig. 3).

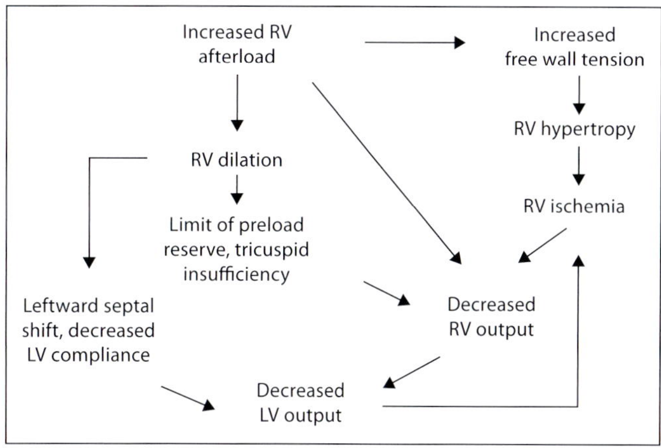

Fig. 3. Main pathophysiological factors involved in right and left heart failure in patients with PH (reproduced from Lankhaar et al. [11] with permission of the publisher).

Effect of Age on Resting Pulmonary Hemodynamics

There is a small decline in resting pulmonary blood flow with age from childhood to older age [30], with wide inter-individual variability at every age. In older adults, resting PVR is higher than in younger adults [31–34], with an approximate doubling from 0.67 ± 0.36 Wood units in early adulthood to 1.20 ± 0.31 Wood units in older adults (61–83 years) [35]. However, the difference in resting mPAP across the range of adult age reported in the literature (up to 83 years) is minimal (<3 mm Hg). Thus, there is no difference in the upper limit of normal in older adults; however, adults over 50 years of age have a considerably higher number of false positives: 1/5,000 <50 years of age will have a resting mPAP ≥25 mm Hg and 1/250 >50-year-old normals will have a resting mPAP ≥25 mm Hg [15 in online supplement table K].

Pulmonary Circulatory Response to Exercise in Normal Adults

On erect dynamic progressive exercise, whether on a treadmill or bicycle ergometer, there is an initial small fall in PVR at the onset of exercise, and it is likely that recruitment is maximal early in exercise [13]. At rest, blood flow is limited in the upper lobes and vessels in the upper lobes will be recruited as CO and pulmonary pressures increase during exercise. This early fall in PVR is not seen during supine exercise, supporting this suggestion.

Small decreases in PVR are seen throughout both steady state [36] and supine progressive exercise in most normals and even in patients with both left heart disease and those with mild PAH [37, 38]. It is thought that this fall reflects further distension of the pulmonary circulation. In patients with severe PAH, the PVR fails to fall or may even rise, though this is a relatively infrequent and limited response as the overloaded RV cannot cope with the increase in afterload [37]. As PAH becomes more severe, the striking abnormality on exercise is an inability to increase CO appropriately and maintain oxygen delivery to the exercising musculature.

In both erect and supine progressive exercise, there is a steady increase in mean pulmonary artery pressure again in response to the increasing CO in younger adults (<50 years), a rise of 1 mm Hg/l increase in CO, which appears to remain constant throughout all loads. It is unknown if there is further recruitment of vessels as pressure increases or whether the increasing volume of blood combined with the variable increase in pulmonary venous pressure as left atrial pressure rises simply leads to further distension at higher COs [13]. At the relatively low mPAP levels seen on maximal exercise in younger normal individuals, it is unlikely that peripheral pulmonary vessels are fully stretched and that compliance would change significantly at higher workloads. We emphasize that the data on compliance and inertance on exercise is very limited and this conclusion is based on earlier work on isolated pulmonary vessels ex vivo [27].

Effect of Age on Pulmonary Circulatory Response to Exercise

In older adults (>60 years), the rate of rise in mPAP/l of CO is increased and has been reported to be a 2.5-mm Hg/l increase in CO based on the small numbers of healthy elderly who have been studied (n = 16) [39]. The increase in the slope of the mPAP/CO relationship is largely explained by a rise in PCWP on exercise, which may reflect decreasing compliance of the LV with age, 1.93 ± 0.94 mm Hg/l of CO in normals over 60 years of age compared to 0.30 ± 0.35 for young normals [40]. Thus, it is unclear if the pattern of PVR changes during progressive exercise in elderly adults differs from that seen in younger adults [41]. There appears to be no description of the changes in pulmonary impedance in the elderly in the literature. However, there is modeling data in men >60 years which suggests that distensibility (compliance) is lower in older men [27], and evidence of decreasing compliance in isolated pulmonary arteries with age [42].

Clinicians need to be aware of these controversies and appreciate the limitations of standard right heart catheterization measurements to assess and quantify right ventricular load at rest and on exercise across the age spectrum [see 35, 43, 44 for more detailed explanations of resistance, distensibility, inertia, and impedance, and 37, 45 for further insight into the current research and potential importance of quantifying right ventricular afterload, right ventricular failure, and the controversies surrounding this field in pulmonary vascular research].

Pulmonary Circulatory Response to Exercise in Pulmonary Vascular Disease

Prior to Dana Point, a rise in mPAP to >30 mm Hg at any workload in any patient no matter the resting mPAP was diagnostic of exercise-induced PH. This diagnostic definition was correctly removed on the basis that we do not have robust data on exercise mPAP responses in normals across all age ranges to identify normal upper limits of mPAP and, thus, identify abnormal responses [1, 15]. However, in a group of patients with scleroderma previously diagnosed with exercise-induced PH over a 3-year period, 19% developed resting PAH and 12% died; therefore, at least a significant minority of these patients had active pulmonary vascular disease [46]. Similarly, Tolle et al. [37], using the original NIH-defined exercise-induced PH as mPAP on exercise >30 mm Hg and an abnormal maximal PVR at maximal exercise, reported a pathological progression from normal mPAP through exercise-induced PAH to resting PAH over 4 years in many patients, suggesting that in the majority of patients exercise-induced PAH is an early phase of the disease. Recently, Kovacs et al. [47] reported that mPAP and PVR in the upper normal range at rest and on exercise is associated with decreased exercise capacity in patients with scleroderma.

Invasive Hemodynamic Methodology

There are many descriptions of the right heart catheterization technique; however, some describe the use of heart catheterization in other situations, e.g. intensive care units, and do not always describe the necessary details and specific techniques required in the investigation of suspected pulmonary vascular disease. There are appropriate descriptions in the literature describing in detail the optimal techniques necessary when investigating pulmonary vascular disease [48]. We will limit our discussion to areas of controversy and issues that surround some of the measurements and variables that are derived.

Safety of Right Heart Catheterization in the Modern Era

The risks of right heart catheterization in experienced units is extremely low and safety concerns should not deter the use of this essential diagnostic and monitoring tool, whose benefits far exceed the risks for the individual patient [49]. In the early days of research in PAH, partly due to the number of patients with advanced end-stage disease and because of a lack of effective therapy, right heart catheterization was seen as risky and repeat catheterization was hard to justify. By following a relatively aggressive program of invasive monitoring, centers can improve patient care and their complication rates for heart catheterization will fall and equal those seen in experienced centers as detailed in the above literature. The literature does not specify the annual number of right heart catheters or vasoreactivity studies an individual clinician or center need to carry out in order to maintain competency. The technique is evolving as catheterization techniques change with changing technology such as ultrasound guidance (table 2).

Table 2. Current techniques and acceptable practices

Technique	Acceptable practice
Venous approach	all approaches (internal jugular, brachial, and femoral) are acceptable – approach operator dependent
Sedation	not essential, use as required, but be aware some agents may decrease filling pressure and hence results
Anticoagulation	can be continued safely, but dependent on patient and venous approach proposed for each individual patient
Measuring CO	thermodilution correlates well with Fick method in majority of patients [50] – be aware of limitations of thermodilution (right to left shunt, low CO, severe tricuspid regurgitation, etc.); ideally both methods should be available in catheter laboratory
Oxygen saturation measurements during right heart catheterization	O_2 saturation from each chamber should be regarded as mandatory; mixed venous saturation has prognostic significance

End-Expiratory Pressure Measurements Are Essential

In theory if major lung disease is absent, at end-expiration pleural pressure is zero and pressure measurements can be referenced to atmospheric pressure. Failure to make all pressure measurements (especially mPAP and PCWP, but also mRA pressure) at the same point in the respiratory cycle will inevitably lead to errors in each specific pressure measurement and in any calculation made from those measurements such as PVR. Unfortunately, some automated catheter pressure measurement systems produce such data without ensuring all measurements are made at the same and appropriate time in the respiratory cycle. Manual analysis of pressure traces and derivation of pressures cannot be overemphasized as the only reliable method to ensure high-quality and consistent data from the catheter laboratory.

Table 3. Conditions in which PCWP will not reflect LV end-diastolic pressure

Situation	Causes/explanation
Conditions in which PCWP is greater than LV end-diastolic pressure	mitral stenosis, left atrial myxoma, pulmonary embolus, mitral valve regurgitation
Catheter tip in upper lung zone	radiological screening to ensure tip in lower lobe artery
Partial occlusion of pulmonary artery	overestimates PCWP: trace often damped and PCWP > RVEDP should be clues; if blood from wedge O_2 saturation not arterial, then confirms not fully wedged.

What Is Pulmonary Capillary Wedge Pressure Measuring?

Inflating a small balloon at the tip of a Swan-Ganz catheter sitting in a small pulmonary artery and measuring the pressure once the trace has stabilized is widely referred to as the PCWP. This is technically a PAOP and does not measure resistance in the pulmonary venous system as would be measured when a small catheter without a balloon is wedged in a small pulmonary arterial branch, i.e. pulmonary artery wedge pressure [16]. It should be understood that neither method measures the pulmonary capillary pressure, though it can be derived from the decay pressure curve when the balloon is inflated [14]. In normal subjects, however, PAOP and pulmonary artery wedge pressure are identical although pulmonary artery wedge pressure is often higher than PAOP in lung disease, reflecting increased venous resistance [51]. We have referred to this measurement as PCWP throughout this chapter as it is the most widely used term, but readers should be aware of the differences in nomenclature used in different papers which can be confusing.

In theory, PCWP should reflect the left atrial pressure, which in the normal heart reflects LV end-diastolic pressure, and thus enable the detection of LV dysfunction and its contribution to PH, i.e. the detection of secondary pulmonary venous hypertension or postcapillary PH. There are a number of situations where the measured PCWP does not reflect LV end-diastolic pressure, and these are outlined in table 3.

What Is Normal Pulmonary Capillary Wedge Pressure?

Unfortunately, as the current guidelines accept a PCWP <15 mm Hg as 'normal', it has obscured the fact that the average PCWP is 8 or 9 mm Hg. The normal range quoted widely in the literature is 4–12 mm Hg. Though it is likely the majority of older individuals with a PCWP >12 mm Hg will have a degree of pulmonary venous hypertension, which is common in elderly populations with extensive comorbidity such as systemic hypertension, the upper limit of normal has varied in the recent literature. Early guidelines suggested an upper limit of normal of 12 mm Hg, but more recently it has been accepted that the upper 95% confidence limit should be 14 mm Hg across adult populations [52].

Exercise Testing in the Catheter Laboratory

Exercise protocols can be divided based on the type of exercise into 'resistive', e.g. hand grip or lifting weights, or 'dynamic', e.g. walking or cycling. The cardiovascular response is different in each type of exercise: in dynamic exercise there are larger increases in CO and only systolic blood pressure changes significantly, whereas in resistive exercise there is less increase in CO and both systolic and diastolic blood pressure increases. We are unaware of any studies demonstrating that one form of exercise is more appropriate in pulmonary vascular disease; however, dynamic exercise is arguably the more relevant for assessing responses to day-to-day activities.

In the catheter laboratory, there are a number of approaches ranging from simply asking the patient to lift weights increasing the heart rate to 85% of the predicted maximum or until breathlessness results in the patient stopping exercise. As an alternative, straight leg raising can be used with similar results. The patient indicates when they are about to stop from breathlessness and hemodynamic measurements are obtained prior to cessation of exercise. These methods are simpler and do not require specialized or expensive equipment; however, the exact workload at each measurement cannot be determined.

A supine bicycle ergometer can be used with progressive incremental increases in load with regular repeat hemodynamic measurements including PCWP at each increment (fig. 4). This approach has the ability to determine precisely the exercise load and pattern of stepwise increases in load. There is no standard exercise protocol for supine ergometry in the literature. As the potential patient population varies widely in age, functional status, and comorbidities,

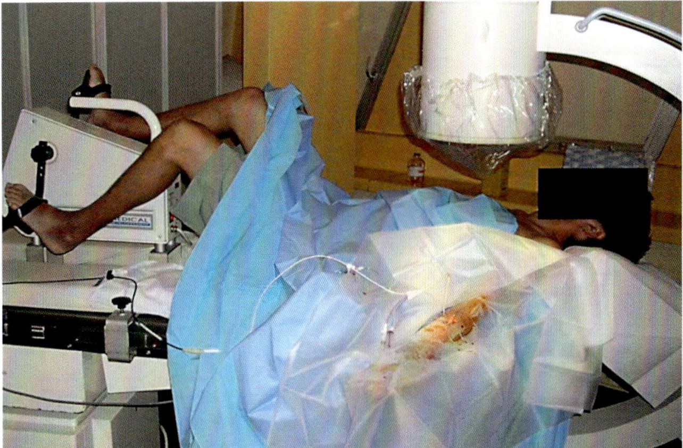

Fig. 4. Patient performing supine bicycle exercise during right heart catheterization.

it is essential that there is flexibility in terms of incremental change in load at each step to ensure the procedure is neither too prolonged nor too onerous for the patient. At first sight, such an approach seems technically challenging; however, with organization and appropriate equipment, it is both feasible and does not consume a great deal of catheter laboratory time.

Role of Exercise Testing in the Catheter Laboratory?

Exercise 'challenge' or 'confrontation' has major diagnostic value; however, this has not been emphasized in the literature as it has been perceived as difficult and complex. As a result, it has not been widely used and its benefits in altering patient management are poorly appreciated. Despite the decision at Dana Point to remove exercise-induced PH as a diagnosis, exercise challenge clearly has a role and one that is likely to develop in the coming years (table 4) [53, 54].

A major benefit of exercise testing at diagnostic right heart catheterization is the detection of an excessive rise in PCWP in patients with resting PCWP <15 mm Hg to confirm a diagnosis of pulmonary venous hypertension or nonsystolic heart failure, as such a diagnosis will lead to a completely different management than that following a diagnosis of PAH.

In patients with a significant pretest probability of pulmonary vascular disease, e.g. a patient with scleroderma reporting increasing exertional dyspnea and whose gas transfer factor (DLCO) has fallen yet the resting mPAP is normal or in the 'gray zone', exercise testing has a clear role.

Table 4. Roles for exercise testing during right heart catheterization

Diagnosis of pulmonary venous hypertension due to diastolic heart failure
Identification of abnormal pulmonary hemodynamic responses to exercise in patients with 'normal' resting pulmonary hemodynamics
Assessment of response to treatment

Even though following Dana Point [1, 15] it is not possible to diagnose PH on exercise, it is possible to use an exercise 'challenge' to determine the individual's hemodynamic response. If mPAP exceeds 30 mm Hg on exercise at mild-to-moderate workloads in a patient under 50 years of age, the response should be considered abnormal, and although a diagnosis of PAH cannot and should not be made, such a patient requires regular monitoring or even further investigation as they are at risk of developing frank PAH in the coming months or years [46]. In patients over 50 years, the upper limit of normal mPAP on mild-to-moderate exercise is less clear; certainly an increase of mPAP to >46 mm Hg is suspicious of an abnormal response and merits further monitoring [15].

As stated previously with supine exercise, PVR is stable or tends to drift down with increasing exercise loads and there is no clear evidence that in older patients the PVR response to exercise is different. Thus, an increase in PVR on exercise, provided the quality of the hemodynamic measurements on exercise is reliable, should also be regarded as highly suspicious [37].

Identifying Pulmonary Hypertension Secondary to Left Heart Disease

With the increasing realization over the last 20 years that PAH is not just a disease of younger adults, pulmonary vascular disease centers are seeing increasing numbers of older patients with PH with comorbidities which increase the risk of left heart disease. When LV systolic function is abnormal, these patients are relatively easy to identify, but in those with diastolic dysfunction the situation is often complex and diagnosis is difficult. When PCWP is raised >15 mm Hg, it is likely 'back pressure' into the pulmonary circulation is present, though a gray area of PCWP of 15–18 mm Hg has been suggested. A TPG of >12 mm Hg [2] is thought to suggest an element of 'reactive' pulmonary

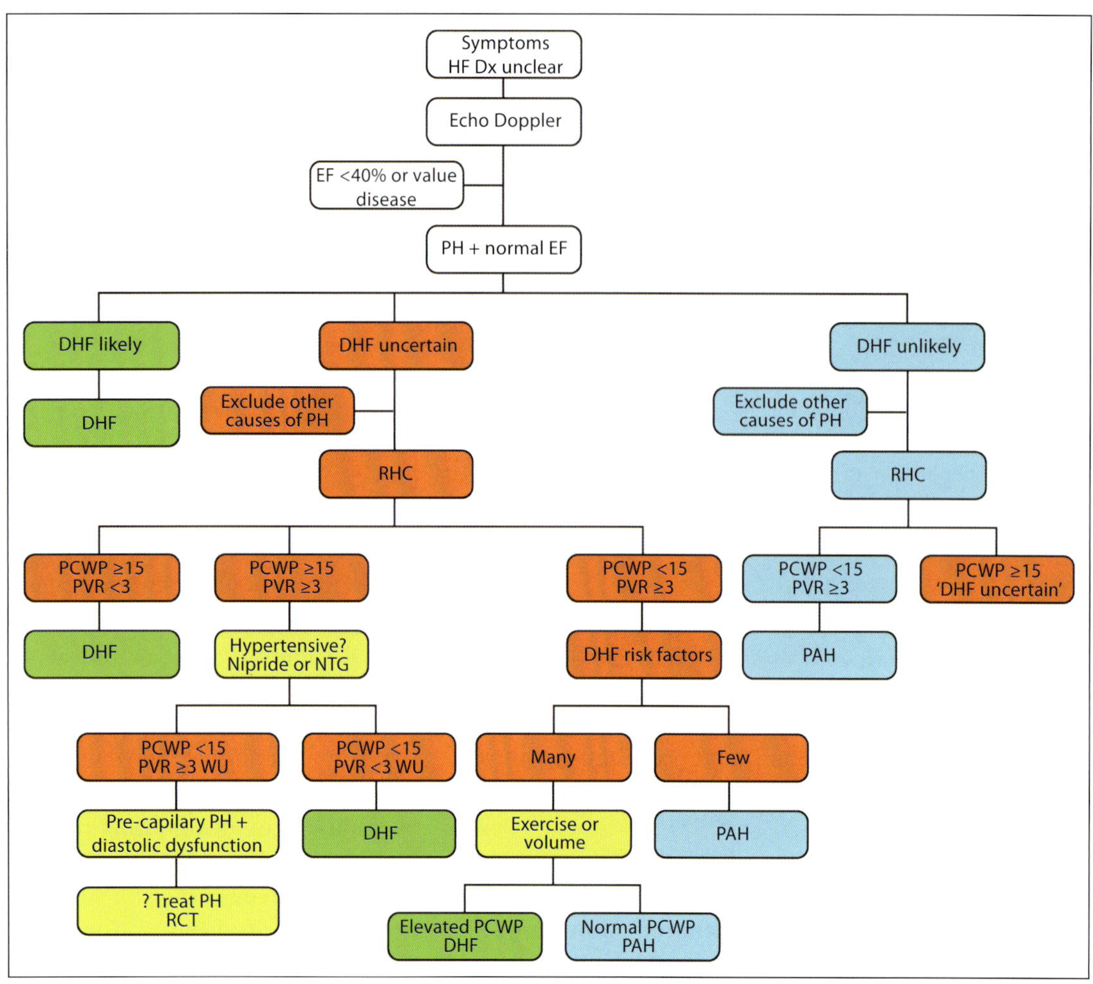

Fig. 5. Diagnostic approach to distinguish between PAH and PH caused by diastolic left heart disease (reproduced from Hoeper et al. [55] with permission of the publisher). DHF = Diastolic heart failure; Dx = diagnosis; EF = ejection fraction; HF = heart failure; NTG = nitroglycerine; OMT = optimized medical therapy; RCT = randomized controlled trial; RHC = right heart catheterization; WU = Wood units.

remodeling and possibly identify patients with disease that may be modifiable with pulmonary vasodilator therapy.

Patients with diastolic dysfunction can have normal PCWP at rest, and it has been proposed that such patients should be challenged by either exercising on the catheter table as discussed earlier or with a fluid challenge [53, 55] (fig. 5). A rapid rise in PCWP to >20 mm Hg suggests left heart dysfunction and vasodilation of the pulmonary circulation is unlikely to improve left heart function.

This area is complex and diagnosis is complicated by the fact that there is evidence that in normals with advanced age, the compliance of the left heart decreases and thus PCWP increases with exercise. The question arises as to what degree of increase in PCWP on exercise is abnormal for each decade of life. Such data is essential, but no reliable population data is available. Similarly, the rate of mPAP rise for each incremental increase in CO varies with age, and is quoted as a 1-mm Hg/l/min increase in CO in those <60 years compared to a 2.5-mm Hg/l/min increase in CO in older individuals [39]. Clearly even with exercise or fluid challenge there will be patients with known left heart disease with very high TPG who presumable have remodeled the pulmonary arterial circulation and may benefit from therapy [55]. However, it is important to remember such patients would not have been recruited into the seminal randomized controlled trials of targeted

Table 5. Current vasodilator reactivity criteria

mPAP	decrease by >10 mm Hg
mPAP	decreases to <40 mm Hg
CO	increase or stable

All three changes are required to be a positive test

pulmonary vasodilator therapy and we do not know the potential benefit or indeed harm of such therapies in this patient group.

Pulmonary Vascular Reactivity Testing

There is a group of patients with PAH who will respond acutely to pulmonary vasodilators and some of these patients have a very good prognosis with high-dose calcium channel blocker therapy [56]. Approximately 13% of patients newly diagnosed with PAH will demonstrate such a response though only a half of these patients will have a long-term sustained response to calcium channel blockers [57]. Criteria to identify a positive response have been recommended [58] and are outlined in table 5.

Current practice for right heart catheterization is to administer a short-acting vasodilator and observe the acute pulmonary hemodynamic response. A number of agents have been used and it is not clear if one agent is more effective than another in identifying this crucial subgroup of patients. Originally, intravenous adenosine was the most widely used agent, but recently inhaled nitric oxide with its very short half-life has been used more frequently – the doses and frequency are given in the table below. A recent paper suggested that inhaled nitric oxide might be more effective than adenosine at identifying individuals with a reactive pulmonary circulation [58]. Alternative agents are intravenous epoprostenol and inhaled iloprost. There is evidence that the acute hemodynamic response to inhaled iloprost is at least as potent as that seen with inhaled nitric oxide [59].

In the absence of clear evidence that one agent is superior, it is appropriate for each PH center to gain experience in using one of the above agents routinely.

Vasoreactivity testing is indicated in idiopathic PAH, heritable PAH, and PAH associated with anorexigen use. The value of acute vasodilator testing in patients with PAH associated with collagen vascular disease is highly questionable as very few patients in this group demonstrate an acute vasodilator response, and other than a few exceptions, it appears that this group of patients is not capable of having a clinically beneficial sustained response to calcium channel blockers [57]. It is not recommended in patients with PH in Dana Point Groups 2, 3, 4, and 5. Patients with evidence of clinical right heart failure or advanced right ventricular dysfunction (raised mRA >12 mm Hg or low cardiac index, <2.0 l/min/kg, WHO functional class IV) should not undergo acute vasodilator challenge as they require aggressive therapy and the negative inotropic effects of calcium channel blockers pose a risk to such patients. Vasoreactivity testing should be carried out only by experienced centers with adequate protocols and technical skills [2] (table 6).

In addition to its central role in diagnosis of PH, right heart catheterization measurements allow assessment of variables that have been demonstrated to have prognostic significance [8]. The measures of cardiac function or, more correctly, those measures that detect a failing RV have the greatest prognostic value, mRA and cardiac index. Mean pulmonary artery pressure is a weak prognostic sign and PVR or PVRI has no useful prognostic value.

Areas Requiring Further Research

Poor Correlation between Pulmonary Hemodynamic Measurements at Rest and Prognosis

It is striking that measures of RV decompensation, cardiac index, and mean right atrial pressure are very powerful prognostic tools, yet standard direct measurements of pulmonary vascular dysfunction, mean pulmonary artery pressure, and PVR have poor prognostic ability.

In addition, despite similar hemodynamics and apparently similar load, the RV can be struggling in one patient and not in another patient. Is this due to different 'hidden' impedance loads on the RV or is it variability between patients in the ability of their RV to cope with a similar load?

With potential therapies to support the RV under investigation, it is crucial to determine for each individual patient whether to add further pulmonary vasodilators with the hope that further improvements in pulmonary vessels to reduce load are achievable, or whether the focus should be on improving RV function as maximal pulmonary vascular response to targeted therapy has already been achieved. We contend that a number of

Table 6. Agents used in pulmonary vasoreactivity testing

Agent	Route	Half-life	Dose range	Increments	Duration
Epoprostenol	intravenous	3 min	2–12 ng/kg/min	2 ng/kg/min	10 min
Adenosine	intravenous	5–10 s	50–350 ug/kg/min	50 ug/kg/min	2 min
Nitric oxide	inhaled	15–30 s	10 or 20 ppm		
Iloprost	inhaled	20–30 min	25 or 50 ug[1]		15 min

[1] The dose of iloprost is the dose in the nebulizer and not the dose delivered to the lungs which is dependent on the nebulizer system used (adapted with addition of iloprost).

fundamental and crucial questions are in urgent need of answers:

(1) What is the range of pulmonary hemodynamic responses to exercise in normals and what is the normal change in impedance on exercise?

(2) How do these exercise hemodynamic responses, including impedance, vary across the decades in normals, including elderly normals?

(3) How does pulmonary vascular disease alter impedance at rest and exercise across the range of pulmonary vascular diseases seen in our practice?

(4) Can we better measure RV afterload and assess RV function both at diagnostic catheterization and when monitoring the effects of therapies to separate out RV responses to therapy from pulmonary vasculature responses?

(5) Can we develop relatively simple and easily repeatable technologies that can be used to monitor and direct patient management not just in large research-oriented PAH centers, but which are applicable in smaller centers where, worldwide, most PAH patients are managed?

Conclusion

Though we have repeatedly highlighted our areas of uncertainty and in some respects ignorance, it is important to understand that invasive pulmonary hemodynamics are essential for diagnosis, assessing prognosis, and monitoring the effect of therapy in pulmonary vascular disease. Other modalities such as echocardiography or MRI provide additional or complementary measurements and even additional functional insights, but cannot replace the central role of invasive hemodynamic measurements which remain the 'gold standard' investigation.

Despite great advances in our insight into pulmonary vascular diseases at the pathological and cell biology level, our limited knowledge of the pathophysiology severely limits our understanding of the response of the pulmonary circulation to these diseases. Currently, as a result of our lack of understanding of the pathophysiology, we cannot explain the variable effects of treatment with pulmonary vasodilator therapy or why changes in functional status correlate poorly with hemodynamic changes. Our understanding of changes in afterload at rest and on exercise and how therapeutic interventions alter these loads on the RV is currently very limited.

Because right heart catheterization is such an important tool, it is essential that it is carried out with precision and with a full understanding of its methodology, pitfalls, and limitations by experienced clinicians.

It is safe, relatively simple, and easy to repeat right heart catheterization, but the reluctance of many physicians to submit patients to repeat hemodynamic monitoring and to repeat exercise testing following therapy further limits our understanding of the pathophysiology of pulmonary vascular disease.

Much of this essential exploration of the pathophysiology of the diseased pulmonary circulation over the coming years will have invasive hemodynamics as a central investigative tool combined with other developing technologies.

References

1 Badesch DB, Champion HC, Sanchez MAG, Hoeper MM, Loyd JE, Manes A, McGoon M, Naeije R, Olschewski H, Oudiz RJ, Torbicki A: Diagnosis and assessment of pulmonary arterial hypertension. J Am Coll Cardiol 2009;54:S55–S66

2 Galie N, Hoeper MM, Humbert M, Torbicki A, Vachiery J-L, Barbera JA, Beghetti M, Corris P, Gaine S, Gibbs JS, Gomez-Sanchez MA, Jondeau G, Klepteko W, Opitz C, Peacock A, Rubin L, Zellweger M, Simonneau G, ESC Committee for Practice Guidelines (CPG): Guidelines for the diagnosis and treatment of pulmonary hypertension: the Task Force for the Diagnosis and Treatment of Pulmonary Hypertension of the European Society of Cardiology (ESC) and the European Respiratory Society (ERS), endorsed by the International Society of Heart and Lung Transplantation (ISHLT). Eur Heart J 2009;30:2493–2537.

3 McLaughlin VV, Archer SL, Badesch DB, Barst RJ, Farber HW, Lindner JR, Mathier MA, McGoon MD, Park MH, Rosenson RS, Rubin LJ, Tapson VF, Varga J, American College of Cardiology Foundation Task Force on Expert Consensus Documents, American Heart Association, American College of Chest Physicians, American Thoracic Society, Inc, Pulmonary Hypertension Association: ACCF/AHA 2009 expert consensus document on pulmonary hypertension – a report of the American College of Cardiology Foundation Task Force on Expert Consensus Documents and the American Heart Association developed in collaboration with the American College of Chest Physicians; American Thoracic Society, Inc.; and the Pulmonary Hypertension Association. J Am Coll Cardiol 2009;53:1573–1619.

4 Rich JD, Shah SJ, Swamy R, Kamp A, Rich S: The inaccuracy of Doppler echocardiography estimates of pulmonary artery pressures in patients with pulmonary hypertension: implications for clinical practice. Chest 2011;139:988–993.

5 Janda S, Shahidi N, Gin K, Swiston J: Diagnostic accuracy of echocardiography for pulmonary hypertension: a systematic review and meta-analysis. Heart 2011;97:612–622.

6 Benza RL, Miller DP, Gomberg-Maitland M, Frantz RP, Foremen AJ, Coffey CS, Frost A, Barst RJ, Badesch DB, Elliott CG, Liou TG, McGoon MD: Predicting survival in pulmonary arterial hypertension: insights from the registry to evaluate early and long term pulmonary arterial hypertension disease management. Circulation 2010;122:164–172.

7 D'Alonzo GE, Barst RJ, Ayres SM, Bergofsky EH, Brundage BH, Detre KM, Fishman AP, Goldring RM, Groves BM, Kernis JT, Levy PS, Pietra GS, Reid LM, Reeves JT, Rich S, Vreim CE, Williams GW, Wu M: Survival in patients with primary pulmonary hypertension. Ann Intern Med 1991;115:343–349.

8 Humbert M, Sitbon O, Chaouat A, Bertocchi M, Habib G, Gressin V, Yaïci A, Weitzenblum E, Cordier JF, Chabot F, Dromer C, Pison C, Reynaud-Gaubert M, Haloun A, Laurent M, Hachulla E, Cottin V, Degano B, Jaïs X, Montani D, Souza R, Simonneau G: Survival in patients with idiopathic, familial and anorexigen-associated pulmonary arterial hypertension in the modern management era. Circulation 2010; 122:156–163.

9 McLaughlin VV, Shillington A, Rich S: Survival in primary pulmonary hypertension: the impact of epoprostenol therapy. Circulation 2002;106:1477–1482.

10 McLaughlin VV, Presberg KW, Doyle RL, Abman SH, McCrory DC, Fortin T, Ahearn G: Prognosis of pulmonary arterial hypertension: ACCP evidence-based clinical practice guidelines. Chest 2004;126:78S–92S.

11 Lankhaar JW, Westerhof N, Faes TJ, Marques KM, Marcus JT, Postmus PE, Vonk-Noodegraaf A: Quantification of right ventricular afterload in patients with and without pulmonary hypertension. Am J Physiol Heart Circ Physiol 2006; 291:H1731–H1737.

12 Davies RJ, Morrell NJ: Molecular mechanisms of PAH. Chest 2008;134:1271–1277.

13 Reeves J, Taylor AE: Pulmonary hemodynamics and fluid exchange in the lungs during exercise; in: Handbook of Physiology. Exercise: Regulation and Integration of Multiple Systems. Bethesda, Am Physiol Soc, 1996, pp 587–613.

14 Chemla D, Castelain V, Herve P, Lecarpentier Y, Brimioulle S: Haemodynamic evaluation of pulmonary hypertension. Eur Respir J 2002;20:1314–1331.

15 Kovacs G, Berghold A, Scheidl S, Olschewski H: Pulmonary arterial pressure during rest and exercise in healthy subjects: a systematic review. Eur Respir J 2009;34:888–894.

16 Pinsky MR: Pulmonary artery occlusion pressure; in Pinsky MR, Brochard L, Mancebo J (eds): Applied Physiology in Intensive Care Medicine. Berlin, Springer, 2009, pp 69–72.

17 Permutt S, Bromberger-Barnea B, Bane HN: Alveolar pressure, pulmonary venous pressure and vascular waterfall. Med Thorac 1962;19:239–260.

18 Naeije R, Huez S: Right ventricular function in pulmonary hypertension: physiological concepts. Eur Heart J Supplements 2007;9:H5–H9.

19 Naeije R: Pulmonary vascular resistance: a meaningless variable. Intensive Care Med 2003; 29:526–529.

20 Castelian V, Chemla D, Humbert M, Sitbon O, Simonneau G, Lecarpentier Y, Herve P: Pulmonary artery pressure-flow relations after prostacyclin in primary pulmonary hypertension. Am J Respir Crit Care Med 2002;165:338–340.

21 Versprille A: Pulmonary vascular resistance. A meaningless variable. Intensive Care Med 1984; 10:51–53.

22 McGregor M, Sniderman A: On pulmonary vascular resistance: the need for more precise definition. Am J Cardiol 1985;55:217–221.

23 Milnor WR: Pulsatile blood flow. N Engl J Med 1972;287:27–34.

24 Westerhof N, Stergiopulos N, Noble MIM (eds): Snapshots of Hemodynamics: An Aid for Clinical Research and Graduate Education, ed 2. New York, Springer, 2010.

25 Huez S, Brimioulle S, Naeije R, Vachiery JL: Feasibility of routine pulmonary arterial impedance measurements in pulmonary hypertension. Chest 2004;125:2121–2128.

26 Castelain V, Herve P, Lecarpentier Y, Duroux P, Simonneau G, Chemla D: Pulmonary artery pulse pressure and wave reflection in chronic pulmonary thromboembolis and primary pulmonary hypertension. J Am Coll Cardiol 2001;37:1085–1092.

27 Reeves JT, Linehan JH, Stenmark KR: Distensibility of the normal human lung circulation during exercise. Am J Physiol Lung Cell Mol Physiol 2005;288:L419–L425.

28 Veolkel NF, Quaife RA, Leinwand LA, Barst RJ, McGoon MD, Meldrum DR, Dupuis J, Long CS, Rubin LJ, Smart FW, Yuichiro JS, Gladwin M, Denholm EM, Gail DB, National Heart Lung Blood Institute Working Group on Cellular Mechanisms of Right Heart Failure: Right ventricular function and failure: report of a National Heart, Lung and Blood Institute Working Group on Cellular and Molecular Mechanisms of Right Heart Failure. Circulation 2006;114:1883–1891.

29 Bogaard HJ, Kohtaro A, Vonk-Noordegraaf A, Voelkel NF: The right ventricle under pressure: cellular and molecular mechanisms of right-heart failure in pulmonary hypertension. Chest 2009;135:794–804.

30 Brandfonbrenner M, Landowne M, Shock NW: Changes in cardiac output with age. Circulation 1955;12:557–566.

31 Granath A, Jonsson B, Strandell T: Circulation in healthy old men studied by right heart catheterization at rest and during exercise in the supine position and sitting position. Acta Med Scand 1964;176:425–446.

32 Granath A, Strandell T: Relationship between output, stroke volume and intracardiac pressures at rest and during exercise in supine position and some anthropometric data in healthy old men. Acta Med Scand 1964;176:447–466.

33 Holmgren A, Jonsson B, Sjostrand T: Circulatory data in normal subjects at rest and during exercise in recumbent position, with special reference to the stroke volume at different work intensities. Acta Physiol Scand 1960;49:343–363.

34 Bevegard S, Holmgren A, Jonsson B: The effect of body position on the circulation at rest and during exercise, with special reference to the influence on stroke volume. Acta Physiol Scand 1960; 49:279–298.

35 Harris P, Heath D: Normal variations in pressure and flow; in: The Human Pulmonary Circulation: Its Form and Function in Health and Disease, ed 3. Edinburgh, Churchill Livingstone, 1986, pp 149–160.

36 Sancetta SM, Ratkia L: Response of pulmonary artery pressure and total pulmonary resistance of untrained convalescent man to prolonged mild steady state exercise. J Clin Invest 1957;36: 1138–1149.
37 Tolle JT, Waxman AB, Van Horn L, Pappagianopolous PP, Systrom DM: Exercise induced pulmonary arterial hypertension. Circulation 2008; 118:2183–2189.
38 Janicki JS, Weber KT, Likoff MJ, Fishman AP: The pressure-flow response of the pulmonary circulation in patients with heart failure and pulmonary vascular disease. Circulation 1985;72: 1270–1278.
39 Reeves J, Dempsey J, Grover R: Pulmonary circulation during exercise; in Weir E, Reeves J (eds): Pulmonary Vascular Physiology and Pathophysiology. New York, Dekker, 1989, pp 107–133.
40 Saggar R, Saggar R, Aboulhosn J, Belperio JA, Zisman DA, Lynch JP III: Diagnosis and hemodynamic assessment of pulmonary arterial hypertension. Seminars Respir Crit Care Med 2009; 30:399–410.
41 Ehrsam RE, Perruchoud A, Oberholzer M, Burkart F, Herzog H: Influence of age on pulmonary haemodynamics at rest and during supine exercise. Clin Sci (Lond) 1983;65:653–660.
42 Harris P, Heath D, Apostopoulus A: Extensibility of the human pulmonary trunk. Br Heart J 1965; 27:651–659.
43 Milnor WR, Conti C, Lewis KB, O'Rourke MF: Pulmonary arterial pulse wave velocity and impedance in man. Circ Res 1969;25:637–649.
44 Milnor WR: Arterial impedance as ventricular afterload. Circ Res 1975;36:565–570.
45 Reeves JT, Groves BM, Turkevich D, Morrison DA, Trapp JA: Right ventricular function in pulmonary hypertension; in Weir E, Reeves J (eds): Pulmonary Vascular Physiology and Pathophysiology. New York, Dekker, 1989, pp 325–345.
46 Condliffe R, Kiely DG, Peacock AJ, Corris P, Gibbs JS, Vrapi F, Das C, Elliot CA, Johnson M, DeSoyza J, Torpy C, Goldsmith K, Hodgkins D, Hughes RJ, Pepke-Zaba J, Coghlan JG: Connective tissue disease-associated pulmonary arterial hypertension in the modern management era. Am J Resp Crit Care Med 2009;179:151–157.
47 Kovacs G, Maier R, Aberer E, Brodmann M, Scheidl S, Tröster N, Hess C, Salmhofer W, Graninger W, Gruenig E, Rubin LJ, Olschewski H: Borderline pulmonary arterial pressure is associated with decreased exercise capacity in scleroderma. Am J Resp Crit Care Med 2009; 180: 881–886.
48 Groves BM, Badesch DB: Cardiac catheterization of patients with pulmonary hypertension; in Peacock AJ, Rubin LJ (eds): Pulmonary Circulation: Diseases and their Treatment, ed 2. London, Arnold, 2004, pp 121–131.
49 Hoeper MM, Lee SH, Voswinckel R, Palazzini M, Jais X, Marinelli A, Barst RJ, Ghorani HA, Jing Z, Optiz C, Seyfarth J, Halank M, McLaughlin V, Oudiz RJ, Ewert R, Wilkens H, Kluge S, Bremer H, Baroke E, Rubin LJ: Complications of right heart catheterization procedures in patients with pulmonary hypertension in experienced centers. J Am Coll Cardiol 2006;48:2546–2552.
50 Hoeper M, Maier R, Tongers J, Niedermeyer J, Hohlfield JM, Hamm M, Fabel H: Determination of cardiac output by the Fick method, thermodilution and acetylene rebreathing in pulmonary hypertension. Am J Resp Crit Care Med 1999; 160:535–541.
51 Naeije R: Pulmonary vascular function; in Peacock AJ, Rubin LJ (eds): Pulmonary Circulation: Diseases and their Treatment, ed 2. London, Arnold, 2004, pp 3–13.
52 Davidson CJ, Bonow RO: Cardiac catheterization; in Libby P, Bonow RO, Mann DL, Zipes DP (eds): Braunwald's Heart Disease: A Textbook of Cardiovascular Medicine, ed 8. Philadelphia, Saunders Elsevier, 2007, p 449.
53 Champion HC, Michelakis ED, Hasssoun PM: Comprehensive invasive and noninvasive approach to the right ventricle-pulmonary circulation unit: state of the art and clinical and research implications. Circulation 2009;120: 992–1007.
54 Naeije R: In defence of exercise stress tests for the diagnosis of pulmonary hypertension. Heart 2011;97:94–95.
55 Hoeper MM, Barbera JA, Channick RN, Hassoun PM, Lang IM, Manes A, Martinez FJ, Naeije R, Olschewski H, Pepke-Zaba J, Redfield MM, Robbins IM, Souza R, Torbicki A, McGoon M: Diagnosis, assessment, and treatment of non-pulmonary arterial hypertension pulmonary hypertension. J Am Coll Cardiol 2009;54:S85–S96.
56 Rich S, Kaufmann E, Levy PS: The effect of high doses of calcium-channel blockers on survival in primary pulmonary hypertension, N Engl J Med 1992;327:76–81.
57 Sitbon O, Humbert M, Xavier Jaïs, Ioos V, Hamid AM, Provencher S, Garcia G, Parent F, Herve P, Simonneau G: Long-term response to calcium channel blockers in idiopathic pulmonary arterial hypertension. Circulation 2005;111:3105–3111.
58 Oliveira EC, Ribeiro AL, Amaral CF: Adenosine for vasoreactivity testing in pulmonary hypertension: a head to head comparison with inhaled nitric oxide. Respir Med 2010;104:606–610.
59 Hoeper MM, Olschewski H, Ghofrani HA, Wilkens H, Winkler J, Borst MM, Niedermeyer J, Fabel H, Seeger W, the German PPH Study Group: A comparison of the acute hemodynamic effects of inhaled nitric oxide and aerosolized iloprost in primary pulmonary hypertension. J Am Coll Cardiol 2000;35:176–182.

Dr. K.F. Whyte
Greenlane Respiratory Service, Auckland City Hospital, Grafton
Private Bag 92024
Auckland 1142 (New Zealand)
Tel. +64 96309943, ext. 25170, E-Mail kenw@adhb.govt.nz

Chapter 4
Humbert M, Souza R, Simonneau G (eds): Pulmonary Vascular Disorders.
Prog Respir Res. Basel, Karger, 2012, vol 41, pp 37–47

Exercise Testing in Pulmonary Arterial Hypertension

Steeve Provencher · Vincent Mainguy

Centre de recherche de l'Institut Universitaire de Cardiologie et de Pneumologie de Québec, Université Laval, Québec, Canada

Abstract
The most significant manifestations of pulmonary arterial hypertension (PAH) are dyspnea, exercise intolerance, and poor quality of life. Mechanisms of exercise intolerance in PAH are clearly multifactorial and involve cardiac, respiratory, and peripheral muscle abnormalities. Exercise capacity is thus a marker of the integrated response of all systems involved in O_2 transport and utilization. As such, the objective measurement of exercise capacity is useful and relevant in the assessment of PAH patients, as it provides benchmarks for disease severity, response to therapy, and disease progression in idiopathic PAH. Over the years, exercise capacity measurement has thus played a major role in patients' evaluation in both clinical trials and PAH clinics. Its responsiveness to pharmacological interventions also permitted the demonstration of efficacy of novel PAH-specific therapies. Its sensitivity to detect improvements following interventions has, however, been challenged in recent combination trials or when used to assess patients with milder disease. The reliability of exercise testing in nonidiopathic PAH also remains to be validated. This review revisits the exercise physiopathology and the clinical relevance of exercise testing in PAH.

Pulmonary arterial hypertension (PAH) is characterized by the progressive increase in pulmonary vascular resistance ultimately leading to right heart failure [1]. The most significant manifestations of this pulmonary artery remodeling and secondary impaired cardiac function are dyspnea, exercise intolerance, and poor quality of life. As such, the objective measurement of exercise capacity is useful and relevant in the assessment of PAH patients, as it provides benchmarks for disease severity, response to therapy, and disease progression. Over the years, exercise capacity measurement has thus played a major role in patients' evaluation in both clinical trials and PAH clinics. While specific guidelines are currently available for the practical aspects of exercise tests [2–5], this review revisits the exercise physiopathology and the clinical relevance of exercise testing in PAH.

Steeve Provencher is a clinical scientist of the Fonds de Recherche en Santé du Québec.

Exercise Physiopathology in Pulmonary Arterial Hypertension

Normal Hemodynamic Response during Exercise

During upright exercise, stroke volume initially increases 20–50% due to enhanced cardiac inotropy and venous return, and then plateau at work rates above approximately 50% of peak oxygen uptake ($\dot{V}o_2$*peak*) [6]. Heart rate linearly rises during an incremental exercise as vagal tone decreases. Enhanced O_2 extraction also contributes to the rise in Vo_2 during exercise. Increases in cardiac output lead to pulmonary vessels distension and recruitment. As a result, pulmonary artery pressure minimally increases in young subjects despite marked increases in pulmonary blood flow (fig. 1) [7]. Even in older subjects, exercise-induced pulmonary hypertension is essentially related to increases in left-heart end-diastolic pressures [7], suggesting that the pulmonary vasculature adaptation during exercise remains normal with aging.

Cardiac Abnormalities during Exercise in Pulmonary Arterial Hypertension

The abnormal and remodeled pulmonary vasculature loses its recruitment and distension capacity, resulting in disproportionate increases in pulmonary artery pressure during exertion (fig. 1) [8]. Exertional limitation in PAH is usually explained by the inability of the overloaded right ventricle to perfuse the lungs and to adapt systemic O_2 delivery to O_2 demand. Indeed, the right ventricle is poorly designed to respond to an increased afterload. As a result, exercising PAH patients exhibit a low stroke volume that fails to increase during exercise [9], such that the increase in cardiac output is mainly achieved through increases in heart rate [10]. However, PAH is also characterized by a failure to increase heart rate to the maximal predicted values, so maximal cardiac output during exercise is limited by both low stroke volume and altered chronotropic response [8–10].

Other Potential Components of Exercise Limitation in Pulmonary Arterial Hypertension

As in other chronic diseases, exercise intolerance in PAH is likely to be multifactorial. In addition to an increase in cardiac output, exercise also requires a global and integrated response of many systems, including peripheral vessels to increase muscle blood flow, the respiratory system for O_2 uptake and CO_2 clearance, blood to carry and deliver O_2, and muscles to generate energy and external work (fig. 2). Numerous observations suggest that exercise limitation in PAH is not simply due to pulmonary hemodynamic impairment [11]. Indeed, PAH is also characterized by increased pulmonary physiologic shunt [12], which in conjunction with decreased mixed venous O_2 saturation, contributes to hypoxemia. However, as the affinity of hemoglobin for O_2 progressively increases as PO_2 decreases, PAH patients are likely to exhibit a lower limit of venous O_2 content at maximal exercise that is comparable to healthy subjects. When maximal cardiac output is limited, decreased arterial O_2 content is thus likely to contribute to exercise intolerance through limitation in peripheral O_2 extraction capacity [13]. Increased dead-space ventilation [12] and hyperventilation [14] markedly increase the respiratory demand both at rest and during exercise. While mechanisms leading to hyperventilation remain poorly understood in PAH, they may include enhanced activation of ergoreceptors and metaboreceptors in skeletal muscles, resulting in sympathetic nervous system activation [15], enhanced chemosensitivity [16–18], and increased central respiratory drive [19, 20].

In other chronic cardiorespiratory disorders, major attention is also placed on skeletal muscle dysfunction. Recently, skeletal muscle abnormalities have also been reported in PAH [21, 22] and include lower proportion of muscle fiber type 1, increased glycolytic enzyme ratio, and less muscle strength and capillarity. Whether these abnormalities participate, in addition to the limited muscle blood flow, to early anaerobic threshold and exercise limitation remains unknown. However, these abnormalities in PAH are partly reversible by exercise training [23, 24]. Rehabilitation also increases exercise capacity in the absence of significant pulmonary hemodynamic changes [25], reinforcing the concept that skeletal muscle abnormalities influence exercise tolerance in these patients. Similarly, recent studies documented decreases in respiratory muscle strength of PAH patients [19, 20]. While maximal inspiratory pressure may be an important determinant of $\dot{V}O_2$ *peak* in congestive heart failure patients [26], it remains unknown whether impaired respiratory muscle strength independently influences exercise capacity in PAH.

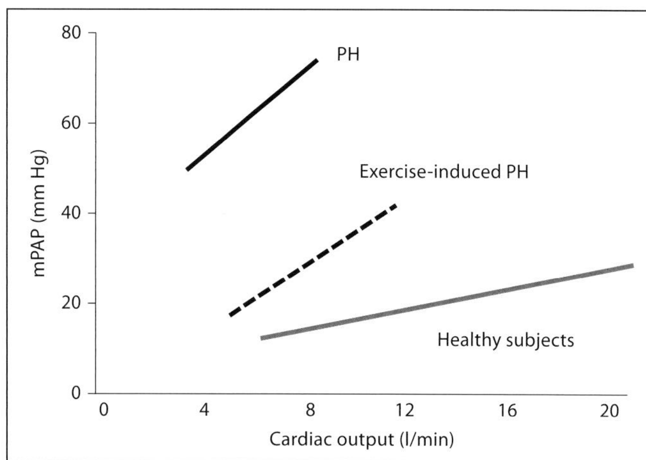

Fig. 1. Pulmonary hemodynamic response during exercise in healthy subjects and in pulmonary hypertensive patients. In healthy subjects, mean pulmonary artery pressure (mPAP) minimally increases during mild-to-moderate exercise despite increases in pulmonary flow because of the pulmonary vessel recruitment and distensibility. Conversely, patients with pulmonary hypertension (PH) exhibit elevated mPAP and disproportionate increases in mPAP during exercise [8]. Some patients may also exhibit normal hemodynamics at rest, but significant increases in mPAP during exercise. Exercise-induced pulmonary hypertension may represent an early sign of pulmonary vessel remodeling. However, approximately 50% of healthy subjects >50 years of age exhibit significant increases in mPAP >30 mm Hg during mild exercise as a result of elevated left heart pressure during exercise. This criterion is thus no longer used to define pulmonary hypertension [1].

Incremental Cardiopulmonary Exercise Test Characteristics in Pulmonary Arterial Hypertension

In patients with limited cardiac reserve, it is reasonable to assume that aerobic exercise capacity is representative of the maximal cardiac output achievable during exercise. Other aspects of the cardiorespiratory maladaptation to exercise

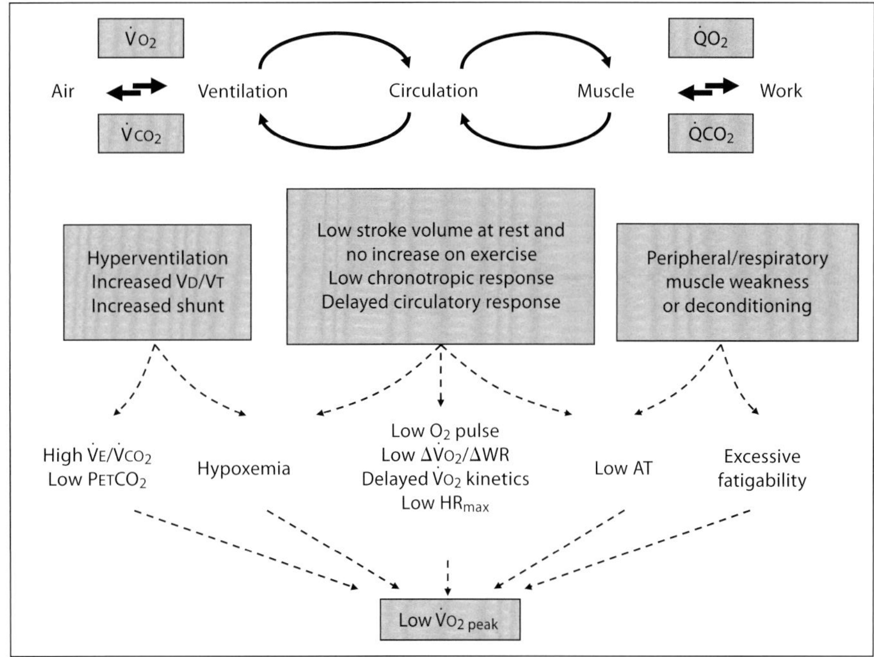

Fig. 2. Schematic overview of the exercise physiopathology in PAH. PAH is characterized by a low stroke volume that fails to increase during exercise, as well as limited chronotropic response. Initial increase in pulmonary flow is also delayed. These abnormalities translate into a low oxygen pulse ($\dot{V}O_2$/heart rate), delayed initial $\dot{V}O_2$ kinetics, and a low maximal heart rate. Because of the limited cardiac output and oxygen delivery, external mechanical work is more dependent on anaerobic metabolism during exercise, resulting in a lower increase in $\dot{V}O_2$ relative to the increase in workload. PAH is also characterized by increased dead-space ventilation, physiologic shunt, and hyperventilation resulting in exercise-induced hypoxemia and nonefficient ventilation (low end-tidal CO_2 and increased minute ventilation in relation to CO_2 production), respectively. More recently, skeletal and respiratory muscle abnormalities have been described. Importantly, the specific contribution of these interrelated cardiac, ventilatory, and peripheral abnormalities on exercise intolerance remain unknown. For example, exercise-induced hypoxemia, low cardiac output, and skeletal muscle abnormalities may all contribute to excessive muscle fatigability, increased perception of effort, and ultimately poor exercise capacity.

described above will also translate into characteristic abnormalities observed during incremental cardiopulmonary exercise testing (CPET) (table 1, fig. 3) [11, 27, 28]. Exercise-induced right-to-left shunt through a patent foramen ovale can also be suspected when abrupt hyperventilation (sudden and sustained increase in end-tidal O_2 and respiratory exchange ratio, with simultaneous decrease in end-tidal CO_2), usually associated with a decline in peripheral O_2 saturation (SpO_2), is observed during exercise [29].

Physiological Response during Walking Tests in Pulmonary Arterial Hypertension

The safety of CPET has been confirmed when performed in appropriately selected PAH patients [11, 12, 28–34]. However, initial concerns about exercise testing in PAH and the incapacity of a significant proportion of patients with advanced disease to complete CPET [31, 35] have led many experts to recommend self-paced submaximal exercise testing to assess functional exercise in PAH as in other debilitating diseases [2]. The 6-min walk test (6MWT) has been widely used in PAH and has the advantages of being simple, easy to administer, reproducible, and potentially better tolerated than CPET [2]. Unlike CPET, walking tests do not provide information on the physiologic mechanism of exercise limitation. Nevertheless, physiologic measurements using portable devices have shown that contrary to healthy subjects, the level of aerobic capacity achieved during a 6MWT is comparable to incremental CPET in PAH [36], as previously reported in moderate-to-severe chronic obstructive pulmonary disease [37]. Moreover, the 6-min walked distance

Table 1. Characteristic abnormalities observed during incremental cardiopulmonary exercise testing in pulmonary arterial hypertension

Cardiorespiratory abnormalities	Consequences during CPET
Low cardiac output	Low maximal workload Low $\dot{V}O_2$ *Peak* Early anaerobic threshold Abnormally low $\Delta\dot{V}O_2/\Delta$workload (representative of a higher than normal dependence on anaerobic metabolism during exercise)
Delayed increase in pulmonary blood flow at the start of exercise	Delayed kinetics in $\dot{V}O_2$ increase during exercise (assessed with mean response time during constant workload exercise)
Low chronotropic reserve	High resting and low maximal heart rates
Low stroke volume at rest and during exercise	Low O_2 pulse
Hyperventilation	Increased $\dot{V}_E/\dot{V}CO_2$ ratio or $\dot{V}_E$–$\dot{V}CO_2$ slope Decreased $P_{ET}CO_2$
Increased dead-space ventilation	
Increased physiologic shunt and low mixed venous oxygen saturation	Exercise-induced hypoxemia
Skeletal muscle abnormalities	Early anaerobic threshold Excessive leg fatigue[1]

$\dot{V}O_2$= Oxygen uptake; $\dot{V}_E$ = minute ventilation; $\dot{V}CO_2$ = carbon dioxide production; $P_{ET}CO_2$ = end-tidal carbon dioxide pressure.
[1] Early leg fatigue and anaerobic threshold are likely to be multifactorial, including low cardiac output and subsequent altered muscle perfusion during exercise, exercise-induced hypoxemia, as well as morphological and functional muscle impairments.

correlates with individuals' $\dot{V}O_2$ *peak* [31, 34, 36], although this relationship presents interindividual variability due to differences in mechanical efficiency [31, 38]. While $\dot{V}O_2$ and O_2 pulse appear to be similar or slightly higher during the 6MWT, CPET is associated with higher V_{CO_2}, minute ventilation, respiratory exchange ratio, and maximal heart rate [36]. This is in keeping with previous reports of later onset and less severe lactic acidosis at the same level of load during walking compared to cycling exercise in other chronic cardiorespiratory diseases. End-exercise SpO_2 is also lower during the 6MWT [36], although mechanisms leading to enhanced exercise-induced hypoxemia during the 6MWT have not been fully elucidated. Finally, the level of exercise ventilation ($V_E/\dot{V}_{CO_2}$ ratio) at anaerobic threshold appeared to be similar during both exercises [36]. Conversely, the kinetics of aerobic and metabolic stress significantly differ during the 6MWT, reaching a plateau after 2–3 min of walking [36]. This steady state condition is representative of the essentially constant walking speed observed during the entire 6MWT [36]. Indeed, previous studies documented that patients modulate their walking velocity to reach their critical walking power, defined as the maximum sustainable walking speed [39]. The 6-min walked distance is thus a marker of patients' sustainable aerobic effort, explaining its high predictive value in many chronic disorders.

The physiological response observed during the incremental shuttle walk test [4] shares many characteristics of the 6MWT and CPET, the kinetics of the cardiorespiratory response being comparable to the one observed during CPET, whereas minute ventilation, respiratory exchange ratio, and end-exercise SpO_2 are comparable with the 6MWT [4, 40]. Other exercise tests such as the endurance shuttle walk test [5], the Naughton-Balke protocol on treadmill [41], and the 6MWT on treadmill [42] have only rarely been used in PAH.

Rationale and Relevance of Exercise Testing in Pulmonary Arterial Hypertension

The main reason why exercise testing is being used in chronic diseases is that exercise tolerance cannot be predicted from resting physiologic parameters, and because subtle abnormalities in cardiac and respiratory systems are more likely

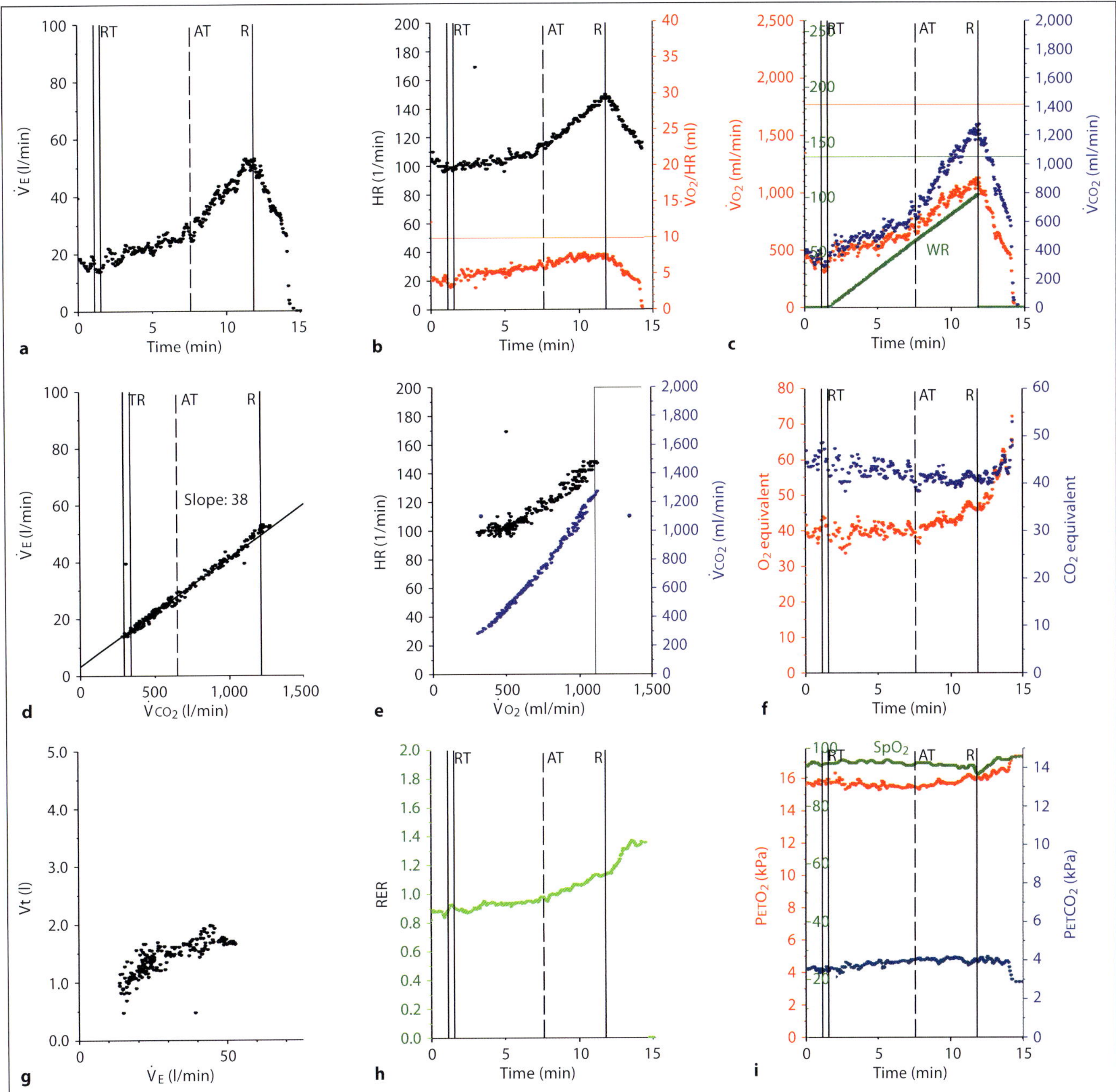

Fig. 3. Typical example of the graphical representation of a cardiopulmonary exercise test in idiopathic PAH. Cardiopulmonary exercise testing in PAH is characterized by a low $\dot{V}O_2$ peak (**c**, **e**) and low maximal workload (**c**). Moreover, $\dot{V}O_2$ increases by approx. 10 ml/min/W in healthy subjects. In this example, a progressive increase in workload up to 100 W was associated with a 800-ml (from 350 to 1,150 ml) increase in $\dot{V}O_2$ only (**c**). This is representative of a higher than normal dependence on anaerobic metabolism during exercise. This limited increase in $\dot{V}O_2$ is associated with a limited chronotropic response and a low oxygen pulse during exercise (**b**). As a result, heart rate does not reach the maximal heart rate predicted despite an abnormally low stroke volume (estimated by a low oxygen pulse). The anaerobic threshold (determined from **a**, **e**, **f** and **i**) occurs at about 60% of the patient's $\dot{V}O_2$ peak, but at about 30% of her predicted $\dot{V}O_2$ peak. Excessive minute ventilation, a marker of hyperventilation and/or increased dead-space ventilation, is documented by the increased $\dot{V}E/\dot{V}CO_2$ slope (**d**), the elevated CO_2 equivalent (**f**) and the low $P_{ET}CO_2$ (**i**). A small decrease in SpO_2 is also observed during exercise (**i**). Exercise-induced hypoxemia is typically worse during walking exercise tests. AT = Anaerobic threshold; HR = heart rate; $P_{ET}CO_2$ = end-tidal CO_2; $P_{ET}O_2$ = end-tidal O_2; RER = respiratory exchange ratio; SpO_2 = peripheral oxygen saturation; $\dot{V}E$ = minute ventilation; $\dot{V}CO_2$ = CO_2 production; $\dot{V}O_2$ = O_2 uptake; Vt = tidal volume.

to be uncovered under high physiological stress during exercise than at rest. In PAH, the relationship between exercise capacity and survival was first documented in an NIH cohort study, in which NYHA functional class was highly predictive of mortality [43]. As described in the previous section, exercise capacity is an objective marker of all the integrative mechanisms involved in O_2 transport and utilization, including maximal cardiac output. As such, the relevance of exercise testing is no longer questioned in PAH and exercise capacity has been used to assess disease severity, prognosis, and response to therapy.

Discriminative Properties of Exercise Tests

Numerous studies have documented the excellent discriminative properties of both CPET and 6MWT in PAH. In fact, exercise tolerance is better correlated with functional class and prognosis than resting hemodynamic parameters. Rhodes et al. [28] first documented the poor prognosis of idiopathic PAH patients with extremely limited exercise capacity on CPET. Among noninvasive parameters, $\dot{V}O_2$ *peak*, peak systolic blood pressure, and peak diastolic blood pressure during exercise also emerged as independent predictors of survival in a larger cohort of idiopathic PAH patients [35]. Optimal cutoff values for $\dot{V}O_2$ *peak* (>10.4 ml/kg/min) and systolic blood pressure (>120 mm Hg) during CPET to predict survival at 12 months were determined using receiver operating characteristic curves. As in congestive heart failure, lower end-tidal CO_2, ventilatory efficiency (assessed by the $\dot{V}E/\dot{V}CO_2$ slope) and maximal heart rate reached during exercise were also associated with an increased risk of mortality on univariate analysis. $\dot{V}O_2$ *peak*, ventilatory efficiency, and O_2 pulse were also found to be predictors of long-term survival in a mixed population of pulmonary hypertensive patients [34].

Many studies have also shown that the 6-min walked distance has excellent discriminative properties in idiopathic PAH [31, 34, 44–46]. Performance in the baseline 6MWT was found to be an independent predictor of survival in the first randomized controlled trial in PAH [47]. Whether exercise-induced desaturation during 6MWT is also related to prognosis remains unknown [48]. While maximal and 'submaximal' testing may be complementary, it remains unknown whether CPET yields additional prognostic information after determination of the 6-min walked distance. Only one study assessed the added value of CPET over 6MWT [34], and suggested that only changes in O_2 pulse during CPET increased the discriminative capacity of 6MWD in a cohort of pulmonary hypertensive patients, whereas $\dot{V}O_2$ *peak* was not independently associated with prognosis. The 6-min walked distance reached on therapy was also shown to be predictive of long-term survival in observational studies [44, 45]. It is noteworthy, however, that except for the recent large-scale registries [49, 50], these results come from monocentric retrospective studies that included both newly diagnosed patients (incidence cases) and those who were diagnosed prior to enrolment (prevalence cases). Nevertheless, the assessment of exercise capacity is now considered a key part of the initial PAH patient evaluation.

Evaluative Properties of Exercise Tests in Pulmonary Arterial Hypertension

Besides its discriminative property for disease severity and patients' prognosis, CPET suffers from a lack of responsiveness following therapeutic intervention in PAH. Indeed, CPET successfully documented improvements in exercise capacity and ventilatory efficiency following PAH-specific therapies in case series [30]. However, it failed to demonstrate clinical benefit in the two randomized controlled trials that used CPET as the primary endpoint [32, 33], whereas the 6MWT was significantly improved. This is in keeping with previous studies documenting that peak exercise capacity is not typically very responsive to intervention (e.g. after pharmacotherapy in chronic obstructive pulmonary disease) [51], especially in the setting of a multicenter randomized controlled trial. Some authors proposed that this lack of responsiveness to therapy was related to increased variability of the CPET measures in less experienced centers [52, 53]. Other explanations may include: (1) the higher incidence of leg fatigue with cycling which can preclude 'cardiorespiratory improvements' to translate into increased exercise tolerance [54]; (2) the CPET duration which if often too short (<6–8 min) in PAH, leading to an earlier lactic acidosis accumulation and a $\dot{V}O_2$ *peak* underestimation due to nonlinearity between O_2 uptake and work load during early exercise.

Conversely, the 6MWT has been successfully used as a primary endpoint in most of the randomized controlled trials in PAH [55]. However, the sensitivity/responsiveness of the 6MWT to clinical changes (i.e. its evaluative properties) in PAH should also be questioned. Indeed, there is commonly some discrepancy between significant clinical improvement and minor changes in 6WMT following therapy. Similarly, only minor improvements in 6MWT (generally <10% from baseline) were observed in trials evaluating novel PAH therapies despite significant clinical efficacy leading to improved survival [55]. This is particularly problematic for patients with a preserved exercise capacity (e.g. 6MWT >450 m) for whom the prognostic relevance of the 6MWT has been questioned [56] and a 'ceiling effect' has been described [56, 57]. In these patients, further improvements become harder to detect because patients are not allowed to run during the 6MWT; as a result, the maximum average speed is no longer representative of changes in patients' maximal cardiac output and $\dot{V}O_2$ peak [38]. Similarly, recent combination therapy trials generally documented smaller changes in the 6-min walked distance in comparison to placebo-controlled trials [84–86]. This potential limited sensitivity to clinical changes may underestimate the true clinical benefit of novel therapies and adversely influence drug development in PAH. In the setting of chronic obstructive pulmonary disease, endurance walking and cycling tests are more responsive to clinical changes than the 6MWT or CPET after therapeutic intervention [51]. While exercise capacity is likely to remain an important end-point in PAH trials because of its independent association with mortality (good discriminative properties) and its easiness of application [58], the validation of a reliable exercise test that is more responsive to clinical changes remains of interest in PAH and is an area still open for research.

Exercise Capacity as a Marker of Health-Related Quality of Life

Exercise capacity and exercise-related symptoms are important factors influencing health-related quality of life. Not surprisingly, physical subscales of quality of life questionnaires have been shown to correlate moderately with the 6-min walked distance in PAH [59–61]. However, although timed walking tests measure the ability to undertake the activities of day-to-day life [87], exercise capacity does not capture the full impact of PAH upon the patient and is not a reliable predictor of health-related quality of life. Exercise capacity is thus complementary to quality of life assessment in both clinical practice and controlled trials.

Exercise Testing as a Screening Tool for Pulmonary Arterial Hypertension

Because dyspnea is an early and cardinal symptom of PAH, exercise testing has been proposed as a screening tool in at-risk populations. Indeed, PAH is rarely diagnosed in asymptomatic patients [62]. Moreover, subtle alterations in ventilatory efficiency, such as higher $\dot{V}E/\dot{V}CO_2$ slope and lower $P_{ET}CO_2$, may be sensitive to early-onset PAH [11, 63]. However, the specificity of these subtle markers is likely to be low in patients with connective tissue disease who frequently have concomitant subclinical interstitial lung disease. More importantly, significant overlap in any of these key parameters was observed when control subjects and PAH patients of the mildest severity were compared [63, 64], suggesting exercise testing may not be sufficiently sensitive enough to distinguish early PAH from normal. Whether exercise echocardiography might be useful in early screening of at-risk populations remains unknown, especially since a significant proportion of exercise-induced pulmonary hypertension will likely be caused by increased left heart end-diastolic pressures in older patients or patients with connective tissue diseases [7].

Interpretability of Exercise Testing in Pulmonary Arterial Hypertension

Exercise tolerance is considered a major marker of PAH severity. However, as for any biomarker of disease severity, relationships are indirect and, therefore, not necessarily tight. Other markers of disease severity should thus be taken into account in the interpretation of exercise testing. Nevertheless, exercise capacity determination guides physicians in decision-making, including the choice of the initial therapy and the timing for more aggressive therapeutic approach such as lung transplant [1].

Exercise Capacity at the Time of Pulmonary Arterial Hypertension Diagnosis

As stated above, baseline exercise capacity is a strong predictor of mortality in PAH. Previous studies described cutoff values (e.g. $\dot{V}O_2$ peak <10.4 ml/kg/min, 6MWT distance <332 m) below which long-term survival was poor [31, 35, 44, 45]. Importantly, these cutoff values categorizing patients into good and bad prognoses were mainly derived from median values of patient cohorts and have little clinical relevance for individuals. Although the 6MWT may be less discriminative among patients walking >450 m [56], exercise capacity should be interpreted as a continuous variable: a better functional status being representative of a better prognosis. It is also worth mentioning that age, height, weight, and sex independently affect the 6MWT in healthy adults [2]. Therefore, these factors should be taken into consideration when interpreting the 6MWT. While equations were developed to predict individuals' 6-min walked distance [65–68], adjusting the 6MWT according to the predicted value did not significantly improve the predicted value of the 6MWT [46], potentially because factors influencing the 6MWT may also influence a patient's prognosis (e.g. age) [49, 50]. Moreover, optimal reference equations from healthy population-based samples are not yet available as current regression equations explain only about 40% of the variance of the 6MWT and were established from studies with small sample sizes [65, 66] or subjects older than 40–50 years [65, 67, 68]. Consequently, the applicability of these equations to younger PAH patients is limited.

Exercise Capacity Observed on Pulmonary Arterial Hypertension Therapy

Exercise tests will generally be repeated after treatment initiation. The primary question is then whether the patient has experienced a clinically significant improvement or worsening. It is noteworthy that the interpretation of changes relies on the reproducibility of the measure, which is excellent for the 6MWT only when patients are tested according to current guidelines [2]. Many observational studies [44, 45] documented that most of the clinical improvements are observed during the first 3–6 months after treatment initiation. These studies, as well as recent large-scale registries [49, 50], also confirmed that exercise capacity reached on therapy is powerfully and independently related to long-term survival in PAH. As a result, many PAH experts now advocate a goal-oriented treatment strategy, adding PAH-specific therapies to reach a certain level of exercise capacity (6MWT generally >400–450 m) on treatment [69]. Although appealing, this strategy needs to be validated in a prospective controlled trial to define which goals will provide the best outcomes for patients, and more importantly, to document the survival benefit associated with such more aggressive treatment strategy.

There has been controversy regarding the relevance of the relative increase in exercise capacity on therapy. Confusion was raised from an observational study that included a very heterogeneous study population with the 6MWT at baseline ranging from 0 to 550 m [45]. The relative increase in the 6MWT was thus more likely to be significant for the very sick patients compared to patients with milder PAH, although the former group remained at a high risk of death. This study reinforced the concept that the absolute 6-min walked distance reached on therapy was of primary importance, and that patients with severe PAH need to have a much greater improvement to have a prognosis similar to those with better exercise capacity at baseline. Nevertheless, relative increases in the 6MWT may be clinically significant in a more homogeneous population or for a given individual [44].

Attempts to define the minimal important difference (MID) in the 6-min walked distance were recently made using distribution-based methods [70]. A MID of 41 m was proposed as a meaningful difference following 12 weeks of therapy. While distribution-based methods estimate the minimal change in an outcome measure based on its variability at baseline and overtime, it does not take into account patients' perception of symptomatic improvement [71]. Indeed, defining MID is complicated because individuals may assess the same benefit differently, or the same individual may change the value placed on a particular benefit based on circumstances. Consequently, the MID representative of clinical improvement may differ from the MID representative of clinical worsening, as it may differ depending on PAH type and severity as well as intervention type (e.g. monotherapy vs. combination therapy) and duration. Thus, the MID in the 6-min walked distance translating to significant changes in survival or patients' perception of well-being remains largely unknown in PAH.

Exercise Testing in Nonidiopathic Pulmonary Arterial Hypertension

The clinical relevance of exercise capacity may differ for patients with other types of pulmonary hypertension who may have considerable comorbidities. In fact, the prognostic value of CPET and the 6MWT has been convincingly validated in idiopathic PAH only. Alterations in exercise capacity may be sensitive to the presence of cardiovascular and pulmonary complications of connective tissue disease [72]. However, these patients are also limited by musculoskeletal dysfunction and pain [73]. Therefore, the validity, reliability, and discriminatory capacity of the 6MWT may be biased by the patients' comorbidities, and the generalizability of the above results is thus currently limited. Nevertheless, two retrospective studies documented that the 6-min walked distance was associated with survival in patients with PAH associated with scleroderma [74, 75]. It remains unknown whether this also applies to other connective tissue diseases. $\dot{V}O_2$ peak [76] and ventilatory efficiency [77] were also documented to be independently related to survival in PAH related to congenital heart defects. Conversely, exercise capacity seems to poorly correlate with survival in PAH associated with HIV infection [78, 79] or portal hypertension [80]. Finally, the 6MWT also appears to be an independent predictor of perioperative mortality as well as long-term survival in nonoperable chronic thromboembolic pulmonary hypertension [81].

The improvement in exercise capacity with PAH therapy may also differ in PAH associated with connective tissue disease. A recent meta-analysis demonstrated that increases in the 6-min walked distance were more limited in patients with PAH associated with scleroderma compared to idiopathic PAH [82]. This is discrepant with observational studies suggesting improved survival with current PAH therapies in these patients [74]. The relationship between hemodynamic impairment and exercise capacity is also not straightforward in chronic thromboembolic pulmonary hypertension in which improvements in pulmonary hemodynamics with therapy were not associated with significant increases in exercise capacity [83]. These results may be explained by a poor therapeutic response in these subsets of patients, or more likely by a weaker relevance of the 6MWT to assess efficacy in other subsets of patients because of older age, increased prevalence of comorbidities, the persistence of severe ventilation-perfusion mismatch due to residual artery obstructions, or the fact that pulmonary vascular resistance does not assess the full impact of pulmonary vessel abnormalities on the right ventricle, especially in the context of chronic thromboembolic pulmonary hypertension. The above limitations thus need to be resolved through further study to assess whether the 6MWT can be reliably used as a surrogate marker of treatment efficacy in nonidiopathic PAH.

Conclusions

Mechanisms of exercise intolerance in PAH are clearly multifactorial and involve cardiac, respiratory, and peripheral muscle abnormalities. Exercise capacity is thus a marker of the integrated response of all systems involved in O_2 transport and utilization. Over the years, exercise testing has been validated for the assessment of disease severity and prognostication, as well as for monitoring response to therapy in idiopathic PAH. Because of its simplicity, reproducibility, noninvasiveness and validity in reflecting PAH severity and disease repercussions on daily living, the 6MWT has been widely incorporated in the routine assessment of PAH patients. Its responsiveness to pharmacological interventions also permitted the demonstration of efficacy of novel PAH-specific therapies. Its sensitivity has, however, been challenged in recent combination trials or when used to assess patients with milder disease. The reliability of exercise testing in nonidiopathic PAH also remains to be validated.

References

1 Galie N, Hoeper MM, Humbert M, Torbicki A, Vachiery JL, Barbera JA, Beghetti M, Corris P, Gaine S, Gibbs JS, Gomez-Sanchez MA, Jondeau G, Klepetko W, Opitz C, Peacock A, Rubin L, Zellweger M, Simonneau G, Vahanian A, Auricchio A, Bax J, Ceconi C, Dean V, Filippatos G, Funck-Brentano C, Hobbs R, Kearney P, McDonagh T, McGregor K, Popescu BA, Reiner Z, Sechtem U, Sirnes PA, Tendera M, Vardas P, Widimsky P, Al Attar N, Andreotti F, Aschermann M, Asteggiano R, Benza R, Berger R, Bonnet D, Delcroix M, Howard L, Kitsiou AN, Lang I, Maggioni A, Nielsen-Kudsk JE, Park M, Perrone-Filardi P, Price S, Domenech MT, Vonk-Noordegraaf A, Zamorano JL: Guidelines for the diagnosis and treatment of pulmonary hypertension: the Task Force for the Diagnosis and Treatment of Pulmonary Hypertension of the European Society of Cardiology (ESC) and the European Respiratory Society (ERS), endorsed by the International Society of Heart and Lung Transplantation (ISHLT). Eur Heart J 2009;30:2493–2537.

2 ATS Committee on Proficiency Standards for Clinical Pulmonary Function Laboratories: ATS statement: guidelines for the six-minute walk test. Am J Respir Crit Care Med 2002;166:111–117.

3 American Thoracic Society, American College of Chest Physicians: ATS/ACCP Statement on cardiopulmonary exercise testing. Am J Respir Crit Care Med 2003;167:211–277.

4 Singh SJ, Morgan MD, Scott S, Walters D, Hardman AE: Development of a shuttle walking test of disability in patients with chronic airways obstruction. Thorax 1992;47:1019–1024.

5 Revill SM, Morgan MD, Singh SJ, Williams J, Hardman AE: The endurance shuttle walk: a new field test for the assessment of endurance capacity in chronic obstructive pulmonary disease. Thorax 1999;54:213–222.

6 Mitchell JH, Blomqvist G: Maximal oxygen uptake. N Engl J Med 1971;284:1018–1022.

7 Kovacs G, Berghold A, Scheidl S, Olschewski H: Pulmonary arterial pressure during rest and exercise in healthy subjects: a systematic review. Eur Respir J 2009;34:888–894.

8 Provencher S, Herve P, Sitbon O, Humbert M, Simonneau G, Chemla D: Changes in exercise haemodynamics during treatment in pulmonary arterial hypertension. Eur Respir J 2008;32:393–398.

9 Groepenhoff H, Holverda S, Marcus JT, Postmus PE, Boonstra A, Vonk-Noordegraaf A: Stroke volume response during exercise measured by acetylene uptake and MRI. Physiol Meas 2007;28:1–11.

10 Provencher S, Chemla D, Herve P, Sitbon O, Humbert M, Simonneau G: Heart rate responses during the 6-minute walk test in pulmonary arterial hypertension. Eur Respir J 2006;27:114–120.

11 Sun XG, Hansen JE, Oudiz RJ, Wasserman K: Exercise pathophysiology in patients with primary pulmonary hypertension. Circulation 2001;104:429–435.

12 Dantzker DR, D'Alonzo GE, Bower JS, Popat K, Crevey BJ: Pulmonary gas exchange during exercise in patients with chronic obliterative pulmonary hypertension. Am Rev Respir Dis 1984;130:412–416.

13 Tolle J, Waxman A, Systrom D: Impaired systemic oxygen extraction at maximum exercise in pulmonary hypertension. Med Sci Sports Exerc 2008;40:3–8.

14 Hoeper MM, Pletz MW, Golpon H, Welte T: Prognostic value of blood gas analyses in patients with idiopathic pulmonary arterial hypertension. Eur Respir J 2007;29:944–950.

15 Velez-Roa S, Ciarka A, Najem B, Vachiery JL, Naeije R, van de Borne P: Increased sympathetic nerve activity in pulmonary artery hypertension. Circulation 2004;110:1308–1312.

16 Ponikowski P, Chua TP, Anker SD, Francis DP, Doehner W, Banasiak W, Poole-Wilson PA, Piepoli MF, Coats AJ: Peripheral chemoreceptor hypersensitivity: an ominous sign in patients with chronic heart failure. Circulation 2001;104:544–549.

17 Clark AL, Poole-Wilson PA, Coats AJ: Exercise limitation in chronic heart failure: central role of the periphery. J Am Coll Cardiol 1996;28:1092–1102.

18 Leimbach WN Jr, Wallin BG, Victor RG, Aylward PE, Sundlof G, Mark AL: Direct evidence from intraneural recordings for increased central sympathetic outflow in patients with heart failure. Circulation 1986;73:913–919.

19 Meyer FJ, Lossnitzer D, Kristen AV, Schoene AM, Kubler W, Katus HA, Borst MM: Respiratory muscle dysfunction in idiopathic pulmonary arterial hypertension. Eur Respir J 2005;25:125–130.
20 Kabitz HJ, Schwoerer A, Bremer HC, Sonntag F, Walterspacher S, Walker D, Schaefer V, Ehlken N, Staehler G, Halank M, Klose H, Ghofrani HA, Hoeper MM, Gruenig E, Windisch W: Impairment of respiratory muscle function in pulmonary hypertension. Clin Sci (Lond) 2008;114: 165–171.
21 Mainguy V, Maltais F, Saey D, Gagnon P, Martel S, Simon M, Provencher S: Peripheral muscle dysfunction in idiopathic pulmonary arterial hypertension. Thorax 2010;65:113–117.
22 Bauer R, Dehnert C, Schoene P, Filusch A, Bartsch P, Borst MM, Katus HA, Meyer FJ: Skeletal muscle dysfunction in patients with idiopathic pulmonary arterial hypertension. Respir Med 2007;101:2366–2369.
23 Mainguy V, Maltais F, Saey D, Gagnon P, Martel S, Simon M, Provencher S: Effects of a rehabilitation program on skeletal muscle function in idiopathic pulmonary arterial hypertension. J Cardiopulm Rehabil Prev 2010;30:319–323.
24 de Man FS, Handoko ML, Groepenhoff H, van 't Hul AJ, Abbink J, Koppers RJ, Grotjohan HP, Twisk JW, Bogaard HJ, Boonstra A, Postmus PE, Westerhof N, van der Laarse WJ, Vonk-Noordegraaf A: Effects of exercise training in patients with idiopathic pulmonary arterial hypertension. Eur Respir J 2009;34:669–675.
25 Mereles D, Ehlken N, Kreuscher S, Ghofrani S, Hoeper MM, Halank M, Meyer FJ, Karger G, Buss J, Juenger J, Holzapfel N, Opitz C, Winkler J, Herth FF, Wilkens H, Katus HA, Olschewski H, Grunig E: Exercise and respiratory training improve exercise capacity and quality of life in patients with severe chronic pulmonary hypertension. Circulation 2006;114:1482–1489.
26 Chua TP, Anker SD, Harrington D, Coats AJ: Inspiratory muscle strength is a determinant of maximum oxygen consumption in chronic heart failure. Br Heart J 1995;74:381–385.
27 Deboeck G, Niset G, Lamotte M, Vachiery JL, Naeije R: Exercise testing in pulmonary arterial hypertension and in chronic heart failure. Eur Respir J 2004;23:747–751.
28 Rhodes J, Barst RJ, Garofano RP, Thoele DG, Gersony WM: Hemodynamic correlates of exercise function in patients with primary pulmonary hypertension. J Am Coll Cardiol 1991; 18:1738–1744.
29 Sun XG, Hansen JE, Oudiz RJ, Wasserman K: Gas exchange detection of exercise-induced right-to-left shunt in patients with primary pulmonary hypertension. Circulation 2002;105:54–60.
30 Wensel R, Opitz CF, Ewert R, Bruch L, Kleber FX: Effects of iloprost inhalation on exercise capacity and ventilatory efficiency in patients with primary pulmonary hypertension. Circulation 2000;101:2388–2392.
31 Miyamoto S, Nagaya N, Satoh T, Kyotani S, Sakamaki F, Fujita M, Nakanishi N, Miyatake K: Clinical correlates and prognostic significance of six-minute walk test in patients with primary pulmonary hypertension. Comparison with cardiopulmonary exercise testing. Am J Respir Crit Care Med 2000;161:487–492.
32 Barst RJ, Langleben D, Frost A, Horn EM, Oudiz R, Shapiro S, McLaughlin V, Hill N, Tapson VF, Robbins IM, Zwicke D, Duncan B, Dixon RA, Frumkin LR: Sitaxsentan therapy for pulmonary arterial hypertension. Am J Respir Crit Care Med 2004;169:441–447.
33 Barst RJ, McGoon M, McLaughlin V, Tapson V, Rich S, Rubin L, Wasserman K, Oudiz R, Shapiro S, Robbins IM, Channick R, Badesch D, Rayburn BK, Flinchbaugh R, Sigman J, Arneson C, Jeffs R: Beraprost therapy for pulmonary arterial hypertension. J Am Coll Cardiol 2003;41:2119–2125.
34 Groepenhoff H, Vonk-Noordegraaf A, Boonstra A, Spreeuwenberg MD, Postmus PE, Bogaard HJ: Exercise testing to estimate survival in pulmonary hypertension. Med Sci Sports Exerc 2008;40:1725–1732.
35 Wensel R, Opitz CF, Anker SD, Winkler J, Hoffken G, Kleber FX, Sharma R, Hummel M, Hetzer R, Ewert R: Assessment of survival in patients with primary pulmonary hypertension: importance of cardiopulmonary exercise testing. Circulation 2002;106:319–324.
36 Deboeck G, Niset G, Vachiery JL, Moraine JJ, Naeije R: Physiological response to the six-minute walk test in pulmonary arterial hypertension. Eur Respir J 2005;26:667–672.
37 Troosters T, Vilaro J, Rabinovich R, Casas A, Barbera JA, Rodriguez-Roisin R, Roca J: Physiological responses to the 6-min walk test in patients with chronic obstructive pulmonary disease. Eur Respir J 2002;20:564–569.
38 Cooper KH: A means of assessing maximal oxygen intake. Correlation between field and treadmill testing. JAMA 1968;203:201–204.
39 Casas A, Vilaro J, Rabinovich R, Mayer A, Barbera JA, Rodriguez-Roisin R, Roca J: Encouraged 6-min walking test indicates maximum sustainable exercise in COPD patients. Chest 2005; 128:55–61.
40 Valli G, Vizza CD, Onorati P, Badagliacca R, Ciuffa R, Poscia R, Brandimarte F, Fedele F, Serra P, Palange P: Pathophysiological adaptations to walking and cycling in primary pulmonary hypertension. Eur J Appl Physiol 2008;102:417–424.
41 Shah SJ, Thenappan T, Rich S, Sur J, Archer SL, Gomberg-Maitland M: Value of exercise treadmill testing in the risk stratification of patients with pulmonary hypertension. Circ Heart Fail 2009;2:278–286.
42 Camargo VM, Martins Bdo C, Jardim C, Fernandes CJ, Hovnanian A, Souza R: Validation of a treadmill six-minute walk test protocol for the evaluation of patients with pulmonary arterial hypertension. J Bras Pneumol 2009;35:423–430.
43 D'Alonzo GE, Barst RJ, Ayres SM, Bergofsky EH, Brundage BH, Detre KM, Fishman AP, Goldring RM, Groves BM, Kernis JT, et al: Survival in patients with primary pulmonary hypertension. Results from a national prospective registry. Ann Intern Med 1991;115:343–349.
44 Provencher S, Sitbon O, Humbert M, Cabrol S, Jais X, Simonneau G: Long-term outcome with first-line bosentan therapy in idiopathic pulmonary arterial hypertension. Eur Heart J 2006;27:589–595.
45 Sitbon O, Humbert M, Nunes H, Parent F, Garcia G, Herve P, Rainisio M, Simonneau G: Long-term intravenous epoprostenol infusion in primary pulmonary hypertension: prognostic factors and survival. J Am Coll Cardiol 2002;40:780–788.
46 Lee WT, Peacock AJ, Johnson MK: The role of percent predicted six-minute walk distance in pulmonary arterial hypertension. Eur Respir J 2010;36:1294–1301.
47 Raymond RJ, Hinderliter AL, Willis PW, Ralph D, Caldwell EJ, Williams W, Ettinger NA, Hill NS, Summer WR, de Boisblanc B, Schwartz T, Koch G, Clayton LM, Jobsis MM, Crow JW, Long W: Echocardiographic predictors of adverse outcomes in primary pulmonary hypertension. J Am Coll Cardiol 2002;39:1214–1219.
48 Paciocco G, Martinez FJ, Bossone E, Pielsticker E, Gillespie B, Rubenfire M: Oxygen desaturation on the six-minute walk test and mortality in untreated primary pulmonary hypertension. Eur Respir J 2001;17:647–652.
49 Humbert M, Sitbon O, Chaouat A, Bertocchi M, Habib G, Gressin V, Yaici A, Weitzenblum E, Cordier JF, Chabot F, Dromer C, Pison C, Reynaud-Gaubert M, Haloun A, Laurent M, Hachulla E, Cottin V, Degano B, Jais X, Montani D, Souza R, Simonneau G: Survival in patients with idiopathic, familial, and anorexigen-associated pulmonary arterial hypertension in the modern management era. Circulation 2010;122:156–163.
50 Benza RL, Miller DP, Gomberg-Maitland M, Frantz RP, Foreman AJ, Coffey CS, Frost A, Barst RJ, Badesch DB, Elliott CG, Liou TG, McGoon MD: Predicting survival in pulmonary arterial hypertension: insights from the Registry to Evaluate Early and Long-Term Pulmonary Arterial Hypertension Disease Management (REVEAL). Circulation 2010;122:164–172.
51 Oga T, Nishimura K, Tsukino M, Hajiro T, Ikeda A, Izumi T: The effects of oxitropium bromide on exercise performance in patients with stable chronic obstructive pulmonary disease. A comparison of three different exercise tests. Am J Respir Crit Care Med 2000;161:1897–1901.
52 Hansen JE, Sun XG, Yasunobu Y, Garafano RP, Gates G, Barst RJ, Wasserman K: Reproducibility of cardiopulmonary exercise measurements in patients with pulmonary arterial hypertension. Chest 2004;126:816–824.
53 Oudiz RJ, Barst RJ, Hansen JE, Sun XG, Garofano R, Wu X, Wasserman K: Cardiopulmonary exercise testing and six-minute walk correlations in pulmonary arterial hypertension. Am J Cardiol 2006;97:123–126.
54 Man WD, Soliman MG, Gearing J, Radford SG, Rafferty GF, Gray BJ, Polkey MI, Moxham J: Symptoms and quadriceps fatigability after walking and cycling in chronic obstructive pulmonary disease. Am J Respir Crit Care Med 2003;168:562–567.
55 Galie N, Manes A, Negro L, Palazzini M, Bacchi-Reggiani ML, Branzi A: A meta-analysis of randomized controlled trials in pulmonary arterial hypertension. Eur Heart J 2009;30:394–403.

56 Degano B, Sitbon O, Savale L, Garcia G, O'Callaghan DS, Jais X, Humbert M, Simonneau G: Characterization of pulmonary arterial hypertension patients walking more than 450 m in 6 min at diagnosis. Chest 2010;137:1297–1303.

57 Frost AE, Langleben D, Oudiz R, Hill N, Horn E, McLaughlin V, Robbins IM, Shapiro S, Tapson VF, Zwicke D, DeMarco T, Schilz R, Rubenfire M, Barst RJ: The 6-min walk test (6MW) as an efficacy endpoint in pulmonary arterial hypertension clinical trials: demonstration of a ceiling effect. Vascul Pharmacol 2005;43:36–39.

58 McLaughlin VV, Badesch DB, Delcroix M, Fleming TR, Gaine SP, Galie N, Gibbs JS, Kim NH, Oudiz RJ, Peacock A, Provencher S, Sitbon O, Tapson VF, Seeger W: End points and clinical trial design in pulmonary arterial hypertension. J Am Coll Cardiol 2009;54:S97–S107.

59 Cenedese E, Speich R, Dorschner L, Ulrich S, Maggiorini M, Jenni R, Fischler M: Measurement of quality of life in pulmonary hypertension and its significance. Eur Respir J 2006;28:808–815.

60 Chua R, Keogh AM, Byth K, O'Loughlin A: Comparison and validation of three measures of quality of life in patients with pulmonary hypertension. Intern Med J 2006;36:705–710.

61 Taichman DB, Shin J, Hud L, Archer-Chicko C, Kaplan S, Sager JS, Gallop R, Christie J, Hansen-Flaschen J, Palevsky H: Health-related quality of life in patients with pulmonary arterial hypertension. Respir Res 2005;6:92.

62 Hachulla E, de Groote P, Gressin V, Sibilia J, Diot E, Carpentier P, Mouthon L, Hatron PY, Jego P, Allanore Y, Tiev KP, Agard C, Cosnes A, Cirstea D, Constans J, Farge D, Viallard JF, Harle JR, Patat F, Imbert B, Kahan A, Cabane J, Clerson P, Guillevin L, Humbert M: The three-year incidence of pulmonary arterial hypertension associated with systemic sclerosis in a multicenter nationwide longitudinal study in France. Arthritis Rheum 2009;60:1831–1839.

63 Yasunobu Y, Oudiz RJ, Sun XG, Hansen JE, Wasserman K: End-tidal PCO_2 abnormality and exercise limitation in patients with primary pulmonary hypertension. Chest 2005;127:1637–1646.

64 Tolle JJ, Waxman AB, Van Horn TL, Pappagianopoulos PP, Systrom DM: Exercise-induced pulmonary arterial hypertension. Circulation 2008;118:2183–2189.

65 Troosters T, Gosselink R, Decramer M: Six minute walking distance in healthy elderly subjects. Eur Respir J 1999;14:270–274.

66 Gibbons WJ, Fruchter N, Sloan S, Levy RD: Reference values for a multiple repetition 6-minute walk test in healthy adults older than 20 years. J Cardiopulm Rehabil 2001;21:87–93.

67 Enright PL, Sherrill DL: Reference equations for the six-minute walk in healthy adults. Am J Respir Crit Care Med 1998;158:1384–1387.

68 Enright PL, McBurnie MA, Bittner V, Tracy RP, McNamara R, Arnold A, Newman AB: The 6-min walk test: a quick measure of functional status in elderly adults. Chest 2003;123:387–398.

69 Hoeper MM, Markevych I, Spiekerkoetter E, Welte T, Niedermeyer J: Goal-oriented treatment and combination therapy for pulmonary arterial hypertension. Eur Respir J 2005;26:858–863.

70 Gilbert C, Brown MC, Cappelleri JC, Carlsson M, McKenna SP: Estimating a minimally important difference in pulmonary arterial hypertension following treatment with sildenafil. Chest 2009;135:137–142.

71 Guyatt GH, Osoba D, Wu AW, Wyrwich KW, Norman GR: Methods to explain the clinical significance of health status measures. Mayo Clin Proc 2002;77:371–383.

72 Kovacs G, Maier R, Aberer E, Brodmann M, Scheidl S, Troster N, Hesse C, Salmhofer W, Graninger W, Gruenig E, Rubin LJ, Olschewski H: Borderline pulmonary arterial pressure is associated with decreased exercise capacity in scleroderma. Am J Respir Crit Care Med 2009;180:881–886.

73 Garin MC, Highland KB, Silver RM, Strange C: Limitations to the 6-minute walk test in interstitial lung disease and pulmonary hypertension in scleroderma. J Rheumatol 2009;36:330–336.

74 Williams MH, Das C, Handler CE, Akram MR, Davar J, Denton CP, Smith CJ, Black CM, Coghlan JG: Systemic sclerosis associated pulmonary hypertension: improved survival in the current era. Heart 2006;92:926–932.

75 Condliffe R, Kiely DG, Peacock AJ, Corris PA, Gibbs JS, Vrapi F, Das C, Elliot CA, Johnson M, DeSoyza J, Torpy C, Goldsmith K, Hodgkins D, Hughes RJ, Pepke-Zaba J, Coghlan JG: Connective tissue disease-associated pulmonary arterial hypertension in the modern treatment era. Am J Respir Crit Care Med 2009;179:151–157.

76 Diller GP, Dimopoulos K, Okonko D, Li W, Babu-Narayan SV, Broberg CS, Johansson B, Bouzas B, Mullen MJ, Poole-Wilson PA, Francis DP, Gatzoulis MA: Exercise intolerance in adult congenital heart disease: comparative severity, correlates, and prognostic implication. Circulation 2005;112:828–835.

77 Dimopoulos K, Okonko DO, Diller GP, Broberg CS, Salukhe TV, Babu-Narayan SV, Li W, Uebing A, Bayne S, Wensel R, Piepoli MF, Poole-Wilson PA, Francis DP, Gatzoulis MA: Abnormal ventilatory response to exercise in adults with congenital heart disease relates to cyanosis and predicts survival. Circulation 2006;113:2796–2802.

78 Nunes H, Humbert M, Sitbon O, Morse JH, Deng Z, Knowles JA, Le Gall C, Parent F, Garcia G, Herve P, Barst RJ, Simonneau G: Prognostic factors for survival in human immunodeficiency virus-associated pulmonary arterial hypertension. Am J Respir Crit Care Med 2003;167:1433–1439.

79 Degano B, Yaici A, Le Pavec J, Savale L, Jais X, Camara B, Humbert M, Simonneau G, Sitbon O: Long-term effects of bosentan in patients with HIV-associated pulmonary arterial hypertension. Eur Respir J 2009;33:92–98.

80 Le Pavec J, Souza R, Herve P, Lebrec D, Savale L, Tcherakian C, Jais X, Yaici A, Humbert M, Simonneau G, Sitbon O: Portopulmonary hypertension: survival and prognostic factors. Am J Respir Crit Care Med 2008;178:637–643.

81 Condliffe R, Kiely DG, Gibbs JS, Corris PA, Peacock AJ, Jenkins DP, Goldsmith K, Coghlan JG, Pepke-Zaba J: Prognostic and aetiological factors in chronic thromboembolic pulmonary hypertension. Eur Respir J 2009;33:332–338.

82 Avouac J, Wipff J, Kahan A, Allanore Y: Effects of oral treatments on exercise capacity in systemic sclerosis related pulmonary arterial hypertension: a meta-analysis of randomised controlled trials. Ann Rheum Dis 2008;67:808–814.

83 Jais X, D'Armini AM, Jansa P, Torbicki A, Delcroix M, Ghofrani HA, Hoeper MM, Lang IM, Mayer E, Pepke-Zaba J, Perchenet L, Morganti A, Simonneau G, Rubin LJ: Bosentan for treatment of inoperable chronic thromboembolic pulmonary hypertension: BENEFIT (Bosentan Effects in Inoperable Forms of Chronic Thromboembolic Pulmonary Hypertension), a randomized, placebo-controlled trial. J Am Coll Cardiol 2008;52:2127–2134.

84 McLaughlin VV, Benza RL, Rubin LJ, Channick RN, Voswinckel R, Tapson VF, Robbins IM, Olschewski H, Rubenfire M, Seeger W: Addition of inhaled treprostinil to oral therapy for pulmonary arterial hypertension: a randomized controlled clinical trial. J Am Coll Cardiol 2010;55:1915–1922.

85 McLaughlin VV, Oudiz RJ, Frost A, Tapson VF, Murali S, Channick RN, Badesch DB, Barst RJ, Hsu HH, Rubin LJ: Randomized study of adding inhaled iloprost to existing bosentan in pulmonary arterial hypertension. Am J Respir Crit Care Med 2006;174:1257–1263.

86 Simonneau G, Rubin LJ, Galiè N, Barst RJ, Fleming TR, Frost AE, Engel PJ, Kramer MR, Burgess G, Collings L, Cossons N, Sitbon O, Badesch DB; PACES Study Group: Addition of sildenafil to long-term intravenous epoprostenol therapy in patients with pulmonary arterial hypertension: a randomized trial. Ann Intern Med 2008;149:521–530.

87 Mainguy V, Provencher S, Maltais F, Malenfant S, Saey D: Assessment of daily life physical activities in pulmonary arterial hypertension. PLoS One 2011;6:e27993.

Steeve Provencher
Centre de Recherche de l'Institut Universitaire de Cardiologie et de Pneumologie de Québec, Service de Pneumologie
2725, chemin Sainte-Foy
Québec (Québec) G1V 4G5 (Canada)
Tel. +1 418 656 4747, E-Mail steve.provencher@criucpq.ulaval.ca

Chapter 5

Humbert M, Souza R, Simonneau G (eds): Pulmonary Vascular Disorders.
Prog Respir Res. Basel, Karger, 2012, vol 41, pp 48–58

Noninvasive Exploration of the Pulmonary Circulation and the Right Heart

Anton Vonk Noordegraaf[a] · Andrew Peacock[b] · Robert Naeije[c]

[a]Department of Pulmonology, VU University Medical Center, Amsterdam, The Netherlands; [b]Scottish Pulmonary Vascular Unit, Regional Heart and Lung Centre, Glasgow, UK; [c]Department of Cardiology, Erasme University, Brussels, Belgium

Abstract

Noninvasive explorations of the pulmonary circulation and the right heart in clinical practice essentially rely on echocardiography, MRI, and CT scanning of the chest. Echocardiography has an established role for the detection, differential diagnosis, and follow-up of pulmonary hypertension. MRI provides excellent 3-dimensional imaging, allowing for measurements of right ventricle volume and mass with great accuracy. In addition, it provides a tool to measure pulmonary artery flow. CT scanning is currently mainly used for the detection of underlying lung disease and the diagnosis of pulmonary thromboembolism. Novel advances in echocardiography and MRI offers the potential to provide measures of right ventricular and pulmonary vascular function in a realistic way.

Noninvasive imaging of the pulmonary circulation and the right heart is indispensable for the early diagnosis, differential diagnosis, and follow-up of pulmonary hypertension [1]. The most commonly used imaging technique is echocardiography, which is widely available, applicable at the bedside, and (relatively) inexpensive. Echocardiography allows for estimations of pulmonary vascular pressures, and right ventricular structure and function, both at rest and at exercise. A limitation of the technique is its operator dependency and, until recently, its inability to provide reliable right ventricular volumetric measurements. Emerging techniques for a more accurate assessment of right ventricular structure and function, and pulmonary arterial morphological changes are MRI and CT scanning.

This chapter provides an overview of imaging techniques in the field of pulmonary arterial hypertension (PAH). Imaging associated with chronic thromboembolic pulmonary hypertension and congenital heart disease will be described in the chapters by Le Gal et al. [pp. 218–225] and Tissot and Beghetti [pp. 122–136], respectively.

Pulmonary Hemodynamics

Pulmonary hypertension is defined by a mean pulmonary artery pressure (PAP) higher than 25 mm Hg [1]. The upper limit of normal of PAP is 20 mm Hg [2]. Accordingly, there is a notion of 'borderline' pulmonary hypertension defined by a PAP higher than 20 mm Hg but lower than 25 mm Hg [1]. However, PAP is a flow-dependent variable. When cardiac output (Q) is increased at exercise in normal subjects, PAP-Q relationships present with an average slope of 1 mm $Hg/l{\bullet}min^{-1}$ in young adults, which increases to 2.5 mm $Hg/l{\bullet}min^{-1}$ in subjects older than 60 years [3]. Furthermore, PAP is influenced by left atrial pressure (LAP). In normal subjects, PAP increases by 1 mm Hg for every 1 mm Hg increase in LAP [3]. The relationships between PAP, LAP, and cardiac output in cardiac or pulmonary diseases are unpredictable; therefore, the obligatory relationship assumed by the pulmonary vascular resistance (PVR) equation, PVR = (PAP – LAP)/Q, cannot be used to evaluate the functional state of the pulmonary circulation at variable flow and/or filling pressures of the left heart [4]. Accordingly, isolated estimates of PAP to define pulmonary hypertension are not sufficient. Both invasive and noninvasive explorations of the pulmonary circulation require estimates of PAP, LAP, and Q, which, in case of uncertain diagnoses, require measurements at several levels of cardiac output during exercise stress tests [5].

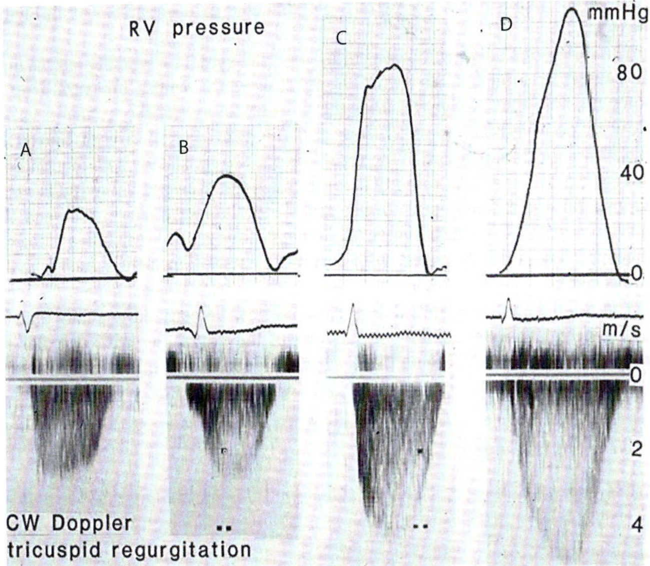

Fig. 1. Tricuspid regurgitation at progressively increased right ventricular (RV) pressures from normal (A) to severe pulmonary hypertension (D). The shape of the tricuspid regurgitation envelope mirrors invasively measured RV pressure. Both signals show late systolic peaking at the highest pressures in D. Pressures can be recalculated at each point of the tricuspid regurgitant wave using the simplified form of the Bernoulli equation.

Echocardiography

PAP can be estimated from the continuous Doppler maximum velocity of tricuspid regurgitation (TRV), in m/s, to calculate a transtricuspid pressure gradient, in mm Hg, using the simplified form of the Bernoulli equation and an estimate of right atrial pressure (RAP) [6]: systolic PAP = 4 × TRV^2 + RAP. The assumptions of this measurement are that systolic pulmonary artery and right ventricular pressures are equal, and that the Bernoulli equation is applicable [7]. RAP is estimated clinically, or, preferably, from the diameter of the inferior vena cava and its inspiratory collapsibility [8] (fig. 1).

Theoretically, mean PAP can be calculated from the estimated systolic PAP derived by echocardiography given the proportionality of pressures in the pulmonary circulation [9]. The main problem with estimates of PAP from TRV is that a good quality signal can be recovered in only 60–90% of patients, especially in the presence of hyperinflated chests, like in obstructive lung diseases, and/or normal or only modestly elevated PAP [7, 10]. Furthermore, the measurement has a poor reputation because of a reported high frequency of false positives and negatives with respect to reference invasive measurements reported in quality-control studies [11, 12]. However, this can probably be improved by the implication of dedicated observers and the implementation of a Bayesian approach with clinical probability algorithms.

The single use of TRV to measure PAP in hypoxia or on exercise has shown increased pulmonary vasoreactivity in family members of PAH patients, independent of identified mutations [13]. This approach combined with estimates of pulmonary flow at exercise has allowed definition of realistic pulmonary vascular mechanics with resistance and compliance determinations that were in good agreement with previous invasive studies [14].

Since PAP is a flow-dependent variable, it is important to couple it with a measurement of cardiac output. Using reference physiological definitions of function helps in the interpretation of images. Cardiac output can be measured from the left ventricular outflow tract (LVOT) diameter and velocity integral (VTI) multiplied by heart rate (HR) [15]: Q = [0.785 × $(LVOT)^2$ × LVOT – VTI] × HR. Perhaps a more useful independent method to estimate mean PAP is based on the pulsed Doppler measurement of the acceleration time (AT) of pulmonary flow (sampled at the right ventricular outflow tract) [18]: mean PAP = 79 – (0.6 × AT) (fig. 2).

Given the importance of a reliable estimate of PAP for the diagnosis of pulmonary hypertension and given the uncertainties encountered with the sampling of good-quality tricuspid regurgitation or pulmonary insufficiency, it is surprising that internal controls based on AT are so uncommonly reported. Moreover, there has been less validation of this method against invasive measurements than reported on the basis of TRV. Accurate estimates of mean PAP are less reliable when AT exceeds 100 ms, the lower limit of normal, and the measurement may need a correction for ejection time at high heart rates [7]. However, there are data suggesting that AT may be more sensitive than tricuspid regurgitation to early or latent pulmonary vasculopathy [19], which may be due to its sensitivity to changes in pulmonary vascular impedance more than PVR [7, 10]. The advantage of the measurement of PAP on the basis of the AT of pulmonary flow is that good quality signals can be obtained [6], independently of the level of PAP. In addition to AT, the shape of the flow wave is of interest, as pulmonary hypertension is associated with a deceleration of flow in late or in mid-systole (notching) [10]. A decreased time to notching has been reported to identify proximal obstruction in patients with chronic thromboembolic pulmonary hypertension and to be of poor prognosis [20].

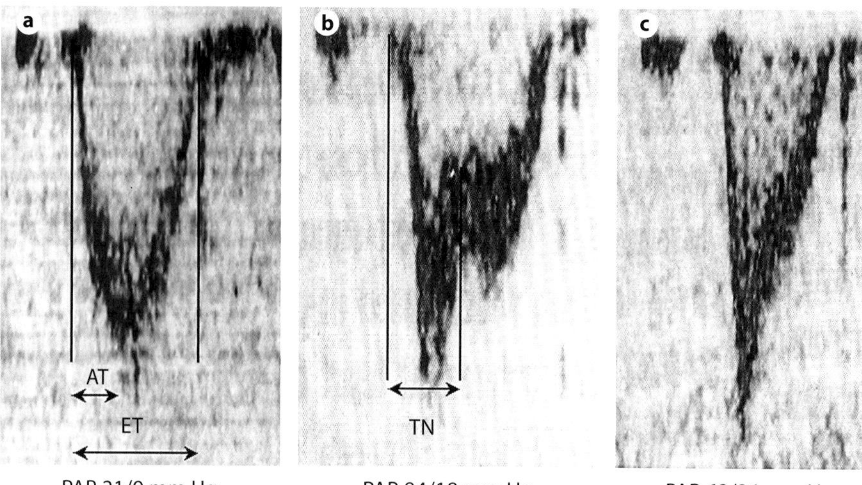

Fig. 2. Pulmonary flow waves in a normal subject (**a**), severe pulmonary hypertension (**b**), and moderate pulmonary hypertension (**c**). Invasively measured PAP are also shown. Pulmonary hypertension is associated with a shortened acceleration time and a late or midsystolic deceleration of flow.

MRI and CT

A standard chest roentgenogram has long been used to diagnose pulmonary hypertension on the basis of a dilatation of the pulmonary arteries, in particular an increase in the diameter of the right descending pulmonary artery [21]. In a total of 98 patients undergoing right heart catheterization, all presenting with a wide range of PAPs, Rich et al. [22] found that a right descending pulmonary artery diameter of more than 18 mm Hg predicted a PAP of more than 20 mm Hg with a sensitivity of 56% and a specificity of 88%, which increased to 75 and 89%, respectively, for severely elevated PAP.

Measurement of the pulmonary artery diameter has also been applied by imaging based on MR and CT scanning, which has the advantage of direct visualization of the main pulmonary artery in a perpendicular plane. An increased ratio of the main pulmonary artery to aortic diameter has been identified as a reliable indication of pulmonary hypertension on both CT [23, 24] and MRI [25]. However, changes in pulmonary artery diameter do not appear to be sensitive to changes in PAP over time [25]. Other clear signs of pulmonary hypertension on CT and MRI are enlargement of the right ventricle, right ventricular hypertrophy, and signs of septal displacement (fig. 3).

Several more advanced MRI estimates of PAP have been proposed. Roeleveld et al. [26] evaluated these methods in a group of 44 patients with established PAH and found poor correlation between catheterization-derived mean PAP and MRI-derived measures, including pulmonary vascular index, acceleration time (defined as time from onset of pulmonary artery forward flow to maximum velocity), and the ratio between acceleration time and ejection time. The only significant correlation between catheterization-based mean PAP and MRI-based measures was for mean pulmonary flow (r = 0.56). Based on these results, it was concluded that at this time, MRI-derived estimates for PAP do not provide a reliable alternative to echocardiography, and *certainly* cannot replace right heart catheterization. Another study examined 59 patients with PAH with both right heart catheterization and phase-contrast MRI comparing different invasive and noninvasive parameters [27]. The measurement that was best correlated to PAP or PVR was the average pulmonary flow velocity (r = 0.86).

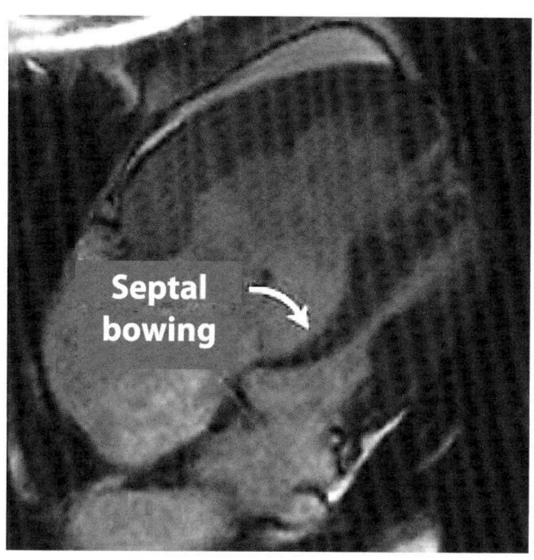

Fig. 3. Long-axis view of the heart of a PAH patient made by MRI showing extensive hypertrophy of the right ventricle and a small volume of the left ventricle due to leftward septal bulging.

However, it remains unclear from this study whether this parameter is just a mere reflection of cardiac output instead of PAP.

Assessment of Right Ventricular Function

The adaptation of ventricular function to afterload is essentially homeometric, allowing initially for maintenance of stroke volume at unchanged end-diastolic or end-systolic dimensions. This is achieved through increased contractility, ideally measured by maximal ventricular elastance and matching afterload, ideally measured by arterial elastance. The heterometric maintenance of stroke volume in the face of increased afterload through increased ventricular dimensions, described in Starling's law of the heart, is achieved by rapid beat-to-beat changes, but eventually will fail with systolic function adaptation [28]. Patients with PAH and no clinical symptomatology of left heart dysfunction may present with a several-fold increase in right ventricular contractility (maximal ventricular elastance) matching increased afterload (arterial elastance) so that right ventricular-arterial coupling is relatively maintained or only slightly decreased [29]. A similar observation of maintained right ventricular-systemic arterial coupling has been reported in an asymptomatic patient with congenitally corrected transposition of the great arteries [30]. Progression of the pulmonary vascular disease is associated with eventual right ventricular-arterial decoupling, leaving no other option to the right ventricle than the Starling mechanism with increased dimensions to maintain flow output in response to peripheral oxygen demand [28]. This pathophysiological scenario of progressive right ventricular-arterial uncoupling in severe pulmonary hypertension (but normal systemic arterial pressure) eventually leads to overt clinical failure with increased right ventricular dimensions, filling pressures, and dysfunction.

Echocardiography

The initial assessment of the right ventricle is based on the measurement of volumes based on linear dimensions and areas obtained from single tomographic echocardiographic planes. The best correlations between single-plane measurements and right ventricular volumes have been obtained with the maximal short axis dimension and the planimetered right ventricular area in the 4-chamber view. The area-length method, which uses an ellipsoidal or pyramidal model, correlates better with right ventricular volume than the Simpson rule. However, this method is based on geometric assumptions, which might not be true in pulmonary hypertension. Right chamber surface areas can be estimated on apical 4-chamber views. The septal displacement caused by the enlarged right ventricle can be quantified by the calculation of an eccentricity index as the ratio of parallel and perpendicular axes on a parasternal short axis view [31] (figure 4).

A commonly used index of systolic function is the right ventricular fractional area change measured in the 4-chamber view, which is calculated as the ratio of systolic to diastolic area. This index is *expected* to correlate with right ventricular ejection fraction (RVEF) in advanced pulmonary hypertension [32]. Both right ventricular fractional area change and ejection fraction relate to contractility, and thus reflect right ventricular-arterial coupling. Another useful measure of systolic function is the tricuspid annual plane systolic excursion (TAPSE), which reflects the longitudinal systolic excursion of the lateral tricuspid annulus towards the apex [33]. The measurement of TAPSE relies on an M mode recording, and as such presents with minimal operator-dependent variability. It has been shown to be a potent predictor of survival in pulmonary hypertension, with a cutoff value of 18 mm and tightly correlated to RVEF [34].

Systolic function of the right ventricle can also be assessed by a tissue Doppler measurement of the tricuspid annulus systolic velocity S wave, which has also been shown to be tightly correlated to TAPSE and RVEF, with values less than 10.5 cm/s indicating right ventricular failure [34]. However, TAPSE and tricuspid annulus S wave are as load-dependent as fractional area change or ejection fraction. Tissue Doppler indices of isovolumic velocity such as maximal right ventricular isovolumic velocity or acceleration may be less load-dependent measurements of contractility [36]. In a large series of patients with either PAH or chronic thromboembolic pulmonary hypertension, right ventricular velocity, with a cutoff value of 9 cm/s, appeared to be a better predictor of survival than any other echocardiographic variable, underscoring the importance of right ventricular systolic function in determining functional state and survival [37].

Tissue Doppler-derived strain and strain-rate measurements of right ventricular systolic function have been developed, but suffer from excessive inter- and intraobserver variability [37, 38]. On the other hand, cardiac output or stroke volumes are indirect but valid indices of right ventricular systolic function as they reflect the adequacy of right ventricular-arterial coupling.

Increased right ventricular afterload is associated with an increase in isovolumic relaxation time and a decreased ratio of transmitral E/A or tissue Doppler E'/A' waves as indices

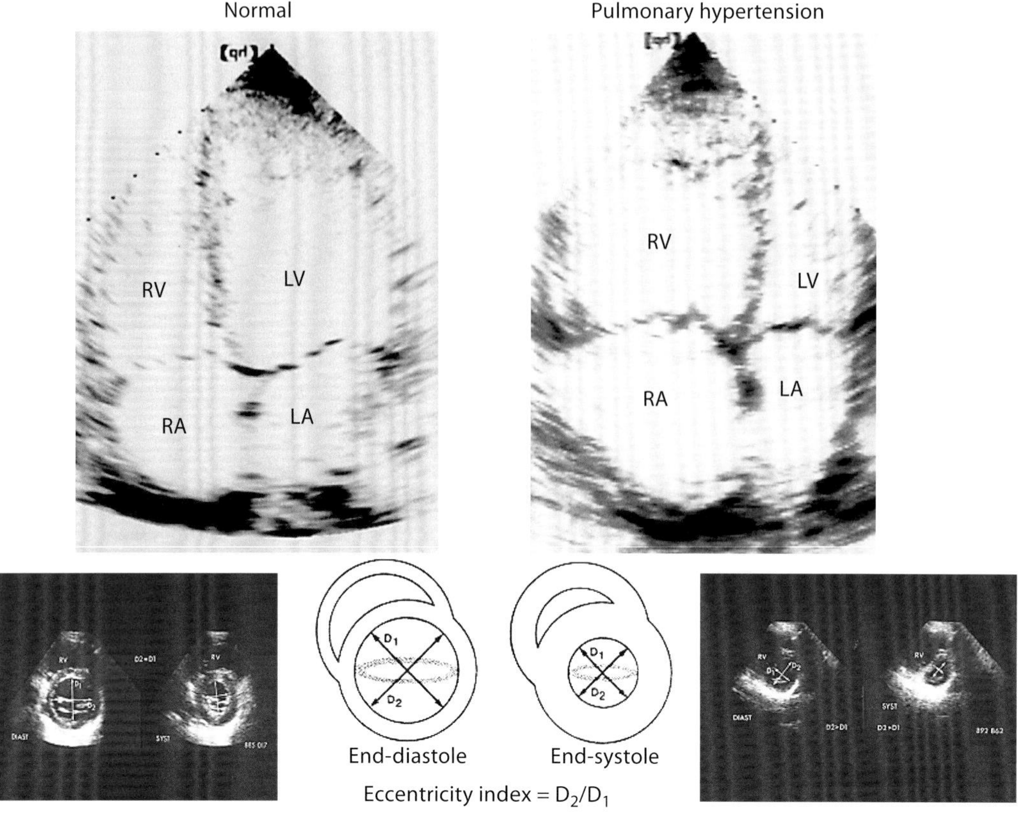

Fig. 4. Apical 4-chamber view showing inflated right heart chambers and a septal shift, and parasternal short-axis view showing an altered eccentricity index in pulmonary hypertension (right) as compared to normal (left).

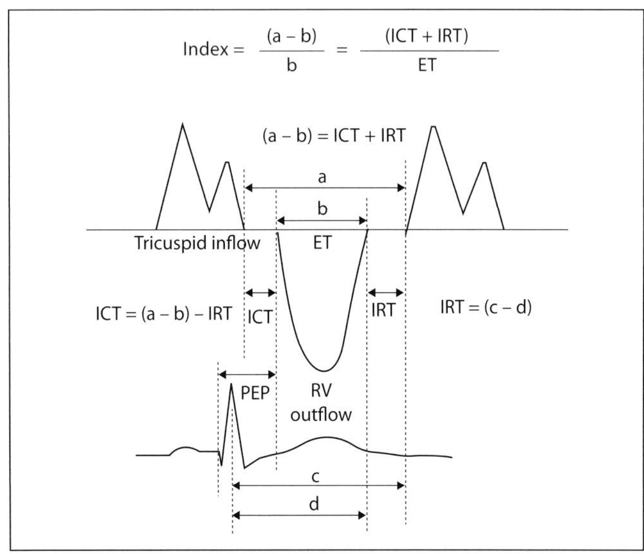

Fig. 5. Calculation of the Tei index. ICT = Isovolumic contraction time; IRT = isovolumic relaxation time; ET = ejection time; PEP = pre-ejection period; RV = right ventricle.

of altered diastolic function [18, 37–40]. These changes are related to increased contractility-related slowing of calcium repumping as well as decreased diastolic compliance because of increased end-diastolic volume and/or competition for space between a dilated right ventricle and left ventricle within a nondistensible pericardium. Diuretic therapy in patients with pulmonary hypertension and right ventricular failure may markedly improve the left ventricle eccentricity index and transmitral E/A as a consequence of decreased septal shift and improved diastolic compliance.

An integrated index of systolic and diastolic function of the right ventricle is offered by the so-called Tei index, which is the ratio of isovolumetric time intervals to ventricular ejection time, calculated from the pulsed wave Doppler derived inflow and outflow durations [41]. The calculation of the Tei index is in figure 5.

It has been recently shown that the lengthening of the isovolumic relaxation period is not the consequence of an abnormal relaxation, but is secondary to an increased contraction period of the right ventricle due to increased right ventricular wall tension [42]. In that respect, the Tei index might be considered more a reflection of abnormal systolic function than of abnormal diastolic function. The normal value of this index is 0.28 ± 0.04. A value greater than 0.88 is associated with a poor prognosis in patients with idiopathic PAH [43].

Pericardial effusion in pulmonary hypertension is explained by increased coronary capillary filtration due to increased right ventricular filling pressures, but increased capillary permeability may also play a role in some systemic diseases. The presence of pericardial fluid is associated with a poor prognosis [44].

MRI

The advantage of MRI over echocardiography is that no geometric assumptions are required, thus allowing accurate measurements of volumes and mass. The principle is that a stack of ECG-triggered transverse images encompassing the right ventricle and central pulmonary arteries is made, from which the 3-dimensional structure of the heart can be derived. In recent years, temporal and spatial resolution have improved further allowing more accurate quantification of global function of both the left and right ventricle and the complex interaction between both ventricles in pulmonary hypertension. The disadvantage is that automatic methods to trace the epi- and endocardial contours are unreliable for the right ventricle, requiring laborious manual tracing of the epi- and endomyocardial contours in order to assess mass and volumes.

The accuracy of MRI for the assessment of right ventricular mass was demonstrated in a study by Calverley et al. [45] showing that right ventricular mass measured by MR corresponds with findings obtained during autopsy studies. Although it was found that right ventricular mass is related to pulmonary arterial pressure, the projected significance of right ventricular mass is unknown [46, 47].

Stroke volume and ejection fraction can be calculated from the end-diastolic and end-systolic volumes. In a study by van Wolferen et al. [47] it was shown that a dilated right ventricle and a low ejection fraction and stroke volume measured at baseline by MRI predicts a poor outcome, whereas a further dilatation of the right ventricle and a further decrease in stroke volume and RVEF is predictive of treatment failure and death. A more simple way to estimate RVEF is to measure the longitudinal or transveral shortening of the myocardium derived from the long-axis or short-axis view, respectively. Both measures closely resemble RVEF [48] (fig. 6).

Diastolic function of the right ventricle can be estimated by end-diastolic volume and can be approximately described by isovolumic relaxation time [49]. Both parameters can be derived from MRI.

Given the relevance of stroke volume in pulmonary hypertension, a simple and accurate method is required to measure stroke volume. Velocity-encoded cine MRI provides such a tool for quantification of stroke volume, pulmonary artery distensibility, and flow tracing of the pulmonary artery flow over time [50]. The major advantage of this method is that precise quantification of the flow per heartbeat of both the right and left ventricle is possible in a reasonably short period of time. Turbulences and vortex flow might induce an error in the assessment of stroke volume from the pulmonary artery in the presence of pulmonary hypertension. For this reason, aortic flow measurements in the absence of an intracardiac shunt are recommended as the most reliable method to assess stroke volume in pulmonary hypertension [51]. A change of 10 ml in stroke volume measured by flow quantification is found to be a clinically meaningful change [52].

By comparing aortic and pulmonary arterial flow, the intracardiac shunt can be quantified by means of MRI. This approach has been successfully used in monitoring shunts in children with a right-to-left and left-to-right intracardiac shunt [53]

Prognostic Relevance and Therapeutic Sensitivity

Several echocardiographic indices of right ventricular function have been shown to be of prognostic relevance in patients with severe pulmonary hypertension. These include pericardial effusion, right atrial size and left ventricle eccentricity index [44], the Tei index [42], TAPSE [34], and isovolumic velocity [37].

An MRI study reported decreased stroke volume, increased right ventricular volume, and decreased left ventricle volume to be of poor prognosis in PAH [47]. Interestingly, in that study right ventricular mass did not have a significant impact on survival. Cutoff values and even the prognostic ability of imaging-derived indices has varied among studies depending on method of analysis and patient populations, but the general trend is in line with the emerging notion that pulmonary hypertension symptomatology and prognosis is predominantly determined by right ventricular function [54, 55]. This is in keeping with invasive measurements in PAH, showing that RAP and cardiac output are the main determinant prognostic factors [55].

Substudies of randomized controlled trials of targeted therapies in PAH have also reported on associated changes

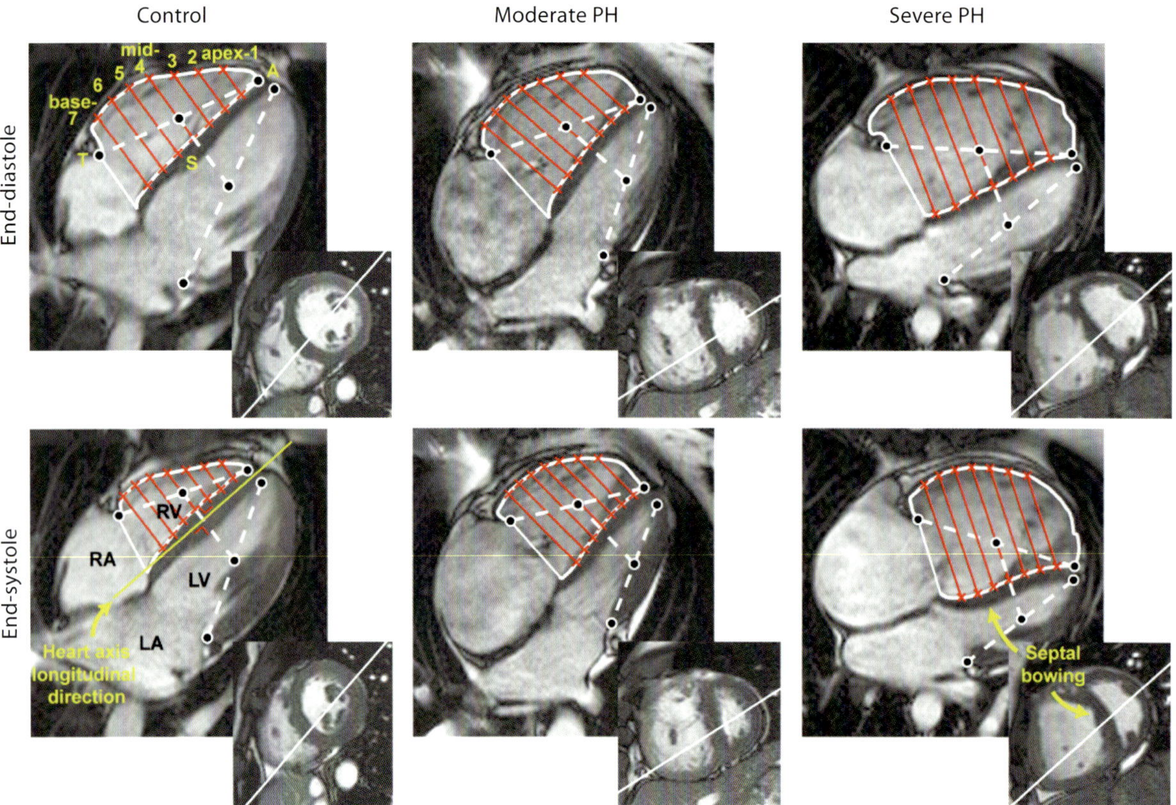

Fig. 6. Long- and short-axis views by MRI of a control, moderate PAH patient, and severe PAH patient showing the longitudinal and transversal displacement during the cardiac cycle (adapted from Kind et al. [48]). PH = Pulmonary hypertension.

in imaging-derived indices. Chronic intravenous epoprostenol improved echocardiographic measurements of right ventricular end-diastolic area, left ventricle eccentricity index, and, somewhat surprisingly, the maximum velocity of tricuspid regurgitation [56]. Chronic oral bosentan improved echocardiographic measurements of the ratio of right ventricular to left ventricle end-diastolic area, inferior vena cava diameter, left ventricle eccentricity index, Tei index, severity of pericardial effusion, right ventricular ejection time, stroke volume, cardiac output, and indices of left ventricle diastolic function [57]. Only a few of these measurements were reported from all the participating centers, raising questions about feasibility. Chronic oral sildenafil decreased MRI-measured right ventricular mass [58]. The clinical significance of this finding is not clear.

It must be stated that the value of imaging indices of the pulmonary circulation and the right ventricular are not only in relation to progress. Changes in imaging measured right ventricular function along with improved clinical state and functional capacity, with or without targeted therapies, are also of major pathophysiological relevance.

Advanced Techniques

It is now becoming apparent that although PAH-specific therapy can reduce PVR, this does not necessarily lead to clinical improvement and prolonged survival unless accompanied by a parallel improvement in right ventricular function [54]. Therefore, adequate monitoring of the right ventricle is of increasing importance for making adequate treatment decisions in time, as has been acknowledged in the recent guidelines [1]. Large studies are required to find the optimal way to monitor the right ventricle. In addition, novel upcoming techniques should be tested for their potential to monitor the disease and to fill in some of the existing knowledge gaps pertaining to PAH pathophysiology. Some of those techniques are briefly discussed below.

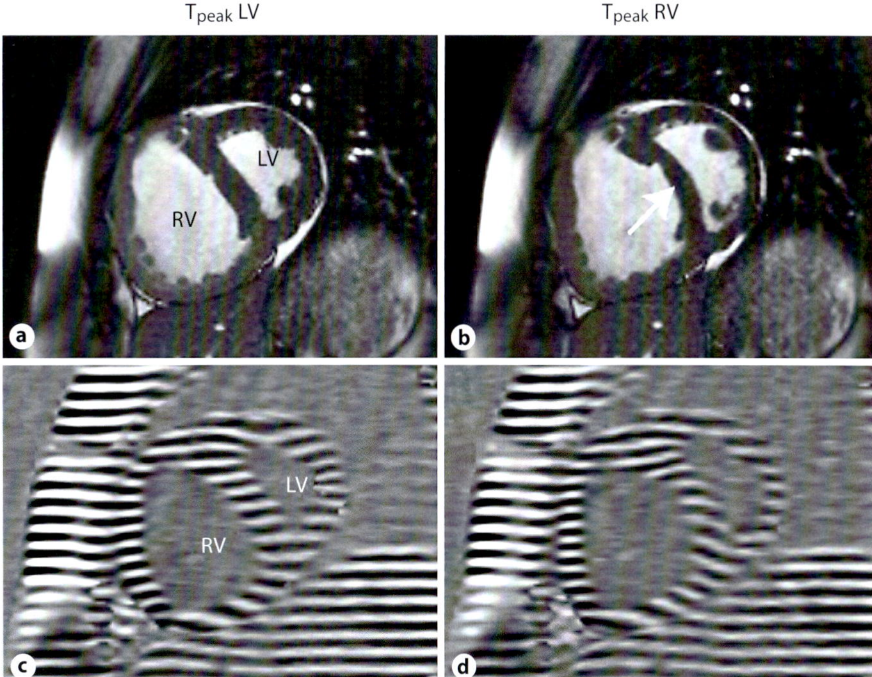

Fig. 7. MRI short-axis and corresponding tagging images. LV = Left ventricle; RV = right ventricle.

Measuring Regional Right Ventricular Structure and Function

During the course of the disease, the shape of the right ventricle alters. This might lead to altered regional patterns of contraction. Insight on regional function can be obtained both by MRI using myocardial tagging and tissue Doppler imaging echocardiography. Tissue Doppler imaging has been introduced to estimate right ventricular function by measuring deformation and velocity of the right ventricular structures during the cardiac cycle. The tissue velocity along a long axis in the 4-chamber view relates to longitudinal shortening and gives a 1-dimensional view of unit velocity at predefined anatomical sites. Several reports show the potential of this technique to measure abnormal strain and relaxation in PAH [38, 59–61].

The MRI alternative to tissue Doppler techniques is myocardial tagging. Tagged MRI, first described by Zerhouni et al. [62], is a noninvasive technique for measuring 3-dimensional motion and deformation in the heart. Tags are regions of tissue, whose longitudinal magnetization has been altered before imaging so that they appear dark in MR images. The changes of these dark areas during the contraction provide information about myocardial shortening. Using tagged MRI, a study conducted in patients with idiopathic PAH showed significant interventricular asynchrony caused by a longer right ventricular systolic contraction time of the right ventricular free wall compared with the septum and left ventricle, which appeared to be the consequence of the large force the right ventricular myocardial fibers must generate to shorten [63]. A corresponding image of 'post-systolic shortening' has been reported using tissue Doppler imaging in a subject with severe pulmonary hypertension developed during high-altitude exposure [64] (fig. 7).

Information about the deposition of collagen in the right ventricular myocardium and especially the presence of fibrotic tissue can be obtained by delayed contrast enhancement, a MRI-based technique using gadolinium contrast. Two studies have independently shown that DCE is present at the insertion points of the septum in PAH patients and that the amount of DCE is related to right ventricular function [65, 66]. Since the insertion points are subject to increased mechanical stress, these findings suggest that mechanical stress may contribute to the occurrence of fibrosis.

Finally, perfusion imaging of the right ventricle is possible to image and quantify regional perfusion. It was shown using this technique that the perfusion reserve is limited in severe PAH, indicating that limited blood supply to the right ventricle might contribute to right ventricular failure [67] (fig. 8).

While this review has focused on imaging of right ventricle structure, function, and pulmonary artery flow, recent

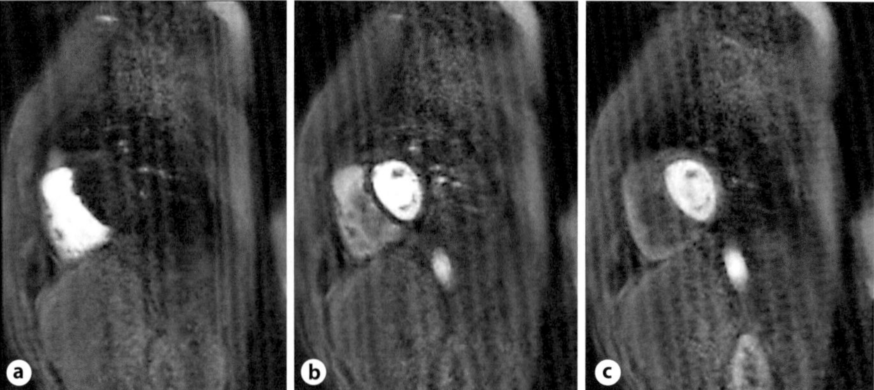

Fig. 8. MR perfusion imaging of the right ventricle. **a** Contrast in right ventricle lumen. **b** Contrast in left ventricle lumen. **c** Contrast in right ventricle myocardium.

molecular insights in heart failure makes molecular imaging an appealing approach. This might allow us to translate preclinical findings to the clinic, looking for the molecular basis for the effects of treatments. Although the possibilities for molecular imaging by MRI and PET scanning have been described [68], the application of these techniques in the field of pulmonary hypertension has been limited thus far [69–71]. Results of these studies show that altered metabolism of the right ventricle and perfusion in PAH can be imaged by means of nuclear techniques and that these results are related to parameters of right ventricular function. The future application of nuclear techniques in the field of pulmonary hypertension is the use of radioligands and iron-tagged tracers allowing molecular imaging of the pulmonary vascular bed and right ventricle by means of PET and MRI.

Conclusions and Future Perspectives

The pivotal role of the right ventricle in determining symptoms and prognosis of pulmonary hypertension has been well recognized in recent years. Careful monitoring of the right ventricle during the course of the disease was therefore recommended in the recent guidelines of PAH. Based on the Starling principles and current literature, the failing right ventricle is characterized by a decrease in stroke volume and an increase in end-systolic and end-diastolic volumes together with an increase in end-diastolic pressure. Stroke volume can be measured accurately by means of MRI. A change of 10 ml over time has been found to be of clinical importance. Changes of right ventricular volume in relation to stroke volume are well described by means of RVEF, which can be estimated from the longitudinal movements (TAPSE) or transverse movements. Improved measurements of contractility are needed for a better assessment of right ventricular-arterial coupling. Upcoming techniques might offer unique insights in the mechanics of right ventricular failure and the underlying mechanisms. At this stage, in spite of insufficient validation against gold standards and inaccuracies, noninvasive imaging techniques offer more than right heart catheterization-derived measurements in this functional description of the right ventricle.

References

1 Galiè N, Hoeper MM, Humbert M, Torbicki A, Vachiery JL, Barbera JA, Beghetti M, Corris P, Gaine S, Gibbs JS, Gomez-Sanchez MA, Jondeau G, Klepetko W, Opitz C, Peacock A, Rubin L, Zellweger M, Simonneau G: Guidelines for the diagnosis and treatment of pulmonary hypertension. Eur Respir J 2009;34:1219–1263.

2 Kovacs G, Berghold A, Scheid S, Olschewski H: Pulmonary artery pressure during rest and exercise in healthy subjects: a systematic review. Eur Respir J 2009;34:888–894.

3 Reeves JT, Dempsey JA, Grover RF: Pulmonary circulation during exercise; in Weir EK, Reeves JT (eds): Pulmonary Vascular Physiology and Physiopathology. New York, Marcel Dekker, 1989, pp 107–133.

4 Naeije R: Pulmonary vascular resistance: a meaningless variable? Intensive Care Med 2003;29:526–529.

5 Naeije R: In defense of exercise stress tests for the diagnosis of pulmonary hypertension. Heart 2011; 97:94–95.

6 Yock PG, Popp RL: Noninvasive estimation of right ventricular systolic pressure by Doppler ultrasound in patients with tricuspid regurgitation. Circulation 1984;70:657–662.

7 Hatle L, Angleson B: Doppler Ultrasound in Cardiology: Physical Principles and Clinical Applications, ed 2. Philadelphia, Lea & Febiger, 1985, pp 252–263.

8 Kircher BJ, Himelman RB, Schiller NB: Noninvasive estimation of right atrial pressure from the inspiratory collapse of the inferior vena cava. Am J Cardiol 1990;66:493–496.

9 Syyed R, Reeves JT, Welsh D, Raeside D, Johnson MK, Peacock AJ: The relationship between the components of pulmonary artery pressure remains constant under all conditions in both health and disease. Chest 2008;133:633–639.

10 Naeije R, Torbicki A: More on the noninvasive diagnosis of pulmonary hypertension. Doppler echocardiography revisited. Eur Respir J 1995;8: 1445–1449.

11 Arcasoy SM, Christie JD, Ferrari VA, Sutton MS, Zisman DA, Blumenthal NP, Pochettino A, Kotloff RM: Echocardiographic assessment of pulmonary hypertension in patients with advanced lung disease. Am J Respir Crit Care Med 2003; 167:735–740.

12 Fisher MR, Forfia PR, Chamera E, et al: Accuracy of Doppler echocardiography in the hemodynamic assessment of pulmonary hypertension. Am J Respir Crit Care Med 2009;179:615–621.

13 Grünig E, Weissmann S, Ehlken N, Fijalkowska A, Fischer C, Fourme T, Galié N, Ghofrani A, Harrison RE, Huez S, Humbert M, Janssen B, Kober J, Koehler R, Machado RD, Mereles D, Naeije R, Olschewski H, Provencher S, Reichenberger F, Retailleau K, Rocchi G, Simonneau G, Torbicki A, Trembath R, Seeger W: Stress-Doppler-echocardiography in relatives of patients with idiopathic and familial pulmonary arterial hypertension: results of a multicenter European analysis of pulmonary artery pressure response to exercise and hypoxia. Circulation 2009;119: 1747–1757.

14 Argiento P, Chesler N, Mulè M, D'Alto M, Bossone E, Unger P, Naeije R: Exercise stress echocardiography for the study of the pulmonary circulation. Eur Respir J 2010;35:1273–1278.

15 Christie J, Sheldahl LM, Tristani FE, Sagar KB, Ptacin MJ, Wann S: Determination of stroke volume and cardiac output during exercise: comparison of two-dimensional and Doppler echocardiography, Fick oximetry, and thermodilution. Circulation 1987;76:539–547.

16 Abbas AE, Fortuin FD, Schiller NB, Appleton CP, Moreno CA, Lester SJ: A simple method for noninvasive estimation of pulmonary vascular resistance. J Am Coll Cardiol 2003;41:1021–1027.

17 Nagueh S, Middleton K, Kopelen H, Zoghbi W, Quinones M: Doppler tissue imaging: a noninvasive technique for evaluation of left ventricular relaxation and estimation of filling pressures. J Am Coll Cardiol 1997;30:1527–1533.

18 Kitabatake A, Inoue M, Asao M, et al: Noninvasive evaluation of pulmonary hypertension by a pulsed Doppler technique. Circulation 1983;68: 302–309.

19 Huez S, Roufosse F, Vachièry JL, Pavelescu A, Derumeaux G, Wautrecht JC, Cogan E, Naeije R: Isolated right ventricular dysfunction in systemic sclerosis: latent pulmonary hypertension? Eur Respir J 2007;30:928–936.

20 Hardziyenka M, Reesink HJ, Bouma BJ, de Bruin-Bon HA, Campian ME, Tanck MW, van den Brink RB, Kloek JJ, Tan HL, Bresser P: A novel echocardiographic predictor of in-hospital mortality and mid-term haemodynamic improvement after pulmonary endarterectomy for chronic thrombo-embolic pulmonary hypertension.Eur Heart J 2007;28:842–849.

21 Abrams HL: Radiologic aspects of increased pulmonary artery pressure and flow: preliminary observations. Stanford Med Bull 1956;14:97–111.

22 Rich S, Chomka E, Hasara L, Hart K, Drizd T, Joo E, Levy PS: The prevalence of pulmonary hypertension in the United States. Chest 1989;96:236–241.

23 Ng CS, Wells AU, Padley SP: A CT sign of chronic pulmonary arterial hypertension: the ratio of main pulmonary artery to aortic diameter. J Thorac Imaging 1999;14:270–278.

24 Heinrich M, Uder M, Tscholl D, Grgic A, Kramann B, Schäfers HJ: CT scan findings in chronic thromboembolic pulmonary hypertension: predictors of hemodynamic improvement after pulmonary thromboendarterectomy. Chest 2005; 127:1606–1613.

25 Boerrigter B, Mauritz GJ, Marcus JT, Helderman F, Postmus PE, Westerhof N, Vonk-Noordegraaf A: Progressive dilatation of the main pulmonary artery is a characteristic of pulmonary arterial hypertension and is not related to changes in pressure. Chest 2010;138:1395–1401.

26 Roeleveld RJ, Marcus JT, Boonstra A, Postmus PE, Marques KM, Bronzwaer JG, Vonk-Noordegraaf A: A comparison of noninvasive MRI-based methods of estimating pulmonary artery pressure in pulmonary hypertension. J Magn Reson Imaging 2005;22:67–72.

27 Sanz J, Kuschnir P, Rius T, et al: Pulmonary arterial hypertension: noninvasive detection with phase-contrast MR imaging. Radiology 2007; 243:70–79.

28 Sagawa K, Maughan L, Suga H, Sunagawa K: Cardiac Contraction and the Pressure-Volume Relationship. New York, Oxford University Press, 1988.

29 Kuehne T, Yilmaz S, Steendijk P, Moore P, Groenink M, Saaed M, Weber O, Higgins CB, Ewert P, Fleck E, Nagel E, Schulze-Neick I, Lange P: Magnetic resonance imaging analysis of right ventricular pressure-volume loops: in vivo validation and clinical application in patients with pulmonary hypertension. Circulation 2004;110: 2010–2016.

30 Wauthy P, Pagnamenta A, Vassali F, Brimioulle S, Naeije R: Right ventricular adaptation to pulmonary hypertension. An interspecies comparison. Am J Physiol Heart Circ Physiol 2004;286: H1441–H1447.

31 Ryan T, Petrovic O, Dillon JC, Feigenbaum H, Conley MJ, Armstrong WF: An echocardiographic index for separation of right ventricular volume and pressure overload. J Am Coll Cardiol 1985;5:918–924.

32 Haddad F, Denault AY, Couture P, Cartier R, Pellerin M, Levesque S, Lambert J, Tardif JC: Right ventricular myocardial performance index predicts perioperative mortality or circulatory failure in high-risk valvular surgery. J Am Soc Echocardiogr 2007;20:1065–1072.

33 Ghio S, Recusani F, Klersy C, Sebastiani R, Laudisa ML, Campana C, Gavazzi A, Tavazzi L: Prognostic usefulness of tricuspid annular planes systolic excursion in patients with congestive heart failure secondary to idiopathic or ischemic dilated cardiomyopathy. Am J Cardiol 2000;85: 837–842.

34 Forfia PR, Fisher MR, Mathai SC, Housten-Harris T, Hemnes AR, Borlaug BA, Chamera E, Corretti MC, Champion HC, Abraham TP, Girgis RE, Hassoun PM: Tricuspid annular displacement predicts survival in pulmonary hypertension. Am J Respir Crit Care Med 2006;174:1034–1041.

35 Saxena N, Rajagopalan N, Edelman K, López-Candales A: Tricuspid annular systolic velocity: a useful measurement in determining right ventricular systolic function regardless of pulmonary artery pressures. Echocardiography 2006; 23:750–755.

36 Vogel M, Schmidt MR, Christiansen SB, Cheung M, White PA, Sorensen K, Redington AN: Validation of myocardial acceleration during isovolumic contraction as a novel non-invasive index of right ventricular contractility. Circulation 2002;105:1693–1699.

37 Ernande L, Cottin V, Leroux PY, Huez S, Mulliez A, Aublet-Cuvelier B, Ovize M, Mornex JF, Cordier JF, Naeije R, Derumeaux G: Prognostic relevance of indices of tight ventricular systolic function in pulmonary hypertension. Heart, submitted.

38 Huez S, Vachiéry JL, Unger P, Brimioulle S, Naeije R: Tissue Doppler imaging evaluation of cardiac adaptation to severe pulmonary hypertension. Am J Cardiol 2007;100:1473–1478.

39 Huez S, Faoro V, Guénard H, Martinot JB, Naeije R: Echocardiographic and tissue Doppler imaging of cardiac adaptation to high altitude in native highlanders versus acclimatized lowlanders. Am J Cardiol 2009;103:1605–1609.

40 Huez S, Retailleau K, Unger P, et al: Right and left ventricular adaptation to hypoxia: a tissue Doppler imaging study. Am J Physiol Heart Circ Physiol 2005;289:H1391–H1398.

41 Tei C, Dujardin K, Hodge D, Bailey KR, McGoon MD, Tajik AJ, Seward SB: Doppler echocardiographic index for assessment of global right ventricular function. J Am Soc Echocardiogr 1996; 9:838–847.

42 Mauritz GJ, Marcus JT, Westerhof N, Postmus PE, Vonk-Noordegraaf A: Prolonged right ventricular post-systolic isovolumic period in pulmonary arterial hypertension is not a reflection of diastolic dysfunction? Heart 2011;97:473–478.

43 Yeo TC, Dujardin KS, Tei C, Mahoney DW, McGoon MD, Seward JB: Value of a Doppler-derived index combining systolic and diastolic time intervals in predicting outcome in primary pulmonary hypertension. Am J Cardiol 1998;82:1071–1076.

44 Raymond RJ, Hinderliter AL, Willis PW, Ralph D, Caldwell EJ, Williams W, Ettinger NA, Hill NS, Summer WR, de Boisblanc B, Schwartz T, Koch G, Clayton LM, Jöbsis MM, Crow JW, Long W: Echocardiographic predictors of adverse outcomes in primary pulmonary hypertension. J Am Coll Cardiol 2002;39:1214–1219.
45 Calverley PM, Howatson R, Flenley DC, Lamb D: Clinicopathological correlations in cor pulmonale. Thorax 1992;47:494–498.
46 Saba TS, Foster J, Cockburn M, Cowan M, Peacock AJ: Ventricular mass index using magnetic resonance imaging accurately estimates pulmonary artery pressure. Eur Respir J 2002;20:1519–1524.
47 Van Wolferen SA, Marcus JT, Boonstra A, Marques KM, Bronzwaer JG, Spreeuwenberg MD, Postmus PE, Vonk-Noordegraaf A: Prognostic value of right ventricular mass, volume, and function in idiopathic pulmonary arterial hypertension. Eur Heart J 2007;28:1250–1257.
48 Kind T, Mauritz GJ, Marcus JT, van de Veerdonk M, Westerhof N, Vonk-Noordegraaf A: Right ventricular ejection fraction is better reflected by transverse rather than longitudinal wall motion in pulmonary hypertension. J Cardiovasc Magn Reson 2010;12:35.
49 Gan CT, Holverda S, Marcus JT, Paulus WJ, Marques KM, Bronzwaer JG, Twisk JW, Boonstra A, Postmus PE, Vonk-Noordegraaf A: Right ventricular diastolic dysfunction and the acute effects of sildenafil in pulmonary hypertension patients. Chest 2007;132:11–17.
50 Kondo C, Caputo GR, Masui T, Foster E, O'Sullivan M, Stulbarg MS, Golden J, Catterjee K, Higgins CB: Pulmonary hypertension: pulmonary flow quantification and flow profile analysis with velocity-encoded cine MR imaging. Radiology 1992;183:751–758.
51 Mauritz GJ, Marcus JT, Boonstra A, Postmus PE, Westerhof N, Vonk-Noordegraaf A: Non-invasive stroke volume assessment in patients with pulmonary arterial hypertension: left-sided data mandatory. J Cardiovasc Magn Reson 2008;10:51.
52 van Wolferen SA, van de Veerdonk MC, Mauritz GJ, Jacobs W, Marcus JT, Marques KM, Bronzwaer JG, Heymans MW, Boonstra A, Postmus PE, Westerhof N, Vonk Noordegraaf A: Clinical significant change of stroke volume in pulmonary hypertension. Chest 2011;139:1003–1009.
53 Beerbaum P, Korperich H, Barth P, Esdorn H, Gieseke J, Meyer H: Noninvasive quantification of left-to-right shunt in pediatric patients: phase-contrast cine magnetic resonance imaging compared with invasive oximetry. Circulation 2001; 103:2476–2482.
54 Champion HC, Michelakis ED, Hassoun PM: Comprehensive invasive and noninvasive approach to the right ventricle-pulmonary circulation unit: state of the art and clinical and research implications. Circulation 2009;120: 992–1007.
55 Humbert M, Sitbon O, Chaouat A, Bertocchi M, Habib G, Gressin V, Yaïci A, Weitzenblum E, Cordier JF, Chabot F, Dromer C, Pison C, Reynaud-Gaubert M, Haloun A, Laurent M, Hachulla E, Cottin V, Degano B, Jaïs X, Montani D, Souza R, Simonneau G: Survival in patients with idiopathic, familial, and anorexigen-associated pulmonary arterial hypertension in the modern management era. Circulation 2010;122:156–163.
56 Hinderliter AL, Willis PW 4th, Barst RJ, Rich S, Rubin LJ, Badesch DB, Groves BM, McGoon MD, Tapson VF, Bourge RC, Brundage BH, Koerner SK, Langleben D, Keller CA, Murali S, Uretsky BF, Koch G, Li S, Clayton LM, Jöbsis MM, Blackburn SD Jr, Crow JW, Long WA: Effects of long-term infusion of prostacyclin (epoprostenol) on echocardiographic measures of right ventricular structure and function in primary pulmonary hypertension. Circulation 1997;95:1479–1486.
57 Galié N, Hinderliter AL, Torbicki A, Fourme T, Simonneau G, Pulido T, Espinola-Zavaleta N, Rocchi G, Manes A, Frantz R, Kurzyna M, Nagueh SF, Barst R, Channick R, Dujardin K, Kronenberg A, Leconte I, Rainisio M, Rubin Ll: Effects of the oral endothelin-receptor antagonist bosentan on echocardiographic and Doppler measures in patients with pulmonary arterial hypertension. J Am Coll Cardiol 2003;41:1380–1386.
58 Wilkins MR, Paul GA, Strange JW, Tunariu N, Gin-Sing W, Banya WA, Westwood MA, Stefanidis A, Ng LL, Pennell DJ, Mohiaddin RH, Nihoyannopoulos P, Gibbs JS: Sildenafil versus Endothelin Receptor Antagonist for Pulmonary Hypertension (SERAPH) study. Am J Respir Crit Care Med 2005;171:1292–1297.
59 Moustapha A, Lim M, Saikia S, Kaushik V, Kang SH, Barasch E: Interrogation of the tricuspid annulus by Doppler tissue imaging in patients with chronic pulmonary hypertension: implications for the assessment of right-ventricular systolic and diastolic function. Cardiology 2001;95:101–104.
60 Caso P, Galderisi M, Cicala S, Cioppa C, D'Andrea A, Lagioia G, Liccardo B, Martiniello AR, Mininni N: Association between myocardial right ventricular relaxation time and pulmonary arterial pressure in chronic obstructive lung disease: analysis by pulsed Doppler tissue imaging. J Am Soc Echocardiogr 2001;14:970–977.
61 Huez S, Vachiéry JL, Naeije R: Improvement in right ventricular function during reversibility testing in pulmonary arterial hypertension: a case report. Cardiovasc Ultrasound 2009;7:9.
62 Zerhouni EA, Parish DM, Rogers WJ, Yang A, Shapiro EP: Human heart: tagging with MR imaging – a method for noninvasive assessment of myocardial motion. Radiology 1988;169:59–63.
63 Marcus JT, Gan CT, Zwanenburg JJ, Boonstra A, Allaart CP, Götte MJ, Vonk-Noordegraaf A: Interventricular mechanical asynchrony in pulmonary arterial hypertension: left-to-right delay in peak shortening is related to right ventricular overload and left ventricular underfilling. J Am Coll Cardiol 2008;51:750–757.
64 Huez S, Faoro V, Vachiery JL, Unger P, Martinot JB, Naeije R: Images in cardiovascular medicine. High-altitude-induced right-heart failure. Circulation 2007;115:e308–e309.
65 Blyth KG, Groenning BA, Martin TN, Foster JE, Mark PB, Dargie HJ, Peacock AJ: Contrast enhanced-cardiovascular magnetic resonance imaging in patients with pulmonary hypertension. Eur Heart J 2005;26:1993–1999.
66 McCann GP, Gan CT, Beek AM, Niessen HW, Vonk Noordegraaf A, van Rossum AC: Extent of MRI delayed enhancement of myocardial mass is related to right ventricular dysfunction in pulmonary artery hypertension. Am J Roentgenol 2007;188:349–355.
67 Vogel-Claussen J, Skrok J, Shehata ML, Singh S, Sibley CT, Boyce DM, Lechtzin N, Girgis RE, Mathai SC, Goldstein TA, Zheng J, Lima JA, Bluemke DA, Hassoun PM: Right and left ventricular myocardial perfusion reserves correlate with right ventricular function and pulmonary hemodynamics in patients with pulmonary arterial hypertension. Radiology 2011;258:119–127.
68 Nagendran J, Michelakis E: MRI: one-stop shop for the comprehensive assessment of pulmonary arterial hypertension? Chest 2007;132:2–5.
69 Kluge R, Barthel H, Pankau H, Seese A, Schauer J, Wirtz H, Seyfarth HJ, Steinbach J, Sabri O, Winkler J: Different mechanisms for changes in glucose uptake of the right and left ventricular myocardium in pulmonary hypertension. J Nucl Med 2005;46:25–31.
70 Oikawa M, Kagaya Y, Otani H, Sakuma M, Demachi J, Suzuki J, Takahashi T, Nawata J, Ido T, Watanabe J, Shirato K: Increased [18F]fluorodeoxyglucose accumulation in right ventricular free wall in patients with pulmonary hypertension and the effect of epoprostenol. J Am Coll Cardiol 2005;45:1849–1855.
71 Gomez A, Bialostozky D, Zajarias A, Santos E, Palomar A, Martinez ML, Sandoval J: Right ventricular ischemia in patients with primary pulmonary hypertension. J Am Coll Cardiol 2001; 38:1137–1142.

A. Vonk Noordegraaf MD PhD
Department of Pulmonology
VU University Medical Center
De Boelelaan 1117, NL–1081 HV Amsterdam (The Netherlands)
Tel: +31 20 444 782, E-Mail a.vonk@vumc.nl

Chapter 6
Humbert M, Souza R, Simonneau G (eds): Pulmonary Vascular Disorders.
Prog Respir Res. Basel, Karger, 2012, vol 41, pp 59–64

Biomarkers in Pulmonary Arterial Hypertension

Rogerio Souza · Susana Hoette · Bruno Dias · Carlos Jardim
Pulmonary Circulation Unit, Heart Institute, University of Sao Paulo Medical School, Sao Paulo, Brazil

Abstract
Together with the improvement of pulmonary arterial hypertension (PAH) management arises the need for adequate surrogate markers for treatment decision and follow-up. In this setting, biomarkers play a definitive role. A number of biomarkers addressing specific features of the different pathophysiological mechanisms of PAH, with the ability to describe disease severity and prognosis, have been described. This chapter reviews the characteristics of the different existing biomarkers as the rationale for their integration as the next step for the evaluation of PAH patients.

A significant improvement in the management of pulmonary arterial hypertension (PAH) has been witnessed over the last 15 years with the development of new treatments that significantly alter the natural course of the disease [1]. Additionally, the possibility of combining drugs in order to further improve the management of PAH patients has become a reality [2–4]. Together, these different treatment alternatives have raised the need for proper efficacy evaluation. Survival should be considered as the ultimate endpoint to be demonstrated when a new intervention is under evaluation; however, it is not easy or even feasible to demonstrate a survival benefit, especially in low prevalence diseases such as PAH.

One way to bypass this significant difficulty is the use of surrogate markers. A surrogate marker should be a reliable substitute for a morbid event, tracking the frequency of such event as an epidemiologic and a therapeutic responder marker [5]. It may also be used as part of a screening algorithm or diagnostic investigation in specific high-risk groups. Many different surrogate markers have been used in PAH, from exercise testing to imaging procedures, passing by biomarkers [6]. The focus of this chapter is on the most used noninvasive biomarkers of PAH.

Uric Acid

Serum uric acid (UA) is the final product of purine degradation and may be elevated in different conditions of impaired oxidative metabolism. It has been demonstrated that UA levels are associated with the hemodynamic profile of pulmonary hypertension (PH) patients [7, 8] as well functional capacity [9]. Two different studies have also demonstrated that higher levels of UA are associated with poorer prognosis. The larger study addressed the significance of UA in PAH and enrolled 90 idiopathic PAH (IPAH) patients (35 males and 55 females), who were diagnosed through right heart catheterization and followed for a mean of 31 months [10]. UA levels were higher in the IPAH group as compared to an age-matched control group and correlated significantly with disease severity, increasing in proportion to the NYHA functional class or pulmonary vascular resistance and decreasing in proportion to cardiac output, without any significant differences between genders.

During follow-up, UA decreased in response to vasodilators and was independently associated with mortality (fig. 1). It is important to take into consideration, however, the many aspects that may interfere with UA levels, such as the presence of renal impairment or the use of diuretic therapy, which may prevent the extrapolation of these finding to some patients.

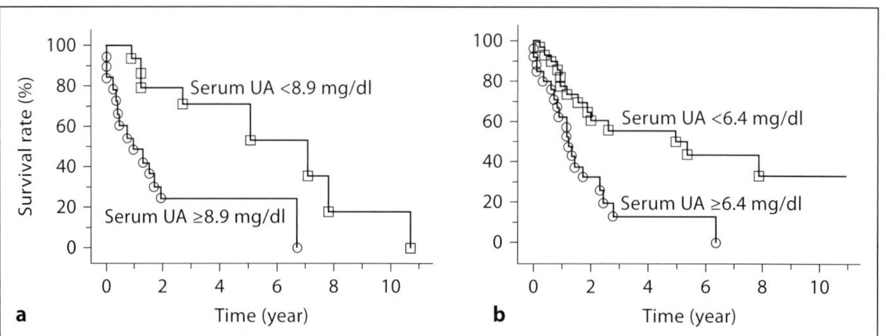

Fig. 1. Kaplan-Meier survival curves according to the median value of serum UA levels in male (**a**) and female (**b**) patients with primary PH. Patients with high serum UA levels had a significantly lower survival rate than those with low serum UA levels (log-rank test, $p < 0.01$) [10].

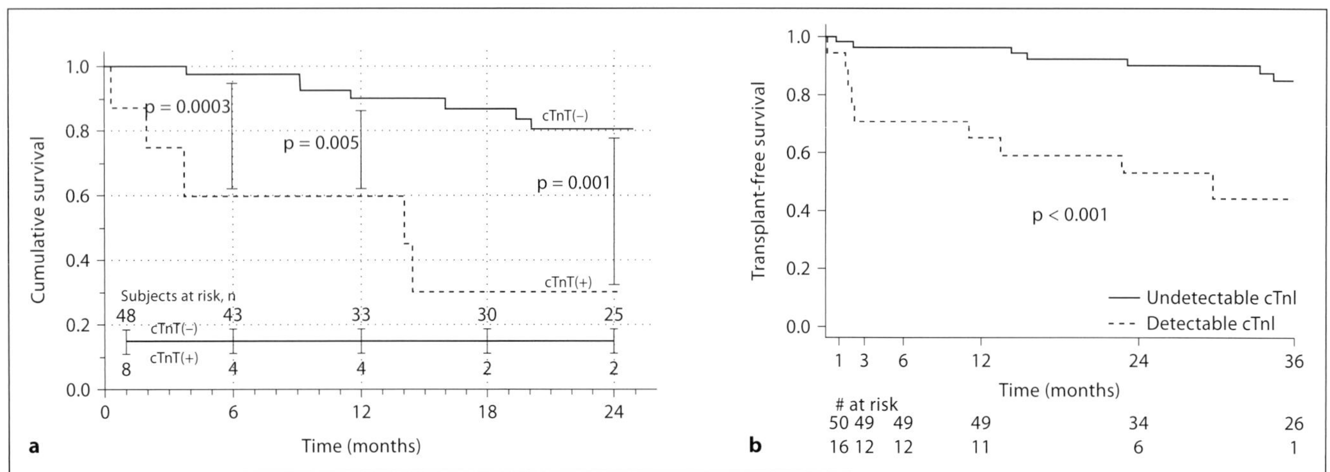

Fig. 2. Kaplan-Meier curves of survival (**a**) and transplant-free survival (**b**) according to the detection of troponin T (**a**) and troponin I (**b**) [12, 13].

Troponins

Troponins are proteins involved in the process of cardiac muscle contraction, modulating calcium-mediated actin and myosin interaction. Many different mechanisms may be associated with cardiac troponin release – from increased wall stress to ischemia [11]. Torbicki et al. [12] evaluated 56 PH patients (51 PAH and 5 patients with chronic thromboembolic PH) and demonstrated that patients with detectable troponin T levels had worse exercise capacity, evaluated by means of 6-min walk test, and a worse 24-month prognosis (fig. 2a). Interestingly, troponin levels became undetectable during the course of successful treatment, but relapsed with disease progression.

More recently, Heresi et al. [13], using a more sensitive assay for detection of troponin I, demonstrated that patients with detectable troponin I walked less at the 6-min walk test and presented more severe functional impairment. Also, 36-month transplant-free survival was significantly lower in patients with detectable troponin I (44 vs. 85%; fig. 2b). Of note, detectable levels of troponin I were found in 25% of the evaluated patients, a much higher proportion when compared to previous studies addressing the role of troponin in PH. If troponins might be considered as 'late markers' of disease severity, this finding raised the question about how much high sensitivity assays might diminish this characteristic of this class of biomarkers.

Asymmetric Dimethylarginine

Asymmetric dimethylarginine (ADMA) is a potent endogenous nitric oxide synthase inhibitor that has been evaluated in different forms of PH [14]. Kielstein et al. [15], evaluating 57 IPAH patients, demonstrated that plasma ADMA levels were higher in patients with IPAH as compared to control

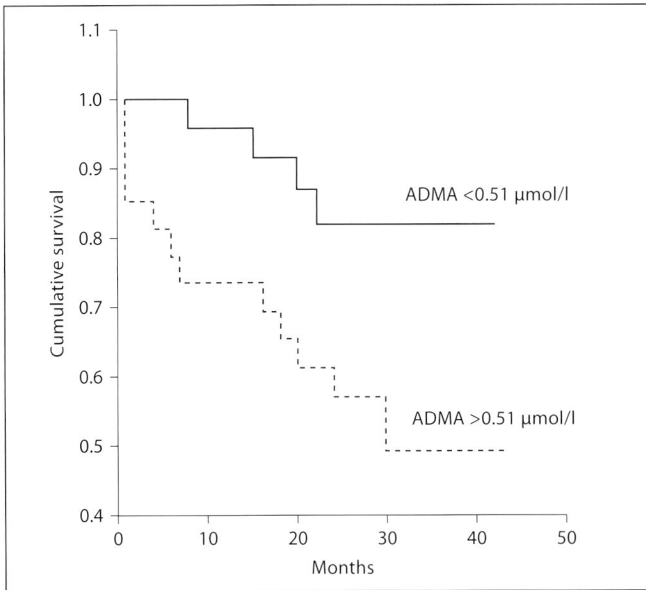

Fig. 3. Survival according to the plasma levels of ADMA [15].

subjects and correlated significantly with the hemodynamic profile, with higher levels denoting worse cardiac function. Furthermore, ADMA levels were independently associated with survival (fig. 3). Similar findings were also demonstrated in a study with 135 patients with chronic thromboembolic PH. Of note, in this later study, ADMA levels dropped to the same range as controls subjects after pulmonary endarterectomy [16].

Endothelin

Endothelin-1 (ET-1) is a potent endogenous vasoconstrictor and smooth-muscle mitogen that is overexpressed in the setting of PH [17]. ET-1 is mainly produced by endothelial cells, with the pulmonary circulation as the most important site of production and clearance. Two different receptors for ETs have been identified: ET receptor A (ET_A) and ET receptor B (ET_B). In the pulmonary vessels, ET_A is expressed on pulmonary smooth-muscle cells, and ET_B is expressed on pulmonary endothelial and smooth-muscle cells. Activation of ET_A or ET_B on pulmonary vascular smooth-muscle cells induces pulmonary vasoconstriction and smooth-muscle cell proliferation [18]. Rubens et al. [19] demonstrated that plasma levels of ET-1 correlate with the hemodynamic profile, with higher levels associated with higher pulmonary vascular resistance and mean pulmonary artery pressure, as with lower cardiac output and lower exercise capacity measured by the 6-min walk distance. In another study, the ratio between ET-1 and ET-3 (another isoform of ET that might be involved in the clearance of ET-1) also correlated with hemodynamics; furthermore, this ratio also was associated to prognosis.

Although ET-1 is recognized as one of the targets for the currently available therapies [20], the concept of using ET levels as guidance to therapy has not been appropriately tested.

D-Dimer and von Willebrand Factor

The presence of prothrombotic mechanisms in the pathogenesis of PH has long been advocated. From endothelial dysfunction to direct platelet activation, many different pathways have been described in this setting [21].

D-dimer is a marker of microvascular thrombosis established for the evaluation of patients with suspected acute pulmonary embolism [22]. In the setting of PAH, it was demonstrated that D-dimer levels were higher than in controls [23] and associated with disease severity [24], although both studies included a remarkably small number of patients.

Plasma von Willebrand factor is a glycoprotein synthetized in endothelial cells and has a direct role in platelet aggregation and adhesion to injured sites. It has been demonstrated that von Willebrand factor is not only elevated in PH, as it correlates to survival [25]. Additionally, a different study demonstrated that von Willebrand factor paralleled the improvement of hemodynamics in a small sample of patients under vasodilator treatment with prostacyclin [26].

Natriuretic Peptides

Pro-brain natriuretic peptide (BNP) is a prohormone, secreted mainly by the ventricles, which is cleaved into N-terminal fragment (NT)-pro-BNP and active BNP in response to stretch of cardiac myocytes. In general, natriuretic peptides have a direct action on kidneys, with consequent natriuresis, and on vascular smooth muscle cells, causing vasodilation; both actions aim to reduce blood pressure and ventricular preload [27].

In PH, BNP levels increase in proportion to the degree of right ventricular dysfunction, as demonstrated in different forms of PH. Nagaya et al. [28] demonstrated that BNP positively correlated with functional class, mean pulmonary arterial pressure, and pulmonary vascular resistance, and correlated negatively with cardiac output. Moreover, baseline and posttreatment levels of BNP were directly associated with survival (fig. 4).

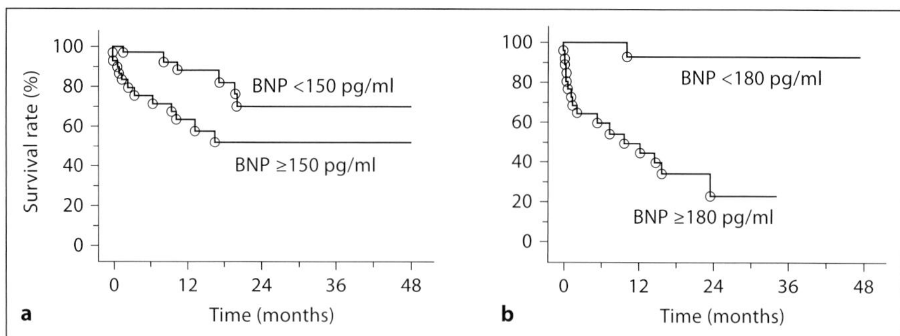

Fig. 4. Kaplan-Meier survival curves according to median value of baseline (**a**) and follow-up (**b**) BNP in patients with IPAH [28].

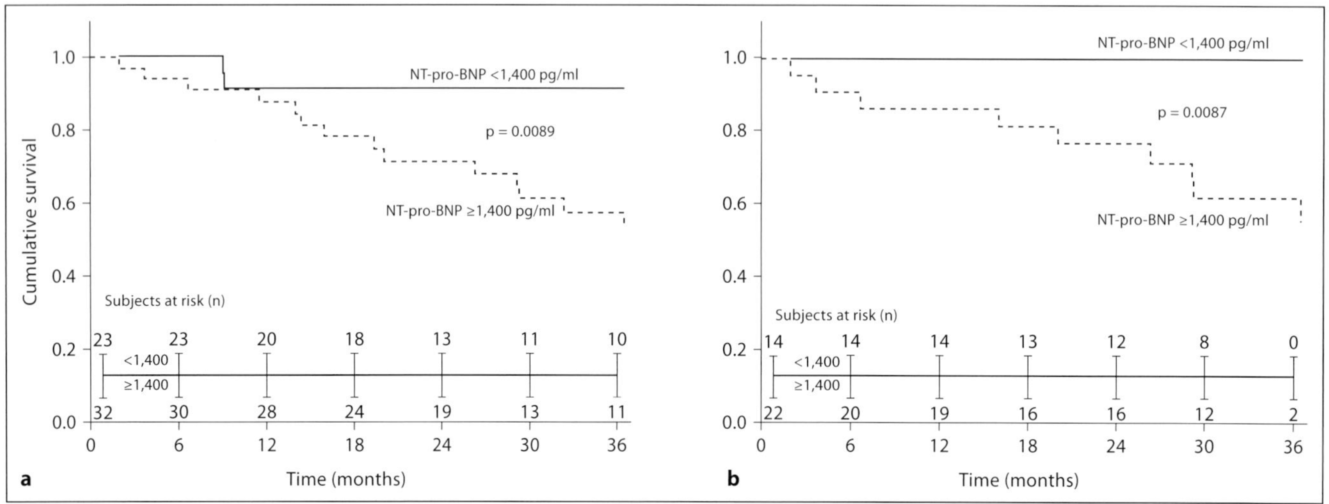

Fig. 5. Cumulative survival estimated by Kaplan-Meier curves was significantly worse at 36 months with initial NT-pro-BNP levels of ≥1,400 pg/ml (dotted line) than NT-pro-BNP levels of <1,400 pg/ml (solid line). Entire study group (**a**) and subgroup with IPAH (**b**) [p = 0.02 for overall group, and p = 0.001 for IPAH (log-rank test)] [35].

Leuchte et al. [29, 30] demonstrated that BNP levels correlated to exercise capacity at baseline and after treatment follow-up.

NT-pro-BNP is highly stable in plasma and has been described as a marker of PH in patients with systemic sclerosis [31]. NT-pro-BNP has been associated with disease severity [32], treatment response [33], and acute hemodynamic response to nitric oxide [34] in the setting of PAH.

Fijalkowska et al. [35], evaluating 55 PH patients (36 IPAH), demonstrated that the baseline levels of NT-pro-BNP were associated with survival (fig. 5).

Leuchte et al. [36] also addressed the potential confounding bias imposed by the presence of renal impairment on the accuracy of NT-pro-BNP as a hemodynamic surrogate in PH. They found that NT-pro-BNP loses its association with hemodynamics in the presence of renal insufficiency, but remains a prognostic indicator while BNP does not, suggesting that NT-pro-BNP might be superior to BNP as a prognostic marker since it accounts for the renal impairment as a consequence of the hemodynamic deterioration. A question that still remains concerns the role of natriuretic peptides in the early phases of PH: since they are a consequence of ventricular overload, they might also be considered as 'late' markers of PH severity in a similar manner to the troponins.

Conclusion

Biomarkers certainly represent a step forward in the evaluation of patients with PH – not only during the diagnostic process, but mainly as prognostic markers and follow-up tools. Nevertheless, thus far not a single biomarker has been able to integrate the multiple mechanisms related to PH development and progression, and it is unlikely that a sole marker will do so in the near future. Therefore, the combination of different biomarkers is the next step for the evaluation of PAH patients. Such combinations, however, cannot be considered trivial: there are many possible combinations and each one of them might be useful to a specific subgroup, but not necessarily applicable to the whole PAH population. Furthermore, proper validation is necessary for any association of biomarkers since a high degree of overlap might exist depending on the chosen markers. Even after taking these difficulties into consideration, the establishment of appropriate routines in the use of biomarkers might represent the way to change the therapeutic approach of an individual PAH patient in a goal-oriented manner.

References

1 Galie N, Manes A, Negro L, Palazzini M, Bacchi-Reggiani ML, Branzi A: A meta-analysis of randomized controlled trials in pulmonary arterial hypertension. Eur Heart J 2009;30:394–403.

2 Simonneau G, Rubin LJ, Galie N, Barst RJ, Fleming TR, Frost AE, Engel PJ, Kramer MR, Burgess G, Collings L, Cossons N, Sitbon O, Badesch DB: Addition of sildenafil to long-term intravenous epoprostenol therapy in patients with pulmonary arterial hypertension: a randomized trial. Ann Intern Med 2008;1498:521–530.

3 McLaughlin VV, Oudiz RJ, Frost A, Tapson VF, Murali S, Channick RN, Badesch DB, Barst RJ, Hsu HH, Rubin LJ: Randomized study of adding inhaled iloprost to existing bosentan in pulmonary arterial hypertension. Am J Respir Crit Care Med 2006;17411:1257–1263.

4 Barst RJ, Gibbs JS, Ghofrani HA, Hoeper MM, McLaughlin VV, Rubin LJ, Sitbon O, Tapson VF, Galie N: Updated evidence-based treatment algorithm in pulmonary arterial hypertension. J Am Coll Cardiol 2009;54(1 suppl):S78–S84.

5 Cohn JN: Introduction to surrogate markers. Circulation 2004;109(25 suppl 1):IV20–IV21.

6 McLaughlin VV, Badesch DB, Delcroix M, Fleming TR, Gaine SP, Galie N, Gibbs JS, Kim NH, Oudiz RJ, Peacock A, Provencher S, Sitbon O, Tapson VF, Seeger W: End points and clinical trial design in pulmonary arterial hypertension. J Am Coll Cardiol 2009;54(1 suppl):S97–S107.

7 Hoeper MM, Hohlfeld JM, Fabel H: Hyperuricaemia in patients with right or left heart failure. Eur Respir J 1999;13:682–685.

8 Voelkel MA, Wynne KM, Badesch DB, Groves BM, Voelkel NF: Hyperuricemia in severe pulmonary hypertension. Chest 2000;117:19–24.

9 Bendayan D, Shitrit D, Ygla M, Huerta M, Fink G, Kramer MR: Hyperuricemia as a prognostic factor in pulmonary arterial hypertension. Respir Med 2003;97:130–133.

10 Nagaya N, Uematsu M, Satoh T, Kyotani S, Sakamaki F, Nakanishi N, Yamagishi M, Kunieda T, Miyatake K: Serum uric acid levels correlate with the severity and the mortality of primary pulmonary hypertension. Am J Respir Crit Care Med 1999;160:487–492.

11 Kociol RD, Pang PS, Gheorghiade M, Fonarow GC, O'Connor CM, Felker GM: Troponin elevation in heart failure prevalence, mechanisms, and clinical implications. J Am Coll Cardiol 2010;56:1071–1078.

12 Torbicki A, Kurzyna M, Kuca P, Fijalkowska A, Sikora J, Florczyk M, Pruszczyk P, Burakowski J, Wawrzynska L: Detectable serum cardiac troponin T as a marker of poor prognosis among patients with chronic precapillary pulmonary hypertension. Circulation 2003;108:844–848.

13 Heresi GA, Tang WH, Aytekin M, Hammel J, Hazen SL, Dweik RA: Sensitive cardiac troponin I predicts poor outcomes in pulmonary arterial hypertension. Eur Respir J 2011, E-pub ahead of print.

14 Zweier JL, Talukder MA: Targeting dimethylarginine dimethylaminohydrolases in pulmonary arterial hypertension: a new approach to improve vascular dysfunction? Circulation 2011;123:1156–1158.

15 Kielstein JT, Bode-Boger SM, Hesse G, Martens-Lobenhoffer J, Takacs A, Fliser D, Hoeper MM: Asymmetrical dimethylarginine in idiopathic pulmonary arterial hypertension. Arterioscler Thromb Vasc Biol 2005;25:1414–1418.

16 Skoro-Sajer N, Mittermayer F, Panzenboeck A, Bonderman D, Sadushi R, Hitsch R, Jakowitsch J, Klepetko W, Kneussl MP, Wolzt M, Lang IM: Asymmetric dimethylarginine is increased in chronic thromboembolic pulmonary hypertension. Am J Respir Crit Care Med 2007;176:1154–1160.

17 Giaid A, Yanagisawa M, Langleben D, Michel RP, Levy R, Shennib H, Kimura S, Masaki T, Duguid WP, Stewart DJ: Expression of endothelin-1 in the lungs of patients with pulmonary hypertension. N Engl J Med 1993;328:1732–1739.

18 Montani D, Souza R, Binkert C, Fischli W, Simonneau G, Clozel M, Humbert M: Endothelin-1/endothelin-3 ratio: a potential prognostic factor of pulmonary arterial hypertension. Chest 2007;131:101–108.

19 Rubens C, Ewert R, Halank M, Wensel R, Orzechowski HD, Schultheiss HP, Hoeffken G: Big endothelin-1 and endothelin-1 plasma levels are correlated with the severity of primary pulmonary hypertension. Chest 2001;120:1562–1569.

20 Humbert M, Sitbon O, Simonneau G: Treatment of pulmonary arterial hypertension. N Engl J Med 2004;351:1425–1436.

21 Farber HW, Loscalzo J: Prothrombotic mechanisms in primary pulmonary hypertension. J Lab Clin Med 1999;134:561–566.

22 Stein PD, Fowler SE, Goodman LR, Gottschalk A, Hales CA, Hull RD, Leeper KV Jr, Popovich J Jr, Quinn DA, Sos TA, Sostman HD, Tapson VF, Wakefield TW, Weg JG, Woodard PK: Multidetector computed tomography for acute pulmonary embolism. N Engl J Med 2006;354:2317–2327.

23 Shitrit D, Bendayan D, Rudensky B, Izbicki G, Huerta M, Fink G, Kramer MR: Elevation of ELISA D-dimer levels in patients with primary pulmonary hypertension. Respiration 2002;69:327–329.

24 Shitrit D, Bendayan D, Bar-Gil-Shitrit A, Huerta M, Rudensky B, Fink G, Kramer MR: Significance of a plasma D-dimer test in patients with primary pulmonary hypertension. Chest 2002;122:1674–1678.

25 Lopes AA, Maeda NY: Circulating von Willebrand factor antigen as a predictor of short-term prognosis in pulmonary hypertension. Chest 1998;114:1276–1282.

26 Veyradier A, Nishikubo T, Humbert M, Wolf M, Sitbon O, Simonneau G, Girma JP, Meyer D: Improvement of von Willebrand factor proteolysis after prostacyclin infusion in severe pulmonary arterial hypertension. Circulation 2000;102:2460–2462.

27 de Lemos JA, McGuire DK, Drazner MH: B-type natriuretic peptide in cardiovascular disease. Lancet 2003;362:316–322.

28 Nagaya N, Nishikimi T, Uematsu M, Satoh T, Kyotani S, Sakamaki F, Kakishita M, Fukushima K, Okano Y, Nakanishi N, Miyatake K, Kangawa K: Plasma brain natriuretic peptide as a prognostic indicator in patients with primary pulmonary hypertension. Circulation 2000;102:865–870.

29 Leuchte HH, Holzapfel M, Baumgartner RA, Ding I, Neurohr C, Vogeser M, Kolbe T, Schwaiblmair M, Behr J: Clinical significance of brain natriuretic peptide in primary pulmonary hypertension. J Am Coll Cardiol 2004;43:764–770.

30 Leuchte HH, Holzapfel M, Baumgartner RA, Neurohr C, Vogeser M, Behr J: Characterization of brain natriuretic peptide in long-term follow-up of pulmonary arterial hypertension. Chest 2005;128:2368–2374.

31 Allanore Y, Borderie D, Meune C, Cabanes L, Weber S, Ekindjian OG, Kahan A: N-terminal pro-brain natriuretic peptide as a diagnostic marker of early pulmonary artery hypertension in patients with systemic sclerosis and effects of calcium-channel blockers. Arthritis Rheum 2003;48:3503–3508.

32 Souza R, Jardim C, Julio Cesar Fernandes C, Silveira Lapa M, Rabelo R, Humbert M: NT-proBNP as a tool to stratify disease severity in pulmonary arterial hypertension. Respir Med 2007;101:69–75.

33 Souza R, Jardim C, Martins B, Cortopassi F, Yaksic M, Rabelo R, Bogossian H: Effect of bosentan treatment on surrogate markers in pulmonary arterial hypertension. Curr Med Res Opin 2005;21:907–911.

34 Souza R, Bogossian HB, Humbert M, Jardim C, Rabelo R, Amato MB, Carvalho CR: N-terminal-pro-brain natriuretic peptide as a haemodynamic marker in idiopathic pulmonary arterial hypertension. Eur Respir J 2005;25:509–513.

35 Fijalkowska A, Kurzyna M, Torbicki A, Szewczyk G, Florczyk M, Pruszczyk P, Szturmowicz M: Serum N-terminal brain natriuretic peptide as a prognostic parameter in patients with pulmonary hypertension. Chest 2006;129:1313–1321.

36 Leuchte HH, El Nounou M, Tuerpe JC, Hartmann B, Baumgartner RA, Vogeser M, Muehling O, Behr J: N-terminal pro-brain natriuretic peptide and renal insufficiency as predictors of mortality in pulmonary hypertension. Chest 2007;131:402–409.

Rogerio Souza, MD, PhD
Pulmonary Circulation Unit
Pulmonary Department, Heart Institute, University of Sao Paulo Medical School
Av. Dr. Eneas de Carvalho Aguiar, 44
Sao Paulo, 05403-000 (Brazil)
Tel. +55 11 26 61 56 95, E-Mail rogerio.souza@incor.usp.br

Chapter 7

Humbert M, Souza R, Simonneau G (eds): Pulmonary Vascular Disorders.
Prog Respir Res. Basel, Karger, 2012, vol 41, pp 65–75

Genetics of Pulmonary Arterial Hypertension and the Concept of Heritable Pulmonary Arterial Hypertension

Barbara Girerd[a–c] · David Montani[a–c] · Azzedine Yaici[a–c] · Mélanie Eyries[d] · Florence Coulet[d] · Florent Soubrier[d] · Marc Humbert[a–c]

[a]Université Paris-Sud, Faculté de Médecine, Kremlin-Bicêtre, [b]AP-HP, Service de Pneumologie et Réanimation Respiratoire, Centre de Référence de l'Hypertension Pulmonaire Sévère, Hôpital Antoine Béclère, Clamart, [c]INSERM U999, Hypertension Artérielle Pulmonaire: Physiopathologie et Innovation Thérapeutique, LabEx LERMIT, Centre Chirurgical Marie-Lannelongue, Le Plessis-Robinson, and [d]Laboratoire d'Oncogénétique et Angiogénétique Moléculaire, Groupe Hospitalier Pitié-Salpétrière, UMRS 956 INSERM, Université Pierre et Marie Curie-Paris 6, Paris, France

Abstract

Germline mutations of *BMPR2* gene (*bone morphogenetic protein receptor type 2*), or more rarely of *ACVRL1* (*activin A receptor type II-like 1*), *ENG* (*endoglin*), and *Smad8* genes have been identified in patients displaying pulmonary arterial hypertension (PAH). *BMPR2, ACVRL1, ENG,* and *Smad8* genes encode proteins involved in the transforming growth factor-β (TGF-β) signaling pathway. This signaling pathway controls growth, differentiation, and apoptosis of various cell types like pulmonary vascular endothelial cells and smooth muscle cells. Mutations in PAH predisposing genes are responsible for abnormal proliferation of pulmonary vascular smooth muscle cells and may promote endothelial cells apoptosis. Such apoptosis might lead to the selection of apoptosis-resistant cells and formation of plexiform lesions, the hallmark of idiopathic PAH. Identification of PAH predisposing genes allows offering genetic testing to PAH patients at risk for heritable disease. Thus, in the French PAH Referral Centre (Hôpital Antoine Béclère, AP-HP, Université Paris Sud 11) genetic screening is proposed to all patients with PAH considered to be idiopathic or due to pulmonary veno-occlusive disease, pulmonary capillary hemangiomatosis, or associated with anorexigen-exposure, irrespectively of the presence or absence of family history. This strategy allowed us to identify and analyze clinical characteristics of PAH patients with a heritable condition, and to offer presymptomatic screening to their relatives. In our center, asymptomatic relative carriers of a *BMPR2* mutation can benefit from a clinical screening (if they wish) because of their high risk of developing PAH.

In 1954, Dresdale et al. [1] first described familial pulmonary arterial hypertension (PAH), suggesting the potential role of genetic defects in the development of the disease. Over the next 50 years, many cases of PAH occurring in a familial context were described. In the French PAH registry, familial PAH accounts for 3.9% of total PAH, forming Group 1 of the Clinical Classification of Pulmonary Hypertension [2–4]. Before the availability of modern genetic tools, we used genealogical studies to understand the genetic transmission of heritable PAH. In 1995, it was known that heritable PAH segregates as an autosomal dominant trait, with an incomplete penetrance (about 20% of mutation carriers develop the disease; fig. 1a). A genetic anticipation phenomenon was suspected, which is characterized by a younger age at PAH diagnosis in subsequent generations [5–8] (fig. 1b). This genetic anticipation phenomenon is well understood in other genetic diseases such as Huntington's disease, Fragile X syndrome, and Steinert's myotonic dystrophy. The usual mechanism for anticipation in these diseases, which is trinucleotide repeat expansions, does not explain the anticipation observed in familial PAH.

In 1997, linkage analysis in affected families allowed Nichols et al. [9] and Morse et al. [10] to localize on chromosome 2 the locus implicated in PAH development. Candidate genes in this region were then identified and mutations in the *BMPR2* (*bone morphogenetic protein receptor type 2*) gene were found in PAH patients [11, 12]. The *BMPR2* gene encodes a receptor which belongs to the transforming growth factor-β (TGF-β) superfamily.

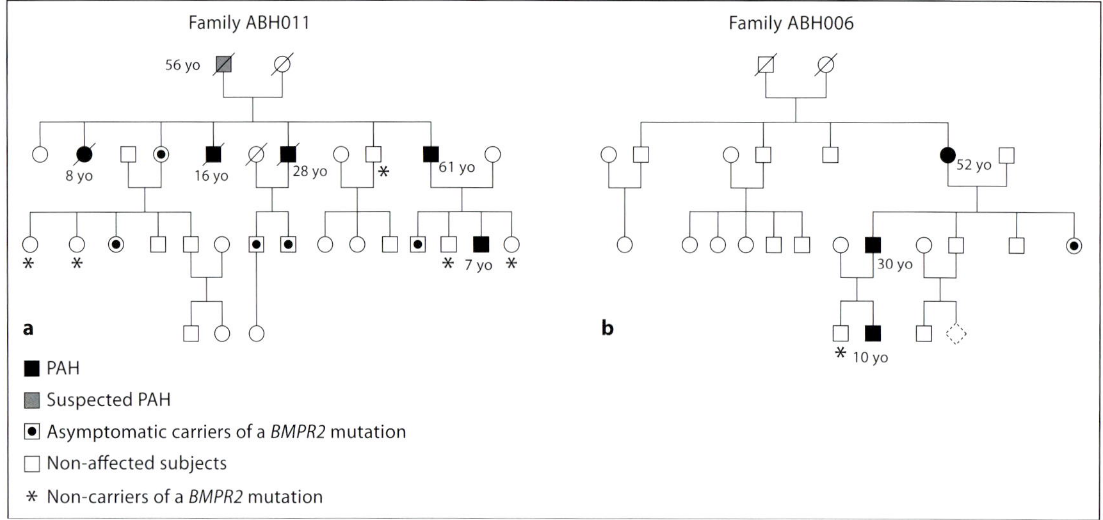

Fig. 1. Genealogical trees of two heritable forms of PAH. We can observe the incomplete penetrance of the familial mutation (**a**) and genetic anticipation of the disease (**b**). yo = Years of age at PAH diagnosis.

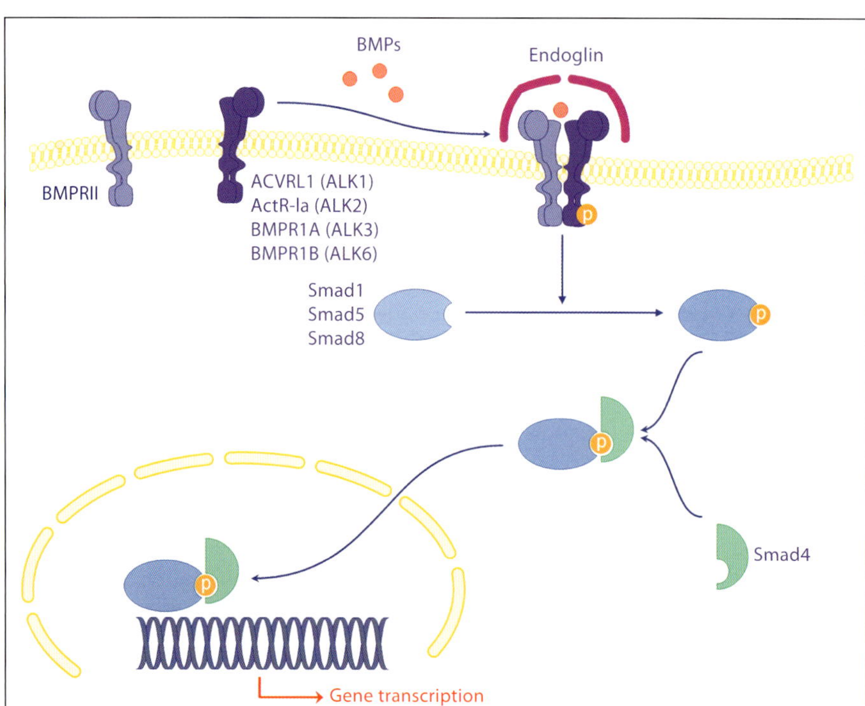

Fig. 2. BMPRII signaling pathway. BMP ligands bind on two type I receptors (ACVRL1, BMPR1A, BMPR1B, ActR-1a) leading to the formation of a heterodimer with two type II receptors (BMPRII, ActR-IIa, ActR-IIb). This complex is stabilized by an accessory protein called endoglin. Following this heteropolymerization, BMPRII receptors phosphorylate type I receptors, resulting in phosphorylation of cytoplasmic proteins called Smads (Smad1, Smad5, and Smad8). These Smad proteins bind with Smad4 in the cytosol, and this new complex is translocated into the nucleus and modulates the expression of target genes.

The development of PAH in patients displaying hereditary hemorrhagic telangiectasia (HHT) led to the identification of two other PAH predisposing genes belonging to the TGF-β superfamily: *activin A receptor type II-like 1 (ACVRL1* or *ALK1)* and *endoglin* (*ENG*; fig. 2). Mutations in the *ACVRL1* and *ENG* genes are infrequent in PAH, but frequently identified in HHT [13–20].

In the latest ESC-ERS guidelines (European Society of Cardiology and the European Respiratory Society) [4, 21–23], patients carrying a mutation of PAH predisposing genes

(*BMPR2*, *ACVRL1*, or *ENG*) and patients with a family history of PAH were grouped under the term 'heritable PAH' in Group 1 of the Clinical Classification of Pulmonary Hypertension.

BMPR2 GENE

Frequency of BMPR2 Mutations

BMPR2 mutations are frequently identified in patients with PAH considered to be idiopathic or occurring in a familial context, but rarely in patients displaying pulmonary veno-occlusive disease (PVOD) or pulmonary capillary hemangiomatosis (PCH), PAH associated with drugs or toxins [24, 25], or PAH associated with congenital heart disease [26].

In the literature, a *BMPR2* mutation is detected in 58–74% of PAH patients with a family history of the disease, and in 3.5–40% of patients with so-called idiopathic PAH [8, 18, 27–32]. PAH patients without family history of the disease and carriers of a *BMPR2* mutation have a genetic form of the disease. These patients could be the first PAH case identified in their family due to the incomplete penetrance of *BMPR2* mutations, ignorance of the medical family history, or de novo mutations.

PVOD and PCH could occur in a familial context, and several *BMPR2* mutations have been identified in these patients [22, 32–34]. However, a *BMPR2* mutation is identified in less than 25% of familial cases of PVOD/PCH.

From BMPR2 Gene to BMPRII Receptor

The *BMPR2* gene is composed of 13 exons. This gene encodes for a BMPRII membrane receptor which belongs to the TGF-β superfamily (fig. 2). This receptor consists of 1,038 amino acids and four different functional domains: a ligand-binding domain, a transmembrane domain, a kinase domain, and a cytoplasmic tail [35]. The BMPRII receptor is conserved between species; however, there is a shorter receptor isoform without a cytoplasmic tail [32, 36, 37]. This receptor was initially described as being involved in the regulation of cell growth and differentiation of bones and cartilages [38, 39]. More recently, it was shown that the BMPRII receptor is involved in the regulation of growth and apoptosis of other cells such as pulmonary smooth muscle cells and pulmonary endothelial cells.

BMPR2 mutations are responsible for a decrease in the BMPRII receptor expression and function, leading to an abnormal proliferation of pulmonary smooth muscle cells [8, 40]. Moreover, this decrease may promote apoptosis of endothelial cells, favoring the emergence of apoptosis-resistant endothelial cells and the formation of plexiform lesions which are specific to PAH [41].

Bone Morphogenetic Protein Signaling Pathway

BMPRII's ligands, the bone morphogenetic proteins (BMPs), are cytokines regulating growth, differentiation, and apoptosis of cells, such as pulmonary smooth muscle cells and pulmonary endothelial cells. Moreover, BMPs play a role in cell differentiation during embryogenesis, and in the maintenance and repair of adult tissues [39, 42, 43]. BMPs bind on two type I receptors (ACVRL1, BMPR1A, BMPR1B, ActR-1a) leading to the formation of a heterodimer with two type II receptors (BMPRII, ActRIIa, ActRIIb). This complex is stabilized by an accessory protein called endoglin. Following this heteropolymerization, type II receptors phosphorylate type I receptors, resulting in phosphorylation of cytoplasmic proteins called Smads (Smad1, Smad5, Smad8). These Smad proteins then bind with Smad4 in the cytosol, and this new complex is translocated into the nucleus and modulates the expression of target genes [43, 44] (fig. 2).

Mutations of the BMPR2 Gene

BMPR2 mutations are described in all exons, except exon 13. Mutation types are missense, truncating, large rearrangement, splice defect, or mutations in the promoter of the gene [22, 31, 45]. They are present only in the heterozygous state; knockout mice for *BMPR2* gene are not viable and die before gastrulation [46]. Two studies published in 2002 by Rudarakanchana et al. [47] and Nishihara et al. [48] showed that *BMPR2* mutations interrupt the signaling pathway BMP/Smad in different ways. Indeed, these authors showed that a substitution of a cysteine in the ligand-binding domain or in the kinase domain reduces the export of the receptor to the cell membrane. In this case, the PAH phenotype is due to haploinsufficiency (the expression of a single copy of the *BMPR2* gene does not allow sufficient cell function). On the contrary, other mutations in the kinase domain allow the translation of a protein able to reach the cell surface, but this protein has lost its ability to phosphorylate type 1 receptors. In this case, PAH phenotype is due to a dominant negative effect of the mutated receptor on wild-type (WT) receptor (the mutated receptor will affect the proper functioning of the nonmutated receptor). Furthermore, receptors encoded by a *BMPR2* gene with missense mutations affecting the BMPRII cytoplasmic tail are able to reach the cell surface, but are unable to activate the Smad pathway [49]. Finally, Austin et al. [50] demonstrated that truncating mutations are degraded by nonsense-mediated decay, a mRNA surveillance mechanism that detects and degrades mRNA transcripts containing premature termination codons, leaving only the WT mRNA detectable. In this case, the PAH phenotype is due to haploinsufficiency. By contrast, missense mutations escape nonsense-mediated decay resulting in stable transcript that may produce dominant negative proteins [51, 52].

Involvement of the BMPRII Receptor in Cellular Function

In situ hybridization has shown that BMPRII receptors are expressed in pulmonary endothelial cells and macrophages, and to a lesser extent in pulmonary smooth muscle cells and fibroblasts [53]. A decrease of BMPRII pulmonary expression in heritable and idiopathic PAH patients compared to controls has been observed [53].

Several research groups are interested in the involvement of the *BMPR2* gene and its mutation in the cellular dysfunction observed in idiopathic and heritable PAH. Studies have shown a decrease in Smads1/5 pathway activity in pulmonary smooth muscle cells of PAH patient carriers or noncarriers of a *BMPR2* mutation [54, 55]. This decrease may lead to reduced ability to inhibit the proliferation of pulmonary smooth muscle cells, explaining in part the development of pulmonary arterial lesions observed in idiopathic and heritable PAH patients. Furthermore, when exposed to VEGF, bFDF, hEGF, and IGF-1, endothelial cells of idiopathic PAH patients proliferate and migrate more than endothelial cells of control subjects [56]. Finally, BMPs may protect endothelial cells from apoptosis [41]. Indeed, it was observed that pulmonary artery endothelial cells with *BMPR2* gene silencing increased the basal level of apoptosis. These results support the hypothesis that mutations in *BMPR2* gene could lead to increase pulmonary endothelial cells apoptosis. This could be a possible initiating mechanism in the pathogenesis of PAH.

Studies of PAH animal models have confirmed the involvement of *BMPR2* mutations in PAH development. Indeed, West et al. [57] showed the development of pulmonary vascular disease in mice expressing a dominant negative form of *BMPR2,* specifically in their pulmonary smooth muscle cells. These mice developed increased pulmonary artery pressure, pulmonary arterial muscularization, and a right ventricular hypertrophy. More recently, Hong et al. [58] showed that deletion of the *BMPR2* gene in pulmonary endothelial cells predisposes mice to the development of PAH. However, these animal models do not reproduce severe PAH as observed in human heritable forms of the disease.

Penetrance of BMPR2 Mutations

Penetrance of *BMPR2* mutations is the frequency of PAH occurrence in *BMPR2* mutation carriers. It was estimated that only 20% of *BMPR2* mutation carriers will develop the disease during their life [32, 59]. Furthermore, BMPRII immunostaining in normal lungs showed that BMPRII expression is prominent on vascular endothelium, with minimal expression in airway and arterial smooth muscles. However, BMPRII is markedly reduced in the peripheral lung of PAH patients, especially in those with a heterozygous *BMPR2* mutation [53]. These findings support the role of the BMPRII receptor in PAH development, but even if a decrease in the expression of BMPRII receptor is necessary, it does not seem sufficient to the development of PAH. Other factors, genetic or environmental, may contribute to disease development.

Anorexigen exposure, particularly to fenfluramine derivatives taken for more than 3 months, is known to be a definite risk factor for PAH. Humbert et al. [24] demonstrated that PAH patients carrying a *BMPR2* mutation had a shorter duration of fenfluramine exposure before illness than PAH patients without identified mutation. These observations may suggest that a *BMPR2* mutation combined with exposure to fenfluramine derivative exposure greatly increases the risk of developing severe PAH [24, 25].

Several studies support the involvement of additional genetic factors in the development of idiopathic and heritable PAH. Hamid et al. [60] showed a decreased of WT *BMPR2* transcripts in LB cell lines from affected carriers of a *BMPR2* mutation compared to unaffected carriers of a *BMPR2* mutation. These findings suggest that levels of expression of WT *BMPR2* allele transcripts is important in the pathogenesis of PAH caused by nonsense-mediated decay mutations. A posttranscriptional mechanism by micro-RNAs (a single-stranded RNA specifically binding to mRNA to guide its degradation) was suspected to be involved in the decreased expression of the WT allele of the *BMPR2* gene [61, 62]. Indeed, Qin et al. [62] demonstrated that the BMPRII receptor is a direct target of miR-21, and also showed that the BMPRII level correlates inversely with the amount of miR-21. Similarly, Brock et al. [61] showed the involvement of miR-17/92 in the recognition and degradation of *BMPR2* mRNA, and demonstrated that the miR-17/92 cluster is modulated by IL-6, a cytokine involved in the pathogenesis of PAH [63–66].

Estrogen metabolites, potent mitogen for smooth muscle cells, are involved in the development of PAH [67, 68]. Indeed, cytochrome P450 1B1 (CYP1B1), which is highly expressed in lungs (likely in endothelial cells) and reduces local concentration of estrogen, is reduced in female PAH patients carrying a *BMPR2* mutation compared to asymptomatic female carriers of a *BMPR2* mutation [67]. Austin et al. [68] demonstrated that there is a fourfold higher penetrance of *BMPR2* mutations among subjects homozygous for the WT genotype (N/N) than those with N/S or S/S genotypes of the *CYP1B1* gene.

Finally, Eddahibi et al. [69] showed that the L-allelic variant of the 5-HTT gene promoter, which is associated with 5-HTT overexpression and increased pulmonary artery smooth muscle cell growth, was present in the homozygous form in 65% of patients, but in only 27% of controls. However, these results on serotonin transporter polymorphisms have not been confirmed in recent studies [70, 71].

Other Genes Involved in the TGF-β Signaling Pathway and the Development of Pulmonary Arterial Hypertension

ACVRL1 and ENG Genes

HHT is characterized by mucocutaneous telangiectases, recurrent epistaxes, and macroscopic arteriovenous malformations, particularly in the pulmonary, hepatic, and cerebral circulation [72]. When present, pulmonary arteriovenous malformations may create clinically significant right-to-left shunts, causing hypoxemia, paradoxical embolism, stroke, and cerebral abscesses. HHT is inherited in an autosomal dominant fashion with late-onset penetrance and nearly complete penetrance (97%) at the age of 60 years [73]. Several genes have been implicated in the pathogenesis of HHT, including activin A receptor type II-like 1 (*ACVRL1* or *ALK-1*) located on chromosome 12, *ENG* on chromosome 9, *MADH4* (encoding *SMAD4*, whereby mutations also lead to juvenile polyposis), and two new loci (HHT3 and HHT4) mapped on chromosomes 5 and 7 [72, 74, 75].

In HHT patients, postcapillary pulmonary hypertension (PH) may develop as a consequence of a hyperkinetic state resulting in a high cardiac output heart failure. However, HHT is also associated with a precapillary pattern of PH that is histologically indistinguishable from idiopathic PAH [76]. The development of PAH in HHT patients allowed for the identification of two other PAH predisposing genes encoding for proteins belonging to the TGF-β superfamily and binding to the BMPRII receptor: the *ACVRL1* gene (or *ALK1)* encoding for a type 1 receptor, and *ENG* encoding an accessory protein (fig. 2). Mutations in these two genes are infrequent in PAH, but are frequently identified in HHT [13–20].

Smad8 Gene

Shintani et al. [77] described a truncating mutation in *Smad8* gene in a 8-year-old boy with idiopathic PAH occurring in a potential familial context. Indeed, two of his brothers and sisters died because of pulmonary diseases at 2 and 13 years of age. The patient's father, a carrier of the *Smad8* mutation, was asymptomatic, suggesting the incomplete penetrance of this mutation. Mutations in the *Smad8* gene have never been described in other cases of PAH or other diseases. Moreover, in our center no *Smad8* mutations were identified in 20 families in whom no mutations in PAH predisposing genes (*BMPR2*, *ACVRL1*, and *ENG*) were identified. The *Smad8* gene encodes for a Smad8 protein, a *receptor-regulated Smad* (R-Smad). This protein is regulated by receptors belonging to the TGF-β superfamily, suggesting a role of this gene in the development of PAH. Indeed, like Smad1 and Smad5, Smad8 is phosphorylated by type I receptors. When Smad8 is phosphorylated, Smad8 associates with the Co-Smad Smad4, and this complex is translocated into the nucleus where it regulates the transcription of target genes (fig. 2). Furthermore, Huang et al. [78] emphasized the potent role of *Smad8* mutations in the PAH development, demonstrating that mice carriers of a *Smad8* mutation had a pulmonary vascular remodeling with a medial thickening of distal pulmonary arteries.

Pulmonary Hypertension and Neurofibromatosis Type 1

Neurofibromatosis type 1 (NF1) or Von Recklinghausen disease, is a genetic disease with an incidence of approximately 1 per 2,500 individuals, and is transmitted as an autosomal dominant and fully penetrant trait with no gender predominance. The *NF1* gene, responsible for NF1, is a tumor suppressor gene encoding for a cytoplasmic protein named neurofibromin. NF1 is characterized by a number of distinct clinical features, including café-au-lait spots, neurofibromas, axillary or groin freckling, bone deformities, learning disabilities, short stature, and macrocephaly. In rare cases, vascular lesions involving medium- and large-sized arteries and veins such as vasculopathy aortic valve stenosis, coarctation of the abdominal aorta, renal artery stenosis, and aneurysms of the cerebral, carotid, renal, vertebral arteries and of the aorta were identified in patients displaying NF1. Malignant tumors such as pheochromocytomas, gliomas, and juvenile chronic myeloid leukemia can also occur in the course of the disease

Precapillary PH is a rare and severe complication of NF1, initially described in patients with advanced parenchymal lung disease which may complicate the course of NF1. In the French Network of Pulmonary Hypertension, we identified 8 patients with NF1 and precapillary PH. All patients were carriers of a *NF1* gene mutation, and no *BMPR2* point mutation or large size rearrangements were identified. We showed that PH occurred late in the course of NF1 (median age 62 years, range: 53–68). At diagnosis of PH, patients had severe hemodynamic impairment and the impact of PH therapy was limited with poor outcomes. Most patients had associated parenchymal lung disease, but some had no or mild lung involvement with disproportionate pulmonary vascular disease [79]. In the literature, plexiform pulmonary arteriopathy similar to that observed in idiopathic PAH was described in NF1. In the most recent update of the PH clinical classification, NF1-associated PH is listed in Group 5, corresponding to a cause of PH with unclear and/or multifactorial mechanisms [3].

Table 1. Key elements of decree 2000-570 (23 June 2000) establishing the conditions for prescribing and conducting reviews of the genetic characteristics of a person and his/her identification by genetic fingerprinting for medical purposes

- Informed consent is mandatory
- The person concerned can refuse to be informed of the genetic results
- Only the prescribing physician is authorized to communicate the test results
- For asymptomatic relatives, the consultation must be carried out by a doctor with clinical and genetic expertise, working in a multidisciplinary team
- Genetic testing may only be undertaken on a minor if he/she or his/her family derives an immediate therapeutic or preventative benefit.

Genetic Counseling and Testing

The establishment of a genetic counseling in the French PAH Referral Center (Hôpital Antoine Béclère, AP-HP, Université Paris Sud 11, Clamart) allows us to offer genetic screening to all patients with PAH considered to be idiopathic or due to PVOD/PCH with or without family history of these diseases, and also to patients with PAH induced by anorexigen exposure. Genetic analysis is performed in the oncogenetics and angiogenetics laboratory of Pitié Salpêtrière Hospital. Genetic counseling follows the recommendations of decree 2000-570 of 23 June 2000, setting the conditions for prescribing and conducting reviews of the genetic characteristics of a person and his identification by genetic fingerprinting for medical purposes and to amend the public health code (table 1).

Genetic screening of the *BMPR2* gene (point mutations and large rearrangements) is proposed to all patients with PAH considered to be idiopathic, or due to PVOD or PCH with or without family history of these diseases, and also to patients with PAH induced by anorexigen exposure. Genetic screening of *ACVRL1* and *ENG* genes (point mutations and large rearrangements) is done in patients with a family history of PAH or PVOD/PCH in whom no mutations in *BMPR2* gene were identified. Moreover, because of a complete penetrance of *ACVRL1* and *ENG* mutations for HHT at an advanced age, personal and family clinical signs of the disease are investigated in all patients and genetic screening of *ACVRL1* and *ENG* genes is done for patients under 30 years of age or when signs of HHT are found. If no mutations in *BMPR2*, *ACVRL1*, and *ENG* genes are identified in patients with a family history of PAH or PVOD/PCH, a search for mutations in the *BMPR2* gene promoter and in *Smad8* gene is made.

This screening strategy allowed us to identify PAH patients with a heritable condition, and therefore the families at risk for this disease. When a mutation in PAH predisposing genes is identified in a patient, genetic counseling and a presymptomatic diagnosis are available for his/her relatives. This presymptomatic diagnosis requires a multidisciplinary approach involving geneticists, pulmonologists, genetic counselors, psychologists, and nurses. During genetic counseling, relatives are informed about their risks of carrying the familial mutation, their risk of developing the disease, and the transmission of the mutation to their progeny. They also have comprehensive information about PAH symptoms, disease characteristics, and the prognosis.

In February 2011, 501 patients underwent genetic counseling. Of the patients we tested, 434 were suffering from PAH (87 with a family history of the disease and 347 without known family history) and 67 were suffering from PVOD or HCP (13 with a family history of the disease). A mutation was identified in 73 patients with a family history of PAH (84%; 69 *BMPR2* mutations and 4 *ACVRL1* mutations) and in 58 patients with PAH considered as idiopathic (17%; 52 *BMPR2* mutations and 6 *ACVRL1* mutations; fig. 3). No mutations were identified in 16% of patients with a family history of PAH (fig. 3). Regarding patients with PVOD or PCH, a *BMPR2* mutation was identified in only 1 patient out of the 54 who had no known family history of the disease (2%), and in 3 patients out of the 13 who had a family history of MVOP/HCP (23%; fig. 3). Moreover, among the 434 PAH patients, 60 had a known history of anorexigen exposure, of which 9 were carriers of a *BMPR2* mutation. Among the 67 PVOD/PCH patients, 3 had a known history of anorexigen exposure, but were not carriers of a *BMPR2* mutation.

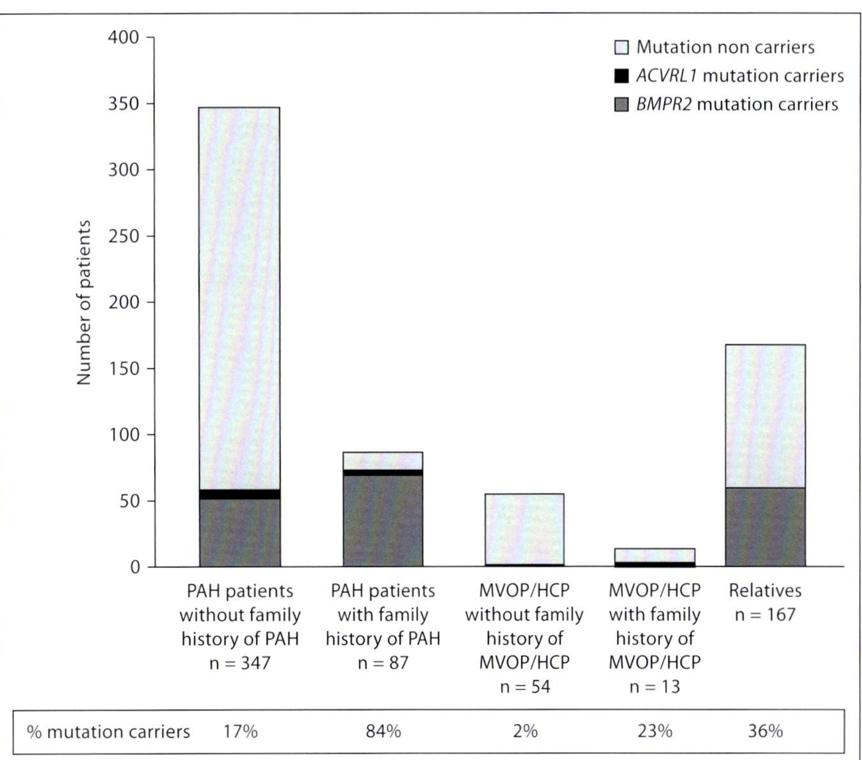

Fig. 3. Frequency of mutations in *BMPR2* and *ACVRL1* genes in patients with PAH considered to be idiopathic or due to PVOD or PCH with or without family history of the disease and also in their relatives.

Furthermore, 167 relatives requested a presymptomatic diagnosis. This allowed us to identify 60 asymptomatic carriers of a mutation in PAH predisposing genes (36%; 59 carriers of a *BMPR2* mutation and 1 carrier of an *ACVRL1* mutation). These asymptomatic carriers are at high risk of developing PAH (fig. 3).

Finally, in the French PAH Referral Center, an *ENG* mutation was identified in 1 PAH patient. This patient was also exposed to dexfenfluramine for a period of 10 months [19].

Interests and Limitations of Genetic Counseling

As we have seen, when a mutation in PAH predisposing genes is identified in a patient, genetic counseling and a presymptomatic diagnosis are available for their relatives. This presymptomatic diagnosis allowed us to identify asymptomatic carriers of the familial mutation who are at high risk of developing PAH. However, because of incomplete penetrance of the *BMPR2* mutations, it is not possible to identify which carrier of a *BMPR2* mutation will develop PAH. Moreover, neither preventive nor curative treatment of the disease is available, and associated factors, genetic or environmental, contributing to the occurrence of PAH in these mutation carriers are still unknown. Thus, genetic testing in relatives can remove the doubt of being a carrier or not of the familial mutation, which can be unbearable. However, mutation carriers will face other fears and uncertainties because among asymptomatic mutation carriers we cannot determine who will develop the disease, the age of onset, or the progression of the disease. Thus, the results of genetic testing among asymptomatic mutation carriers may have a psychological impact, with feelings of guilt, fear, and anxiety, and these individuals will think of illness and death at the slightest dyspnea. The study of our cohort did reveal, however, that the result of genetic testing also has an impact on relatives who do not carry the familial mutation, with feelings of guilt, anger, cowardice, injustice, and abandonment. For all these reasons, presymptomatic diagnosis in PAH is controversial and is a subject of debate. However, it was shown that early treatment of the disease may improve clinical characteristics of PAH patients and could prevent deterioration [82–84].

Presymptomatic screening can be interesting because clinical follow-up of asymptomatic carriers of a *BMPR2* mutation could lead to early diagnosis of the disease in high-risk relatives. Therefore, in the French PAH Referral Center, we offer to all asymptomatic mutation carriers a program to detect the disease in an early phase. This clinical screening includes a clinical examination, an electrocardiogram, and an echocardiogram every 1–3 years or when disease symptoms occur (particularly dyspnea, chest pain, and discomfort). However, the arguments for this recommendation are not validated and a hospital research program [Programme Hospitalier de Recherche Clinique (PHRC) DELPHI-2] will soon start in order to help us to better organize the management of presymptomatic mutation carriers.

The identification of a *BMPR2* mutation in an asymptomatic subject may also lead to consider a request for prenatal diagnosis or preimplantation diagnosis. These two techniques are used to avoid the birth of an individual with a mutation causing a serious disease. Prenatal diagnosis allows determining in utero if the fetus is carrier of the familial mutation. If a mutation is found, a medical abortion could be proposed. Preimplantation diagnosis is a medically assisted reproduction with selection and implantation of embryos who are not carriers of the familial mutation. These techniques are used in other diseases such as Huntington's disease or cystic fibrosis, but they are still a subject of debate in PAH because of the low penetrance of *BMPR2* mutations. Due to the incomplete penetrance of *BMPR2* mutations and the potential impact of abortion on parents, our group is in favor of the technique of preimplantation diagnosis in heritable PAH after collegial discussion. Currently, preimplantation diagnosis is not proposed when the woman carries the familial mutation because of the risk of occurrence of the disease in case of pregnancy and our ignorance of the effect of ovarian stimulation in females with a *BMPR2* mutation.

Characteristics of Patients Displaying Heritable Pulmonary Arterial Hypertension

Characteristics of Patients Carrying a BMPR2 Mutation

The analysis of clinical, functional, and hemodynamic characteristics of PAH patients indicates that PAH patients carrying a *BMPR2* mutation develop the disease 10 years earlier than noncarriers and have a more severe hemodynamic compromise at diagnosis [27, 28, 76]. A recent report by Austin et al. [50] suggested that this may only be the case for females. However, we found in our largest cohort that this is also the case for male PAH patients [85].

Moreover, we observed a trend for more severe prognosis of the disease in males, and particularly in those carrying a *BMPR2* mutation [82, 83, 85]. Austin et al. [50] showed an implication of *BMPR2* mutation types (missense, truncating, large rearrangement, or splice defect) in the phenotypic development of the disease. This result was not confirmed in our cohort [85]. Finally, PAH mostly occurs in females irrespective of *BMPR2* mutation status. To explain overrepresentation of PAH female patients, it was suggested that estrogens and estrogen metabolism might participate in the pathogenesis of PAH [67, 68].

Characteristics of Patients Carrying an ACVRL1 Mutation

The analysis of clinical, functional, and hemodynamic characteristics of PAH patients carrying an *ACVRL1* mutation indicates that these patients are significantly younger at PAH diagnosis as compared with PAH patients carrying a *BMPR2* mutation and PAH patients without identified mutation [76]. PAH patients carrying an *ACVRL1* mutation have better hemodynamic status at diagnosis than *BMPR2* mutation carriers, but have shorter survival when compared with other patients despite similar treatment [76]. These observations suggest more rapid disease progression in *ACVRL1* mutation carriers [76]. Although *ACVRL1* mutations predispose to HHT, PAH may develop in *ACVRL1* mutation carriers without obvious manifestations of HHT. Thus, PAH may be the first or only manifestation of HHT [76].

Perspectives

Some heritable PAH, PVOD, and PCH remain without biomolecular explanations. Indeed, no mutations in PAH predisposing genes were identified in 16% of PAH patients with familial history of the disease or in 75% of PVOD/PCH patients with familial history of PVOD/PCH. These observations suggest that other genes may be involved in PAH/PVOD/PCH development, or that current techniques do not allow the identification of all abnormalities in genes known to predispose to PAH. In order to identify new genes potentially implicated in the PAH development, a genome-wide association study was set up. This study consists of analyzing and comparing genomes of controls and PAH patients in order to find an association of one or more haplotype with the disease.

Conclusion

To date, it is well known that *BMPR2*, *ACVRL1*, and *ENG* mutations predispose to PAH development, and a lot of studies allowed us to understand the implication of these mutations in the pathophysiology of this rare disease. Genetic counseling is an important activity of the PAH French Network. Thus, in the French PAH Referral Center, genetic screening is proposed to all patients with PAH considered to be idiopathic, or due to PVOD or PCH with or without family history of these diseases, and also to patients with PAH induced by anorexigen exposure. This allowed us to identify PAH patients with a heritable condition, analyze their clinical characteristics, and offer presymptomatic screening to their relatives. In our center, asymptomatic relatives carrying a *BMPR2* mutation could benefit from a clinical screening, if they wish, because of their high risk to develop PAH.

Acknowledgements

We thank the association HTAP France for its support.

References

1 Dresdale DT, Michtom RJ, Schultz M: Recent studies in primary pulmonary hypertension, including pharmacodynamic observations on pulmonary vascular resistance. Bull NY Acad Med 1954;30:195–207.

2 Humbert M, Sitbon O, Chaouat A, et al: Pulmonary arterial hypertension in France: results from a national registry. Am J Respir Crit Care Med 2006;173:1023–1030.

3 Simonneau G, Robbins IM, Beghetti M, et al: Updated clinical classification of pulmonary hypertension. J Am Coll Cardiol 2009;54(1 suppl): S43–S54.

4 Galie N, Hoeper MM, Humbert M, et al: Guidelines for the diagnosis and treatment of pulmonary hypertension. Eur Respir J 2009;34:1219–1263.

5 Loyd JE, Primm RK, Newman JH: Familial primary pulmonary hypertension: clinical patterns. Am Rev Respir Dis 1984;129:194–197.

6 Loyd J, Butler MG, Foround TM, Conneally PM, Philips JA, Newman JH: Genetic anticipation and abnormal gender ratio at birth in familial primary pulmonary hypertension. Am J Respir Crit Care Med 1995;152:93–97.

7 Sztrymf B, Yaici A, Girerd B, Humbert M: Genes and pulmonary arterial hypertension. Respiration 2007;74:123–132.

8 Machado RD, Eickelberg O, Elliott CG, et al: Genetics and genomics of pulmonary arterial hypertension. J Am Coll Cardiol 2009;54(1 suppl): S32–S42.

9 Nichols WC, Koller DL, Slovis B, et al: Localization of the gene for familial primary pulmonary hypertension to chromosome 2q31–32. Nat Genet 1997;15:277–280.

10 Morse JH, Jones AC, Barst RJ, Hodge SE, Wilhelmsen KC, Nygaard TG: Mapping of familial primary pulmonary hypertension locus (PPH1) to chromosome 2q31-q32. Circulation 1997;95:2603–2606.

11 Lane KB, Machado RD, Pauciulo MW, et al: Heterozygous germline mutations in BMPR2, encoding a TGF-beta receptor, cause familial primary pulmonary hypertension. The International PPH Consortium. Nat Genet 2000;26:81–84.

12 Deng Z, Morse JH, Slager SL, et al: Familial primary pulmonary hypertension (gene PPH1) is caused by mutations in the bone morphogenetic protein receptor-II gene. Am J Hum Genet 2000;67:737–744.

13 Trembath RC, Thomson JR, Machado RD, et al: Clinical and molecular genetic features of pulmonary hypertension in patients with hereditary hemorrhagic telangiectasia. N Engl J Med 2001; 345:325–334.

14 Harrison RE, Flanagan JA, Sankelo M, et al: Molecular and functional analysis identifies ALK-1 as the predominant cause of pulmonary hypertension related to hereditary haemorrhagic telangiectasia. J Med Genet 2003;40:865–871.

15 Harrison RE, Berger R, Haworth SG, et al: Transforming growth factor-beta receptor mutations and pulmonary arterial hypertension in childhood. Circulation 2005;111:435–441.

16 Abdalla SA, Gallione CJ, Barst RJ, et al: Primary pulmonary hypertension in families with hereditary haemorrhagic telangiectasia. Eur Respir J 2004;23:373–377.

17 Fujiwara M, Yagi H, Matsuoka R, et al: Implications of mutations of activin receptor-like kinase 1 gene (ALK1) in addition to bone morphogenetic protein receptor II gene (BMPR2) in children with pulmonary arterial hypertension. Circ J 2008;72:127–133.

18 Girerd B, Montani D, Coulet F, et al: Clinical outcomes of pulmonary arterial hypertension in patients carrying an ACVRL1 (ALK1) mutation. Am J Respir Crit Care Med 2010;181:851–861.

19 Chaouat A, Coulet F, Favre C, et al: Endoglin germline mutation in a patient with hereditary haemorrhagic telangiectasia and dexfenfluramine associated pulmonary arterial hypertension. Thorax 2004;59:446–448.

20 Smoot LB, Obler D, McElhinney D, et al: Clinical features of pulmonary arterial hypertension in young people with an ALK1 mutation and hereditary hemorrhagic Telangiectasia. Arch Dis Child 2009;94:506–511.

21 Galie N, Hoeper MM, Humbert M, et al: Guidelines for the diagnosis and treatment of pulmonary hypertension: the Task Force for the Diagnosis and Treatment of Pulmonary Hypertension of the European Society of Cardiology (ESC) and the European Respiratory Society (ERS), endorsed by the International Society of Heart and Lung Transplantation (ISHLT). Eur Heart J 2009;30:2493–2537.

22 Aldred MA, Vijayakrishnan J, James V, et al: BMPR2 gene rearrangements account for a significant proportion of mutations in familial and idiopathic pulmonary arterial hypertension. Hum Mutat 2006;27:212–213.

23 Montani D, O'Callaghan D, Jaïs X, et al: Implementing the ESC/ERS pulmonary hypertension guidelines: real-life cases from a national referral centre. Eur Respir Rev 2009;18:231–249.

24 Humbert M, Deng Z, Simonneau G, et al: BMPR2 germline mutations in pulmonary hypertension associated with fenfluramine derivatives. Eur Respir J 2002;20:518–523.

25 Souza R, Humbert M, Sztrymf B, et al: Pulmonary arterial hypertension associated with fenfluramine exposure: report of 109 cases. Eur Respir J 2008;31:343–348.

26 Roberts KE, McElroy JJ, Wong WPK, et al: BMPR2 mutations in pulmonary arterial hypertension with congenital heart disease. Eur Respir J 2004;24:371–374.

27 Sztrymf B, Coulet F, Girerd B, et al: Clinical outcomes of pulmonary arterial hypertension in carriers of BMPR2 mutation. Am J Respir Crit Care Med 2008;177:1377–1383.

28 Rosenzweig EB, Morse JH, Knowles JA, et al: Clinical implications of determining BMPR2 mutation status in a large cohort of children and adults with pulmonary arterial hypertension. J Heart Lung Transplant 2008;27:668–674.

29 Humbert M: Update in pulmonary hypertension 2008. Am J Respir Crit Care Med 2009 in press.

30 Aldred MA, Machado RD, James V, Morrell NW, Trembath RC. Characterization of the BMPR2 5′-untranslated region and a novel mutation in pulmonary hypertension. Am J Respir Crit Care Med 2007;176:819–824.

31 Cogan JD, Pauciulo MW, Batchman AP, et al: High frequency of BMPR2 exonic deletions/duplications in familial pulmonary arterial hypertension. Am J Respir Crit Care Med 2006;174:590–598.
32 Machado RD, Aldred MA, James V, et al: Mutations of the TGF-beta type II receptor BMPR2 in pulmonary arterial hypertension. Hum Mutat 2006;27:121–132.
33 Montani D, Achouh L, Dorfmuller P, et al: Pulmonary veno-occlusive disease: clinical, functional, radiologic, and hemodynamic characteristics and outcome of 24 cases confirmed by histology. Medicine (Baltimore) 2008;87:220–233.
34 Runo JR, Vnencak-Jones CL, Prince M, et al: Pulmonary veno-occlusive disease caused by an inherited mutation in bone morphogenetic protein receptor II. Am J Respir Crit Care Med 2003;167:889–894.
35 Durrington HJ, Morrell NW: What we know and what we would like to know about genetics and pulmonary arterial hypertension. Int J Clin Pract Suppl 2009;161:11–16.
36 Wong WK, Knowles JA, Morse JH. Bone morphogenetic protein receptor type II C-terminus interacts with c-Src: implication for a role in pulmonary arterial hypertension. Am J Respir Cell Mol Biol 2005;33:438–446.
37 Foletta V, Lim M, Soosairajah J, et al: Direct signaling by the BMP type II receptor via the cytoskeletal regulator LIMK1. J Cell Biol 2003;162:1089–1098.
38 Fujii M, Takeda K, Imamura T, et al: Roles of bone morphogenetic protein type I receptors and smad proteins in osteoblast and chondroblast differentiation. Mol Biol Cell 1999;10:3801–3813.
39 Miyazono K, Maeda S, Imamura T: BMP receptor signaling: transcriptional targets, regulation of signals, and signaling cross-talk. Cytokine Growth Factor Rev 2005;16:251–263.
40 Valdimarsdottir G, Goumans MJ, Rosendahl A, et al: Stimulation of Id1 expression by bone morphogenetic protein is sufficient and necessary for bone morphogenetic protein-induced activation of endothelial cells. Circulation 2002;106:2263–2270.
41 Teichert-Kuliszewska K, Kutryk M, Kuliszewski M, et al: Bone morphogenetic protein receptor-2 signaling promotes pulmonary arterial endothelial cell survival: implications for loss-of-function mutations in the pathogenesis of pulmonary hypertension. Circ Res 2006;98: 209–217.
42 Kawabata M, Imamura T, Miyazono K: Signal transduction by bone morphogenetic proteins. Cytokine Growth Factor Rev 1998;9:49–61.
43 Massagué J, Chen Y. Controlling TGF-beta signaling. Genes Dev 2000;14:627–644.
44 Attisano L, Wrana J: Signal transduction by the TGF-beta superfamily. Science 2002;296:1646–1647.
45 Wang H, Li W, Zhang W, et al: Novel promoter and exon mutations of the BMPR2 gene in Chinese patients with pulmonary arterial hypertension. Eur J Hum Genet 2009;17:1063–1069.
46 Beppu H, Kawabata M, Hamamoto T, et al: BMP type II receptor is required for gastrulation and early development of mouse embryos. Dev Biol 2000;221:249–258.
47 Rudarakanchana N, Flanagan JA, Chen H, et al: Functional analysis of bone morphogenetic protein type II receptor mutations underlying primary pulmonary hypertension. Hum Mol Genet 2002;11:1517–1525.
48 Nishihara A, Watabe T, Imamura T, Miyazono K: Functional heterogeneity of bone morphogenetic protein receptor-II mutants found in patients with primary pulmonary hypertension. Mol Biol Cell 2002;13:3055–3063.
49 Yu P, Beppu H, Kawai N, Li E, Bloch K: Bone morphogenetic protein (BMP) type II receptor deletion reveals BMP ligand-specific gain of signaling in pulmonary artery smooth muscle cells. J Biol Chem 2005;280:24443–24450.
50 Austin ED, Phillips JA, Cogan JD, et al: Truncating and missense BMPR2 mutations differentially affect the severity of heritable pulmonary arterial hypertension. Respir Res 2009;10:87.
51 Kuzmiak H, Maquat L: Applying nonsense-mediated mRNA decay research to the clinic: progress and challenges. Trends Mol Med 2006; 12:306–316.
52 Harries L, Bingham C, Bellanne-Chantelot C, Hattersley A, Ellard S. The position of premature termination codons in the hepatocyte nuclear factor -1 beta gene determines susceptibility to nonsense-mediated decay. Hum Genet 2005; 118:214–24.
53 Atkinson C, Stewart S, Upton PD, et al: Primary pulmonary hypertension is associated with reduced pulmonary vascular expression of type II bone morphogenetic protein receptor. Circulation 2002;105:1672–1678.
54 Morrell N, Yang X, Upton PD, et al: Altered growth responses of pulmonary artery smooth muscle cells from patients with primary pulmonary hypertension to transforming growth factor-beta1 and bone morphogenetic proteins. Circulation 2001;104:790–795.
55 Yang X, Long L, Southwood M, et al: Dysfunctional Smad signaling contributes to abnormal smooth muscle cell proliferation in familial pulmonary arterial hypertension. Circ Res 2005;96:1053–1063.
56 Masri F, Xu W, Comhair S, et al: Hyperproliferative apoptosis-resistant endothelial cells in idiopathic pulmonary arterial hypertension. Am J Physiol Lung Cell Mol Physiol 2007;293:L548–L554.
57 West J, Fagan K, Steudel W, et al: Pulmonary hypertension in transgenic mice expressing a dominant-negative BMPRII gene in smooth muscle. Circ Res 2004;94:1109–1114.
58 Hong K, Lee Y, Lee E, et al: Genetic ablation of the BMPR2 gene in pulmonary endothelium is sufficient to predispose to pulmonary arterial hypertension. Circulation 2008;118:722–730.
59 Newman JH, Wheeler L, Lane KB, et al: Mutation in the gene for bone morphogenetic protein receptor II as a cause of primary pulmonary hypertension in a large kindred. N Engl J Med 2001;345:319–324.
60 Hamid R, Cogan J, Hedges L, et al: Penetrance of pulmonary arterial hypertension is modulated by the expression of normal BMPR2 allele. Hum Mutat 2009;30:649–654.
61 Brock M, Trenkmann M, Gay R, et al: Interleukin-6 modulates the expression of the bone morphogenic protein receptor type II through a novel STAT3-microRNA cluster 17/92 pathway. Circ Res 2009;104:1184–1191.
62 Qin W, Zhao B, Shi Y, Yao C, Jin L, Jin Y: BMPRII is a direct target of miR-21. Acta Biochim Biophys Sin (Shanghai) 2009;41:618–623.
63 Selimovic N, Bergh C, Andersson B, Sakiniene E, Carlsten H, Rundqvist B: Growth factors and interleukin-6 across the lung circulation in pulmonary hypertension. Eur Respir J 2009;34:662–668.
64 Savale L, Tu L, Rideau D, et al: Impact of interleukin-6 on hypoxia-induced pulmonary hypertension and lung inflammation in mice. Respir Res 2009;10:6.
65 Steiner M, Syrkina O, Kolliputi N, Mark E, Hales C, Waxman A: Interleukin-6 overexpression induces pulmonary hypertension. Circ Res 2009;104:236–244, 28p following 244.
66 Chaouat A, Savale L, Chouaid C, et al: Role for interleukin-6 in COPD-related pulmonary hypertension. Chest 2009;136:678–687.
67 West J, Cogan J, Geraci M, et al: Gene expression in BMPR2 mutation carriers with and without evidence of pulmonary arterial hypertension suggests pathways relevant to disease penetrance. BMC Med Genomics 2008;1:45.
68 Austin ED, Cogan JD, West JD, et al: Alterations in oestrogen metabolism: implications for higher penetrance of familial pulmonary arterial hypertension in females. Eur Respir J 2009;34:1093–1099.
69 Eddahibi S, Humbert M, Fadel E, et al: Serotonin transporter overexpression is responsible for pulmonary artery smooth muscle hyperplasia in primary pulmonary hypertension. J Clin Invest 2001;108:1141–1150.
70 Willers E, Newman J, Loyd J, et al: Serotonin transporter polymorphisms in familial and idiopathic pulmonary arterial hypertension. Am J Respir Crit Care Med 2006;173:798–802.
71 Machado RD, Koehler R, Glissmeyer E, et al: Genetic association of the serotonin transporter in pulmonary arterial hypertension. Am J Respir Crit Care Med 2006;173:793–797.
72 Govani FS, Shovlin CL: Hereditary haemorrhagic telangiectasia: a clinical and scientific review. Eur J Hum Genet 2009;17:860–871.
73 Plauchu H, de Chadarévian J, Bideau A, Robert J: Age-related clinical profile of hereditary hemorrhagic telangiectasia in an epidemiologically recruited population. Am J Med Genet 1989;32:291–297.

74 Gallione CJ, Repetto GM, Legius E, et al: A combined syndrome of juvenile polyposis and hereditary haemorrhagic telangiectasia associated with mutations in MADH4 (SMAD4). Lancet 2004;363:852–859.
75 Cole SG, Begbie ME, Wallace GM, Shovlin CL: A new locus for hereditary haemorrhagic telangiectasia (HHT3) maps to chromosome 5. J Med Genet 2005;42:577–582.
76 Girerd B, Montani D, Coulet F, et al: Clinical outcomes of pulmonary arterial hypertension in patients carrying an ACVRL1 (ALK1) mutation. Am J Respir Crit Care Med 2010;181:851–861.
77 Shintani M, Yagi H, Nakayama T, Saji T, Matsuoka R: A new nonsense mutation of SMAD8 associated with pulmonary arterial hypertension. J Med Genet 2009;46:331–337.
78 Huang Z, Wang DG, Ihida-Stansbury K, Jones PL, Martin JF: Defective pulmonary vascular remodeling in Smad8 mutant mice. Hum Mol Genet 2009;18:2791–2801.
79 Montani D, Coulet F, Girerd B, et al: Pulmonary hypertension in patients with neurofibromatosis type I: from clinical observation to therapeutic perspectives drawn from molecular insights. Medicine (Baltimore) 2011;90:201–211.
80 Samuels N, Berkman N, Milgalter E, Bar-Ziv J, Amir G, Kramer MR: Pulmonary hypertension secondary to neurofibromatosis: intimal fibrosis versus thromboembolism. Thorax 1999;54:858–859.
81 Stewart DR, Cogan JD, Kramer MR, et al: Is pulmonary arterial hypertension in neurofibromatosis type 1 secondary to a plexogenic arteriopathy? Chest 2007;132:798–808.
82 Humbert M, Sitbon O, Chaouat A, et al: Survival in patients with idiopathic, familial, and anorexigen-associated pulmonary arterial hypertension in the modern management era. Circulation 2010;122:156–163.
83 Humbert M, Sitbon O, Yaici A, et al: Survival in incident and prevalent cohorts of patients with pulmonary arterial hypertension. Eur Respir J 2010;36:549–555.
84 Galie N, Rubin L, Hoeper M, et al: Treatment of patients with mildly symptomatic pulmonary arterial hypertension with bosentan (EARLY study): a double-blind, randomised controlled trial. Lancet 2008;371:2093–2100.
85 Girerd B, Montani D, Eyries M, et al: Absence of influence of gender and BMPR2 mutation type on clinical phenotypes of pulmonary arterial hypertension. Respir Res 2010;11:73.

Marc Humbert, MD, PhD
Université Paris-Sud 11, Service de Pneumologie et Réanimation Respiratoire
Hôpital Antoine-Béclère, 157, Rue de la Porte de Trivaux
FR–92140 Clamart (France)
Tel. +331 4537 4772; E-Mail marc.humbert@abc.aphp.fr

Chapter 8

Humbert M, Souza R, Simonneau G (eds): Pulmonary Vascular Disorders.
Prog Respir Res. Basel, Karger, 2012, vol 41, pp 76–84

Drug- and Toxin-Induced Pulmonary Arterial Hypertension

Laura Price[a] · Kim Bouillon[b] · S. John Wort[a] · Marc Humbert[c]

[a]Royal Brompton Hospital, Department of Critical Care, National Heart and Lung Institute, and [b]University College London, Department of Epidemiology and Public Health, London, UK; [c]Université Paris-Sud 11, Centre National de Référence de l'Hypertension Artérielle Pulmonaire, Service de Pneumologie et Réanimation Respiratoire, Hôpital Antoine-Béclère, Assistance Publique, Hôpitaux de Paris, Clamart, France

Abstract

Pulmonary arterial hypertension (PAH) is a progressive disease leading to remodeling of small pulmonary arteries. The exact pathogenesis of PAH is uncertain; however, several risk factors are likely to contribute. These include inflammatory 'hits', such as a viral infection, and inherited disorders in vascular cell growth, such as a mutation in the bone morphogenetic protein receptor type 2 gene. It has also become apparent, first through early associations and later with larger epidemiological studies, that the use of certain drugs and toxins are important in triggering PAH, especially in susceptible individuals. One of the earliest observations of drug-related PAH followed use of the stimulant appetite suppressant aminorex fumarate. Similar associations have also been reported, especially in other stimulant anorectics such as the serotonin reuptake inhibitor dexfenfluramine, as well as a range of other agents, including illegal substances. Agents are described to cause 'isolated PAH', or PAH as part of a multisystem process, such as that which followed toxic oil syndrome in the 1980s. Furthermore, some substances specifically lead to pulmonary veno-occlusive disease. All these agents have been recently categorized according to the strength of their association with PAH. Clinicians should be aware of the associations of exposure of these drugs with PAH.

Pulmonary arterial hypertension (PAH) is a progressive disease leading to remodeling of the small pulmonary arteries, resulting in an increase in pulmonary vascular resistance and premature death from right heart failure [1]. PAH and pulmonary veno-occlusive disease (PVOD), are classified in Groups 1 and 1', respectively, of the updated clinical classification of pulmonary hypertension (see table 2 in Montani and Simonneau [this vol., p. 2]) [2], and the conditions within these groups have similarities in terms of clinical manifestations, hemodynamic measures, pathological changes, and treatment. Their common histopathological features include pulmonary artery medial hypertrophy, intimal thickening, adventitial fibrosis, and plexiform lesions (in PVOD, the vascular changes predominate in small postcapillary pulmonary venules; fig. 1). Although the pathogenesis of these conditions is not fully understood, it is thought that several risk factors trigger the onset of the disease and/or worsen its progression, and these may include drugs and toxins (tables 1 and 2) [2]. Cases that are clearly precipitated by a drug or toxin are termed 'drug- and toxin-induced PAH'.

The identification of drugs and toxins as risk factors for PAH poses a great challenge to both the physician and the epidemiologist: their role in pathogenesis may be suggested from the drug and social history, and the setting up of cohort or case-control studies from large patient databases is important to assess the probability of causality. Drugs and toxins associated with PAH are listed in table 1 [2]. Agents have been described as contributing to pulmonary vascular disease as an isolated process or as part of a multisystem disorder. This chapter will review the principle drugs and toxins that have been implicated in PAH and PVOD. It should also be noted that some agents are likely to contribute to the pathophysiology of persistent pulmonary hypertension of the newborn, but a detailed description of this is beyond the scope of this article.

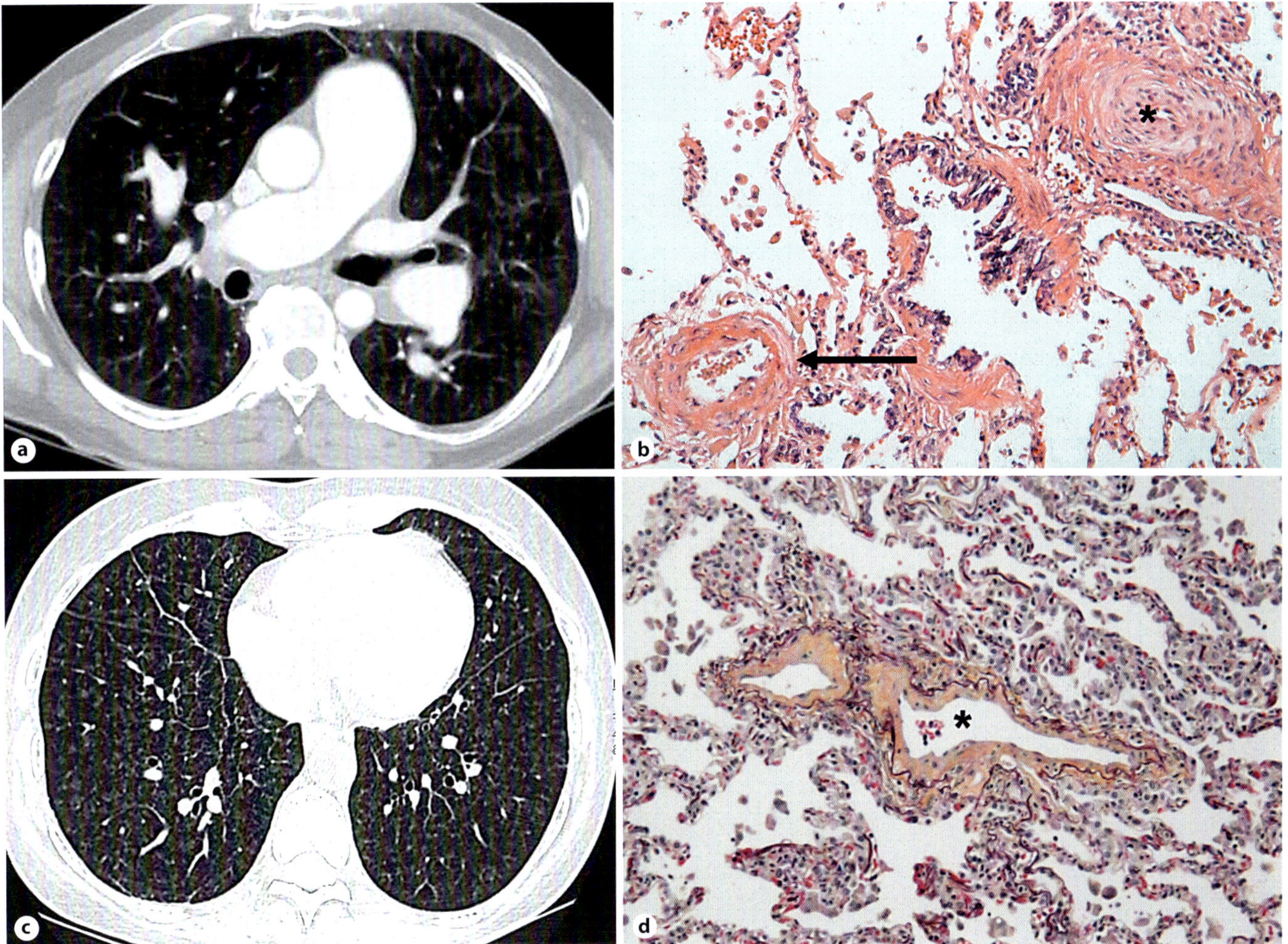

Fig. 1. Presentations of idiopathic PAH and PVOD. **a** High-resolution contrast CT showing enlargement of the central pulmonary artery and mosaic attenuation perfusion abnormality in idiopathic PAH. **b** Pathological examination of lung tissue in idiopathic PAH shows marked medial hypertrophy (arrow) and plexiform lesions (*). **c** High-resolution chest CT shows nodular centrilobular ground-glass opacities and septal lines in PVOD. **d** Pathological examination of lung tissue in PVOD shows narrowing of small pulmonary veins (* = the lumens of the pulmonary veins). Images supplied by Drs. David Montani, Peter Dorfmüller, Sophie Maitre, Dominique Musset, Gerald Simonneau, and Marc Humbert (Universite Paris-Sud 11, Hopital Antoine Beclere, Clamart, France).

Proposed Pathological Mechanisms in Drug- and Toxin-Induced Pulmonary Arterial Hypertension

There are little data on cellular mechanisms for most proposed drugs and toxins contributing to PAH. An exception may be that of the activation of serotoninergic signaling associated with stimulant appetite suppressants and other agents: serotonin [5- hydroxytryptamine (5-HT)] is a direct pulmonary vasoconstrictor and an active mitogen for smooth muscle cells, and plasma levels are elevated in PAH where abnormal handling by platelets is likely [3]. The active metabolite of dexfenfluramine is a 5-HT 2B receptor agonist, and it has been shown that PAH development requires activation of 5-HT 2B receptors [4]. Although these agents do inhibit serotonin reuptake, it is not always the case that plasma serotonin levels are increased following their use [5]. They are also thought to interact with serotonin transporters in the lung: aminorex and fenfluramine act as serotonin transporter substrates, thereby increasing extracellular serotonin [6]. Fenfluramines [7] and pergolide [8] have also been shown to cause inhibition of voltage-gated K[+] channels in pulmonary arterial smooth muscle cells, leading to vasoconstriction. The contribution of sympathomimetic agents (including stimulant anorectics and

Table 1. Drugs and toxins related to pulmonary hypertension

Drugs and toxins associated with PAH
Appetite suppressants
Aminorex
Fenfluramine
Dexfenfluramines
Benfluorex
Propylhexedrine
Phendimetrazine
Mazindol
Phenylpropanolamine
Diethylpropion
Other drugs
Thalidomide
Cyclophosphamide
Bevacizumab
Dasatinib
Pergolide
Phenformin
Leflunomide
Interferon-α_2
Alglucerase
Substance abuse
4-methyl-aminorex
Methamphetamine
Cocaine
Toluene
Herbal preparations
Hypericum perforatum (Saint John's wort)
Pyrrolizidine alkaloids
Drugs associated with PVOD
Mitomycin-C
BCNU
Cyclophosphamide
Bleomycin
MOPP/COPP
Substances associated with systemic diseases
Toxic rapeseed oil
L-tryptophan

drugs of abuse) to PAH pathophysiology is unclear, with proposed mechanisms including pulmonary vasoconstriction, fenfluramine-like effects, toxic endothelial injury, vasculitis, and dysregulation of mediators of vascular tone. It is also likely that the contribution of drugs and toxins represents a single step in the multifaceted pathological process

Table 2. Risk of pulmonary arterial hypertension associated with a selection of drugs and toxins

Definite	Likely	Possible
Toxic rapeseed oil	Amphetamines	St John's Wort
Aminorex	Methamphetamines	Cocaine
Fenfluramine	L-tryptophan	Phenylpropanolamine
Dexfenfluramine		Chemotherapeutic agents
		Selective serotonin reuptake inhibitors

that leads to PAH in susceptible individuals, such as those with a predisposing genetic tendency such as a mutation in bone morphogenetic protein receptor type 2 (see chapter by Girerd et al. [pp. 65–75]).

Drugs Associated with Isolated Pulmonary Arterial Hypertension

Appetite Suppressants

Aminorex Fumarate

Aminorex fumarate structurally resembles adrenaline and ephedrine (fig. 2), and is a potent appetite suppressant and central stimulant. Its use in the 1960s led to an outbreak of rapidly progressive PAH (then termed primary pulmonary hypertension), with a median exposure-to-onset time, when known, of 8 months (ranging from 3 weeks to over 1 year), as first described in a Swiss medical clinic [9]. A collaborative study identified 582 cases of PAH, of which 61% had used aminorex [10], and it was withdrawn from Switzerland in 1968. The incidence of PAH in patients who had used aminorex was shown to be about 0.2% overall [11] and related to the amount of drug taken. Furthermore, if discontinued early enough, a regression of PAH could be seen [12].

Fenfluramines

The fenfluramines (DL-fenfluramine and its analogue dexfenfluramine; fig. 2) are serotonin reuptake inhibitors and were widely used obesity medications. Early reports associated their use with PAH, with time from exposure to onset of symptoms varying from 3 months to 8 years [13–15]. In 1993, a French 5-year retrospective review of 73 PAH patients found that 20% had been exposed to fenfluramines [16]. A multicenter case-control study conducted in 1992, the International Primary Pulmonary Hypertension Study (IPPHS), found a strong association

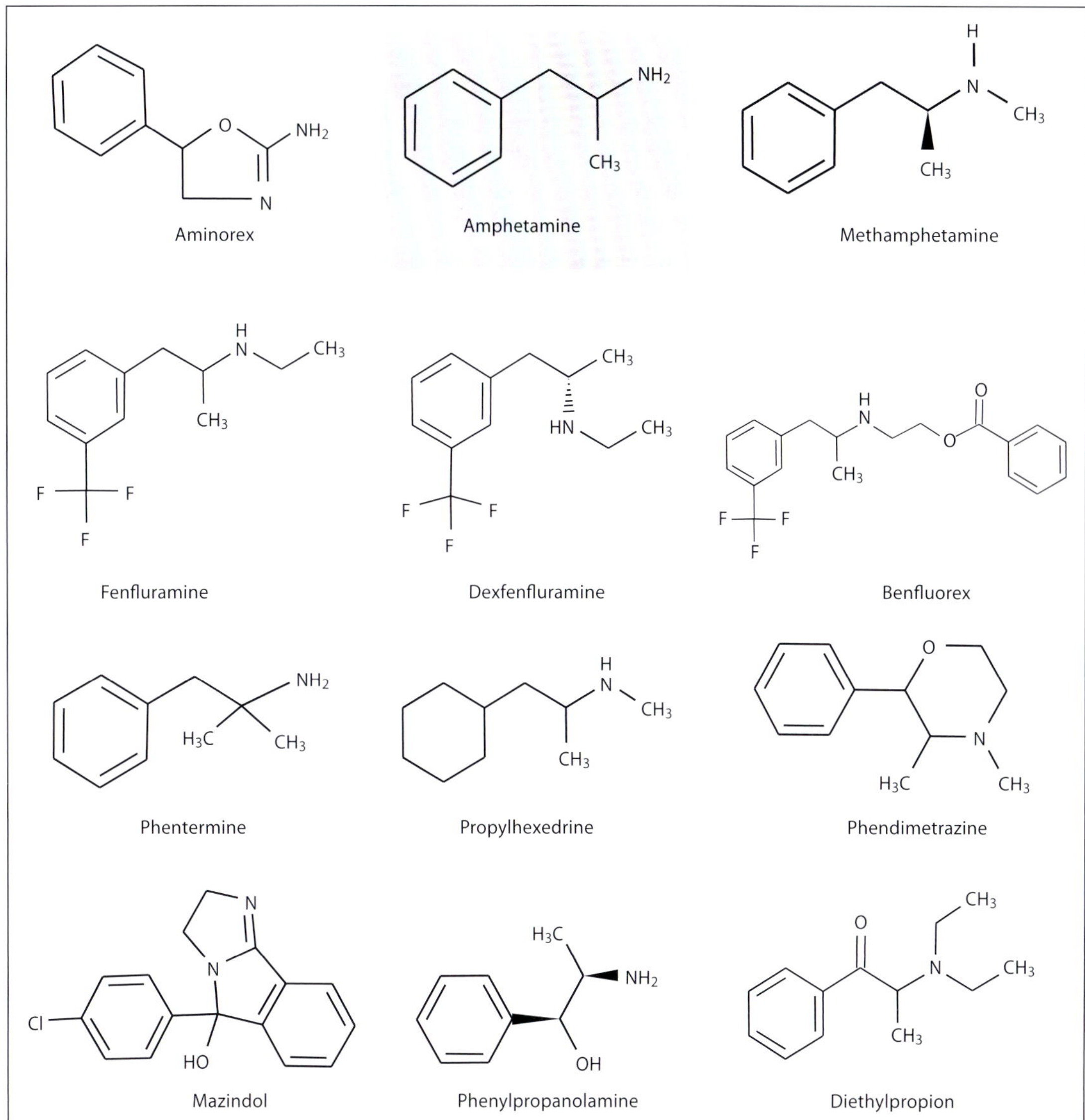

Fig. 2. Chemical structures of drugs associated with PAH.

between these appetite suppressants and PAH, with an OR (relative risk estimate) of 6.3 (95% CI: 3.0–13.20). The risk increased with duration of use (OR: 23.1 for more than 3 months; 95% CI: 6.9–77.7) and decreased after cessation of use [17]; therefore, the agents were withdrawn from France. In the UK, these cases were less common, and were thought to reflect a difference in prescribing of appetite suppressants [18].

Despite the IPPHS results, dexfenfluramine was approved for prescription use by the Food and Drug Administration in the US: case reports of fenfluramine-induced PAH followed in 1997 [19]. Additionally, a significant number of patients took the off-label combination of fenfluramine and phentermine, commonly called 'Fen-Phen'. Following the important association of valvular heart disease made with fenfluramine-phentermine [20], these agents were removed from worldwide use in 1997. Since their removal, several American [Surveillance of North American Pulmonary Hypertension (SNAP) [21], Surveillance of Pulmonary Hypertension in America (SOPHIA) [22]] and European [23, 24] observational studies have shown an association between the use of fenfluramine or dexfenfluramine and PAH, consistent with the IPPHS results [17]. More recently, analysis of the large French National PAH Registry has shown that 9.5% of patients have had a history of anorexigen exposure, mainly to fenfluramine derivatives for more than 6 months [24].

Survival implications are probably that there is no difference between patients with fenfluramine-induced PAH and those with idiopathic and heritable PAH [23], although a smaller US study did suggest that survival was worse in patients with fenfluramine-induced PAH compared to those with idiopathic or heritable PAH (median 1.2 vs. 4.1 years) [25]. Bone morphogenetic protein receptor type II mutations were found in around 10–20% of fenfluramine-induced PAH, emphasizing the possible relevance of genetic background in the occurrence of this complication [23].

Other Appetite Suppressants

Other agents that have been implicated in PAH include propylhexedrine, phendimetrazine, mazindol, phenylpropanolamine, and diethylpropion. They are mostly amphetamine-like appetite suppressants (fig. 2). It is of interest because one of the patients whose PAH followed diethylpropion use was later shown to also have a mutation of bone morphogenetic protein receptor type 2 [26].

Other Drugs

Benfluorex

Benfluorex was marketed as an adjunctive drug for patients with hypertriglyceridemia or for obese diabetics. It is structurally similar to fenfluramine (fig. 2), and has been used off-license as a slimming aid. A relationship between benfluorex use and PAH was suggested after cases of PAH surfacing following 3 months to 10 years of use in obese diabetic females [27]; however, a strong causal relationship with PAH has not yet been confirmed by larger studies. This has importantly, however, been the case with benfluorex in valvular heart disease following two major studies, resulting in its withdrawal from the market in some countries (including France and Portugal). A large cohort of diabetic patients exposed to benfluorex were followed over a 2-year period: those exposed were shown to have a significantly increased risk of aortic and mitral valvular insufficiency [28]. Furthermore, a case-control study looking specifically at 'unexplained' versus 'explained' (e.g. rheumatic) cases of mitral regurgitation in exposed patients showed a definite association with benfluorex exposure in those unexplained cases [29]. Therefore, given these clear associations in valvular heart disease, the risk of previous exposure to benfluorex in causing PAH should be formally assessed in well-designed studies using large patient databases [27].

Pergolide

Pergolide is an ergot alkaloid dopamine 1- and 2-receptor agonist used in Parkinson's disease. It has been associated with valvulopathies, and has recently been linked with a case of reversible PAH following 4 years of pergolide use [30].

Phenformin

Phenformin is a biguanide antidiabetic drug, known to cause severe lactic acidosis. In 1973, 2 cases of pulmonary hypertension were reportedly associated with phenformin treatment [31], and the drug was withdrawn from the US market in 1977. No such associations have been described with metformin.

Thalidomide

Thalidomide is an immunomodulatory agent used in combination with dexamethasone in multiple myeloma therapy. There have been several reports suggesting an association between thalidomide use and pulmonary hypertension [63, 64]. The mechanisms for this are not clear, although thalidomide is known to increase the risk of venous thromboembolism.

Cyclophosphamide

Cyclophosphamide, when used as combination chemotherapy to treat neuroblastoma and myelomonocytic leukemia, has been reported to precipitate PAH in children, confirmed as a plexogenic arteriopathy histologically, without evidence of cardiopulmonary malignancy, pulmonary vein involvement, lung fibrosis, or portal hypertension [32, 33]. The reader should be reminded, however, that cyclophosphamide has been successfully used in the treatment of PAH, complicating the course of systemic lupus erythematosus and mixed connective disease [34].

Interferon-α2

Interferon-α2 is an immunomodulator widely used in hepatitis and high-risk melanoma. Jochmann et al. [65] described a 40-year-old woman who developed a severe PAH 30 months after initiation of interferon-α2 for adjuvant treatment of spreading melanoma. Symptoms and echographic signs improved after its discontinuation. This association has been previously observed by Al-Zahrani et al. [66].

Growth Factor Inhibitors

There have been sporadic reports of growth factor inhibitors, used as part of cancer chemotherapy regimens, causing PAH. These include bevacizumab, the recombinant antivascular endothelial growth factor monoclonal antibody used to treat ovarian cancer (although notably these patients were also given cyclophosphamide) [35], and dasatinib, a tyrosine kinase inhibitor approved for treatment of chronic myeloid leukemia. In the case of dasatinib, several cases of confirmed PAH have been reported, with right ventricular size and systolic function returning to normal after stopping the agent, e.g. at 6 weeks [36] and 6 months [37]. More recently, cases of persistent PAH have been reported in dasatinib-treated patients (Montani and Humbert, submitted). It is relevant that imatinib, another tyrosine kinase inhibitor, has been studied in the treatment of idiopathic PAH [38].

Illicit Drugs

There are several known and probably many unknown illicit drugs (and their constituents) that may contribute to PAH. The importance of taking a full social and detailed drug history, including all nonprescription and street drugs, must be stressed. It may be difficult to disentangle the role of the product used from contaminants such as talc, and from that of emboli associated with intravenous drug use.

Amphetamine Derivatives

Amphetamines and methamphetamines are central nervous system stimulants (fig. 2). Amphetamines were first marked for rhinitis and asthma in the 1920s, and approved uses today include narcolepsy and attention deficit hyperactivity disorder. Although these are now controlled substances, illicit use of amphetamines and methamphetamines ('crystal meth') is prevalent. These agents may be inhaled or taken orally or by intravenous injection. A case report in 1993 described a 33-year-old man who developed PAH and died from right ventricular failure 26 months after presentation following a 10-year history of methamphetamine inhalation [39]. A recent retrospective study of 340 patients with PAH showed a significant association between these substances and idiopathic PAH compared to those with PAH and a known risk factor, with methamphetamine use being especially prevalent [40].

Cocaine

Cocaine blocks the release and reuptake of catecholamines and serotonin. It was originally developed as an anesthetic, and is now mostly used medically as a topical vasoconstrictor to facilitate nasal surgery. It is a popular drug of abuse and may be smoked, inhaled, or injected, and is associated with several well-described medical complications including myocardial infarction and stroke, and specifically pulmonary complications including alveolar hemorrhage, interstitial pneumonitis/fibrosis, and intra-alveolar edema [41]. Cocaine has been implicated in PAH: a reduction in pulmonary transfer factor is seen in cocaine smokers [42], and reversible pulmonary vasoconstriction is reported with its use [43]. Furthermore, histological studies have shown that medial hypertrophy of muscular pulmonary arteries occurs in cocaine smokers, which is unrelated to interstitial lung abnormalities such as foreign particle microembolization [42].

Other Substances

In the early 1980s, severe clinical pulmonary hypertension was reported in boys with a history of chronic glue (toluene) abuse for 6 months or more [44]. It is also of concern that 3,4-methylenedioxymethamphetamine (MDMA, 'ecstasy'), another common abused recreational drug, causes valvular myocardial cell proliferation through binding to and activating 5-HT 2B receptors in vitro similar to that induced by fenfluramine [45], although the nature of its abuse is not regular daily use.

Herbal Preparations

Hypericum perforatum

Hypericum perforatum (Saint John's wort) is a plant extract which is licensed in Europe for treating depression and anxiety. Recently, the SOPHIA study showed an association between Saint John's wort use and PAH with an OR of 3.6 (95% CI: 1.0–13.0 vs. chronic thromboembolic pulmonary hypertension) [22], thus classifying it in the 'possible' category [2].

Pyrrolizidine Alkaloids

Pyrrolizidine is a heterocyclic organic compound that forms the central chemical structure of a variety of alkaloids known collectively as pyrrolizidine alkaloids. They are hepatotoxic plants that can also cause pulmonary arterial endothelial injury leading to PAH in animals. They are named differently according to the species of plants geni *Crotalaria* and *Senecio*. Monocrotaline is found in *Crotalaria spectabilis* and fulvine in *Crotalaria fulva* [46]. Monocrotaline-induced PAH in rats is a well-described inflammatory model. In *Senecio jacobaea*, several alkaloids are found – in particular seneciphylline. Leaves and seeds of these plants are used for the preparation of bush teas, which are consumed by indigenous population for medicinal and other purposes. To our knowledge, just one case of PAH suspected to be related to the ingestion of pyrrolizidine alkaloids has been reported. In this case, a 66-year-old woman took several herbal remedies including comfrey (*Symphytum officinale*), known to contain pyrrolizidine alkaloids [47].

Drugs Associated with Pulmonary Veno-Occlusive Disease

Mitomycin-C

Mitomycin-C is used in combination as chemotherapy for solid tumors. There are case reports of histologically confirmed PVOD occurring in patients treated for metastatic cervical carcinoma [48, 49], metastatic gastric adenocarcinoma [50] and non-small cell lung cancer [51, 52]. It may also cause interstitial lung disease and hemolytic-uremia syndrome.

Other Chemotherapy Regimens

Several other regimens have been shown to induce PVOD. These include BCNU (carmustine) for treatment of glioma [53], cyclophosphamide and etoposide with autologous bone marrow transplantation for neuroblastoma [54], bleomycin for lymphocytic lymphoma [55], and MOPP and COPP or MOPP alone regimens for Hodgkin's disease [53].

It may be difficult to pick out the causality of PVOD in these complex cases, as pulmonary vascular disease may reflect the malignancy itself (e.g. Hodgkin's lymphoma [56]) as well as other types of drug-induced lung disease (e.g. mitomycin may induce interstitial pneumonitis). Furthermore, PVOD may develop following radiotherapy without any chemotherapy [57] or allogeneic bone marrow transplantation after total body irradiation [58]. Finally, a lung biopsy may be indicated to classify pulmonary hypertension in this setting, although this is likely to be contraindicated due to the very high risk.

Drugs and Toxins Associated with Systemic Diseases

Toxic Rapeseed Oil

A well-documented toxic association with pulmonary hypertension followed the ingestion of toxic oil in Spain in 1981 [59], in which contaminants of illegally refined food oil led to a syndrome of acute respiratory distress syndrome with eosinophilia and myalgia, and to pulmonary hypertension in 20% of hospitalized patients 2–4 months from onset. The causal contaminant was thought to be 3-phenylamino-1,2-propanediol (DEPAP) or related compounds. Toxic oil syndrome was defined as a clinical syndrome occurring within 8 months of exposure, and it affected 20,000 people, leading to over 300 deaths [59]. PAH was also found in 8% of longer-term survivors, with pathological changes of medial hypertrophy, intimal fibrosis, and plexiform lesions, with early perivascular inflammatory cell infiltrates [60].

L-Tryptophan

L-tryptophan is an essential amino acid used as a dietary supplement. It has been associated with eosinophilia-myalgia syndrome, and has been withdrawn from use [61]. Other clinical manifestations include pulmonary involvement (interstitial infiltrates and pleural effusions) and pulmonary hypertension. Lung biopsies of symptomatic patients 1–9 months after taking L-tryptophan showed both interstitial inflammatory infiltrate with lymphocytes and small numbers of eosinophils, and vascular changes with arterial and arteriolar medial hypertrophy [62].

Summary of the Key Issues

- Drugs and toxins related to PAH have been classified by an international expert group as 'definite', 'likely', 'possible', or 'unlikely', based on the strength of their association and their probable causal role (table 2). Several drugs and toxins listed in this chapter have not yet been categorized because of lack of evidence.
- Drugs and toxins can be associated with PAH, PVOD, or systemic diseases.
- Other than for those 'definite' risk factors, it is difficult to evaluate the role of drugs and toxins in the occurrence of PAH. This may relate to several factors, including individual susceptibility, concomitant medication, initial disease or even insidious underlying idiopathic PAH. Notably in oncology, several drugs are given concomitantly, and patients can be exposed to several lines of combination chemotherapy as well as other potentially attributable therapies during follow-up.
- When pulmonary hypertension is diagnosed, it is essential to conduct an exhaustive and systematic investigation to establish a list of prescribed and nonprescribed medications, herbal preparations, supplementary diets, and illicit drugs. This may involve establishing a certain level of trust with some patients.
- When a suspected drug or toxin was discontinued early enough, a regression of pulmonary hypertension and

right ventricular hypertrophy has been observed, at least in some reported cases.

- The risk of future epidemics of PAH due to drugs or toxins persists, as well as the unknown risk from as yet unidentified drugs and toxins. For the time being, certain amphetamine-like appetite suppressants are commonly found in over-the-counter cold and allergy remedies.
- Physicians should be encouraged to notify their appropriate regulatory authority and publish case reports when they suspect a drug/toxin of causing of PAH. These actions are particularly important when a drug is seldom used, which is the case for treatment for a rare disease.

References

1 Chin KM, Rubin LJ: Pulmonary arterial hypertension. J Am Coll Cardiol 2008;51:1527–1538.
2 Simonneau G, Robbins IM, Beghetti M, Channick RN, Delcroix M, Denton CP, et al: Updated clinical classification of pulmonary hypertension. J Am Coll Cardiol 2009;54(1 suppl):S43–S54.
3 Herve P, Launay JM, Scrobohaci ML, Brenot F, Simonneau G, Petitpretz P, et al: Increased plasma serotonin in primary pulmonary hypertension. Am J Med 1995;99:249–254.
4 Launay JM, Herve P, Peoc'h K, Tournois C, Callebert J, Nebigil CG, et al: Function of the serotonin 5-hydroxytryptamine 2B receptor in pulmonary hypertension. Nat Med 2002;8: 1129–1135.
5 Rothman RB, Redmon JB, Raatz SK, Kwong CA, Swanson JE, Bantle JP: Chronic treatment with phentermine combined with fenfluramine lowers plasma serotonin. Am J Cardiol 2000;85:913–915.
6 Rothman RB, Ayestas MA, Dersch CM, Baumann MH: Aminorex, fenfluramine, and chlorphentermine are serotonin transporter substrates. Implications for primary pulmonary hypertension. Circulation 1999;100:869–875.
7 Weir EK, Reeve HL, Huang JM, Michelakis E, Nelson DP, Hampl V, et al: Anorexic agents aminorex, fenfluramine, and dexfenfluramine inhibit potassium current in rat pulmonary vascular smooth muscle and cause pulmonary vasoconstriction. Circulation 1996;94:2216–2220.
8 Hong Z, Smith AJ, Archer SL, Wu XC, Nelson DP, Peterson D, et al: Pergolide is an inhibitor of voltage-gated potassium channels, including Kv1.5, and causes pulmonary vasoconstriction. Circulation 2005;112:1494–1499.
9 Follath F, Burkart F, Schweizer W: Drug-induced pulmonary hypertension? Br Med J 1971;1:265–266.
10 Greiser E: Epidemiologic studies on the relation between use of appetite depressants and primary vascular pulmonary hypertension (in German). Internist (Berl) 1973;14:437–442.
11 Olivari MT: Primary pulmonary hypertension. Am J Med Sci 1991;302:185–198.
12 Loogen F, Worth H, Schwan G, Goeckenjan G, Losse B, Horstkotte D: Long-term follow-up of pulmonary hypertension in patients with and without anorectic drug intake. Cor Vasa 1985;27:111–124.
13 Douglas JG, Munro JF, Kitchin AH, Muir AL, Proudfoot AT: Pulmonary hypertension and fenfluramine. Br Med J (Clin Res Ed) 1981;283:881–883.
14 McMurray J, Bloomfield P, Miller HC: Irreversible pulmonary hypertension after treatment with fenfluramine. Br Med J (Clin Res Ed) 1986;292:239–240.
15 Roche N, Labrune S, Braun JM, Huchon GJ: Pulmonary hypertension and dexfenfluramine. Lancet 1992;339:436–437.
16 Brenot F, Herve P, Petitpretz P, Parent F, Duroux P, Simonneau G: Primary pulmonary hypertension and fenfluramine use. Br Heart J 1993;70: 537–541.
17 Abenhaim L, Moride Y, Brenot F, Rich S, Benichou J, Kurz X, et al: Appetite-suppressant drugs and the risk of primary pulmonary hypertension. International Primary Pulmonary Hypertension Study Group. N Engl J Med 1996;335: 609–616.
18 Thomas SH, Butt AY, Corris PA, Egan JJ, Higenbottam TW, Madden BP, et al: Appetite suppressants and primary pulmonary hypertension in the United Kingdom. Br Heart J 1995;74:660–663.
19 Mark EJ, Patalas ED, Chang HT, Evans RJ, Kessler SC: Fatal pulmonary hypertension associated with short-term use of fenfluramine and phentermine. N Engl J Med 1997;337:602–606.
20 Connolly HM, Crary JL, McGoon MD, Hensrud DD, Edwards BS, Edwards WD, et al: Valvular heart disease associated with fenfluramine-phentermine. N Engl J Med 1997;337:581–588.
21 Rich S, Rubin L, Walker AM, Schneeweiss S, Abenhaim L: Anorexigens and pulmonary hypertension in the United States: results from the surveillance of North American pulmonary hypertension. Chest 2000;117:870–874.
22 Walker AM, Langleben D, Korelitz JJ, Rich S, Rubin LJ, Strom BL, et al: Temporal trends and drug exposures in pulmonary hypertension: an American experience. Am Heart J 2006;152:521–526.
23 Souza R, Humbert M, Sztrymf B, Jais X, Yaici A, Le Pavec J, et al: Pulmonary arterial hypertension associated with fenfluramine exposure: report of 109 cases. Eur Respir J 2008;31:343–348.
24 Humbert M, Sitbon O, Chaouat A, Bertocchi M, Habib G, Gressin V, et al: Pulmonary arterial hypertension in France: results from a national registry. Am J Respir Crit Care Med 2006;173: 1023–1030.
25 Rich S, Shillington A, McLaughlin V: Comparison of survival in patients with pulmonary hypertension associated with fenfluramine to patients with primary pulmonary hypertension. Am J Cardiol 2003;92:1366–1368.
26 Abramowicz MJ, Van Haecke P, Demedts M, Delcroix M: Primary pulmonary hypertension after amfepramone (diethylpropion) with BMPR2 mutation. Eur Respir J 2003;22:560–562.
27 Boutet K, Frachon I, Jobic Y, Gut-Gobert C, Leroyer C, Carlhant-Kowalski D, et al: Fenfluramine-like cardiovascular side-effects of benfluorex. Eur Respir J 2009;33:684–688.
28 Weill A, Paita M, Tuppin P, Fagot JP, Neumann A, Simon D, et al: Benfluorex and valvular heart disease: a cohort study of a million people with diabetes mellitus. Pharmacoepidemiol Drug Saf 2010;19:1256–1262.
29 Frachon I, Etienne Y, Jobic Y, Le Gal G, Humbert M, Leroyer C: Benfluorex and unexplained valvular heart disease: a case-control study. PLoS One 2010;5:e10128.
30 Evrard F, Dupuis M, Muller T, Jacquerye P: Isolated pulmonary hypertension and pergolide (in French). Rev Neurol (Paris) 2008;164:278–279.
31 Fahlen M, Bergman H, Helder G, Ryden L, Wallentin I, Zettergren L: Phenformin and pulmonary hypertension. Br Heart J 1973;35:824–828.
32 Bentur L, Cullinane C, Wilson P, Greenberg M, O'Brodovich H, Silver MM: Fatal pulmonary arterial occlusive vascular disease following chemotherapy in a 9-month-old infant. Hum Pathol 1991;22:1295–1298.
33 Vaksmann G, Nelken B, Deshildre A, Rey C: Pulmonary arterial occlusive disease following chemotherapy and bone marrow transplantation for leukaemia. Eur J Pediatr 2002;161:247–249.
34 Sanchez O, Sitbon O, Jais X, Simonneau G, Humbert M: Immunosuppressive therapy in connective tissue diseases-associated pulmonary arterial hypertension. Chest 2006;130:182–189.

35 Garcia AA, Hirte H, Fleming G, Yang D, Tsao-Wei DD, Roman L, et al: Phase II clinical trial of bevacizumab and low-dose metronomic oral cyclophosphamide in recurrent ovarian cancer: a trial of the California, Chicago, and Princess Margaret Hospital phase II consortia. J Clin Oncol 2008;26:76–82.
36 Rasheed W, Flaim B, Seymour JF: Reversible severe pulmonary hypertension secondary to dasatinib in a patient with chronic myeloid leukemia. Leuk Res 2009;33:861–864.
37 Mattei D, Feola M, Orzan F, Mordini N, Rapezzi D, Gallamini A: Reversible dasatinib-induced pulmonary arterial hypertension and right ventricle failure in a previously allografted CML patient. Bone Marrow Transplant 2009;43:967–968.
38 Souza R, Sitbon O, Parent F, Simonneau G, Humbert M: Long term imatinib treatment in pulmonary arterial hypertension. Thorax 2006;61:736.
39 Schaiberger PH, Kennedy TC, Miller FC, Gal J, Petty TL: Pulmonary hypertension associated with long-term inhalation of 'crank' methamphetamine. Chest 1993;104:614–616.
40 Chin KM, Channick RN, Rubin LJ: Is methamphetamine use associated with idiopathic pulmonary arterial hypertension? Chest 2006; 130:1657–1663.
41 Bailey ME, Fraire AE, Greenberg SD, Barnard J, Cagle PT: Pulmonary histopathology in cocaine abusers. Hum Pathol 1994;25:203–207.
42 Murray RJ, Smialek JE, Golle M, Albin RJ: Pulmonary artery medial hypertrophy in cocaine users without foreign particle microembolization. Chest 1989;96:1050–1053.
43 Collazos J, Martinez E, Fernandez A, Mayo J: Acute, reversible pulmonary hypertension associated with cocaine use. Respir Med 1996;90:171–174.
44 Devathasan G, Low D, Teoh PC, Wan SH, Wong PK: Complications of chronic glue (toluene) abuse in adolescents. Aust NZ J Med 1984;14:39–43.
45 Setola V, Hufeisen SJ, Grande-Allen KJ, Vesely I, Glennon RA, Blough B, et al: 3,4-methylenedioxymethamphetamine (MDMA, 'ecstasy') induces fenfluramine-like proliferative actions on human cardiac valvular interstitial cells in vitro. Mol Pharmacol 2003;63:1223–1229.
46 Kay JM: Dietary pulmonary hypertension. Thorax 1994;49(Suppl):S33–S38.
47 Gyorik S, Stricker H: Severe pulmonary hypertension possibly due to pyrrolizidine alkaloids in polyphytotherapy. Swiss Med Wkly 2009;139: 210–211.
48 Joselson R, Warnock M: Pulmonary veno-occlusive disease after chemotherapy. Hum Pathol 1983;14:88–91.
49 Knight BK, Rose AG: Pulmonary veno-occlusive disease after chemotherapy. Thorax 1985;40:874–875.
50 Waldhorn RE, Tsou E, Smith FP, Kerwin DM: Pulmonary veno-occlusive disease associated with microangiopathic hemolytic anemia and chemotherapy of gastric adenocarcinoma. Med Pediatr Oncol 1984;12:394–396.
51 Vansteenkiste JF, Bomans P, Verbeken EK, et al: Fatal pulmonary veno-occlusive disease possibly related to gemcitabine. Lung Cancer 2001;31:83–85.
52 Gagnadoux F, Capron F, Lebeau B: Pulmonary veno-occlusive disease after neoadjuvant mitomycin chemotherapy and surgery for lung carcinoma. Lung Cancer 2002;36:213–215.
53 Lombard CM, Churg A, Winokur S: Pulmonary veno-occlusive disease following therapy for malignant neoplasms. Chest 1987;92:871–876.
54 Trobaugh-Lotrario AD, Greffe B, Deterding R, Deutsch G, Quinones R: Pulmonary veno-occlusive disease after autologous bone marrow transplant in a child with stage IV neuroblastoma: case report and literature review. J Pediatr Hematol Oncol 2003;25:405–409.
55 Rose AG: Pulmonary veno-occlusive disease due to bleomycin therapy for lymphoma. Case reports. S Afr Med J 1983;64:636–638.
56 Capewell SJ, Wright AJ, Ellis DA: Pulmonary veno-occlusive disease in association with Hodgkin's disease. Thorax 1984;39:554–555.
57 Kramer MR, Estenne M, Berkman N, Antoine M, de Francquen P, Lipski A, et al: Radiation-induced pulmonary veno-occlusive disease. Chest 1993;104:1282–1284.
58 Williams LM, Fussell S, Veith RW, Nelson S, Mason CM: Pulmonary veno-occlusive disease in an adult following bone marrow transplantation. Case report and review of the literature. Chest 1996;109:1388–1391.
59 Posada de la Paz M, Philen RM, Borda AI: Toxic oil syndrome: the perspective after 20 years. Epidemiol Rev 2001;23:231–247.
60 Gomez-Sanchez MA, Mestre de Juan MJ, Gomez-Pajuelo C, Lopez JI, Diaz de Atauri MJ, Martinez-Tello FJ: Pulmonary hypertension due to toxic oil syndrome. A clinicopathologic study. Chest 1989;95:325–331.
61 Kilbourne EM: Eosinophilia-myalgia syndrome: coming to grips with a new illness. Epidemiol Rev 1992;14:16–36.
62 Tazelaar HD, Myers JL, Drage CW, King TE Jr, Aguayo S, Colby TV: Pulmonary disease associated with L-tryptophan-induced eosinophilic myalgia syndrome. Clinical and pathologic features. Chest 1990;97:1032–1036.
63 Antonioli E, Nozzoli C, Gianfaldoni G, et al: Pulmonary hypertension related to thalidomide therapy in refractory multiple myeloma. Ann Oncol 2005;16:1849–1850.
64 Hattori Y, Shimoda M, Okamoto S, et al: Pulmonary hypertension and thalidomide therapy in multiple myeloma. Br J Haematol 2005;128:885–887.
65 Jochmann N, Kiecker F, Borges AC, et al: Long-term therapy of interferon-alpha induced pulmonary arterial hypertension with different PDE-5 inhibitors: a case report. Cardiovasc Ultrasound 2005;3:26.
66 Al-Zahrani H, Gupta V, Minden MD, et al: Vascular events associated with alpha interferon therapy. Leuk Lymphoma 2003;44:471–475.

Marc Humbert, MD, PhD
Hôpital Antoine-Béclère, Service de Pneumologie
Assistance Publique – Hôpitaux de Paris, Université Paris-Sud 11
157 rue de la Porte de Trivaux, FR–92140 Clamart (France)
Tel. +33 1 45 37 47 72, E-Mail marc.humbert@abc.aphp.fr

Chapter 9

Humbert M, Souza R, Simonneau G (eds): Pulmonary Vascular Disorders.
Prog Respir Res. Basel, Karger, 2012, vol 41, pp 85–93

Idiopathic Pulmonary Arterial Hypertension and Its Prognosis in the Modern Management Era in Developed and Developing Countries

Xin Jiang[a] · Marc Humbert[b] · Zhi-Cheng Jing[a]

[a]Department of Cardio-Pulmonary Circulation, Shanghai Pulmonary Hospital, Tongji University School of Medicine, Shanghai, PR China; [b]Université Paris-Sud, Faculté de Médecine, Le Kremlin-Bicêtre, Service de Pneumologie, Hôpital Antoine Béclère, Assistance-Publique Hôpitaux de Paris, Clamart, INSERM U999, Clamart, France

Abstract

Idiopathic pulmonary arterial hypertension (IPAH) is a rare and severe disease characterized by a progressive increase of pulmonary vascular resistance without demonstrable cause, always leading to right ventricular failure and premature death. Up to now, nearly all the knowledge about IPAH, including epidemiology, demographics, clinical features, diagnosis, treatment, and prognosis, came from the large-scale registries or clinical studies in Western and developed countries. However, little is known about the status of patient with IPAH in Eastern and developing countries. Most recently, a new registry study aimed to investigate the clinical characteristics of patients with WHO Group 1 pulmonary arterial hypertension in the modern therapeutic era was performed at 9 pulmonary hypertension centers in China. This chapter reviews those large-scale registries and conducts a detail comparison of clinical characteristics of IPAH between developed and developing countries.

Idiopathic pulmonary arterial hypertension (IPAH), formerly referred to as primary pulmonary hypertension, is a rare and severe disease characterized by a progressive increase of pulmonary vascular resistance without demonstrable cause, always leading to right ventricular failure and premature death [1–3]. Since the publication of epidemiologic and survival data for patients with primary pulmonary hypertension in the NIH registry before pulmonary arterial hypertension (PAH)-specific therapies [4, 5], there has been significant progress in our understanding of the pathophysiology of PAH [6, 7] and its diagnosis [8, 9]. In recent years, three large academic observational registries from France[10], the United States [the single-center (Chicago) Pulmonary Hypertension Connection] [11], and Scotland [12] have reported country- and institutional-specific epidemiologic trends of PAH. More recently, a multicenter observational registry (54 US sites), the Registry to Evaluate Early and Long-Term PAH Disease Management (REVEAL) [13], has enrolled a large number of patients with PAH. Baseline data in the modern era for WHO Group I PAH patients presented in recent publications have a changing picture compared with the previous NIH registry [14, 15].

Advances in the management of PAH, including the assessment of patients with objective parameters and novel medical therapies, have led to improved survival in PAH, as observed in a meta-analysis of randomized controlled trials [16] and multicenter registries [17–19]. Moreover, improved survival has been identified in long-term follow-up of patients with IPAH enrolled in clinical trials and open-label studies by comparison with the NIH equation [20, 21]. However, almost all of those encouraging data were performed in Western and developed countries.

Registries of Pulmonary Arterial Hypertension in China

In 2007, a pioneer registry study in an Asian population was undertaken by Jing et al. [22]. Their study reviewed 72 patients with IPAH or familial/heritable PAH from 1999 to 2004; only 20 of these patients underwent right heart catheterization. The study reported similar demographic features, but a poorer prognosis compared with the NIH registry data. Although modern diagnostic strategies and treatment options have been available in China since 2006, the similarities and differences between patients with IPAH in Western countries and China are still unclear.

To define the clinical characteristics of the Chinese patients with WHO Group 1 PAH, and to compare these data with current Western registries, we initiated a new registry and retrospectively collected patients diagnosed as WHO Group 1 PAH from 9 pulmonary hypertension centers between May 2008 and May 2011. In this registry, a total of 1,165 patients were diagnosed as Group 1 PAH. Of these, 132 pediatric patients and 77 patients with incomplete diagnostic right heart catheterization data were excluded, and 956 adult patients were included. The patients came from 31 of the 34 provinces in China and were well distributed geographically. This registry is the first large-scale academic study to describe the baseline characteristics of patients with WHO Group 1 PAH among a population in a developing and Asian country. Our results demonstrate several striking differences between Chinese PAH patients and Western PAH patients enrolled in registries in the modern therapy era.

Diagnostic and Therapeutic Status of Pulmonary Arterial Hypertension in Modern China

Diagnostic Catheterization

Since the modern classification and diagnostic strategies were introduced in China after 2004, right heart catheterization, instead of echocardiography, is being performed by more and more centers to establish the diagnosis of pulmonary hypertension. In the majority of pulmonary hypertension centers, cardiopulmonary hemodynamics were recorded by a Swan-Ganz or pigtail catheter and cardiac output was measured by the thermodilution technique (for patients without intracardiac shunts) or indirect Fick method (for patients with intracardiac shunts).

Acute Pulmonary Vasodilator Testing

Acute pulmonary vasodilator testing is a critical procedure for screening patients who might have a sustained benefit from long-term and high-dose calcium channel blockers (CCBs). The screening agents recommended by recent guidelines include inhaled nitric oxide, intravenous epoprostenol, or adenosine. In clinical practice, inhaled nitric oxide was preferred in the majority of pulmonary hypertension centers in Western countries [23] due to its characteristics of a very short half-life and selectivity to pulmonary circulation. However, inhaled nitric oxide and intravenous epoprostenol were not available in China, and inhaled iloprost and intravenous adenosine were the choice for acute pulmonary vasodilator testing.

We identified the comparable effects of inhaled iloprost and intravenous adenosine for screening long-term responders of CCBs [24]. For all patients suspected of having IPAH, an acute pulmonary vasodilator challenge is performed during right heart catheterization with inhaled iloprost or intravenous stepwise up-titrated adenosine. A positive vasodilator response is defined as a reduction of mean pulmonary arterial pressure (mPAP) greater than 10 mm Hg leading to a value less than 40 mm Hg, with normal or high cardiac output.

Exclusion of Other Etiologies of Pulmonary Hypertension Idiopathic Pulmonary Arterial Hypertension

To establish the diagnosis of IPAH, patients with known severe pulmonary parenchymal disease (defined as a forced vital capacity or total lung capacity <70% of predicted, or forced expiratory volume in 1 s <60% of predicted), pulmonary interstitial disease (defined by high-resolution CT and a severely impaired pulmonary diffusion function: diffusion capacity for carbon monoxide of the lung <70% of predicted), left heart disease (pulmonary capillary wedge pressure or left ventricular end diastolic pressure >15 mm Hg measured by right heart catheterization), or chronic pulmonary embolism (revealed by pulmonary angiography or CT, pulmonary angiography, or ventilation/perfusion lung scan) were excluded because they are prone to develop another type of pulmonary hypertension. Furthermore, to ensure a homogeneous population of IPAH, patients with severe chronic pulmonary parenchymal disease with an out-of-proportion elevated PAP (mPAP >40 mm Hg) were also classified as Group 3 pulmonary hypertension.

Treatments

PAH-specific drugs were not available in mainland China until 2006, about a 14-year delay from when the first PAH-specific drug, epoprostenol (Floran), was launched in the United States. Up to now, only three drugs, oral bosentan, ambrisentan, and inhaled iloprost, are approved for the treatment of severe PAH in WHO functional classes III or IV. Moreover, intravenous prostanoids are still not available in mainland China and phosphodiesterase type 5 (PDE5) inhibitors can only be used off-label in patients with PAH. Additionally, these PAH-specific drugs are not yet reimbursable by the government or insurance in China; therefore, the expensive cost for these drugs is a very important issue which could influence the therapeutic choice for both doctors and patients.

Comparison of Idioathic Pulmonary Arterial Hypertension in Developed and Developing Countries

Epidemiology

A review of incident cases in Belgium as part of a case-control study of IPAH with anorexigen use concluded that the annual incidence in Belgian inhabitants aged 18–70 years was 1.7 per million inhabitants [25]. Similarly, the estimated incidence of IPAH in Israel between 1988 and 1997 was estimated to be 1.4 cases per million inhabitants [26]. The French registry enrolled patients between 2002 and 2003, and concluded that its lower-bound estimates of incidence and prevalence of PAH was 2.4 and 15 cases per million adult inhabitants, respectively, and the low estimate for prevalence of IPAH was 5.9 cases per million inhabitants [10]. The low estimate for incidence of adult IPAH and familial PAH in the United States based on the REVEAL registry is 1.1 cases per million inhabitants [15]. For all adult patients in Group 1 PAH, the incidence is 2.3 cases per million. Matched to the French registry enrollment criteria (i.e. pulmonary capillary wedge pressure <15 mm Hg), the incidence of adult patients with IPAH or familial PAH in Group 1 PAH is 0.9 and 2.0 per million, respectively. The low estimate for adult prevalence for Group 1 PAH is 12.4 in REVEAL. Given the recognition that not all patients with PAH are included in the registry studies, the real numbers of incidence and prevalence of IPAH and PAH might be underestimated.

In contrast, the epidemiology of IPAH and PAH is still unknown in China as well as other developing countries because no perspective or nation-wide registry data could be used in calculation. The initiation of a national registry should be based on establishing completed networks of pulmonary hypertension.

Demographics

The first NIH registry showed that IPAH often affected young women (mean age of 36.4 years, with a female-to-male ratio of 1.7:1), and only 9% of the patients were older than 60 years. Race and ethnicity of the cohort were similar to those of the general population. However, the demographic pictures were partly changed in the recent French and US REVEAL registries. In these two large registries, IPAH was the leading etiology of WHO Group 1 PAH (39.2% in France and 46.2% in USA) and, as in prior studies, disease was seen more commonly in women (63% in France and 80% in USA). The mean age of patients with IPAH was 53 ± 16 and 50 ± 15 years in the France and USA, respectively, which is older than that seen in prior series.

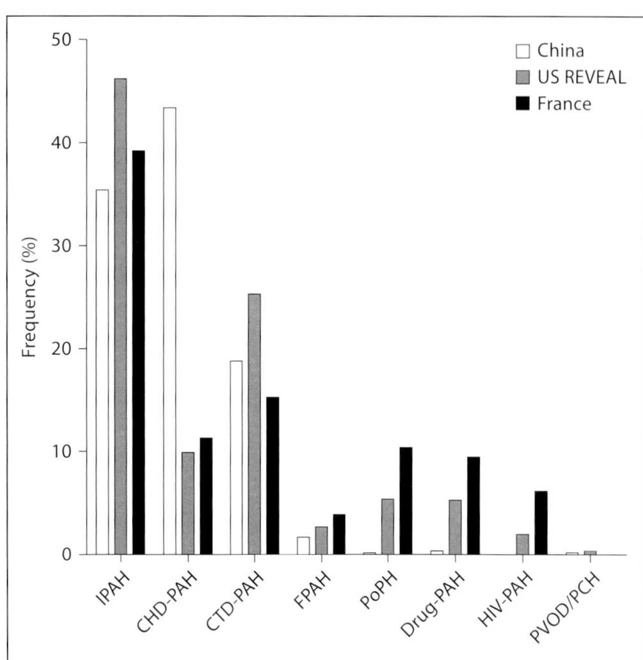

Fig. 1. Etiologies of patients with PAH in China, US REVEAL, and France. CHD-PAH = Congenital heart disease associated with PAH; CTD-PAH = connective tissue disease associated with PAH; Drug-PAH = drug-induced PAH; FPAH = familial PAH; HIV-PAH = human immunodeficiency virus infection-related PAH; PoPH = portopulmonary hypertension; PVOD/PCH = pulmonary veno-occlusive disease/pulmonary capillary hemangiomatosis.

Although data specific to IPAH were not available, 20–25% of patients with PAH of any form in these registries were older than 60 years, and some patients were diagnosed in their eighties.

In the new Chinese multicenter registry, 338 of 956 (35.4%) adults in WHO Group 1 PAH were diagnosed as IPAH. In contrast to Western countries, congenital heart disease associated with PAH, but not IPAH, was the leading cause for WHO Group 1 PAH (43.4%). In contrast, only 11.3% of the patients in the French registry and 9.9% in the US REVEAL study had congenital heart disease-related PAH (fig. 1). This dramatic difference might be attributed to delayed diagnosis and delayed surgical or interventional repair in China due to low awareness of cardiac malformation or unaffordable costs for patients with left-to-right cardiac or noncardiac shunts. The mean age of the Chinese adult patients with PAH and IPAH was 36 ± 13 years and 38 ± 13 years, respectively, which was younger than that of US REVEAL and French PAH patients, but still similar with the previous Chinese registry (36 ± 12 years) (fig. 2). The female preponderance in PAH (70%) and IPAH

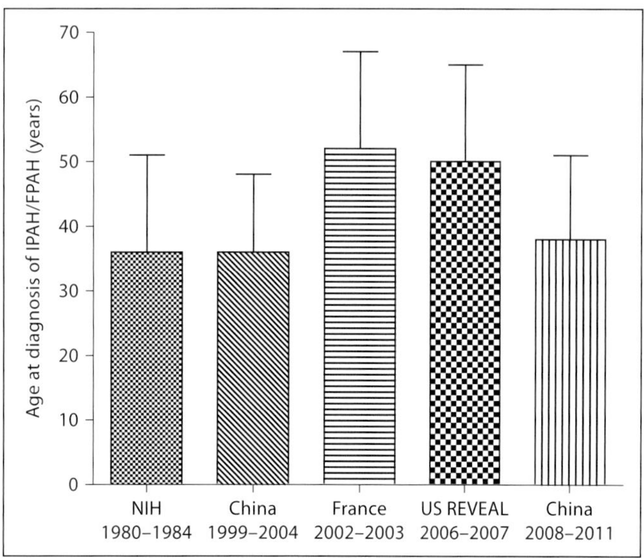

Fig. 2. Comparison of the age at diagnosis in patients with IPAH/FPAH among registries from different regions and different therapeutic eras. China (1999–2004) indicates the first monocenter registry including primary pulmonary hypertension and familiar PAH patients in era of only conventional treatment used in clinical practice. China (2008–2011) indicates the new multicenter registry including the WHO Group 1 PAH patients in the era when several PAH-specific drugs were available. France shows the data from the national registry in France and enrolled patients of Group 1 PAH. NIH shows the first national registry in the USA and the patients enrolled with primary pulmonary hypertension. US REVEAL shows data for enrolled patients of Group 1 PAH.

(70%) was comparable to that recorded in the French and US REVEAL registries. The time from symptom onset to diagnostic right heart catheterization was also significantly delayed in the PAH (median: 30 months) and in IPAH (median: 24 months) patients, which was much more delayed compared with that of the REVEAL registry (median: 14 months in Group 1 PAH patients).

Functional Class and 6-Min Walking Distance

As there is still no method to detect IPAH in the early stage, functional class was severely impaired in patients of the French, US REVEAL, and new Chinese registries, with 75, 55, and 66% of the patients in functional class III or IV at diagnosis, respectively. Accordingly, the mean 6-min walk distances were also decreased significantly in those registries, with only 328, 374, and 353 m in the French, US, and Chinese registries, respectively. The impaired functional class and 6-min walk distances were similar to the NIH study, suggesting little change over time in the severity of PAH at time of diagnosis.

Hemodynamics

Right heart catheterization was performed in all patients in the US REVEAL and new Chinese registries, and in 96% of the patients in the French registry at the time of diagnosis. Cardiopulmonary hemodynamic parameters were severely compromised in all three registries, demonstrated as markedly elevated PAP and pulmonary vascular resistance, and reduced cardiac index. Compared with the French and US REVEAL registries, Chinese patients with IPAH had a higher mPAP (63 ± 15 vs. 52 ± 13 and 56 ± 14 mm Hg) and pulmonary vascular resistance index (27 ± 12 vs. 23 ± 11 and 23 ± 10 Wood•m^2). The reason for these differences of severity of hemodynamic compromise is still unknown. The other hemodynamic parameters were comparable between Chinese patients and Western registries, e.g. right atrial pressure, pulmonary capillary wedge pressure and cardiac index (table 1).

Acute pulmonary vasoreactivity testing was conducted in all hemodynamically stable patients with IPAH to screen the potent responders to long-term therapy of CCBs. The acute responders account for 10.2% in French Group 1 PAH patients, 10.3% in US REVEAL IPAH patients, and 5.0% in Chinese IPAH patients. The relatively lower acute response rate may be due to the more severe hemodynamic compromise in Chinese IPAH patients because higher mPAP at baseline suggests a lower probability of reaching 40 mm Hg after acute vasodilator challenge.

Comorbid Conditions

Obesity (defined as BMI above 30) was observed in 14.8, 33.3, and 1.5% of Group 1 PAH patients in the French, US REVEAL, and new Chinese registries, respectively. In terms of patients with IPAH, obesity was observed in 38.4% in the US REVEAL registry and 2.1% in the Chinese registry. The proportion of obesity was similar to that of the adult population in those countries [27, 28]. The significantly lower prevalence of obesity in the Chinese population is mainly due to ethnic, nutritional, and socioeconomic factors compared with Western countries. As a result of the lower incidence of obesity, the suspicion of anorexigen exposure in Chinese patients was dramatically lower than the Western registries. Moreover, compared with the US REVEAL registry, significantly fewer comorbid conditions like cardiovascular disease and renal insufficiency, both in number and frequency, were identified in Chinese IPAH patients (table 2). This difference was partially due to more elderly and obese patients being enrolled in the REVEAL study.

Table 1. Comparison of clinical and hemodynamic characteristics in PAH and IPAH among China, the USA (REVEAL), and France

Characteristic	Overall Group 1 PAH			IPAH		
	China (n = 956)	USA (n = 2,525)	France (n = 674)	China (n = 383)	USA (n = 1,166)	France (n = 259)
Female, %	70	80	65	70	83	62
Age, years	36±13	50±14	50±15	38±13	50±15	52±15
Obesity (BMI ≥30), %	1.5	33.3	14.8	2.1	38.4	–
Median time from symptom onset to diagnosis, months	30	14	–	24	–	–
WHO FC III/IV, %	53.6	56	75	66	55	81
6MWD, m	378±125	366±126	329±109	353±127	374±129	328±112
mPAP, mm Hg	63±20	51±14	55±15	63±15	52±13	56±14
mRAP, mm Hg	8±5	9±6	8±5	8±6	10±6	9±5
PCWP, mm Hg	9±3	9±4	8±3	8±	9±4	8±3
CI, $l/min/m^2$	2.5±0.9	2.4±0.8	2.5±0.8	2.2±0.8	2.2±0.8	2.3±0.7
PVRI, Wood•m^2	25±14	21±13	21±10	27±12	23 ±11	23±10
SvO_2, %	66±12	63±10	63±9	60±11	62±10	61±10
Acute vasodilator responders, %	2.8	10.2	5.8	5.0	–	10.3

Values are means ± SD unless otherwise indicated. CI = Cardiac index; mRAP = mean right atrial pressure; 6MWD = 6-min walking distance; PCWP = pulmonary capillary wedge pressure; PVRI = pulmonary vascular resistance index; SvO_2 = mixed venous blood oxygen saturation.

Medications at Enrollment

Remarkable advances have been achieved in elucidating the pathogenesis of PAH since the mid-1990s, leading to the development of disease-targeted therapies for this condition. Up to now, over 10 agents from 3 well-established pathways have been used in clinical practice in Western countries. The majority of patients could be treated by different drugs or combinations according to the recommended therapeutic strategies in recent guidelines. The REVEAL registry firstly provides important insights into current treatment patterns in United States. Among the 2,704 Group 1 PAH patients, 266 received no PAH-specific drugs (9.8%), 1,008 were on two or more drugs, and 183 were on three or more drugs. Of the 2,438 patients on any PAH treatment, 624 were taking CCBs. Of these, 212 (34.0%) were on CCBs specifically for PAH. Among the 1,335 patients for whom results of a vasodilator challenge were known at enrollment, 136 were vasodilator responders and 55 of the responders (40.4%) were on CCBs for PAH. Among patients on endothelin receptor antagonists at enrollment, 953 were on bosentan, 89 on ambrisentan, and 106 on sitaxsentan. Among patients on PDE5 inhibitors, 1,147 were on sildenafil and 47 were on tadalafil. A total of 1,012 patients were treated with a prostacyclin analog: treprostinil was given intravenously, subcutaneously, in inhaled form, and orally for 159, 112, 28, and 9 patients, respectively; 237 patients received inhaled iloprost; and 480 were treated with intravenous epoprostenol sodium. Additionally, only a small proportion of patients enrolled were participating in randomized clinical trials, with more patients participating in open-label extension studies. Treatment with prostanoids increased with disease severity, as assessed by functional class. The most commonly used analog was intravenous epoprostenol, with smaller numbers of patients receiving inhaled iloprost or intravenously or subcutaneously administered treprostinil.

In the new Chinese registry, a total of 27 WHO Group 1 PAH patients were identified as acute responders. Among them, 17 patients with IPAH were on high-dose CCB monotherapy (diltiazem 240–720 mg/day). The other 10 acute responders with congenital heart disease or connective tissue diseases were treated with low-dose CCBs (diltiazem 60–180 mg/day) and PAH-specific drugs. In addition, patients with a 20% decrease in mPAP and 30% decrease in pulmonary vascular resistance in the acute vasoreactivity test were also treated with low-dose CCBs (diltiazem 60–180 mg/day) combined with PAH-specific drugs. After exclusion of the 27 acute responders, 226 (23.6%) patients were taking no PAH therapies,

Table 2. Comparison of comorbid conditions in PAH and IPAH between China and the USA (REVEAL)

Comorbid condition	Group 1 PAH		IPAH	
	US REVEAL (n = 2,438)	China (n = 956)	US REVEAL (n = 1,114)	China (n = 338)
Hypertension	980 (40.2)	44 (4.6)	466 (41.8)	10 (3.0)
Diabetes	293 (12.0)	16 (1.6)	158 (14.2)	4 (1.2)
Ischemic cardiovascular event[1]	227 (9.3)	15 (1.6)	114 (10.2)	8 (2.4)
Chronic parenchymal disease[2]	533 (21.9)	29 (3.0)	258 (23.2)	5 (1.5)
Renal insufficiency	109 (4.9)	8 (0.8)	48 (4.3)	2 (0.6)
Thyroid disease[3]	527 (21.6)	10 (1.0)	227 (20.4)	1 (0.3)
Cirrhosis	151 (6.2)	4 (0.4)	20 (1.8)	1 (0.3)
History of VTE[4]	313 (12.8)	11 (1.2)	164 (14.7)	0 (0)
Cancer	148 (6.1)	5 (0.5)	69 (6.2)	1 (0.3)

All values are presented as numbers of patients (%).
[1] Includes patients with the comorbid conditions coronary artery disease and/or cerebral infarction diagnosed by angiography or CT scan.
[2] Includes patients with obstructive lung disease, reactive airways disease, and chronic obstructive pulmonary disease in the US-based REVEAL study, and those defined as having chronic bronchitis, bronchiectasis, mild interstitial lung disease, mild obstructive lung disease, and lung tuberculosis in the current study.
[3] Includes patients with the comorbid conditions hypothyroidism or hyperthyroidism.
[4]Includes patients with an episode of pulmonary embolism and/or deep venous thrombosis.

476 (49.8%) were on monotherapy, and 227 (23.7%) were taking two or more drugs. Of the 511 patients in WHO functional classes III or IV, 127 (24.9%) were taking combinations of PAH-specific drugs, while 122 (23.9%) were not taking any PAH-specific medications. Among patients taking PAH-specific therapies, PDE5 inhibitors were the most commonly prescribed agents [506 patients (53.0%), 361 of whom were taking sildenafil and 145 taking vardenafil]. Prostanoids were used in monotherapy or combination regimens in 192 patients (21.1%), 83 of whom were taking inhaled iloprost and 109 oral beraprost, while 124 patients (13.0%) were taking an endothelin receptor antagonist (bosentan). A total of 219 patients (22.9%) were participating in clinical trials at the time of enrollment; of these, 197 (20.6%) were in randomized and blinded clinical trials. In patients with IPAH and connective tissue disease-associated PAH (CTD-PAH), 118 of 338 (34.9%) and 58 of 180 (32.2%), respectively, were enrolled in clinical trials. Among patients with congenital heart diseases, 35 of 415 (8.4%) were treated with PAH-specific drugs in clinical trials, all of whom were repaired patients (table 3).

Compared with Western registries, only a small proportion of patients was treated with combinations of PAH-specific drugs in the present study, in particular a combination of inhaled prostanoids. However, the available data on medication use reflect only the initial status of treatment. Many patients have to decrease the dosage or switch combination therapy to monotherapy, or even stop PAH-specific drugs due to their high cost. The percentages of patients receiving adequate long-term targeted therapies were definitely much lower than the initial percentages at enrollment. In addition, nearly one fourth of the total Group 1 PAH patients and nearly half of the IPAH patients were enrolled in clinical trials. Given the huge economic burden of long-term PAH-specific treatment, entering clinical trials has become a very important method of offering PAH patients an opportunity to receive potential PAH-targeted drugs.

Prognosis

IPAH has been considered a progressive and often fatal disease. In the first NIH registry of 194 patients with primary pulmonary hypertension between July 1981 and December 1985, the estimated median survival of these patients was 2.8 years and the estimated 1-, 3- and 5-year survival rates were 68, 48, and 34%, respectively. Over the past decade, new treatments for PAH, such the use of prostanoids, endothelin receptor antagonists, and PDE5 inhibitors, have brought about dramatic improvements in clinical outcomes, and it is

Table 3. Conventional and PAH-specific medications taken by Chinese patients with PAH following diagnostic right heart catheterization

Medications	Total (n = 956)	IPAH (n = 338)
Conventional therapies	730 (76.4)	294 (87.0)
Diuretics	624 (65.3)	248 (73.4)
Warfarin	314 (32.8)	149 (44.1)
Oxygen	190 (19.9)	56 (16.6)
Digoxin	493 (51.6)	203 (60.1)
CCBs	80 (8.4)	35 (10.4)
PAH-specific therapies	702 (73.4)	182 (89.2)
ERA (bosentan)	124 (13.0)	51 (15.1)
Prostanoids	192 (21.1)	53 (15.7)
Iloprost	83 (8.7)	25 (7.4)
Beraprost	109 (11.4)	28 (8.3)
PDE5 inhibitors	506 (53.0)	167 (49.4)
Sildenafil	361 (37.8)	124 (36.7)
Vardenafil	145 (15.2)	43 (12.7)
Combination therapy	227 (23.7)	74 (21.9)
Clinical trials	219 (22.9)	118 (34.9)
Placebo-controlled	197 (20.6)	106 (31.4)

All values are presented as numbers of patients (%). The medications listed were those recorded for patients on discharge from our center. The patients' compliance with the medications was unknown. Medications recorded in less than 5% of the overall study population were excluded from the analysis.
ERA = Endothelin receptor antagonist.

clear that newer PAH-specific drugs can significantly alter the natural history of the disease. In the modern treatment era (referring to the time when PAH-specific drugs were available; thus, the beginning of the modern treatments era can be different for each country), improved survival has been demonstrated in those registries. In prevalent idiopathic, familial and anorexigen associated PAH, 1-, 2-, and 3-year survival rates in the French registry were 89, 77, and 69%. This was higher than in incident patients who were characterized by 1-, 2-, and 3-year survival rates of 89, 68, and 55%. With the advent of modern treatment in the United States, the 1-year estimate of survival of the overall Group 1 PAH was 91% in the REVEAL registry. Although the detailed survival data in patients with IPAH in the modern United States is still not available as the patients enrolled in the REVEAL registry are to be followed up to 2014, the increased survival rate in Group 1 PAH could partly reflect the improved survival in IPAH subgroup because nearly half of the patients of Group 1 PAH in REVEAL registry were IPAH.

In China, the modern therapy era for PAH started with the launch of bosentan and iloprost in 2006. We previously reported a registry and survival study of Chinese patients with IPAH in 2007. In this cohort study, 1- and 3-year survival estimates were only 68 and 39%, respectively, which were similar to those recorded by the US NIH registry in the 1980s. Lack of effective treatment was the main cause of poor survival in this study. With the introduction of right heart catheterization and a targeted treatment approach, the survival and the quality of life of patients with PAH have improved gradually in China. More recently, Zhang et al. [29] reported a retrospective study to evaluate the new survival data of IPAH and CTD-PAH when a majority of patients could access only inadequate PAH-specific therapies. In this study, a total 173 patients with IPAH and 103 patients with CTD-PAH were collected from 5 centers in China. During a median follow-up of 2.75 years, there were 25 deaths in IPAH and 22 deaths in CTD-PAH. Cardiovascular causes (heart failure or sudden death) accounted for 90% of the deaths in the IPAH patients. The 1-, 2-, and 3-year survival rates of patients with IPAH were estimated to be 92.1, 80.1, and 75.1%, respectively. These new survival data in IPAH demonstrated a marked improvement compared with the survival in the era lacking PAH-specific therapies in China. Furthermore, the new survival rates seemed to be even better than that of the French registry, despite that the majority of patients with IPAH in China could only receive inadequate PAH-specific therapies. The primary reason for better survival in China may due to the younger age and less cardiovascular comorbidities.

Conclusion

Recent registries give us a chance to compare the clinical characteristics of IPAH in developed and developing countries, and also in Western and Eastern populations. The differences of age at diagnosis, exercise capacity, hemodynamics, comorbidities, medications, and survival are quite important for better understanding the overall status of IPAH throughout the world, and are also useful for instituting global diagnostic and therapeutic strategies for IPAH. A new pulmonary hypertension community needs to be established to collaborate in the design of a more representative and meaningful study, and thereby enhance the quality of PAH care in both developed and developing countries [30].

Key Points

- IPAH is a rare but severe disease with a quite poor natural history.
- The demographic and clinical characteristics of PAH in developed and developing countries were not of the same status.
- IPAH is the leading cause of WHO Group 1 PAH in Western countries. In contrast, PAH associated with congenital heart disease is the leading cause in China.
- Chinese patients with IPAH are younger, but with more severe hemodynamic compromise than those patients in Western countries.
- The comorbid conditions in Chinese patients with IPAH are much lower than those patients in Western countries. The dramatic differences are perhaps due to the younger age and lower percentage of obesity of Chinese patients.
- Compared with Western countries, more patients with IPAH cannot receive PAH-specific drugs and fewer patients received combinational therapies in China due to economic considerations.
- Although 1-, 2-, and 3-year survival of IPAH improved in both Western countries and China, death still can only be delayed for years in majority patients.

References

1 Farber HW, Loscalzo J: Pulmonary arterial hypertension. N Engl J Med 2004;351:1655–1665.
2 Rubin LJ, Badesch DB: Evaluation and management of the patient with pulmonary arterial hypertension. Ann Intern Med 2005;143:282–292.
3 Simonneau G, Robbins IM, Beghetti M, Channick RN, Delcroix M, Denton CP, Elliott CG, Gaine SP, Gladwin MT, Jing ZC, Krowka MJ, Langleben D, Nakanishi N, Souza R: Updated clinical classification of pulmonary hypertension. J Am Coll Cardiol 2009;54:S43–S54.
4 Rich S, Dantzker DR, Ayres SM, Bergofsky EH, Brundage BH, Detre KM, Fishman AP, Goldring RM, Groves BM, Koerner SK, Levy PC, Reid LM, Vreim CE, Williams GW: Primary pulmonary hypertension. A national prospective study. Ann Intern Med 1987;107:216–223.
5 D'Alonzo GE, Barst RJ, Ayres SM, Bergofsky EH, Brundage BH, Detre KM, Fishman AP, Goldring RM, Groves BM, Kernis JT, Levy PS, Pietra GG, Reid LM, Reeves JT, Rich S, Vreim CE, Williams GW, Wu M: Survival in patients with primary pulmonary hypertension. Results from a national prospective registry. Ann Intern Med 1991;115:343–349.
6 Morrell NW, Adnot S, Archer SL, Dupuis J, Jones PL, MacLean MR, McMurtry IF, Stenmark KR, Thistlethwaite PA, Weissmann N, Yuan JX, Weir EK: Cellular and molecular basis of pulmonary arterial hypertension. J Am Coll Cardiol 2009;54:S20–S31.
7 Tuder RM, Abman SH, Braun T, Capron F, Stevens T, Thistlethwaite PA, Haworth SG: Development and pathology of pulmonary hypertension. J Am Coll Cardiol 2009;54:S3–S9.
8 Galiè N, Hoeper M, Humbert M, Torbicki A, Vachiery JL, Barbera JA, Beghetti M, Corris P, Gaine S, Gibbs JS, Gomez-Sanchez MA, Jondeau G, Klepetko W, Opitz C, Peacock A, Rubin L, Zellweger M, Simonneau G. ESC Committee for Practice Guidelines (CPG): Guidelines on diagnosis and treatment of pulmonary hypertension: the Task Force on Diagnosis and Treatment of Pulmonary Hypertension of the European Society of Cardiology (ESC) and the European Respiratory Society (ERS). Eur Heart J 2009;30:2493–2537.
9 McLaughlin VV, Archer SL, Badesch DB, Barst RJ, Farber HW, Lindner JR, Mathier MA, McGoon MD, Park MH, Rosenson RS, Rubin LJ, Tapson VF, Varga J: ACCF/AHA 2009 expert consensus document on pulmonary hypertension: a report of the American College of Cardiology Foundation Task Force on Expert Consensus Documents and the American Heart Association developed in collaboration with the American College of Chest Physicians; American Thoracic Society, Inc.; and the Pulmonary Hypertension Association. J Am Coll Cardiol 2009;53:1573–2619.
10 Humbert M, Sitbon O, Chaouat A, Bertocchi M, Habib G, Gressin V, Yaici A, Weitzenblum E, Cordier JF, Chabot F, Dromer C, Pison C, Reynaud-Gaubert M, Haloun A, Laurent M, Hachulla E, Simonneau G: Pulmonary arterial hypertension in France: results from a national registry. Am J Respir Crit Care Med 2006;173:1023–1030.
11 Thenappan T, Shah SJ, Rich S, Gomberg-Maitland M: A USA-based registry for pulmonary arterial hypertension: 1982–2006. Eur Respir J 2007;30:1103–1110.
12 Peacock AJ, Murphy NF, McMurray JJ, Caballero L, Stewart S: An epidemiological study of pulmonary arterial hypertension. Eur Respir J 2007;30:104–109.
13 McGoon MD, Krichman A, Farber HW, Barst RJ, Raskob GE, Liou TG, Miller DP, Feldkircher K, Giles S: Design of the REVEAL registry for US patients with pulmonary arterial hypertension. Mayo Clin Proc 2008;83:923–931.
14 Badesch DB, Raskob GE, Elliott CG, Krichman AM, Farber HW, Frost AE, Barst RJ, Benza RL, Liou TG, Turner M, Giles S, Feldkircher K, Miller DP, McGoon MD: Pulmonary arterial hypertension: baseline characteristics from the REVEAL registry. Chest 2010;137:376–387.
15 Frost AE, Badesch DB, Barst RJ, Benza RL, Elliott CG, Farber HW, Krichman A, Liou TG, Raskob GE, Wason P, Feldkircher K, Turner M, McGoon MD: The changing picture of pulmonary arterial hypertension (PAH) patients in the United States: how the REVEAL registry differs from historic and non-US contemporary registries. Chest 2011;139:128–137.
16 Galiè N, Palazzini M, Manes A: Pulmonary arterial hypertension: from the kingdom of the near-dead to multiple clinical trial meta-analyses. Eur Heart J 2010;31:2080–2086.
17 Humbert M, Sitbon O, Yaïci A, Montani D, O'Callaghan DS, Jaïs X, Parent F, Savale L, Natali D, Günther S, Chaouat A, Chabot F, Cordier JF, Habib G, Gressin V, Jing ZC, Souza R, Simonneau G, French Pulmonary Arterial Hypertension Network: Survival in incident and prevalent cohorts of patients with pulmonary arterial hypertension. Eur Respir J 2010;36:549–555.
18 Humbert M, Sitbon O, Chaouat A, Bertocchi M, Habib G, Gressin V, Yaïci A, Weitzenblum E, Cordier JF, Chabot F, Dromer C, Pison C, Reynaud-Gaubert M, Haloun A, Laurent M, Hachulla E, Cottin V, Degano B, Jaïs X, Montani D, Souza R, Simonneau G: Survival in patients with idiopathic, familial, and anorexigen-associated pulmonary arterial hypertension in the modern management era. Circulation 2010;122:156–163.
19 Benza RL, Miller DP, Gomberg-Maitland M, Frantz RP, Foreman AJ, Coffey CS, Frost A, Barst RJ, Badesch DB, Elliott CG, Liou TG, McGoon MD: Predicting survival in pulmonary arterial hypertension: insights from the Registry to Evaluate Early and Long-Term Pulmonary Arterial Hypertension Disease Management (REVEAL). Circulation 2010;122:164–172.
20 McLaughlin VV, Sitbon O, Badesch DB, Barst RJ, Black C, Galiè N, Rainisio M, Simonneau G, Rubin LJ: Survival with first-line bosentan in patients with primary pulmonary hypertension. Eur Respir J 2005;25:244–249.

21 Sitbon O, McLaughlin VV, Badesch DB, Barst RJ, Black C, Galiè N, Humbert M, Rainisio M, Rubin LJ, Simonneau G: Survival in patients with class III idiopathic pulmonary arterial hypertension treated with first line oral bosentan compared with an historical cohort of patients started on intravenous epoprostenol. Thorax 2005;60:1025–1030.
22 Jing ZC, Xu XQ, Han ZY, Wu Y, Deng KW, Wang H, Wang ZW, Cheng XS, Xu B, Hu SS, Hui RT, Yang YJ: Registry and survival study in Chinese patients with idiopathic and familial pulmonary arterial hypertension. Chest 2007;132:373–379.
23 Hoeper MM, Lee SH, Voswinckel R, Palazzini M, Jais X, Marinelli A, Barst RJ, Ghofrani HA, Jing ZC, Opitz C, Seyfarth HJ, Halank M, McLaughlin V, Oudiz RJ, Ewert R, Wilkens H, Kluge S, Bremer HC, Baroke E, Rubin LJ: Complications of right heart catheterization procedures in patients with pulmonary hypertension in experienced centers. J Am Coll Cardiol 2006;48:2546–2552.
24 Jing ZC, Jiang X, Han ZY, Xu XQ, Wang Y, Wu Y, Lv H, Ma CR, Yang YJ, Pu JL: Iloprost for pulmonary vasodilator testing in idiopathic pulmonary arterial hypertension. Eur Respir J 2009;33:1354–1360.
25 Abenhaim L, Moride Y, Brenot F, Rich S, Benichou J, Kurz X, Higenbottam T, Oakley C, Wouters E, Aubier M, Simonneau G, Bégaud B: Appetite-suppressant drugs and the risk of primary pulmonary hypertension. International Primary Pulmonary Hypertension Study Group. N Engl J Med 1996;335:609–616.
26 Appelbaum L, Yigla M, Bendayan D, Reichart N, Fink G, Priel I, Schwartz Y, Richman P, Picard E, Goldman S, Kramer MR: Primary pulmonary hypertension in Israel: a national survey. Chest 2001;119:1801–1806.
27 Ford ES, Mokdad AH: Epidemiology of obesity in the Western hemisphere. J Clin Endocrinol Metab 2008;93:S1–S8.
28 Wu Y: Overweight and obesity in China. BMJ 2006;333:362–363.
29 Zhang R, Dai LZ, Xie WP, Yu ZX, Wu BX, Pan L, Yuan P, Jiang X, He J, Humbert M, Jing ZC: Survival of Chinese patients with pulmonary arterial hypertension in the modern treatment era. Chest 2011;140:301–309.
30 Gomberg-Maitland M, Michelakis ED: A global pulmonary arterial hypertension registry: is it needed? Is it feasible? Pulmonary vascular disease: the global perspective. Chest 2010;137:95S–101S.

Prof. Zhi-Cheng Jing, MD
Department of Cardio-Pulmonary Circulation, Shanghai Pulmonary Hospital, Tongji University School of Medicine
507 Zhengmin Road
Shanghai, 200433 (PR China)
Tel: +86 21 65115006 2110, E-Mail jingzhicheng@gmail.com

Chapter 10

Humbert M, Souza R, Simonneau G (eds): Pulmonary Vascular Disorders.
Prog Respir Res. Basel, Karger, 2012, vol 41, pp 94–104

Pulmonary Arterial Hypertension Complicating Connective Tissue Disorders

Jérôme Le Pavec[a] · Paul M. Hassoun[b]

[a]Université Paris-Sud 11, Service de Pneumologie et Réanimation Respiratoire, Hôpital Antoine Béclère, Assistance Publique Hôpitaux de Paris, Clamart, France; [b]Division of Pulmonary and Critical Care Medicine, Johns Hopkins University School of Medicine, Baltimore, Md., USA

Abstract

Connective tissue diseases (CTD) are commonly complicated by pulmonary arterial hypertension (PAH) which is often the leading cause of death in this population. Despite recent advances in therapy for PAH in general, the response to treatment in patients with CTD, particularly patients with scleroderma-associated PAH (SSc-PAH), has been quite discouraging. This chapter reviews the pathophysiology, clinical manifestations, and current and promising therapy for CTD-associated PAH with a particular focus on SSc-PAH. The lack of clinical response to modern therapies may merely reflect the limitations of traditionally employed PAH outcome measures in CTD-associated PAH patients or highlight the heterogeneity of the disease manifestations within this group of patients. Importantly, since involvement of vital organs other than the lung, such as the gastrointestinal tract and the kidneys (particularly in SSc-PAH), may limit candidacy for lung transplantation, new therapies that target abnormal cellular proliferation in the pulmonary vasculature that are currently under investigation may be of particular relevance in this syndrome.

Pulmonary arterial hypertension (PAH), defined as a mean pulmonary arterial pressure greater than 25 mm Hg in the absence of elevation of the pulmonary capillary wedge pressure, is a cause of significant morbidity and mortality [1, 2]. PAH includes a heterogeneous group of clinical entities sharing similar pathological changes such as idiopathic (IPAH) and heritable PAH (associated with known or presumed gene defects), and PAH associated with other diseases or conditions such as connective tissue diseases [CTD, e.g. systemic sclerosis, systemic lupus erythematosus (SLE), and mixed connective tissue disease (MCTD)], portopulmonary hypertension, HIV infection, drugs, and toxins [3]. PAH is characterized by increased pulmonary vascular resistance due to remodeling and occlusion of the small pulmonary arterioles. Left untreated, PAH leads irremediably to right ventricular hypertrophy, pressure overload, and failure resulting in death within 2–3 years [2].

While the mechanisms involved in the pathogenesis of PAH are vastly unknown, there are several lines of evidence implicating autoimmunity in the development of the pulmonary vascular changes, including the presence of circulating autoantibodies [4], proinflammatory cytokines (e.g. IL-1 and IL-6) [5], and association of PAH with autoimmune diseases such as systemic sclerosis (SSc) and SLE. From a pathologic standpoint, the pulmonary vascular lesions in PAH associated with SSc (SSc-PAH) are indistinguishable from those present in IPAH (with the exception of a higher rate of veno-occlusive disease in SSc-PAH [6]), although the two diseases have quite divergent outcomes and response to therapy. Survival is significantly worse in SSc-PAH compared to IPAH despite the use of modern medical therapy [7–9]. While there are serologic and pathologic features suggestive of inflammation in both IPAH and SSc-PAH, it is likely that inflammatory pathways and autoimmunity, as well as fibrotic processes, are more pronounced in SSc-PAH and may explain survival discrepancies between the two syndromes and a differential response to therapy [8–10]. Other CTD such as SLE, MCTD, and to a lesser extent rheumatoid arthritis (RA), dermatomyositis, and Sjögren's syndrome, can also be complicated by PAH and will be discussed separately in this chapter.

Systemic Sclerosis-Associated Pulmonary Arterial Hypertension

SSc is a heterogeneous disorder characterized by dysfunction of the endothelium, dysregulation of fibroblasts resulting in excessive production of collagen, and abnormalities of the immune system [11]. These processes lead to progressive fibrosis of the skin and internal organs resulting in premature organ failure and death. Although the etiology of SSc is unknown, genetic and environmental factors are thought to contribute to host susceptibility [12]. Whether presenting in the limited or diffuse form, SSc is a systemic disease with the potential for multiple organ involvement, including the gastrointestinal, cardiac, renal, and pulmonary systems [11]. However, SSc-PAH has emerged as a leading cause of mortality [13, 14]. Although remarkable advances have been achieved in elucidating the pathogenesis of PAH over the past two decades, leading to the development of disease-targeted therapies for IPAH, the response to therapy is suboptimal in SSc-PAH and survival remains very poor [7–9, 15].

Prevalence and Incidence

In prospective studies using right heart catheterization for diagnosis, the prevalence of SSc-PAH is between 7.8 and 12% [16, 17]. With an estimated prevalence of SSc in the USA of about 240 cases per million and a conservative PAH prevalence of 10% among these patients, the estimated overall prevalence of SSc-PAH is around 24 individuals per million, which represents 5–10 times the number of patients affected by IPAH [18]. In the French PAH registry, CTD (mainly represented by SSc) accounts for 15.3% of PAH cases [19], while in the US registry CTD accounts for about 25% and SSc-PAH for about 17% of all PAH cases [20]. In a large single US center registry, the proportion of SSc-PAH is about 30% of all PAH patients [21]. The higher prevalence of SSc in the USA [22] probably accounts for a somewhat higher prevalence of SSc-PAH in the USA compared to France. In a recent prospective study, the estimated incidence of PAH among patients with SSc was 0.61 cases per 100 patient-years [15].

Pathophysiology

Inflammation plays a significant role in IPAH and SSc-PAH. Macrophages, T and B lymphocytes, and dendritic cells are found around plexiform lesions [23]. Levels of macrophage inflammatory protein-1α, IL-1β and IL-6, growth differentiation factor-15, and P-selectin are increased in severe IPAH [23]. Involvement of leukocytes, macrophages, and lymphocytes, initially described in the complex vascular lesions of IPAH [24], is also a prominent feature in CTD-associated PAH [6].

A role for autoimmunity is suggested by the presence of a number of autoantibodies in the serum of SSc patients, including classic autoantibodies such as anticentromere, antitopoisomerase 1, anti-RNA-polymerase III, antifibrillarin (U3 small nucleolar RNP), anti-Th/To, and anti-PM/Scl, and more recently antifibrillarin 1, anti-matrix metalloproteinases 1–3, anti-PDGF, anti-nag-2 (nonsteroidal anti-inflammatory drug-activated gene), antifibroblast, and anti-endothelial cell antibodies [25]. Antibodies have also been reported in SSc-PAH including fibrin-bound tissue plasminogen activator in patients with limited cutaneous SSc and in IPAH patients with HLA-DQ7 antigen [26] and antitopoisomerase II-α antibodies, particularly in association with HLA-B35 antigen [27]. Anti-endothelial cell antibodies can activate endothelial cells, induce the expression of adhesion molecules, and trigger apoptosis [28]. In vitro, autoantibodies from patients with CTD (anti-U1-RNP and anti-ds-DNA) can upregulate adhesion molecules and histocompatibility complex class II molecules on human pulmonary arterial endothelial cells [29], suggesting that inflammation could lead to pulmonary proliferative vasculopathy. Fibroblasts are found in the remodeled neointimal layer in both SSc-PAH and IPAH. Thus, the detection of antifibroblast antibodies in the serum of SSc-PAH and IPAH patients [30] has significant pathogenic importance since these antibodies can activate fibroblasts and induce collagen synthesis, contributing potentially directly to the remodeling process. They induce a proadhesive and proinflammatory response in normal fibroblasts, and have distinct reactivity profiles in IPAH and SSc-PAH, as assessed by immunoblotting [31]. Several fibroblast antigens recognized by serum IgG from IPAH and SSc-PAH patients have been identified thus far, including proteins involved in regulation of cytoskeletal function, cell contraction, cell and oxidative stress, cell energy metabolism, and other key cellular pathways [31].

Riemakesten et al. [32] recently demonstrated that functional immunity directed at the angiotensin II type 1 receptor and endothelin-1 type A receptor were commonly found in patients with SSc, particularly in patients with the diffuse form, and were associated with more severe disease manifestations and late complications, including pulmonary hypertension, lung fibrosis, and digital ulcers. Of particular interest is that both angiotensin II type 1 receptor and endothelin-1 type A receptor antibodies stimulate phosphorylation of ERK1/2 and increase TGF-β transcripts in cultured microvascular endothelial cells, effects which were blocked with specific receptor antagonists. Thus, these antibodies may contribute to disease pathogenesis and could potentially serve as biomarkers. These studies also highlight the potential benefit of specifically targeting the renin-angiotensin and endothelin systems in SSc.

Despite limited statistical power, several studies have suggested a number of candidate genes in association with SSc in different populations: a variant in the promoter of CCL2 (MCP-1) [33]; two variants in CD19 [34]; a promoter and coding polymorphism in TNF-α [35]; a variant in the promoter of IL-1α gene [36]; a 3-SNP haplotype in IL-10 [37]; a polymorphism in the CTGF promoter region [38]; the interferon regulatory factor 5 rs2004640 GT substitution [39]; the STAT4 rs7574865 single nucleotide polymorphism [39]; and a potassium voltage-gated channel, shaker-related subfamily, member 5 (KCN5) gene polymorphism [40]. Thus, there is compelling data supporting a genetic basis for SSc. Despite these recent advances in genetics, little is known about genetic involvement in SSc-PAH [41]. Mutations in the gene coding for bone morphogenetic protein receptor 2 (a member of the TGF-β receptor family) have not been detected in two small cohorts of SSc-PAH [41, 42]. An association between an endoglin gene polymorphism and SSc-PAH was reported by Wipff et al. [40], who demonstrated a significant lower frequency of the 6-base insertion in intron 7 (6bINS) of endoglin in SSc-PAH patients as compared to controls or patients with SSc but no PAH. Endoglin, a homodimeric membrane glycoprotein primarily present on human vascular endothelium, is part of the TGF-β receptor complex. Endoglin mutations are known causes of hereditary hemorrhagic telangiectasia and have been rarely identified in PAH patients [43, 44]. However, raised levels of endoglin have recently been identified in SSc-PAH patients, suggesting a role for endoglin in SSc vasculopathy [45]. These promising genetic studies will need validation in larger cohorts.

Vascular changes occur at an early stage in SSc and include apoptosis [46], endothelial cell activation with increased expression of cell adhesion molecules, inflammatory cell recruitment, a procoagulant state [47], intimal proliferation, and adventitial fibrosis leading to vessel obliteration. Endothelial injury is reflected by increased levels of soluble cell adhesion molecules, disturbances of angiogenesis as reflected by increased levels of circulating vascular endothelial growth factor (VEGF) [48, 49], and presence of angiostatic factors [49]. Thus, the role of dysregulated angiogenesis in SSc-PAH, whether driven by the inflammatory process or other mechanisms, is a predominant feature of the disease and may represent an ideal target for potential therapy.

Risk Factors

Several clinical markers are associated with an increased risk of developing PAH in the setting of SSc, including limited skin involvement [50–52], disease duration of more than 10 years [51], late age of onset of SSc [50], severity [52] or duration [53] of Raynaud's phenomenon, and reduced nailfold capillary density [51, 54]. Several investigators have emphasized the pivotal role of an isolated reduction in DLCO or a progressive decline of DLCO as an independent predictor for subsequent PAH [50, 52]. While the decrease in DLCO is likely the result of progressive pulmonary vascular remodeling over time, it is interesting to note that this alteration is significantly more pronounced in SSc-PAH compared to IPAH patients [8], perhaps suggesting more profound small vessel remodeling in the former compared to the latter patients.

Clinical Features

Typically, patients with SSc-PAH are predominantly women, have limited sclerosis, are older, and have seemingly less severe hemodynamic impairment compared to IPAH patients [8]. Like in IPAH, clinical symptoms are nonspecific, including dyspnea, functional limitations which may be more severe than in IPAH due not only to older age, but also to frequent involvement of the musculoskeletal system in these patients. SSc-PAH patients also tend to have other organ involvement, such as renal dysfunction and intrinsic heart disease.

Indeed, patients with SSc (even in the absence of PAH) tend to have depressed right ventricular function [55, 56] and left ventricular systolic as well as diastolic dysfunction [57]. Like IPAH patients, SSc-PAH patients have severe right ventricular dysfunction at time of presentation, but have more severely depressed right ventricular contractility compared to IPAH patients [58]. In addition, SSc-PAH patients tend to have more commonly left ventricle diastolic dysfunction and a high prevalence of pericardial effusion (34% compared to 13% for IPAH) [8]. In both groups, pericardial effusion portends a particularly poor prognosis [8]. SSc-PAH patients also have more severe hormonal and metabolic dysfunction such as high levels of N-terminal brain natriuretic peptide (N-TproBNP) [59] and hyponatremia [60]. Both N-TproBNP and hyponatremia have been shown, at baseline and with serial changes (for N-TproBNP) [59], to correlate with survival in PAH [59, 60].

Early Diagnosis

Because the prevalence of PAH in SSc is high, this population may be considered at risk and therefore worthy of a specific diagnostic approach to detect the presence of disease at an earlier stage when therapeutic intervention may potentially improve outcome. An algorithm for detection of PAH in patients with SSc may be helpful if based on a combination of symptoms and screening echocardiography. In a large French study encompassing 21 referral centers, patients with SSc with tricuspid regurgitation velocity (TRV) jet by transthoracic echocardiography greater than 3 m/s, or between 2.5 and 3 m/s if accompanied by unexplained dyspnea, were systematically referred for right heart catheterization. This approach allowed detection of incident cases of SSc-PAH with less severe disease (as judged on hemodynamic data) compared with patients with known disease. Therefore, unexplained dyspnea should prompt a search for PAH in these patients, in particular in the setting of a low single-breath DLCO or declining DLCO over time, echocardiographic findings suggestive of the disease (elevated TRV jet or dilated right ventricle or atrium), or elevated levels of N-TproBNP (see below) [17]. However, whether early diagnosis and treatment of SSc-PAH patients improves outcomes is still uncertain [61]; this issue should be addressed in properly designed studies in order to control for confounders such as lead time bias.

Prognosis

Compared with IPAH, SSc-PAH patients are almost four times more likely to die from their disease [8]. Moreover, outcomes in SSc-PAH remain worse than those in PAH associated with other CTD [7, 62]. At a time of broader treatment availability, and despite substantial improvements in other PAH categories, 3-year survival remains below 60% [7, 8, 15, 16, 62, 63]. Markers of worse prognosis include male gender [62], late age at diagnosis [62], pericardial effusion [8], functional severity based on New York Heart Association (NYHA) functional class [62], right heart dysfunction [8, 16, 64], hyponatremia [60], and renal dysfunction [64]. We recently demonstrated that measures of right ventricular afterload, both proximal and distal vascular resistance (pulmonary arterial capacitance as estimated by stroke volume divided by pulmonary artery pulse pressure and pulmonary vascular resistance, respectively) independently predict survival in SSc-PAH [64]. We also recently demonstrated that for patients with PAH admitted to the hospital for treatment of right ventricular failure, hyponatremia and low systolic blood pressure upon admission, and a diagnosis of CTD are the main prognostic factors for in-hospital mortality. In addition, the short-term outcomes after discharge are poor and remarkably worse in patients with underlying CTD or renal impairment [65].

Pulmonary Arterial Hypertension Associated with Other Connective Tissue Diseases

PAH can complicate any CTD, most frequently SSc as discussed above, but also SLE, MCTD, RA, or other diseases such as Sjögren's syndrome and dermatomyositis.

Systemic Lupus Erythematosus

There are many reasons for a pulmonary vascular involvement in SLE. Like in SSc, there is evidence of endothelial dysfunction in SLE with a potential consequent imbalance between vasodilators and vasoconstrictors. Endothelin levels are high in patients with SLE and particularly in those patients with pulmonary hypertension. Release of endothelin-1 from cultured endothelial cells in response to exposure to serum from SLE patients correlates with levels of anti-endothelial cell antibodies and immune complexes [66]. Other causes of pulmonary vascular disease that may lead to pulmonary hypertension in SLE include recurrent thromboembolic disease, in particular in patients with a hypercoagulable state from antiphospholipid antibodies (such as anticardiolipin antibody present in up to 10% of patients with SLE) [67], pulmonary vasculitis, and parenchymal disease (including interstitial lung disease and the shrinking lung syndrome from myositis of the diaphragm). Combined vasculitis and chronic hypoxia are frequent contributing offenders in these syndromes. In addition, pulmonary venous hypertension can be a consequence of left ventricular dysfunction, myocarditis, or Libman-Sacks endocarditis.

The prevalence of PAH in SLE is unclear, but is likely less than in SSc, affecting about 0.5–14% of the patients with SLE in a large review of the literature encompassing over 100 patients [68]. The patients are predominantly female (90%), young (average age of 33 at time of diagnosis), and often suffer from Raynaud's phenomenon (underscoring a generalized endothelial dysfunction in these patients with SLE and pulmonary hypertension). The pathological lesions are often indistinguishable from IPAH or SSc-PAH lesions, with intimal hyperplasia, smooth muscle cell hypertrophy, and medial thickening. Survival, which was thought to be quite poor (25–50% at 2 years) even compared to SSc-PAH in studies antedating specific pulmonary hypertension treatment, is now estimated at 75% [62].

Mixed Connective Tissue Disease
Patients with MCTD have clinical features which overlap those of SSc, SLE, RA, and polymyositis. The exact prevalence of PAH in MCTD is unknown and has been reported to be as high as 50% [69]. PAH in these patients may occasionally respond to immunosuppressive drugs [70].

Rheumatoid Arthritis
Both the prevalence and impact of pulmonary hypertension in patients with RA is not well known. PAH is, however, a rather rare complication of RA.

Primary Sjögren's Syndrome
Although primary Sjögren's syndrome (pSS) is a relatively common autoimmune disease with glandular and extraglandular manifestations, it is very rarely complicated by PAH. In a recent review by Launay et al. [71] of 28 well-characterized patients with pSS and PAH, the mean age at diagnosis of PAH of these almost exclusively female patients (27/28) was 50 years. Patients had severe functional class (III and IV) and hemodynamic impairment. Standard therapy (with endothelin receptor antagonists, phosphodiesterase inhibitors, or prostanoids) was typically ineffective despite an initial improvement. Some patients were reported to respond to immunosuppressive treatment. However, conclusion regarding treatment is limited by the small size of this case report. The survival rate was low (66% at 3 years).

Therapies for Connective Tissue Disease-Pulmonary Arterial Hypertension

Evidence of chronically impaired endothelial function [72–74] affecting vascular tone and remodeling has been the basis for current therapy of PAH. Vasodilator therapy using high-dose calcium channel blockers is an effective long-term therapy [75], but only for a minority of patients (less than 7% [76] of IPAH patients) who demonstrate acute vasodilation (e.g. to nitric oxide or adenosine) during hemodynamic testing, and an even smaller number of patients with PAH related to CTD who typically fail to show a vasodilator response to acute testing (only about 2.6% responders in that group in one large study) [19]. In addition, long-term response to calcium channel blockers remains very rare in patients with CTD [77]. Therefore, high-dose calcium channel therapy is usually not indicated for patients with PAH associated with CTD such as SSc-PAH, although most patients often receive these drugs at low dosage, typically for Raynaud's syndrome.

General Measures
General guidelines for the treatment of PAH recommend the use of supplemental oxygen in patients who are hypoxic at rest or with exercise, and in patients who have evidence of oxygen desaturation at night (which may not be uncommon in CTD patients). Loop diuretics are often used for the management of volume overload and in overt right heart failure. Finally, digoxin has been suggested in a small series as an adjunct therapy specifically for the management of symptomatic right heart failure where treatment resulted in modest increases in cardiac output as well as a decrease in circulating norepinephrine [78].

Anti-Inflammatory Drugs
As discussed above, it has been increasingly recognized that inflammation may play a significant role in various types of pulmonary hypertension, including IPAH and PAH associated with CTD. Interestingly, some patients with severe PAH associated with some forms of CTD (such as SLE, pSS, and MCTD) have had dramatic improvement of their pulmonary vascular disease with corticosteroids and/or immunosuppressive therapy [70], emphasizing the relevance of inflammation in these subsets of patients. However, this has not been the case for patients with SSc-PAH whose PAH is usually refractory to immunosuppressive drugs [70].

Prostaglandins
Prostacyclin (epoprostenol), on the other hand, has potent pulmonary vasodilator as well as antiplatelet aggregating and antiproliferative properties [79], and has proven effective in improving exercise capacity, cardiopulmonary hemodynamics, NYHA functional class, symptoms, and survival in patients with PAH when given by continuous infusion [80–82]. In SSc-PAH, continuous intravenous epoprostenol marginally improves exercise capacity and hemodynamics [83], compared to conventional therapy, and may have long-term beneficial effects [84], although a clear effect on survival in these patients has yet to be demonstrated.

Treprostinil, an analogue of epoprostenol suitable for continuous subcutaneous administration, has modest effects on symptoms and hemodynamics in PAH [85]. In a small study of 16 patients (among whom 6 had CTD-related PAH), recently FDA-approved intravenous treprostinil was shown to improve hemodynamics, 6-min walk distance (6MWD), functional class, and hemodynamics after 12 weeks of therapy [86]. Although the safety profile of this drug is similar to intravenous epoprostenol, required maintenance doses are usually twice as much as for epoprostenol. However, for patients with SSc-PAH, the lack of requirement of ice packing and less frequent mixing of the drug offer obvious advantages.

Several reports of pulmonary edema in SSc-PAH patients treated with prostaglandin derivatives, both in acute and chronic settings, have raised the suspicion of increased prevalence of veno-occlusive disease in these patients [87, 88] and concern about the usefulness of these drugs for this entity. Nevertheless, intravenous prostaglandin therapy remains an option for patients with SSc-PAH with NYHA class IV. Considering the frequent digital problems and disabilities that these patients often experience, this form of therapy can be quite challenging and may increase the already heavy burden of disease in these patients. In summary, both epoprostenol and treprostinil are FDA approved for PAH, but are cumbersome therapies requiring continuous parenteral administration with the attendant numerous adverse effects (e.g. infection and possibility of pump failure [89]), which make these drugs less than ideal.

Endothelin Receptor Antagonists

Randomized placebo-controlled trials of 12–16 weeks' duration demonstrated a beneficial effect of bosentan therapy on functional class, 6MWD, time to clinical worsening, and hemodynamics in PAH [90, 91]. In these studies, roughly one fifth of the population consisted of SSc-PAH patients, while a large majority had a diagnosis of IPAH. A subgroup analysis, performed by Rubin et al. [91] reported a nonsignificant trend towards a positive treatment effect on 6MWD among the SSc-PAH patients treated with bosentan compared to placebo. At most, bosentan therapy prevented deterioration in these patients (as assessed by an increase of 3 m in the 6 MWD in the treated group compared to a decrease of 40 m in the placebo group). This less than optimal effect of therapy in patients with SSc-PAH is unclear, but may be related to the severity of PAH at time of presentation as well as other factors such as, hypothetically, more severe right ventricular and pulmonary vascular dysfunction, as compared to patients with other forms of PAH (e.g. IPAH).

In an analysis of patients with associated PAH related to CTD (e.g. patients with lupus, overlap syndrome, and other rheumatological disorders) included in randomized clinical trials of bosentan, there was a trend toward improvement in 6MWD and improved survival compared to historical cohorts [92]. Single-center experience suggests that the long-term outcome of first-line bosentan monotherapy is inferior in SSc-PAH compared to IPAH patients, with no change in functional class and worse survival in the former group [63]. Since endothelin-1 appears to play an important pathogenic role in the development of SSc-PAH, contributing to vascular damage and fibrosis, inhibiting endothelin-1 remains a rational and viable therapeutic strategy for these patients. In fact, in a small study of 35 patients with SSc (10 of whom had SSc-PAH), bosentan treatment appeared to reduce endothelial cell (as determined by endothelial soluble serum factors such as ICAM-1, VCAM-1, P-selectin, and PECAM-1) and T cell subset (assessed by expression of lymphocyte function-associated antigen-1, very late antigen-4, and L-selectin on CD3 T cells) activation [93]. Aside from improving pulmonary hypertension, endothelin-1 receptor antagonists (specifically bosentan) cause significant reductions in the occurrence of new digital ulcerations, but do not heal preexisting ulcers [94].

In an effort to target the vasoconstrictive effects of endothelin while preserving its vasodilatory action, selective endothelin-A receptor antagonists have been developed. Sitaxsentan, which was only approved in Europe for treatment of PAH, improved exercise capacity (i.e. change in peak Vo_2 at week 12, which was the main end point of the study) [95]. Elevation in liver enzymes was noted in 10% of patients at the higher dose tested (300 mgs orally once daily). Patients with PAH associated with CTD represented less than a quarter of the study group. A post-hoc analysis of 42 patients (33 patients who received the drug and 9 patients who received placebo) with CTD-PAH demonstrated improved exercise capacity, quality of life, and hemodynamics with sitaxsentan, although elevated liver enzymes were reported in 2 patients [96]. However, this drug was recently removed from the market due to significant hepatotoxicity and death in a few patients. A large placebo-controlled randomized trial of ambrisentan, the only currently FDA-approved selective endothelin receptor antagonist, improved 6MWD in PAH patients at week 12 of treatment; however, the effect was larger in patients with IPAH compared to patients with CTD-PAH (range of 50–60 vs. 15–23 m, respectively) [97]. Ambrisentan is generally well tolerated, although peripheral edema (in up to 20% of patients [97]) and congestive heart failure have been reported.

Phosphodiesterase Inhibitors

Sildenafil, a phosphodiesterase type V inhibitor that reduces the catabolism of cGMP thereby enhancing the cellular effects mediated by nitric oxide, has become a widely used and highly efficacious therapy for PAH. A large clinical trial showed that sildenafil therapy led to an improvement in the 6MWD in patients with IPAH and PAH related to CTD or repaired congenital heart disease (patients were predominantly functional class II or III) at all three doses tested (20, 40, and 80 mg, given three times a day) [98]. Since there were no significant differences in clinical effects and time to clinical worsening at week 12 between the doses, the FDA recommended a dose of 20 mg three times a day. In a post-hoc subgroup analysis of 84 patients with PAH related to CTD (45% of whom had SSc-PAH), data from the SUPER study suggest that sildenafil at a dose of 20 mg improved exercise capacity (6MWD), hemodynamic measures, and functional class after 12 weeks of therapy [99]. However, for reasons that remain unclear (but in part related to the limitations of the study such as post-hoc subgroup analysis), there was no effect for the dose of 80 mg three times a day on hemodynamics in this subgroup of patients with CTD-related PAH [99]. For this reason and because of the potential of increased side effects (such as bleeding from arteriovenous malformations) at high doses, a sildenafil dosage of 20 mg three times a day is recommended for SSc-PAH patients (and perhaps patients with PAH associated with other forms of CTD) as standard therapy. Higher doses are occasionally attempted in case of limited response. The impact of long-term sildenafil therapy on survival in these patients remains to be determined. Finally, tadalafil, another phosphodiesterase inhibitor, has now been shown to be effective for PAH [100]. Subgroup analysis, however, has not been performed, thus its effects on CTD-PAH remain unclear. Tadalafil has the advantage over sildenafil of single daily dosage.

Combination Therapy

It is now common practice to add drugs when patients fail to improve on monotherapy. Adding inhaled iloprost to patients receiving bosentan has been shown to be beneficial in a small randomized trial. Combining inhaled iloprost with sildenafil is mechanistically appealing and anecdotally efficacious [101, 102] as these drugs target separate potentially synergistic pathways. Several multicenter trials are now exploring the efficacy of various combinations of two oral drugs or one oral and one inhaled drug. The results of the PACES trial demonstrate that adding sildenafil (at a dose of 80 mg three times a day) to intravenous epoprostenol improves exercise capacity, hemodynamic measurements, time to clinical worsening, and quality of life [103]. About 21% of these patients had CTD, including 11% with SSc-PAH. Although no specific subgroup analysis is provided, improvement was apparently mainly in patients with IPAH. In a smaller single-center clinical trial, adding sildenafil to patients with IPAH or SSc-PAH after they failed initial monotherapy with bosentan demonstrated that combination therapy improved the 6MWD and functional class in IPAH patients. The outcome in patients with SSc-PAH was less favorable, although combination therapy may have halted clinical deterioration. In addition, there were more side effects reported in the SSc-PAH compared to the IPAH patients, including hepatotoxicity that developed after addition of sildenafil to bosentan monotherapy [104].

Anticoagulation

The rationale for the use of anticoagulation in severe PAH is based on pathologic evidence of pulmonary thromboembolic arterial disease and thrombosis in situ in patients with IPAH [105] and two clinical studies (a retrospective analysis [106] and a small nonrandomized prospective study [75]) demonstrating a significant beneficial effect of anticoagulation on survival in IPAH. Based essentially on these findings, anticoagulation is routinely recommended in the treatment of IPAH patients. The role of anticoagulation in other forms of PAH, in particular in SSc-PAH or other forms of CTD, is much less clear. Theoretically, there is potential for increased bleeding in patients with CTD, particularly with SSc where intestinal telangiectasias may be common. An unpublished review of our experience with anticoagulation in over 100 patients with SSc-PAH suggests that less than 50% of these patients remain on long-term anticoagulation therapy. The reason for discontinuing anticoagulation in these patients is often related to occult bleeding in the gastrointestinal tract. In our experience, the source of bleeding is often difficult to diagnose.

Tyrosine Kinase Inhibitors

The finding that there is pathologically aberrant proliferation of endothelial and smooth muscle cells in PAH, as well increased expression of secreted growth factors such as VEGF and bFGF, has caused a paradigm shift in treatment strategies for this disease as some investigators have likened this condition to a neoplastic process reminiscent of advanced solid tumors [107]. As a result, antineoplastic drugs have been tested in experimental models [108, 109] and some patients [110, 111]. Two strategies are currently tested for treatment of PAH: disruption of PDGF signaling and disruption of the VEGF signaling pathway. A phase II multicenter trial to evaluate the safety, tolerability, and efficacy of imatinib in patients with PAH recently demonstrated that imatinib is well tolerated. However, there was no significant change in 6MWD (primary end point), although there was a significant decrease in pulmonary vascular resistance and an increase in cardiac output in imatinib-treated patients versus placebo [112]. Whether these new antineoplastic drugs with antityrosine kinase activity will have a role in PAH associated with CTD such as SSc-PAH (where there is evidence for both dysregulated proliferation and increased expression of growth factors such as VEGF) remains to be determined. Of note is that a single case report has suggested significant improvement in right ventricular function in response to imatinib treatment in a SSc-PAH patient [113]. Also of note is that imatinib is currently being investigated for SSc-related interstitial lung disease.

Lung Transplantation

Lung transplantation is typically offered as a last resort to patients with PAH who fail medical therapy. Although CTD is not an absolute contraindication to lung transplantation, patients with CTD often have associated morbidity and organ dysfunction other than the lung that place them at a specifically high risk for lung transplantation. The involvement of the esophagus with severe motility disorder and gastroesophageal reflux in patients with SSc is an example of specific risk that surgeons do not take lightly because of the enhanced postoperative potential of aspiration and damage to the recipient lung. For these reasons, patients with SSc-PAH are often denied the lung transplantation option. However, the results of two recent studies [114, 115] suggest that lung transplantation, in carefully selected patients, may represent a viable therapeutic option in patients with end-stage lung dysfunction resulting from SSc. Transplant experts now suggest that candidates for transplantation should be evaluated on an individual basis.

Conclusion

Pulmonary hypertension is a common complication of CTD, particularly SSc where it has a significantly worse outcome compared to other diseases (such as IPAH) within Group 1 of the WHO classification. In addition, modern therapy for PAH appears to be of limited value in SSc-PAH. Similarly, currently available markers of disease severity or response to therapy in SSc-PAH and other CTD are either limited or lacking. Therefore, there is an urgent need to identify potential genetic causes and novel physiologic, molecular, and imaging biomarkers that will allow a better understanding of the underlying pathogenesis and serve as reliable tools to monitor therapy in this devastating syndrome.

References

1 Badesch DB, Champion HC, Sanchez MA, Hoeper MM, Loyd JE, Manes A, McGoon M, Naeije R, Olschewski H, Oudiz RJ, Torbicki A: Diagnosis and assessment of pulmonary arterial hypertension. J Am Coll Cardiol 2009;54:S55–S66.

2 D'Alonzo GE, Barst RJ, Ayres SM, Bergofsky EH, Brundage BH, Detre KM, Fishman AP, Goldring RM, Groves BM, Kernis JT, et al: Survival in patients with primary pulmonary hypertension. Results from a national prospective registry. Ann Intern Med 1991;115:343–349.

3 Simonneau G, Robbins IM, Beghetti M, Channick RN, Delcroix M, Denton CP, Elliott CG, Gaine SP, Gladwin MT, Jing ZC, Krowka MJ, Langleben D, Nakanishi N, Souza R: Updated clinical classification of pulmonary hypertension. J Am Coll Cardiol 2009;54:S43–S54.

4 Isern RA, Yaneva M, Weiner E, Parke A, Rothfield N, Dantzker D, Rich S, Arnett FC: Autoantibodies in patients with primary pulmonary hypertension: association with anti-Ku. Am J Med 1992;93:307–312.

5 Humbert M, Monti G, Brenot F, Sitbon O, Portier A, Grangeot-Keros L, Duroux P, Galanaud P, Simonneau G, Emilie D: Increased interleukin-1 and interleukin-6 serum concentrations in severe primary pulmonary hypertension. Am J Respir Crit Care Med 1995;151:1628–1631.

6 Dorfmüller P, Humbert M, Perros F, Sanchez O, Simonneau G, Müller KM, Capron F: Fibrous remodeling of the pulmonary venous system in pulmonary arterial hypertension associated with connective tissue diseases. Hum Pathol 2007;38:893–902.

7 Chung L, Liu J, Parsons L, Hassoun PM, McGoon M, Badesch DB, Miller DP, Nicolls MR, Zamanian RT: Characterization of connective tissue disease-associated pulmonary arterial hypertension from REVEAL: identifying systemic sclerosis as a unique phenotype. Chest;138:1383–1394.

8 Fisher MR, Mathai SC, Champion HC, Girgis RE, Housten-Harris T, Hummers L, Krishnan JA, Wigley F, Hassoun PM: Clinical differences between idiopathic and scleroderma-related pulmonary hypertension. Arthritis Rheum 2006;54:3043–3050.

9 Kawut SM, Taichman DB, Archer-Chicko CL, Palevsky HI, Kimmel SE: Hemodynamics and survival in patients with pulmonary arterial hypertension related to systemic sclerosis. Chest 2003;123:344–350.

10 Le Pavec J, Humbert M, Mouthon L, Hassoun PM: Systemic sclerosis-associated pulmonary arterial hypertension. Am J Respir Crit Care Med;181:1285–1293.

11 Jimenez SA, Derk CT: Following the molecular pathways toward an understanding of the pathogenesis of systemic sclerosis. Ann Intern Med 2004;140:37–50.

12 Tan FK: Systemic sclerosis: the susceptible host (genetics and environment). Rheum Dis Clin North Am 2003;29:211–237.

13 Steen VD, Medsger TA: Changes in causes of death in systemic sclerosis, 1972–2002. Ann Rheum Dis 2007;66:940–944.

14 Tyndall AJ, Bannert B, Vonk M, Airo P, Cozzi F, Carreira PE, Bancel DF, Allanore Y, Muller-Ladner U, Distler O, Iannone F, Pellerito R, Pileckyte M, Miniati I, Ananieva L, Gurman AB, Damjanov N, Mueller A, Valentini G, Riemekasten G, Tikly M, Hummers L, Henriques MJ, Caramaschi P, Scheja A, Rozman B, Ton E, Kumanovics G, Coleiro B, Feierl E, Szucs G, Von Muhlen CA, Riccieri V, Novak S, Chizzolini C, Kotulska A, Denton C, Coelho PC, Kotter I, Simsek I, de la Pena Lefebvre PG, Hachulla E, Seibold JR, Rednic S, Stork J, Morovic-Vergles J, Walker UA: Causes and risk factors for death in systemic sclerosis: a study from the EULAR Scleroderma Trials and Research (EUSTAR) database. Ann Rheum Dis 2010;69:1809–1815.

15 Hachulla E, Launay D, Mouthon L, Sitbon O, Berezne A, Guillevin L, Hatron PY, Simonneau G, Clerson P, Humbert M: Is pulmonary arterial hypertension really a late complication of systemic sclerosis? Chest 2009;136:1211–1219.

16 Mukerjee D, St George D, Coleiro B, Knight C, Denton CP, Davar J, Black CM, Coghlan JG: Prevalence and outcome in systemic sclerosis associated pulmonary arterial hypertension: application of a registry approach. Ann Rheum Dis 2003;62:1088–1093.

17 Hachulla E, Gressin V, Guillevin L, Carpentier P, Diot E, Sibilia J, Kahan A, Cabane J, Frances C, Launay D, Mouthon L, Allanore Y, Tiev KP, Clerson P, de Groote P, Humbert M: Early detection of pulmonary arterial hypertension in systemic sclerosis: a French nationwide prospective multicenter study. Arthritis Rheum 2005;52:3792–3800.
18 Gaine SP, Rubin LJ: Primary pulmonary hypertension. Lancet 1998;352:719–725.
19 Humbert M, Sitbon O, Chaouat A, Bertocchi M, Habib G, Gressin V, Yaici A, Weitzenblum E, Cordier JF, Chabot F, Dromer C, Pison C, Reynaud-Gaubert M, Haloun A, Laurent M, Hachulla E, Simonneau G: Pulmonary arterial hypertension in France: results from a national registry. Am J Respir Crit Care Med 2006;173:1023–1030.
20 Badesch DB, Raskob GE, Elliott CG, Krichman AM, Farber HW, Frost AE, Barst RJ, Benza RL, Liou TG, Turner M, Giles S, Feldkircher K, Miller DP, McGoon MD: Pulmonary arterial hypertension: baseline characteristics from the REVEAL Registry. Chest 2010;137:376–387.
21 Thenappan T, Shah SJ, Rich S, Gomberg-Maitland M: A USA-based registry for pulmonary arterial hypertension: 1982–2006. Eur Respir J 2007;30:1103–1110.
22 Mayes MD, Lacey JV Jr, Beebe-Dimmer J, Gillespie BW, Cooper B, Laing TJ, Schottenfeld D: Prevalence, incidence, survival, and disease characteristics of systemic sclerosis in a large US population. Arthritis Rheum 2003;48:2246–2255.
23 Hassoun PM: Pulmonary arterial hypertension complicating connective tissue diseases. Semin Respir Crit Care Med 2009;30:429–439.
24 Tuder RM, Groves B, Badesch DB, Voelkel NF: Exuberant endothelial cell growth and elements of inflammation are present in plexiform lesions of pulmonary hypertension. Am J Pathol 1994;144:275–285.
25 Gabrielli A, Svegliati S, Moroncini G, Avvedimento EV: Pathogenic autoantibodies in systemic sclerosis. Curr Opin Immunol 2007;19:640–645.
26 Morse JH, Barst RJ, Fotino M, Zhang Y, Flaster E, Gharavi AE, Fritzler MJ, Dominguez M, Angles-Cano E: Primary pulmonary hypertension, tissue plasminogen activator antibodies, and HLA-DQ7. Am J Respir Crit Care Med 1997;155:274–278.
27 Grigolo B, Mazzetti I, Meliconi R, Bazzi S, Scorza R, Candela M, Gabrielli A, Facchini A: Anti-topoisomerase II alpha autoantibodies in systemic sclerosis-association with pulmonary hypertension and HLA-B35. Clin Exp Immunol 2000;121:539–543.
28 Nicolls MR, Taraseviciene-Stewart L, Rai PR, Badesch DB, Voelkel NF: Autoimmunity and pulmonary hypertension: a perspective. Eur Respir J 2005;26:1110–1118.
29 Okawa-Takatsuji M, Aotsuka S, Fujinami M, Uwatoko S, Kinoshita M, Sumiya M: Up-regulation of intercellular adhesion molecule-1 (ICAM-1), endothelial leucocyte adhesion molecule-1 (ELAM-1) and class II MHC molecules on pulmonary artery endothelial cells by antibodies against U1-ribonucleoprotein. Clin Exp Immunol 1999;116:174–180.
30 Tamby MC, Humbert M, Guilpain P, Servettaz A, Dupin N, Christner JJ, Simonneau G, Fermanian J, Weill B, Guillevin L, Mouthon L: Antibodies to fibroblasts in idiopathic and scleroderma-associated pulmonary hypertension. Eur Respir J 2006;28:799–807.
31 Terrier B, Tamby MC, Camoin L, Guilpain P, Broussard C, Bussone G, Yaici A, Hotellier F, Simonneau G, Guillevin L, Humbert M, Mouthon L: Identification of target antigens of antifibroblast antibodies in pulmonary arterial hypertension. Am J Respir Crit Care Med 2008;177:1128–1134.
32 Riemekasten G, Philippe A, Nather M, Slowinski T, Muller DN, Heidecke H, Matucci-Cerinic M, Czirjak L, Lukitsch I, Becker M, Kill A, van Laar JM, Catar R, Luft FC, Burmester GR, Hegner B, Dragun D: Involvement of functional autoantibodies against vascular receptors in systemic sclerosis. Ann Rheum Dis 2011;70:530–536.
33 Karrer S, Bosserhoff AK, Weiderer P, Distler O, Landthaler M, Szeimies RM, Müller-Ladner U, Scholmerich J, Hellerbrand C: The –2518 promotor polymorphism in the MCP-1 gene is associated with systemic sclerosis. J Invest Dermatol 2005;124:92–98.
34 Tsuchiya N, Kuroki K, Fujimoto M, Murakami Y, Tedder TF, Tokunaga K, Takehara K, Sato S: Association of a functional CD19 polymorphism with susceptibility to systemic sclerosis. Arthritis Rheum 2004;50:4002–4007.
35 Tolusso B, Fabris M, Caporali R, Cuomo G, Isola M, Soldano F, Montecucco C, Valentini G, Ferraccioli G: –238 and +489 TNF-alpha along with TNF-RII gene polymorphisms associate with the diffuse phenotype in patients with systemic sclerosis. Immunol Lett 2005;96:103–108.
36 Hutyrova B, Lukac J, Bosak V, Buc M, du Bois R, Petrek M: Interleukin 1alpha single-nucleotide polymorphism associated with systemic sclerosis. J Rheumatol 2004;31:81–84.
37 Crilly A, Hamilton J, Clark CJ, Jardine A, Madhok R: Analysis of the 5′ flanking region of the interleukin 10 gene in patients with systemic sclerosis. Rheumatology (Oxford) 2003;42:1295–1298.
38 Fonseca C, Lindahl GE, Ponticos M, Sestini P, Renzoni EA, Holmes AM, Spagnolo P, Pantelidis P, Leoni P, McHugh N, Stock CJ, Shi-Wen X, Denton CP, Black CM, Welsh KI, du Bois RM, Abraham DJ: A polymorphism in the CTGF promoter region associated with systemic sclerosis. N Engl J Med 2007;357:1210–1220.
39 Dieude P, Guedj M, Wipff J, Ruiz B, Hachulla E, Diot E, Granel B, Sibilia J, Tiev K, Mouthon L, Cracowski JL, Carpentier PH, Amoura Z, Fajardy I, Avouac J, Meyer O, Kahan A, Boileau C, Allanore Y: STAT4 is a genetic risk factor for systemic sclerosis having additive effects with IRF5 on disease susceptibility and related pulmonary fibrosis. Arthritis Rheum 2009;60:2472–2479.
40 Wipff J, Kahan A, Hachulla E, Sibilia J, Cabane J, Meyer O, Mouthon L, Guillevin L, Junien C, Boileau C, Allanore Y: Association between an endoglin gene polymorphism and systemic sclerosis-related pulmonary arterial hypertension. Rheumatology (Oxford) 2007;46:622–625.
41 Morse J, Barst R, Horn E, Cuervo N, Deng Z, Knowles J: Pulmonary hypertension in scleroderma spectrum of disease: lack of bone morphogenetic protein receptor 2 mutations. J Rheumatol 2002;29:2379–2381.
42 Tew MB, Arnett FC, Reveille JD, Tan FK: Mutations of bone morphogenetic protein receptor type II are not found in patients with pulmonary hypertension and underlying connective tissue diseases. Arthritis Rheum 2002;46:2829–2830.
43 Harrison RE, Flanagan JA, Sankelo M, Abdalla SA, Rowell J, Machado RD, Elliott CG, Robbins IM, Olschewski H, McLaughlin V, Gruenig E, Kermeen F, Halme M, Raisanen-Sokolowski A, Laitinen T, Morrell NW, Trembath RC: Molecular and functional analysis identifies ALK-1 as the predominant cause of pulmonary hypertension related to hereditary haemorrhagic telangiectasia. J Med Genet 2003;40:865–871.
44 Machado RD, Eickelberg O, Elliott CG, Geraci MW, Hanaoka M, Loyd JE, Newman JH, Phillips JA 3rd, Soubrier F, Trembath RC, Chung WK: Genetics and genomics of pulmonary arterial hypertension. J Am Coll Cardiol 2009;54:S32–S42.
45 Coral-Alvarado PX, Garces MF, Caminos JE, Iglesias-Gamarra A, Restrepo JF, Quintana G: Serum endoglin levels in patients suffering from systemic sclerosis and elevated systolic pulmonary arterial pressure. Int J Rheumatol 2010;2010:pii 969383.
46 Sgonc R, Gruschwitz MS, Boeck G, Sepp N, Gruber J, Wick G: Endothelial cell apoptosis in systemic sclerosis is induced by antibody-dependent cell-mediated cytotoxicity via CD95. Arthritis Rheum 2000;43:2550–2562.
47 Cerinic MM, Valentini G, Sorano GG, D'Angelo S, Cuomo G, Fenu L, Generini S, Cinotti S, Morfini M, Pignone A, Guiducci S, Del Rosso A, Kalfin R, Das D, Marongiu F: Blood coagulation, fibrinolysis, and markers of endothelial dysfunction in systemic sclerosis. Semin Arthritis Rheum 2003;32:285–295.
48 Choi JJ, Min DJ, Cho ML, Min SY, Kim SJ, Lee SS, Park KS, Seo YI, Kim WU, Park SH, Cho CS: Elevated vascular endothelial growth factor in systemic sclerosis. J Rheumatol 2003;30:1529–1533.
49 Distler O, Del Rosso A, Giacomelli R, Cipriani P, Conforti ML, Guiducci S, Gay RE, Michel BA, Bruhlmann P, Müller-Ladner U, Gay S, Matucci-Cerinic M: Angiogenic and angiostatic factors in systemic sclerosis: increased levels of vascular endothelial growth factor are a feature of the earliest disease stages and are associated with the absence of fingertip ulcers. Arthritis Res 2002;4:R11.
50 Chang B, Schachna L, White B, Wigley FM, Wise RA: Natural history of mild-moderate pulmonary hypertension and the risk factors for severe pulmonary hypertension in scleroderma. J Rheumatol 2006;33:269–274.
51 Cox SR, Walker JG, Coleman M, Rischmueller M, Proudman S, Smith MD, Ahern MJ, Roberts-Thomson PJ: Isolated pulmonary hypertension in scleroderma. Intern Med J 2005;35:28–33.

52 Steen V, Medsger TA Jr: Predictors of isolated pulmonary hypertension in patients with systemic sclerosis and limited cutaneous involvement. Arthritis Rheum 2003;48:516–522.

53 Plastiras SC, Karadimitrakis SP, Kampolis C, Moutsopoulos HM, Tzelepis GE: Determinants of pulmonary arterial hypertension in scleroderma. Semin Arthritis Rheum 2007;36:392–396.

54 Ong YY, Nikoloutsopoulos T, Bond CP, Smith MD, Ahern MJ, Roberts-Thomson PJ: Decreased nailfold capillary density in limited scleroderma with pulmonary hypertension. Asian Pac J Allergy Immunol 1998;16:81–86.

55 Hsiao SH, Lee CY, Chang SM, Lin SK, Liu CP: Right heart function in scleroderma: insights from myocardial Doppler tissue imaging. J Am Soc Echocardiogr 2006;19:507–514.

56 Lee CY, Chang SM, Hsiao SH, Tseng JC, Lin SK, Liu CP: Right heart function and scleroderma: insights from tricuspid annular plane systolic excursion. Echocardiography 2007;24:118–125.

57 Meune C, Avouac J, Wahbi K, Cabanes L, Wipff J, Mouthon L, Guillevin L, Kahan A, Allanore Y: Cardiac involvement in systemic sclerosis assessed by tissue-Doppler echocardiography during routine care: a controlled study of 100 consecutive patients. Arthritis Rheum 2008;58:1803–1809.

58 Overbeek MJ, Lankhaar JW, Westerhof N, Voskuyl AE, Boonstra A, Bronzwaer JG, Marques KM, Smit EF, Dijkmans BA, Vonk-Noordegraaf A: Right ventricular contractility in systemic sclerosis-associated and idiopathic pulmonary arterial hypertension. Eur Respir J 2008;31:1160–1166.

59 Williams MH, Handler CE, Akram R, Smith CJ, Das C, Smee J, Nair D, Denton CP, Black CM, Coghlan JG: Role of N-terminal brain natriuretic peptide (N-TproBNP) in scleroderma-associated pulmonary arterial hypertension. Eur Heart J 2006;27:1485–1494.

60 Forfia PR, Mathai SC, Fisher MR, Housten-Harris T, Hemnes AR, Champion HC, Girgis RE, Hassoun PM: Hyponatremia predicts right heart failure and poor survival in pulmonary arterial hypertension. Am J Respir Crit Care Med 2008;177:1364–1369.

61 Williams MH, Das C, Handler CE, Akram MR, Davar J, Denton CP, Smith CJ, Black CM, Coghlan JG: Systemic sclerosis associated pulmonary hypertension: improved survival in the current era. Heart 2006;92:926–932.

62 Condliffe R, Kiely DG, Peacock AJ, Corris PA, Gibbs JS, Vrapi F, Das C, Elliot CA, Johnson M, DeSoyza J, Torpy C, Goldsmith K, Hodgkins D, Hughes RJ, Pepke-Zaba J, Coghlan JG: Connective tissue disease-associated pulmonary arterial hypertension in the modern treatment era. Am J Respir Crit Care Med 2009;179:151–157.

63 Girgis RE, Mathai SC, Krishnan JA, Wigley FM, Hassoun PM: Long-term outcome of bosentan treatment in idiopathic pulmonary arterial hypertension and pulmonary arterial hypertension associated with the scleroderma spectrum of diseases. J Heart Lung Transplant 2005;24:1626–1631.

64 Campo A, Mathai SC, Le Pavec J, Zaiman AL, Hummers LK, Boyce D, Housten T, Champion HC, Lechtzin N, Wigley FM, Girgis RE, Hassoun PM: Hemodynamic predictors of survival in scleroderma-related pulmonary arterial hypertension. Am J Respir Crit Care Med 2010;82:252–260.

65 Campo A, Mathai SC, Le Pavec J, Zaiman AL, Hummers LK, Boyce D, Housten T, Lechtzin N, Chami H, Girgis RE, Hassoun PM: Outcomes of hospitalization for right heart failure in pulmonary arterial hypertension. Eur Respir J 2011;38:359–367.

66 Yoshio T, Masuyama J, Mimori A, Takeda A, Minota S, Kano S: Endothelin-1 release from cultured endothelial cells induced by sera from patients with systemic lupus erythematosus. Ann Rheum Dis 1995;54:361–365.

67 Pope J: An update in pulmonary hypertension in systemic lupus erythematosus – do we need to know about it? Lupus 2008;17:274–277.

68 Haas C: Pulmonary hypertension associated with systemic lupus erythematosus (in French). Bull Acad Natl Med 2004;188:985–997, discussion 997.

69 Sullivan WD, Hurst DJ, Harmon CE, Esther JH, Agia GA, Maltby JD, Lillard SB, Held CN, Wolfe JF, Sunderrajan EV, et al: A prospective evaluation emphasizing pulmonary involvement in patients with mixed connective tissue disease. Medicine (Baltimore) 1984;63:92–107.

70 Sanchez O, Sitbon O, Jais X, Simonneau G, Humbert M: Immunosuppressive therapy in connective tissue diseases-associated pulmonary arterial hypertension. Chest 2006;130:182–189.

71 Launay D, Hachulla E, Hatron PY, Jais X, Simonneau G, Humbert M: Pulmonary arterial hypertension: a rare complication of primary Sjogren syndrome: report of 9 new cases and review of the literature. Medicine (Baltimore) 2007;86:299–315.

72 Giaid A, Saleh D: Reduced expression of endothelial nitric oxide synthase in the lungs of patients with pulmonary hypertension. N Engl J Med 1995;333:214–221.

73 Giaid A, Yanagisawa M, Langleben D, Michel RP, Levy R, Shennib H, Kimura S, Masaki T, Duguid WP, Stewart DJ: Expression of endothelin-1 in the lungs of patients with pulmonary hypertension. N Engl J Med 1993;328:1732–1739.

74 Tuder RM, Cool CD, Geraci MW, Wang J, Abman SH, Wright L, Badesch D, Voelkel NF: Prostacyclin synthase expression is decreased in lungs from patients with severe pulmonary hypertension. Am J Respir Crit Care Med 1999;159:1925–1932.

75 Rich S, Kaufmann E, Levy PS: The effect of high doses of calcium-channel blockers on survival in primary pulmonary hypertension. N Engl J Med 1992;327:76–81.

76 Sitbon O, Humbert M, Jais X, Ioos V, Hamid AM, Provencher S, Garcia G, Parent F, Herve P, Simonneau G: Long-term response to calcium channel blockers in idiopathic pulmonary arterial hypertension. Circulation 2005;111:3105–3111.

77 Montani D, Savale L, Natali D, Jais X, Herve P, Garcia G, Humbert M, Simonneau G, Sitbon O: Long-term response to calcium-channel blockers in non-idiopathic pulmonary arterial hypertension. Eur Heart J 2010;31:1898–1907.

78 Rich S, Seidlitz M, Dodin E, Osimani D, Judd D, Genthner D, McLaughlin V, Francis G: The short-term effects of digoxin in patients with right ventricular dysfunction from pulmonary hypertension. Chest 1998;114:787–792.

79 Vane JR, Anggard EE, Botting RM: Regulatory functions of the vascular endothelium. N Engl J Med 1990;323:27–36.

80 Barst RJ, Rubin LJ, Long WA, McGoon MD, Rich S, Badesch DB, Groves BM, Tapson VF, Bourge RC, Brundage BH, et al: A comparison of continuous intravenous epoprostenol (prostacyclin) with conventional therapy for primary pulmonary hypertension. The Primary Pulmonary Hypertension Study Group. N Engl J Med 1996;334:296–302.

81 McLaughlin VV, Genthner DE, Panella MM, Rich S: Reduction in pulmonary vascular resistance with long-term epoprostenol (prostacyclin) therapy in primary pulmonary hypertension. N Engl J Med 1998;338:273–277.

82 Rubin LJ, Mendoza J, Hood M, McGoon M, Barst R, Williams WB, Diehl JH, Crow J, Long W: Treatment of primary pulmonary hypertension with continuous intravenous prostacyclin (epoprostenol). Results of a randomized trial. Ann Intern Med 1990;112:485–491.

83 Badesch DB, Tapson VF, McGoon MD, Brundage BH, Rubin LJ, Wigley FM, Rich S, Barst RJ, Barrett PS, Kral KM, Jobsis MM, Loyd JE, Murali S, Frost A, Girgis R, Bourge RC, Ralph DD, Elliott CG, Hill NS, Langleben D, Schilz RJ, McLaughlin VV, Robbins IM, Groves BM, Shapiro S, Medsger TA Jr: Continuous intravenous epoprostenol for pulmonary hypertension due to the scleroderma spectrum of disease. A randomized, controlled trial. Ann Intern Med 2000;132:425–434.

84 Badesch DB, McGoon MD, Barst RJ, Tapson VF, Rubin LJ, Wigley FM, Kral KM, Raphiou IH, Crater GD: Longterm survival among patients with scleroderma-associated pulmonary arterial hypertension treated with intravenous epoprostenol. J Rheumatol 2009;36:2244–2249.

85 Simonneau G, Barst RJ, Galie N, Naeije R, Rich S, Bourge RC, Keogh A, Oudiz R, Frost A, Blackburn SD, Crow JW, Rubin LJ: Continuous subcutaneous infusion of treprostinil, a prostacyclin analogue, in patients with pulmonary arterial hypertension: a double-blind, randomized, placebo-controlled trial. Am J Respir Crit Care Med 2002;165:800–804.

86 Tapson VF, Gomberg-Maitland M, McLaughlin VV, Benza RL, Widlitz AC, Krichman A, Barst RJ: Safety and efficacy of IV treprostinil for pulmonary arterial hypertension: a prospective, multicenter, open-label, 12-week trial. Chest 2006;129:683–688.

87 Farber HW, Graven KK, Kokolski G, Korn JH: Pulmonary edema during acute infusion of epoprostenol in a patient with pulmonary hypertension and limited scleroderma. J Rheumatol 1999;26:1195–1196.
88 Palmer SM, Robinson LJ, Wang A, Gossage JR, Bashore T, Tapson VF: Massive pulmonary edema and death after prostacyclin infusion in a patient with pulmonary veno-occlusive disease. Chest 1998;113:237–240.
89 Galie N, Manes A, Branzi A: Emerging medical therapies for pulmonary arterial hypertension. Prog Cardiovasc Dis 2002;45:213–224.
90 Channick RN, Simonneau G, Sitbon O, Robbins IM, Frost A, Tapson VF, Badesch DB, Roux S, Rainisio M, Bodin F, Rubin LJ: Effects of the dual endothelin-receptor antagonist bosentan in patients with pulmonary hypertension: a randomised placebo-controlled study. Lancet 2001;358:1119–1123.
91 Rubin LJ, Badesch DB, Barst RJ, Galie N, Black CM, Keogh A, Pulido T, Frost A, Roux S, Leconte I, Landzberg M, Simonneau G: Bosentan therapy for pulmonary arterial hypertension. N Engl J Med 2002;346:896–903.
92 Denton CP, Humbert M, Rubin L, Black CM: Bosentan treatment for pulmonary arterial hypertension related to connective tissue disease: a subgroup analysis of the pivotal clinical trials and their open-label extensions. Ann Rheum Dis 2006;65:1336–1340.
93 Iannone F, Riccardi MT, Guiducci S, Bizzoca R, Cinelli M, Matucci-Cerinic M, Lapadula G: Bosentan regulates the expression of adhesion molecules on circulating T cells and serum soluble adhesion molecules in systemic sclerosis-associated pulmonary arterial hypertension. Ann Rheum Dis 2008;67:1121–1126.
94 Jain M, Varga J: Bosentan for the treatment of systemic sclerosis-associated pulmonary arterial hypertension, pulmonary fibrosis and digital ulcers. Expert Opin Pharmacother 2006;7:1487–1501.
95 Barst RJ, Langleben D, Frost A, Horn EM, Oudiz R, Shapiro S, McLaughlin V, Hill N, Tapson VF, Robbins IM, Zwicke D, Duncan B, Dixon RA, Frumkin LR: Sitaxsentan therapy for pulmonary arterial hypertension. Am J Respir Crit Care Med 2004;169:441–447.
96 Girgis RE, Frost AE, Hill NS, Horn EM, Langleben D, McLaughlin VV, Oudiz RJ, Robbins IM, Seibold JR, Shapiro S, Tapson VF, Barst RJ: Selective endothelin A receptor antagonism with sitaxsentan for pulmonary arterial hypertension associated with connective tissue disease. Ann Rheum Dis 2007;66:1467–1472.
97 Galie N, Olschewski H, Oudiz RJ, Torres F, Frost A, Ghofrani HA, Badesch DB, McGoon MD, McLaughlin VV, Roecker EB, Gerber MJ, Dufton C, Wiens BL, Rubin LJ: Ambrisentan for the treatment of pulmonary arterial hypertension: results of the ambrisentan in pulmonary arterial hypertension, randomized, double-blind, placebo-controlled, multicenter, efficacy (ARIES) study 1 and 2. Circulation 2008;117:3010–3019.
98 Galie N, Ghofrani HA, Torbicki A, Barst RJ, Rubin LJ, Badesch D, Fleming T, Parpia T, Burgess G, Branzi A, Grimminger F, Kurzyna M, Simonneau G: Sildenafil citrate therapy for pulmonary arterial hypertension. N Engl J Med 2005;353:2148–2157.
99 Badesch DB, Hill NS, Burgess G, Rubin LJ, Barst RJ, Galie N, Simonneau G: Sildenafil for pulmonary arterial hypertension associated with connective tissue disease. J Rheumatol 2007;34:2417–2422.
100 Galie N, Brundage BH, Ghofrani HA, Oudiz RJ, Simonneau G, Safdar Z, Shapiro S, White RJ, Chan M, Beardsworth A, Frumkin L, Barst RJ: Tadalafil therapy for pulmonary arterial hypertension. Circulation 2009;119:2894–2903.
101 McLaughlin VV, Oudiz RJ, Frost A, Tapson VF, Murali S, Channick RN, Badesch DB, Barst RJ, Hsu HH, Rubin LJ: Randomized study of adding inhaled iloprost to existing bosentan in pulmonary arterial hypertension. Am J Respir Crit Care Med 2006;174:1257–1263.
102 Hoeper MM, Faulenbach C, Golpon H, Winkler J, Welte T, Niedermeyer J: Combination therapy with bosentan and sildenafil in idiopathic pulmonary arterial hypertension. Eur Respir J 2004;24:1007–1010.
103 Simonneau G, Rubin LJ, Galie N, Barst RJ, Fleming TR, Frost AE, Engel PJ, Kramer MR, Burgess G, Collings L, Cossons N, Sitbon O, Badesch DB: Addition of sildenafil to long-term intravenous epoprostenol therapy in patients with pulmonary arterial hypertension: a randomized trial. Ann Intern Med 2008;149:521–530.
104 Mathai SC, Girgis RE, Fisher MR, Champion HC, Housten-Harris T, Zaiman A, Hassoun PM: Addition of sildenafil to bosentan monotherapy in pulmonary arterial hypertension. Eur Respir J 2007;29:469–475.
105 Pietra GG: Histopathology of primary pulmonary hypertension. Chest 1994;105:2S-6S.
106 Fuster V, Steele PM, Edwards WD, Gersh BJ, McGoon MD, Frye RL: Primary pulmonary hypertension: natural history and the importance of thrombosis. Circulation 1984;70:580–587.
107 Adnot S: Lessons learned from cancer may help in the treatment of pulmonary hypertension. J Clin Invest 2005;115:1461–1463.
108 Schermuly RT, Dony E, Ghofrani HA, Pullamsetti S, Savai R, Roth M, Sydykov A, Lai YJ, Weissmann N, Seeger W, Grimminger F: Reversal of experimental pulmonary hypertension by PDGF inhibition. J Clin Invest 2005;115:2811–2821.
109 Moreno-Vinasco L, Gomberg-Maitland M, Maitland ML, Desai AA, Singleton PA, Sammani S, Sam L, Liu Y, Husain AN, Lang RM, Ratain MJ, Lussier YA, Garcia JG: Genomic assessment of a multikinase inhibitor, sorafenib, in a rodent model of pulmonary hypertension. Physiol Genomics 2008;33:278–291.
110 Ghofrani HA, Seeger W, Grimminger F: Imatinib for the treatment of pulmonary arterial hypertension. N Engl J Med 2005;353:1412–1413.
111 Patterson KC, Weissmann A, Ahmadi T, Farber HW: Imatinib mesylate in the treatment of refractory idiopathic pulmonary arterial hypertension. Ann Intern Med 2006;145:152–153.
112 Ghofrani HA, Morrell NW, Hoeper MM, Olschewski H, Peacock AJ, Barst RJ, Shapiro S, Golpon H, Toshner M, Grimminger F, Pascoe S: Imatinib in pulmonary arterial hypertension patients with inadequate response to established therapy. Am J Respir Crit Care Med 2010;182:1171–1177.
113 ten Freyhaus H, Dumitrescu D, Bovenschulte H, Erdmann E, Rosenkranz S: Significant improvement of right ventricular function by imatinib mesylate in scleroderma-associated pulmonary arterial hypertension. Clin Res Cardiol 2009;98:265–267.
114 Schachna L, Medsger TA Jr, Dauber JH, Wigley FM, Braunstein NA, White B, Steen VD, Conte JV, Yang SC, McCurry KR, Borja MC, Plaskon DE, Orens JB, Gelber AC: Lung transplantation in scleroderma compared with idiopathic pulmonary fibrosis and idiopathic pulmonary arterial hypertension. Arthritis Rheum 2006;54:3954–3961.
115 Shitrit D, Amital A, Peled N, Raviv Y, Medalion B, Saute M, Kramer MR: Lung transplantation in patients with scleroderma: case series, review of the literature, and criteria for transplantation. Clin Transplant 2009;23:178–183.

Paul M. Hassoun
Division of Pulmonary and Critical Care Medicine, Johns Hopkins University Department of Medicine
1830 East Monument Street, Room 530
Baltimore, MD 21287 (USA)
Tel. +1 410 614 5158, E-Mail phassoun@jhmi.edu

Chapter 11

Humbert M, Souza R, Simonneau G (eds): Pulmonary Vascular Disorders.
Prog Respir Res. Basel, Karger, 2012, vol 41, pp 105–112

Pulmonary Arterial Hypertension and HIV and Other Viral Infections

Bruno Degano[a] · Séverine Valmary[b] · Olivier Sitbon[c] · Marc Humbert[c]

Departments of [a]Physiology and [b]Pathology, CHU Jean Minjoz, Besançon, [c]Department of Pneomonology, Hôpital Antoine Béclère, Clamart, France

Abstract

HIV is an independent risk factor for development of pulmonary arterial hypertension (PAH). PAH can complicate the course of HIV infection regardless of the route of HIV transmission, the stage of HIV infection, and the degree of immunosuppression. The clinical presentation and underlying pathology of PAH associated with HIV infection (PAH-HIV) are similar to those encountered in other forms of PAH, although there are data suggesting a greater inflammatory component in the HIV-related form. Although beneficial effects of antiretroviral treatments on established PAH-HIV still remain to be proven, these treatments seem to have led to a tenfold decrease over the last decade, mainly through higher CD4 cell counts and lower immune activation in HIV-infected patients. The prostacyclin epoprostenol is indicated in PAH-HIV patients in functional class IV. Treatment with the oral dual endothelin receptor antagonist bosentan benefit patients with PAH-HIV without adversely affecting the control of HIV infection, and in one series resulted in functional and hemodynamic normalization in 20% of the patients. Another virus, human herpesvirus-8 (HHV-8), has also been suggested to trigger the development of PAH. However, recent data strongly suggest that human γ-herpesviruses, and in particular HHV-8, are unlikely to play a role in the pathogenesis of PAH.

Pulmonary arterial hypertension (PAH) constitutes a heterogeneous group of clinical entities sharing similar pathologic features. Beside the idiopathic form of the disease, PAH has been subcategorized as heritable PAH and PAH associated with other diseases. Among these diseases, infection by HIV has been established as an independent risk factor for the development of PAH [1, 2]. Another virus, human herpesvirus-8 (HHV-8), has also been suggested to trigger the development of PAH [3].

Epidemiologic evidence to determine whether a virus is causally related to a disease depends on strength of association, specificity, temporality, consistency, reproducibility, biologic gradient, biologic plausibility, and experimental evidence [4]. The following chapter will examine the current knowledge about involvement of HIV and the two human γ-herpesviruses [HHV-8 and Epstein-Barr virus (EBV)] in the pathophysiology of PAH.

HIV Infection and Pulmonary Arterial Hypertension

HIV infection has been associated with both infectious and noninfectious complications. With the advent of highly active antiretroviral therapy (HAART) and specific chemoprophylactic drugs, prolonged survival has allowed noninfectious complications of HIV to gain greater recognition and attention. PAH is one of these complications [1, 2, 5].

Epidemiology of Pulmonary Arterial Hypertension in HIV-Infected Patients

Demographic Features of Patients with Pulmonary Arterial Hypertension-HIV

PAH-HIV has been described in both HIV-1 and HIV-2 infection [6]. There is no apparent correlation between the severity of PAH and the stage of HIV infection or the degree of immunodeficiency [6, 7]. Unlike idiopathic PAH, which is more common in women than in men (ratio of males to females 1:1.7), males are more frequently affected by PAH-

HIV (ratio of males to females 1.2:1) [2, 6–8]. PAH-HIV arises regardless of the route of HIV infection [1, 6, 7, 9–11]. Most studies have reported a higher proportion of patients with HIV acquired from intravenous drug use among PAH-HIV patients compared to HIV-infected patients without PAH [2, 9, 12]. Although the role of intravenous drug use as an independent risk factor of PAH has been ruled out [10], recently published results support an additive effect of cocaine to HIV-infection in the development of pulmonary arteriopathy through enhancement of endothelial dysfunction and proliferation of pulmonary smooth muscle cells [13].

Incidence and Prevalence of PAH-HIV in HIV-Infected Patients

In the French PAH Registry, PAH-HIV represented around 7% of all the reported cases of PAH [2]. Initial studies in the early 1990s – a time when therapy with HAART was not yet available – indicated a prevalence of 0.5% (95% CI: 0.10–0.90) [14]. In the current HAART era, a prospective study conducted with more than 7,500 HIV-infected patients found a prevalence of 0.46% (95% CI: 0.32–0.64) [9]. Although the prevalence of PAH-HIV seems to have not changed in recent years, recent data from the Swiss HIV Cohort Study indicate that the incidence declined from 0.21% in 1995 to only 0.03% in 2006 [12]. This decrease in incidence may be related to improvements in HAART and corresponding higher CD4 cell counts and lower immune activation [12].

Pathophysiology

Pathology

In PAH-HIV, the pathological aspect of the affected vessels share broad similarities with all other forms of PAH [15]. Plexiform lesions are found in approximately 80% of cases of PAH-HIV. Pulmonary vein involvement, a hallmark of pulmonary veno-occlusive disease, is observed in only approximately 7% of patients [15]. There is often a significant inflammatory infiltrate surrounding the pulmonary vessels of patients with PAH-HIV, which is more apparent than that seen in idiopathic PAH [16].

Genetic Predisposition in PAH-HIV

Heterozygous germline mutations in the bone morphogenetic protein receptor 2 (*BMPR2*) have been identified in more than 70% of patients with familial PAH, and also in up to 25% of patients with apparently sporadic idiopathic PAH [17]. In PAH-HIV, no *BMPR2* mutation of any kind has been identified [6]. Of note, the HIV-1 tat protein (transcriptional transactivator) represses *BMPR2* gene expression in human macrophages in vitro, thus interfering with transcriptional regulation of BMP and *BMPR2* [18]. It might therefore be possible that *BMPR2* protein downregulation may participate in PAH in HIV-infected individuals.

HIV Infection

Although HIV is present in inflammatory cells in the lungs, HIV-1 nucleic acid and HIV-1 p24 antigen have not been detected in the complex pulmonary lesions of patients with PAH-HIV [19]. However, viral proteins and their interactions with molecular partners in the infected host may promote apoptosis, growth, and proliferation. Excessive production of endothelin-1 (ET-1) has been implicated in endothelial cell dysfunction and in the pathogenesis of PAH [20, 21]. In the setting of HIV infection, HIV-related proteins may affect ET-1 production, not only by endothelial cells but also by inflammatory cells [22]. Glycoprotein 120, a viral protein necessary for the binding and entry of HIV into macrophages, targets human lung endothelial cells, increases markers of apoptosis, and stimulates the secretion of ET-1 [23].

Infection with HIV induces a chronic inflammatory state and persistent immune activation and dysregulation that induce the release of proinflammatory cytokines and growth factors, which may be implicated in the pathogenesis of PAH. Increased expression of platelet-derived growth factor (PDGF), a potent stimulus of smooth muscle cell and fibroblast growth and migration, has been noted in lung tissue from patients with PAH-HIV [24]. Similarly, vascular endothelial growth factor A produced by T cells infected by HIV induces vascular permeability and endothelial cell proliferation, and has therefore been implicated in the development of vasculopathy in HIV-infected patients [25].

The negative factor (*nef*) antigen, critical for the maintenance of HIV viral loads and host cell signaling interactions, has been localized to multiple pulmonary and vascular cell types in HIV-infected patients [19]. In vitro, human endothelial cells exposed to *nef* demonstrate increased apoptosis followed by proliferation [19]. In a comparison of primates infected with a chimeric *nef* virion (SHIV: chimeric viral construct containing the *nef* gene of HIV in a SIV backbone) and those infected with constructs containing the native SIV *nef* allele, complex plexiform-like lesions were found exclusively in animals infected with SHIV [19]. The pattern of *nef* expression in patients with PAH-HIV was found to be similar to that seen in SHIV-infected primates, suggesting that *nef* may play a role in the development of PAH in HIV-infected individuals [19]. In human monocyte-derived macrophages, *nef* activates the secretion of macrophage inflammatory protein-1, IL-1β, IL-6, and TNF-α [26]. An increase in IL-1β and IL-6 serum concentrations has been demonstrated in patients with PAH [27]. The effects of these cytokines on pulmonary vascular vessels could be direct or partly indirect and mediated by PDGF. PDGF production is upregulated by IL-1β, and PDGF appears to be able to promote IL-1β synthesis by macrophages, suggesting a self-perpetuating loop between these two cytokines.

Synergic Role of HIV Infection and Cocaine

As PAH-HIV is more common in intravenous drug users than nonusers, the role of cocaine in the development of pulmonary vascular dysfunction has been examined. Dhillon et al. [13] have shown an additive role of HIV infection and cocaine on vascular cell dysfunction, with alteration in expression of tight junction proteins in pulmonary endothelial cells and enhanced proliferation of pulmonary smooth muscle cells through modulation of the PDGF/PDGF-receptor axis. The nature of the relationship of HIV infection with PDGF (each driving the other) and increased viral replication in the presence of cocaine may allow for a constant source of viral proteins and PDGF [13].

Clinical Presentation and Diagnosis of PAH in HIV-Infected Patients

Detection

The major presenting symptoms of PAH in HIV-infected patients arise as a result of right ventricular dysfunction [6]. These symptoms are nonspecific and could relate to a number of underlying conditions, especially in HIV-infected individuals. A detection algorithm based on dyspnea and transthoracic Doppler echocardiography has recently been proposed (fig. 1) [9].

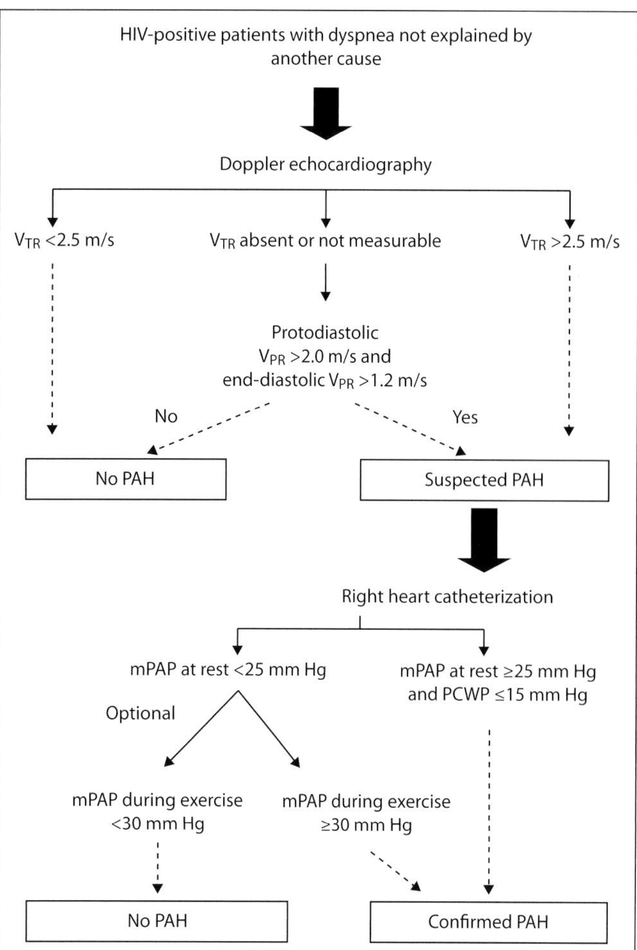

Fig. 1. Diagnostic algorithm based on clinical symptoms of dyspnea, transthoracic Doppler echocardiography, and right heart catheterization. mPAP = Mean pulmonary arterial pressure; PCWP = pulmonary capillary wedge pressure; V_{PR} = peak velocity of pulmonary regurgitation; V_{TR} = peak velocity of tricuspid regurgitation. Reproduced from Sitbon et al. [9].

Characterization

Diagnosis of PAH. The false positive rate from Doppler echocardiography for PAH diagnosis in HIV-infected patients was reported to be as high as 72% when the algorithm presented in figure 1 was used [9]. Therefore, right heart catheterization remains the standard for diagnosing PAH, as well as for evaluating hemodynamic status and response to treatment [9].

HIV-Infected Patients with Portal Hypertension. A history of viral hepatitis is found in about half the PAH-HIV patients in many series [28]. Some of these patients present with cirrhosis and, therefore, with portal hypertension at the time of PAH diagnosis. As they have two associated risk factors for PAH – namely, portal hypertension and HIV infection – these patients are generally excluded from reports on PAH-HIV [6]. This situation is, however, not unusual, representing about 4% of all PAH patients from the French registry [2].

Pulmonary Veno-Occlusive Disease. Pulmonary veno-occlusive disease has been described as a cause of PAH in HIV-infected patients [16]. Several features in the setting of severe PAH support the diagnosis of pulmonary veno-occlusive disease. Examination of lung parenchyma on CT scan provides evidence of septal lines, centrilobular ground-

Table 1. Summary of data from studies of patients with PAH-HIV

	Year	Age at diagnosis years	Duration of HIV infection, years	CD4+ <200/ mm^3, n (%)	HAART at diagnosis n (%)	Median survival months	Survival at 1/2/3 years, %
Speich et al. [14]	1991	30±5	–	3 (50)	0	8.5	–
Petitpretz et al. [8]	1994	32±5	5 ± 2	12 (60)	0	–	53/53/24
Opravil et al. [1]	1997	30[1]	–	12 (63)	6 (32)	15.6	58/32/21
Nunes et al. [6]	2003	34±6	6.4 ± 3.7	42 (51)	39 (48)	~36	73/60/47
Zuber et al. [11]	2004	34.4[1]	7.7[1]	28 (60)	19 (40)	32.4	–
Opravil and Sereni [12]	2008	43[1]	–	–	13 (68)	55.2	90/~75/~65
Degano et al. [7]	2010	41[1]	11.1[1]	18 (23)	64 (84)	>64	88/84/72

[1] Median.

glass opacities, and lymph node enlargement. Low diffusing lung capacity of carbon monoxide is typically measured, and alveolar hemorrhage may be found on bronchoalveolar lavage [20, 21].

Survival and Prognostic Factors
Survival data from several studies of patients with PAH-HIV are summarized in table 1. The presence of PAH is an independent risk factor of mortality in patients with HIV infection [1]. In a majority of cases, death has been reported to be causally related to PAH rather than other complications of HIV infection [8]. In a recent report, we showed that prognosis in PAH-HIV in the current therapeutic era is mainly related to CD4+ lymphocyte count and cardiac function [7].

Treatments
In patients with PAH-HIV, the current guidelines recommend to consider the same treatment algorithm as in patients with idiopathic PAH, taking into consideration comorbidities and drug-drug interactions [20, 21].

Effects of Antiretroviral Therapy on Pulmonary Arterial Hypertension-HIV
In the HAART era, a large majority of PAH-HIV patients are diagnosed while on HAART (table 1), showing that although effective against HIV, this treatment does not prevent PAH [12]. Most results concerning the effects of HAART on functional and hemodynamic parameters in PAH-HIV are based on indirect and retrospective data, and are somehow controversial. Pellicelli et al. [29] reported an accelerated course of PAH in two HIV patients receiving HAART. In a study by Barbaro et al. [30], significant improvements in exercise capacity were seen in PAH-HIV patients after 12 weeks of HAART alone, but hemodynamic parameters were not improved. By contrast, HAART was shown to improve right ventricular systolic pressure over right atrial pressure gradient (evaluated by cardiac echo Doppler) in a retrospective analysis of 35 patients from the Swiss HIV Cohort Study [11]. In this study, HAART significantly decreased mortality due to PAH as well as to other causes, and the authors therefore recommended treating all PAH-HIV patients with HAART, irrespective of their CD4+ lymphocyte counts [11].

Recently published data from animal models have shown that protease inhibitors (PIs) may reverse or attenuate the progression of pulmonary hypertension (PH) induced in rats by monocrotaline injection [31]. PIs given to these animals inhibited Akt phosphorylation in proximal pulmonary arteries and decreased the number of muscularized pulmonary vessels. In addition, PIs inhibited PDGF-induced phosphorylation of Akt in cultured pulmonary artery smooth muscle cells and blocked pulmonary artery smooth muscle cell proliferation. These results support the ability of PIs to interfere with pulmonary vascular remodeling, at least in the inflammatory monocrotaline pulmonary hypertension model [31].

Nonspecific Supportive Therapies
Nonspecific supportive therapies in PAH include supplemental oxygen, anticoagulants, and oral vasodilators. Treatment with oral anticoagulants is recommended as background therapy in patients with idiopathic PAH, but their use in PAH-HIV needs to be considered in light of the risk of thrombocytopenia and associated hepatic disease frequently seen in these patients, and of the potential for drug interactions, particularly with some PIs [20, 21].

Calcium Channel Blockers
Indication for high doses of calcium channel blockers in PAH is strictly limited to patients with acute pulmonary vasodilator response, a situation rarely encountered in patients with PAH-HIV. Moreover, the use of calcium channel blockers in PAH-HIV has been associated with drug-drug interaction with antiretroviral therapies [32].

Specific Pulmonary Arterial Hypertension Therapies
Prostacyclin and Prostacyclin Analogues. Treatment with intravenous epoprostenol in PAH-HIV has been shown to result in a significant and sustained improvement in exercise capacity and hemodynamics [6]. However, continuous intravenous infusion is associated with a risk of catheter-related sepsis, particularly in HIV-positive patients who present with immunosuppression. Nebulized prostacyclin analogs may overcome the limitations of intravenous administration, but there are very few data regarding these compounds in PAH-HIV. Similarly, subcutaneous treprostinil was shown to be effective on functional parameters only in a very limited number of PAH-HIV patients, and its usefulness in this indication remains to be proven [33].

Inhibitors of Type 5 Phosphodiesterase Inhibitors. There are currently no controlled trials of type 5 phosphodiesterase (PDE5) inhibitors in PAH-HIV. Some case studies indicate that sildenafil may improve mean pulmonary arterial pressure, dyspnea, NYHA functional class, and exercise capacity [16]. PDE5 inhibitors are largely metabolized by cytochrome P450 3A4 and there is a potential for drug interactions when coadministered with a number of antiretroviral therapies, particularly PIs, resulting in increases in serum PDE5 inhibitors levels. The coadministration of PDE5 inhibitors with potent CYP3A4 inhibitors, including ritonavir, is contraindicated [34].

Oral Endothelin Receptor Antagonists. In the prospective, open-label BREATHE-4 study, Sitbon et al. [35] showed that treatment of PAH-HIV patients with the dual ET-1 receptor antagonist bosentan improved functional and hemodynamic parameters compared with baseline. Barbaro et al. [30] showed that treatment of PAH-HIV patients with bosentan plus HAART resulted in significant hemodynamic improvements compared with patients treated with HAART alone. A retrospective study showed a long-term beneficial effect of bosentan on functional and hemodynamic parameters without impacting control of HIV infection [28]. Notably, bosentan resulted in functional and hemodynamic normalization in 10 of the 59 patients in this series [28]. The selective ERA ambrisentan has demonstrated efficacy on symptoms, exercise capacity, hemodynamics, and time to clinical worsening in patients with PAH-HIV [36].

Pulmonary Arterial Hypertension and γ-Herpes Viruses

Some diseases (such as connective tissue diseases, portal hypertension, and/or HIV infection) and/or conditions (such as genetic mutations known to be associated with PAH) are associated with a higher prevalence of PAH than in the general population. Nevertheless, PAH occurs in a minority of subjects with these underlying diseases or conditions. Therefore, the question arises as to whether an additional factor can trigger the development of PAH.

Human Herpesvirus-8 in Pulmonary Arterial Hypertension
Cool et al. [3] have suggested that HHV-8 should act as a 'second hit' in the development of PAH. Their evidence for HHV-8 infection in idiopathic PAH stemmed from polymerase chain reaction (PCR) and immunohistochemical analysis that revealed the presence of the HHV-8 genome and proteins in plexiform lesions and cells outside these lesions [3]. However, several other groups using similar techniques have subsequently failed to show the presence of HHV-8 in lung lesions of PAH [37, 38].

Rationale for a Putative Role of a γ-Herpesvirus in Pulmonary Arterial Hypertension
The initial hypothesis that γ-herpesviruses may play a role in PAH comes from clinical observations. Patients with severe PAH and multicentric Castleman's disease, an angioproliferative disorder associated with HHV-8 infection in which IL-6 is produced in large quantities in the germinal centers of hyperplastic lymph nodes, may experience complete resolution of PAH after successful treatment of Castleman's disease [39]. Thus, HHV-8 has been suggested to be a common inciting agent for both diseases.

Another clinical observation has been the histologic similarities between the plexiform lesions of PAH and the characteristic endothelial abnormalities of Kaposi's sarcoma [3]. In addition, infection of primary pulmonary microvascular cells by HHV-8 alters the expression of genes perceived as important in the pathophysiology of PAH, including BMP pathway genes and a variety of mediators including IL-6 [40]. Increased production of IL-6 might be a pathophysiological link between γ-herpesviruses and PAH. Interestingly, the two known γ-herpesviruses, HHV-8 and EBV, each lead

– although by different mechanisms – to an increased production of IL-6 [41].

Some data from animal models also indicate that the murine γ-herpesvirus γHV68, a vasculotropic virus closely related to both HHV-8 and EBV, can mediate neointimal lesions and pulmonary hypertension in mice [42].

Controversy about a Role for Human Herpesvirus-8 in Pulmonary Arterial Hypertension

The seroprevalence of HHV-8 in PAH patients has been found to be similar to that of healthy controls. Although serologic tests are unlikely to reflect organ-specific HHV-8 infection in patients, these results argue against an association between PAH and HHV-8 [43].

In contrast to the relatively poor sensitivity of serologic tests, PCR is very sensitive in detecting the virus in DNA samples from infected lesions, particularly Kaposi's sarcoma [38]. Nevertheless, this extremely sensitive technique is prone to cross-contamination. This is probably the reason why several reports have described the presence of HHV-8 DNA in tissue samples of patients with sarcoidosis, multiple myeloma, Waldenström macroglobulinemia, atheromatous lesions, and pemphigus [38]. The negativity of PCR found by many authors in PAH goes strongly against any presence of HHV-8 in the examined pulmonary lesions, while positivity found by others might possibly be due to other factors including contamination [38].

One of the best tools to detect HHV-8 in tissues is immunohistochemistry with anti-latent nuclear antigen-1 (LANA-1) antibodies [38]. The LANA-1 protein is expressed in the nucleus of infected cells. Immunohistochemistry is sensitive, and the presence of a positive nuclear stippling pattern is highly specific. In our hands, none of 34 lung tissues from PAH patients gave a positive 'stippling' staining with anti-LANA-1, and all PCR examinations were negative, although DNA extraction from formalin-fixed tissues was reliable [38].

The Epstein-Barr Virus Hypothesis in Pulmonary Arterial Hypertension

It was suggested that the discrepancy between positive immunostaining found by some authors and the negativity of PCR analyzed in the same tissue samples could be due to the presence of another γ-herpesvirus or of a yet-to-be-discovered herpesvirus [44]. Although it is closely related to the murine γ-herpesvirus γHV68, which can induce PAH in mice, EBV has never been associated with PAH in the literature. In a recent study, we failed to detect EBV antigens in any cell type of our samples [38].

Is There a Putative Role for Other Viruses?

Interferon (IFN) is produced in response to the presence in a cell of a viral genome. Human pulmonary artery smooth muscle cells are stimulated to release ET-1 by the combination of TNF-α and the type II INF-γ. It has recently been reported that human pulmonary artery smooth muscle cells release high levels of ET-1 when stimulated with INF-β, especially when the cells are cotreated with TNF-α. Therefore, it remains plausible that viruses may trigger the development of pulmonary lesions through induction of ET-1 production via type I IFN, although viruses may be absent in end-stage PAH (which correspond to most of the studied lung fragments).

Conclusion

A role for HIV in the development of PAH is clear, although the exact role of HIV in this pathology remains unclear. The implication of HHV-8 has been suggested, but the implication of this virus seems very unlikely. Nevertheless, a role for viral infection, especially at the early stage of the disease, seems difficult to definitively rule out.

References

1 Opravil M, Pechere M, Speich R, Joller-Jemelka HI, Jenni R, Russi EW, Hirschel B, Luthy R: HIV-associated primary pulmonary hypertension. A case control study. Swiss HIV Cohort Study. Am J Respir Crit Care Med 1997;155:990–995.

2 Humbert M, Sitbon O, Chaouat A, Bertocchi M, Habib G, Gressin V, Yaici A, Weitzenblum E, Cordier JF, Chabot F, Dromer C, Pison C, Reynaud-Gaubert M, Haloun A, Laurent M, Hachulla E, Simonneau G: Pulmonary arterial hypertension in France: results from a national registry. Am J Respir Crit Care Med 2006;173:1023–1030.

3 Cool CD, Rai PR, Yeager ME, Hernandez-Saavedra D, Serls AE, Bull TM, Geraci MW, Brown KK, Routes JM, Tuder RM, Voelkel NF: Expression of human herpesvirus 8 in primary pulmonary hypertension. N Engl J Med 2003;349:1113–1122.

4 Tarte K, Chang Y, Klein B: Kaposi's sarcoma-associated herpesvirus and multiple myeloma: lack of criteria for causality. Blood 1999;93:3159–3163, discussion 3163–3164.

5 Kim KK, Factor SM: Membranoproliferative glomerulonephritis and plexogenic pulmonary arteriopathy in a homosexual man with acquired immunodeficiency syndrome. Hum Pathol 1987;18:1293–1296.

6 Nunes H, Humbert M, Sitbon O, Morse JH, Deng Z, Knowles JA, Le Gall C, Parent F, Garcia G, Herve P, Barst RJ, Simonneau G: Prognostic factors for survival in human immunodeficiency virus-associated pulmonary arterial hypertension. Am J Respir Crit Care Med 2003;167:1433–1439.

7 Degano B, Guillaume M, Savale L, Montani D, Jais X, Yaici A, Le Pavec J, Humbert M, Simonneau G, Sitbon O: HIV-associated pulmonary arterial hypertension: survival and prognostic factors in the modern therapeutic era. AIDS 2010;24:67–75.

8 Petitpretz P, Brenot F, Azarian R, Parent F, Rain B, Herve P, Simonneau G: Pulmonary hypertension in patients with human immunodeficiency virus infection. Comparison with primary pulmonary hypertension. Circulation 1994;89:2722–2727.

9 Sitbon O, Lascoux-Combe C, Delfraissy JF, Yeni PG, Raffi F, De Zuttere D, Gressin V, Clerson P, Sereni D, Simonneau G: Prevalence of HIV-related pulmonary arterial hypertension in the current antiretroviral therapy era. Am J Respir Crit Care Med 2008;177:108–113.

10 Hsue PY, Deeks SG, Farah HH, Palav S, Ahmed SY, Schnell A, Ellman AB, Huang L, Dollard SC, Martin JN: Role of HIV and human herpesvirus-8 infection in pulmonary arterial hypertension. AIDS 2008;22:825–833.

11 Zuber JP, Calmy A, Evison JM, Hasse B, Schiffer V, Wagels T, Nuesch R, Magenta L, Ledergerber B, Jenni R, Speich R, Opravil M: Pulmonary arterial hypertension related to HIV infection: improved hemodynamics and survival associated with antiretroviral therapy. Clin Infect Dis 2004;38:1178–1185.

12 Opravil M, Sereni D: Natural history of HIV-associated pulmonary arterial hypertension: trends in the HAART era. AIDS 2008;22(suppl 3):S35–S40.

13 Dhillon NK, Li F, Xue B, Tawfik O, Morgello S, Buch S, O'Brien Ladner A: Effect of cocaine on HIV-mediated pulmonary endothelial and smooth muscle dysfunction. Am J Respir Cell Mol Biol 2011;45:40–52.

14 Speich R, Jenni R, Opravil M, Pfab M, Russi EW: Primary pulmonary hypertension in HIV infection. Chest 1991;100:1268–1271.

15 Pietra GG, Capron F, Stewart S, Leone O, Humbert M, Robbins IM, Reid LM, Tuder RM: Pathologic assessment of vasculopathies in pulmonary hypertension. J Am Coll Cardiol 2004;43:25S–32S.

16 Degano B, Sitbon O, Simonneau G: Pulmonary arterial hypertension and HIV infection. Semin Respir Crit Care Med 2009;30:440–447.

17 Sztrymf B, Coulet F, Girerd B, Yaici A, Jais X, Sitbon O, Montani D, Souza R, Simonneau G, Soubrier F, Humbert M: Clinical outcomes of pulmonary arterial hypertension in carriers of BMPR2 mutation. Am J Respir Crit Care Med 2008;177:1377–1383.

18 Caldwell RL, Gadipatti R, Lane KB, Shepherd VL: HIV-1 TAT represses transcription of the bone morphogenic protein receptor-2 in U937 monocytic cells. J Leukoc Biol 2006;79:192–201.

19 Marecki JC, Cool CD, Parr JE, Beckey VE, Luciw PA, Tarantal AF, Carville A, Shannon RP, Cota-Gomez A, Tuder RM, Voelkel NF, Flores SC: HIV-1 Nef is associated with complex pulmonary vascular lesions in SHIV-nef-infected macaques. Am J Respir Crit Care Med 2006;174:437–445.

20 Galie N, Hoeper MM, Humbert M, Torbicki A, Vachiery JL, Barbera JA, Beghetti M, Corris P, Gaine S, Gibbs JS, Gomez-Sanchez MA, Jondeau G, Klepetko W, Opitz C, Peacock A, Rubin L, Zellweger M, Simonneau G, Vahanian A, Auricchio A, Bax J, Ceconi C, Dean V, Filippatos G, Funck-Brentano C, Hobbs R, Kearney P, McDonagh T, McGregor K, Popescu BA, Reiner Z, Sechtem U, Sirnes PA, Tendera M, Vardas P, Widimsky P, Al Attar N, Andreotti F, Aschermann M, Asteggiano R, Benza R, Berger R, Bonnet D, Delcroix M, Howard L, Kitsiou AN, Lang I, Maggioni A, Nielsen-Kudsk JE, Park M, Perrone-Filardi P, Price S, Domenech MT, Vonk-Noordegraaf A, Zamorano JL: Guidelines for the diagnosis and treatment of pulmonary hypertension: the Task Force for the Diagnosis and Treatment of Pulmonary Hypertension of the European Society of Cardiology (ESC) and the European Respiratory Society (ERS), endorsed by the International Society of Heart and Lung Transplantation (ISHLT). Eur Heart J 2009;30:2493–2537.

21 Galie N, Hoeper MM, Humbert M, Torbicki A, Vachiery JL, Barbera JA, Beghetti M, Corris P, Gaine S, Gibbs JS, Gomez-Sanchez MA, Jondeau G, Klepetko W, Opitz C, Peacock A, Rubin L, Zellweger M, Simonneau G: Guidelines for the diagnosis and treatment of pulmonary hypertension. Eur Respir J 2009;34:1219–1263.

22 Humbert M: Mediators involved in HIV-related pulmonary arterial hypertension. AIDS 2008;22(suppl 3):S41–S47.

23 Kanmogne GD, Primeaux C, Grammas P: HIV-1 gp120 proteins alter tight junction protein expression and brain endothelial cell permeability: implications for the pathogenesis of HIV-associated dementia. J Neuropathol Exp Neurol 2005;64:498–505.

24 Humbert M, Monti G, Fartoukh M, Magnan A, Brenot F, Rain B, Capron F, Galanaud P, Duroux P, Simonneau G, Emilie D: Platelet-derived growth factor expression in primary pulmonary hypertension: comparison of HIV seropositive and HIV seronegative patients. Eur Respir J 1998;11:554–559.

25 Ascherl G, Hohenadl C, Schatz O, Shumay E, Bogner J, Eckhart L, Tschachler E, Monini P, Ensoli B, Sturzl M: Infection with human immunodeficiency virus-1 increases expression of vascular endothelial cell growth factor in T cells: implications for acquired immunodeficiency syndrome-associated vasculopathy. Blood 1999;93:4232–4241.

26 Olivetta E, Percario Z, Fiorucci G: HIV-1 Nef induces the release of inflammatory factors from human monocytes/macrophages: involvement of Nef endocytotic signals and NF-kappaB activation. J Immunol 2003;170:1716–1727.

27 Humbert M, Monti G, Brenot F, Sitbon O, Portier A, Grangeot-Keros L, Duroux P, Galanaud P, Simonneau G, Emilie D: Increased interleukin-1 and interleukin-6 serum concentrations in severe primary pulmonary hypertension. Am J Respir Crit Care Med 1995;151:1628–1631.

28 Degano B, Yaici A, Le Pavec J, Savale L, Jais X, Camara B, Humbert M, Simonneau G, Sitbon O: Long-term effects of bosentan in patients with HIV-associated pulmonary arterial hypertension. Eur Respir J 2009;33:92–98.

29 Pellicelli AM, Palmieri F, D'Ambrosio C, Rianda A, Boumis E, Girardi E, Antonucci G, D'Amato C, Borgia MC: Role of human immunodeficiency virus in primary pulmonary hypertension – case reports. Angiology 1998;49:1005–1011.

30 Barbaro G, Lucchini A, Pellicelli AM, Grisorio B, Giancaspro G, Barbarini G: Highly active antiretroviral therapy compared with HAART and bosentan in combination in patients with HIV-associated pulmonary hypertension. Heart 2006;92:1164–1166.

31 Gary-Bobo G, Houssaini A, Amsellem V, Rideau D, Pacaud P, Perrin A, Bregeon J, Marcos E, Dubois-Rande JL, Sitbon O, Savale L, Adnot S: Effects of HIV protease inhibitors on progression of monocrotaline- and hypoxia-induced pulmonary hypertension in rats. Circulation 2010;122:1937–1947.

32 Glesby MJ, Aberg JA, Kendall MA, Fichtenbaum CJ, Hafner R, Hall S, Grosskopf N, Zolopa AR, Gerber JG: Pharmacokinetic interactions between indinavir plus ritonavir and calcium channel blockers. Clin Pharmacol Ther 2005;78:143–153.

33 Degano B, Sitbon O, Simonneau G: Pulmonary arterial hypertension and HIV infection. Semin Respir Crit Care Med 2009;30:440–447.

34 Sildenafil Summary of Product Characteristics. http://emc.medicines.org.uk/emc/assets/c/html/DisplayDoc.asp?DocumentID=17443#CONTRAINDICATIONS.

35 Sitbon O, Gressin V, Speich R, Macdonald PS, Opravil M, Cooper DA, Fourme T, Humbert M, Delfraissy JF, Simonneau G: Bosentan for the treatment of human immunodeficiency virus-associated pulmonary arterial hypertension. Am J Respir Crit Care Med 2004;170:1212–1217.

36 Galie N, Olschewski H, Oudiz RJ, Torres F, Frost A, Ghofrani HA, Badesch DB, McGoon MD, McLaughlin VV, Roecker EB, Gerber MJ, Dufton C, Wiens BL, Rubin LJ: Ambrisentan for the treatment of pulmonary arterial hypertension: results of the ambrisentan in pulmonary arterial hypertension, randomized, double-blind, placebo-controlled, multicenter, efficacy (ARIES) study 1 and 2. Circulation 2008;117:3010–3019.

37 Henke-Gendo C, Mengel M, Hoeper MM, Alkharsah K, Schulz TF: Absence of Kaposi's sarcoma-associated herpesvirus in patients with pulmonary arterial hypertension. Am J Respir Crit Care Med 2005;172:1581–1585.
38 Valmary S, Dorfmuller P, Montani D, Humbert M, Brousset P, Degano B: Human gamma-herpesviruses EBV and HHV-8 are not detected in the lungs of patients with severe pulmonary arterial hypertension. Chest 2011;139:1310–1316.
39 Montani D, Achouh L, Marcelin AG, Viard JP, Hermine O, Canioni D, Sitbon O, Simonneau G, Humbert M: Reversibility of pulmonary arterial hypertension in HIV/HHV8-associated Castleman's disease. Eur Respir J 2005;26:969–972.
40 Bull TM, Meadows CA, Coldren CD, Moore M, Sotto-Santiago SM, Nana-Sinkam SP, Campbell TB, Geraci MW: Human herpesvirus-8 infection of primary pulmonary microvascular endothelial cells. Am J Respir Cell Mol Biol 2008;39:706–716.
41 Kwun HJ, da Silva SR, Shah IM, Blake N, Moore PS, Chang Y: Kaposi's sarcoma-associated herpesvirus latency-associated nuclear antigen 1 mimics Epstein-Barr virus EBNA1 immune evasion through central repeat domain effects on protein processing. J Virol 2007;81:8225–8235.
42 Spiekerkoetter E, Alvira CM, Kim YM, Bruneau A, Pricola KL, Wang L, Ambartsumian N, Rabinovitch M: Reactivation of gammaHV68 induces neointimal lesions in pulmonary arteries of S100A4/Mts1-overexpressing mice in association with degradation of elastin. Am J Physiol Lung Cell Mol Physiol 2008;294:L276–L289.
43 Montani D, Marcelin AG, Sitbon O, Calvez V, Simonneau G, Humbert M: Human herpes virus 8 in HIV and non-HIV infected patients with pulmonary arterial hypertension in France. AIDS 2005;19:1239–1240.
44 Katano H, Hogaboam CM: Herpesvirus-associated pulmonary hypertension? Am J Respir Crit Care Med 2005;172:1485–1486.

Bruno Degano, MD, PhD
Explorations Fonctionnelles-Physiologie
CHU Jean Minjoz
FR–25030 Besançon Cedex (France)
Tel. +33 3 81 21 18 07, E-Mail bruno.degano@univ-fcomte.fr

Chapter 12
Humbert M, Souza R, Simonneau G (eds): Pulmonary Vascular Disorders.
Prog Respir Res. Basel, Karger, 2012, vol 41, pp 113–121

Portopulmonary Hypertension and Hepatopulmonary Syndrome

Laurent Savale[a–c] · Philippe Hervé[a–c] · Olivier Sitbon[a–c]

[a]Université Paris-Sud, Faculté de Médecine, Kremlin-Bicêtre, [b]Centre de Référence de l'Hypertension Pulmonaire Sévère, Service de Pneumologie et Réanimation Respiratoire, Hôpital Antoine Béclère (AP-HP), Clamart, [c]INSERM U999, Hypertension Artérielle Pulmonaire: Physiopathologie et Innovation Thérapeutique, Le Plessis Robinson, France

Abstract

Liver disease and/or portal hypertension may have major consequences on pulmonary vasculature. Two distinct vascular disorders associated with this condition are described: hepatopulmonary syndrome (HPS), which is characterized by intrapulmonary vascular dilatation, and portopulmonary hypertension (PoPH), which is characterized by a high level of pulmonary vascular resistance due to pulmonary vascular remodeling. The trigger of these two diseases is the same, but the pathophysiological mechanisms that lead to these diseases are not well understood. Both are independent predictive factors of survival, justifying that screening for these two disorders should be systematically undertaken in symptomatic patients and in all orthotopic liver transplantation candidates. Resolution of HPS is common after liver transplantation. In contrast, the evolution of PoPH after transplantation is often unpredictable. The treatment strategies most commonly employed for PoPH patients are based on data from pharmacological studies and clinical experiences of populations with other forms of pulmonary arterial hypertension.

Chronic liver dysfunction may have major consequences on the pulmonary vasculature. Portal hypertension, more than liver disease by itself, may lead to pulmonary endothelial dysfunction which can favor pulmonary vascular remodeling, neoangiogenesis, and vascular tone dysfunction. In portal hypertension, with or without liver dysfunction, the pulmonary vascular endothelium can be directly injured by cytokines and growth factors coming from the gut and shunting both the liver and portal system. Two pulmonary vascular diseases associated with portal hypertension can be distinguished: portopulmonary hypertension (PoPH) and hepatopulmonary syndrome (HPS). PoPH is characterized by vascular remodeling of small muscular pulmonary arteries leading to increased pulmonary vascular resistance (PVR) and ultimately right heart failure. In contrast, the HPS is characterized by neoangiogenesis and vasodilatation of pulmonary capillaries leading to substantially altered gas exchange. These two pulmonary vascular diseases can affect functional outcome and prognosis of patients with portal hypertension irrespective of the liver function status. Because they determine the management of the patient, these pulmonary vascular diseases should be routinely screened in patients in whom orthotopic liver transplantation (OLT) is indicated. Similarly, it is crucial to consider these diseases in symptomatic patients. This chapter explores possible relevant etiological factors and summarizes current diagnostic and therapeutic approaches for these two vascular conditions associated with portal hypertension (table 1).

Portopulmonary Hypertension

Definition and Epidemiology of Portopulmonary Hypertension

Diagnostic criteria of PoPH include a mean pulmonary arterial pressure (mPAP) ≥25 mm Hg with a normal mean pulmonary artery occlusion pressure (i.e. <15 mm Hg) and a PVR ≥240 dynes•s•cm^{-5}, associated with evidence of portal hypertension (confirmed by measurement of transhepatic gradient or suggested by the presence of splenomegaly, thrombocytopenia, esophageal varices, portal-to-systemic shunts, or portal vein abnormalities) [1]. As a consequence, right heart catheterization is mandatory to definitively establish the diagnosis of PoPH. Calculation of PVR is of major importance in order to exclude passive elevation of

Table 1. Physiopathological, clinical, and management distinctions between HPS and PoPH

	HPS	PoPH
Trigger of the vascular disease	abnormal angiogenesis of the pulmonary microcirculation induced by chronic liver disease and/or portal hypertension	
	– damage of the endothelium directly injured by constituents of venous blood arising in the liver and portal system – imbalance between pro- and antiangiogenic factors within the lung – imbalance of vasoconstrictive and vasodilatory mediators – systemic and local inflammation – high cardiac output due to portal hypertension may promote vascular remodeling	
Location of the vasculopathy	precapillary and capillary vessels	pulmonary artery of small caliber
Histopathological features	– dilatation of precapillary and capillary vessels – neoangiogenesis – precapillary arteriovenous communications	– endothelial cell proliferation – smooth muscle cell hypertrophy – in situ thrombosis
Physiopathological features	abnormalities of gas exchange leading to hypoxemia due to: – alveolar ventilation-perfusion imbalance – intrapulmonary shunt – diffusion-perfusion defect	increased PVR leading to right heart failure
Clinical impact	Both are independent predictive factors of survival	
Medical therapy	no medical therapy	specific treatment of pulmonary hypertension with specific considerations
OLT	OLT is the best option to reverse severe HPS	OLT should not be considered as a treatment for PoPH

pulmonary pressures. Indeed, portal hypertension is frequently associated with hyperkinetic status and/or fluid overload that can favor passive and moderate elevation of pulmonary pressures without elevation of PVR [2].

In the literature, the prevalence of PoPH ranges from 0.5–5% in patients with portal hypertension with or without cirrhosis [3–5]. In the French PAH Registry, portal hypertension is the third common risk factor associated with PAH, and represents 10% of the overall PAH population [6]. In the US registry, 5.1% of patients with PAH were identified as having portal hypertension [7]. Females with liver disease have a higher risk of developing PoPH, which suggests that hormonal factors may play a role in its pathogenesis [8, 9]. A higher prevalence of autoimmune liver disease among patients with PoPH in comparison to the overall population with cirrhosis has also been reported, suggesting that dysregulated immunity may be pathogenetically relevant [8, 10].

Physiopathology of Portopulmonary Hypertension

Pathological lesions observed in the lungs of patients with PoPH are similar to those seen in patients with idiopathic PAH. Plexiform lesions of small pulmonary arteries associated with medial hypertrophy with or without intimal fibrosis are typically observed in these patients [11].

Portal hypertension, rather than the liver disease by itself, is responsible for pulmonary vascular disorders described in liver diseases. One hypothesis that has been proposed is that toxic substances from the digestive tract, that are normally cleared by hepatic metabolism, bypass the liver via portosystemic shunts and directly damage the pulmonary vascular endothelium [2]. In cirrhosis, plasma concentrations of some vasoactive mediators such as proinflammatory cytokines or growth factors are increased. A local imbalance of vasoconstrictive and vasodilatory mediators, due to endothelial dysfunction, is also likely to be pathophysiologically relevant, as in idiopathic PAH. A lower expression of the endothelial nitric oxide synthase (NOS) associated with an overexpression of endothelin-1 (ET-1) in the pulmonary vessels could favor pulmonary vascular remodeling leading to increased PVR in susceptible patients. It was also suggested that the high cardiac output typically observed in patients with portal hypertension may promote pulmonary vascular remodeling on its own by inducing shear stress lesions.

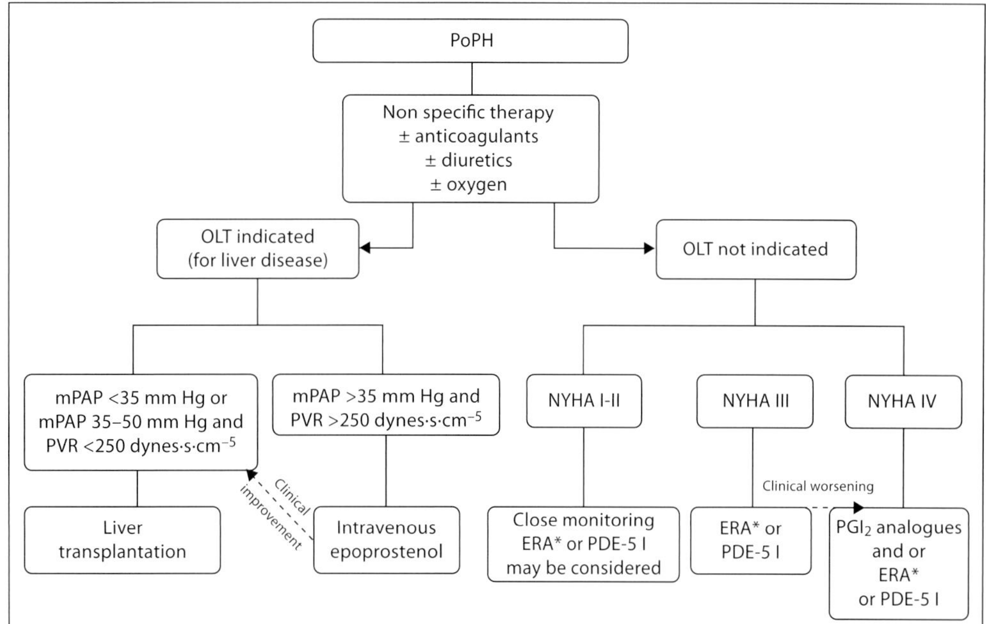

Fig. 1. Management of PoPH (from Savale et al. [65]). * Endothelin receptor antagonists (ERA) should only be considered for patients without evidence of severe hepatocellular insufficiency.

Finally, it is likely that there are genetic factors that could favor the occurrence of PoPH. For example, genetic polymorphisms in estrogen metabolism and other signaling pathways, in particular those associated with cellular growth and apoptosis, also seem to play a role in the development of the disease [12].

Management of Portopulmonary Hypertension (fig. 1)
The treatment strategies most commonly applied in patients with PoPH are based on data from pharmacological studies and clinical experience in patients with other forms of PAH. In contrast to other types of associated PAH, patients with PoPH have been excluded from the large clinical trials in PAH and there is no controlled study accessing PAH-specific therapies in PoPH patients exclusively. The majority of data on treatment of PoPH, therefore, is derived from small series and case reports. However, significant differences exist between PoPH and other PAH subtypes which may impact the efficacy and tolerability of PAH-specific therapies. In particular, the potential for potent vasodilator treatments to worsen portal hypertension via a direct action on the splanchnic circulation remains a significant concern.

Conventional Therapy
The use of diuretics is advocated for control of symptomatic fluid overload, and supplementary oxygen is routinely prescribed in order to maintain arterial oxygen saturation above 90%. In patients with cirrhosis, anticoagulants are not usually administered when there is severe hepatocellular insufficiency and/or thrombocytopenia due to hypersplenism. The use of β-adrenergic receptor blockers, which are widely employed for prophylaxis of gastrointestinal hemorrhage from esophageal varices, may be associated with significant worsening of exercise capacity and pulmonary hemodynamics in the setting of PoPH, and are generally contraindicated [13]. Instead, ligation of esophageal varices is preferred in patients deemed to be at high risk of bleeding. There is also no place for transjugular intrahepatic portosystemic shunt placement in the setting of PoPH because this procedure may acutely augment cardiac preload and potentially aggravate pulmonary hypertension and precipitate right ventricular failure [14].

Endothelin Receptor Antagonists
There is evidence to suggest that ET-1 not only plays an important role in the pathogenesis of PoPH, but may also be etiologically relevant in portal hypertension and hepatic fibrotic remodeling [15–18]. These observations form the basis for the hypothesis that antagonism of ET-1 may be beneficial in PoPH patients. Bosentan is an orally active ET-1 receptor antagonist that is approved for use in different forms of PAH [19]. There are now a number of reports also suggesting that bosentan is well tolerated and effective in patients with severe PoPH [20–23]. Hoeper et al. [24] showed that treatment with bosentan is efficacious in PoPH patients with Child-Pugh class A cirrhosis. A recently published

observational study has reported the effects of ambrisentan, a selective ET-1 A receptor antagonist, in 13 patients with moderate-to-severe PoPH. Treatment was associated with a significant reduction in mPAP and PVR without adverse effects on liver function tests [25]. However, there has been no prospective study assessing the efficacy and safety of ET-1 receptor antagonists in patients with advanced liver disease, mainly due to safety concerns regarding impaired drug metabolism.

To date, there are no data on the plasma levels of ET-1 receptor antagonists according to the severity of liver disease. However, pharmacological studies indicate that mild cirrhosis does not influence the metabolism of bosentan [26]. Despite these encouraging findings, the risk/benefit ratio of the use of ET-1 receptor antagonists in patients with liver diseases must be evaluated on a case-by-case basis. Furthermore, given the risk to increase liver enzymes with the use of ET-1 receptor antagonists, clinicians must be particularly cautious when utilizing these agents in patients with PoPH.

Phosphodiesterase Type-5 Inhibitors

NO is an endothelium-derived potent vasodilator that exerts its effects on pulmonary vascular tone through increased production of the intracellular second messenger cyclic guanosine 5′-monophospate (cGMP). The effects of cGMP are regulated by the enzyme phosphodiesterase type-5 (PDE-5). Sildenafil is a potent and selective inhibitor of PDE-5 that promotes vasodilatation and antiproliferative activity that has been granted regulatory approval in different forms of PAH [27].

No placebo-controlled randomized study of PDE-5 inhibitors in PoPH has been conducted to date. However, three small retrospective studies evaluating the impact of sildenafil treatment in PoPH patients have been published [28–30]. Overall, treatment with this agent has been shown to favorably impact a number of relevant clinical endpoints, including 6-min walk distance, NYHA functional class, and pulmonary hemodynamics, without increasing the number of significant adverse events. However, it is important to note that two of these studies evaluated only OLT candidates, thus limiting the extrapolation of data to PoPH patients in general. Furthermore, target doses of sildenafil employed in two of the studies were higher than those recommended in published guidelines (50 mg t.i.d.) [28, 30], while the third compared the impact of doses ranging from 60 to 400 mg per day [29]. This suggests that higher doses of this drug may possibly confer additional improvements in functional status and hemodynamic indices. In general, treatment was well tolerated in participants from these series, with adverse events being reported no more frequently than in other PAH populations. However, PDE-5 inhibitors should nonetheless be employed with caution in PoPH patients, particularly as some experts have suggested this approach may increase splanchnic blood flow resulting in worsening of portal hypertension [31].

Prostaglandin Analogues

No controlled clinical trial has been conducted with this agent in PoPH to date. However, numerous case series have reported positive effects on exercise capacity and pulmonary hemodynamics with epoprostenol administration in selected patients [32, 33], and it is often employed as a therapeutic bridge to enable OLT to be performed. Krowka et al. [34] showed that in a cohort of moderate-to-severe PoPH patients, chronic epoprostenol therapy conferred significant and durable improvements in PVR, mPAP, and cardiac output. However, treatment is burdensome and may be associated with severe catheter-related bloodstream infections [35]. In addition, some cases of progressive splenomegaly, with worsening thrombocytopenia and leukopenia have been reported with the use of intravenous epoprostenol treatment in patients with PoPH [36]. This finding may limit the usefulness of epoprostenol in those patients.

The use of other more stable prostacyclin analogues has also been the focus of study in PoPH. A case of successful treatment with intravenous iloprost (which has a longer half-life than epoprostenol) used as a bridge to OLT in a patient with severe PoPH has been described [37]. Treatment with aerosolized iloprost, administered by multiple daily inhalations, has also been attempted [38, 39]. Recently, Melgosa et al. [40] reported that 12 months of aerosolized iloprost treatment was associated with overall improvement in functional class and exercise capacity in a cohort of 21 patients. A multicenter observational open-label study evaluating the safety and efficacy of treprostinil, a prostanoid delivered by continuous subcutaneous infusion, to facilitate OLT in patients with PoPH is also underway.

Portopulmonary Hypertension and Orthotopic Liver Transplantation

PoPH dramatically increases the peri- and postoperative risk of OLT. Moreover, the outcome of PoPH after OLT is uncertain and varies from one patient to another. Only rarely have cases of improvement in pulmonary hypertension been reported after OLT, and there is no pathophysiological evidence to support this approach. Indeed, in patients with PoPH who do undergo OLT, it is likely that any significant reductions in mPAP that are observed postoperatively are due to decreases in cardiac output rather than a reversal of the pathologic mechanisms that drive intrinsic pulmonary vasculopathy. Moreover, residual PAH after OLT may lead to acute right failure and a dramatically increased risk of peri- and postoperative mortality [10]. For this reason OLT should not be considered as a treatment for PoPH in any case, unlike hepatopulmonary syndrome.

If a patient has an indication for OLT in relation to the severity of underlying liver disease, it is recommended to detect pulmonary hypertension by systematic echocardiography performed during the pretransplantation assessment [1]. If PoPH is suspected (systolic pulmonary pressure >50 mm Hg), right heart catheterization is mandatory in order to definitively establish the diagnosis and assess the severity of the pulmonary vascular disease to appreciate the peri- and postoperative risk of mortality. In their meta-analysis, Krowka et al. [41] reported a mortality rate of 100% due to pulmonary hypertension in patients with a preoperative mPAP >50 mm Hg and a mortality rate of 50% among those with mPAP of 35–50 mm Hg and a PVR >250 dynes•s•cm^{-5}. Data from this analysis have been used to assist physicians in decision making with respect to pulmonary hemodynamics for patients with PoPH being considered for OLT [42]. If hemodynamic data represent too high a risk for OLT, bridge therapy for PAH should be considered. Epoprostenol remains the most evaluated treatment in this indication even though some case reports have reported the efficacy of oral therapy in this situation. If specific PAH treatment significantly improves hemodynamic status, OLT can be reconsidered. However, no study has investigated the survival of patients transplanted under treatment for PAH.

Survival of Patients with Portopulmonary Hypertension
Estimates of survival in patients with PoPH have varied widely among published studies. The US Registry to Evaluate Early and Long-Term PAH Disease Management (REVEAL) database, in which data from more than 2,700 patients were collected, identified PoPH as an independent predictor of increased mortality among PAH patients (HR: 3.6; 95% CI: 2.4–5.4) [7]. In contrast, Le Pavec et al. [10] found that 1-, 3-, and 5-year survival rates were 88, 75, and 68%, respectively, among patients followed at the French National Referral Centre, suggesting that these patients may in fact have less severe outcomes. Poorer prognosis was associated with cirrhosis with Child-Pugh class B or C, high right atrial pressure, and low cardiac index. Differences in the severity of liver disease at the time of first assessment among the different series may in part explain the discordance of findings.

The impact of specific PAH treatment on survival in PoPH has not been clearly demonstrated because of the lack of prospective studies. In a retrospective analysis of 74 patients, treatment of PAH, followed or not followed by OLT, was associated with an improved outcome [43]. By contrast, others observed no survival differences when outcomes of patients receiving long-term epoprostenol were compared to those not receiving this form of therapy [44]. Similarly, among PoPH patients followed at the French National Referral Center, use of specific PAH treatments also failed to improve the overall outcome [45]. Interestingly, treated patients who had milder disease (defined as either those with Child-Pugh A cirrhosis or portal hypertension without cirrhosis) had a statistically significant survival advantage compared to untreated patients.

Hepatopulmonary Syndrome

Definition and Frequency of Hepatopulmonary Syndrome
HPS is defined as a defect in arterial oxygenation induced by intrapulmonary vascular dilatations associated with hepatic disease. The ERS Task Force has defined the criteria for HPS by the following triad: portal hypertension with or without cirrhosis, increased alveolar-arterial gradient for oxygen (PA-aO_2) in ambient air greater than or equal to 15 mm Hg or greater than or equal to 20 mm Hg in patients more than 64 years of age with or without hypoxemia, and intrapulmonary vascular dilations at the capillaries [1]. Calculation of PA-aO_2 is one of the most sensitive approaches for the detection of early arterial deoxygenation, as PA-aO_2 can increase before arterial oxygen tension (PaO_2) itself becomes abnormally low.

The reported frequency of HPS in patients with liver cirrhosis is between 4 and 80% [1, 46]. The differing incidence is primarily due to heterogeneity of the applied diagnostic criteria and study populations.

The ERS task force has proposed a classification staging the severity of the pulmonary hypertension according to the severity of the hypoxemia:

- Mild: PaO_2 >80 mm Hg
- Moderate: PaO_2 <80 to 60 mm Hg
- Severe (PaO_2 <60 to 50 mm Hg)
- Very severe: PaO_2 <50 mm Hg.

Physiopathology of Hepatopulmonary Syndrome
HPS is characterized pathologically by the presence of diffuse precapillary and capillary bed dilatations that result in diffusion-perfusion abnormalities in which unsaturated

venous blood passes through dilated vessels and is inadequately saturated with oxygen because of a combination of high-flow perfusion and increased depth for diffusion [47]. Dysregulation of vascular signaling pathways may lead to pulmonary vascular dilatation and neoangiogenesis in patients who develop hepatopulmonary syndrome. Physiopathological triggers are the same as in PoPH, but the consequences on the pulmonary vasculature are different because of the distinct anatomical location of angiogenic activity within the pulmonary vascular bed. The remodeling process in HPS involves more distal vessels: the vascular abnormalities include increased numbers of dilated precapillary and capillary vessels and precapillary arteriovenous communications [48]. Although PoPH and HPS show contrasting hemodynamics profiles, the coexistence of these two distinct complications in patients with portal hypertension has been reported [49].

Signaling Pathway Dysregulation Leading to Vascular Abnormalities in Hepatopulmonary Syndrome

In cirrhosis, the development of portosystemic shunts, the dramatic decrease in the phagocytic capacity of the liver, and the frequent bacterial translocation allow inflammatory and angiogenic cytokines, circulating bacteria, or bacterial endotoxins to enter the pulmonary circulation, damage the pulmonary endothelium, and induce extensive recruitment of pulmonary intravascular macrophages [50]. The accumulation of intravascular macrophages probably plays a key role in the physiopathology of HPS [51]. Activated and accumulated in HPS pulmonary arteries and drawn by elevated levels of plasma endotoxin and lung monocyte chemoattractant protein-1, these macrophages express inducible NOS, vascular endothelial growth factor, and platelet-derived growth factor.

NO has been shown to play a pivotal role in HPS, probably mediating downstream signaling in response to these angiogenic factors. Overproduction of NO may result from the overexpression of endothelial NOS caused by shear stress and overexpression of inducible NOS in pulmonary intravascular macrophages [50]. In an animal model of HPS, treatment with L-NAME, a NO synthase inhibitor, prevented and reversed development of the pulmonary vascular disease [50]. However, prevention of intravascular macrophage accumulation induced by hepatic liver, with anti-inflammatory treatment such as pentoxifylline or TNF inhibitors, reversed and prevented HPS in rats by decreasing overexpression of inducible NOS and overproduction of NO [52].

Experimental HPS after common bile duct ligation in rats is also accompanied by increased lung vascular endothelial ET-1 type B receptor (ET_B) expression and increased circulating levels of ET-1. The onset of HPS is hypothesized to be triggered by ET-1/ET_B receptor activation of endothelial NOS-derived NO production in the pulmonary endothelium [53]. There is also evidence to suggest that ET-1 not only plays an important role in the pathogenesis of vascular diseases associated with liver diseases, but may also be etiologically relevant in portal hypertension and hepatic fibrotic remodeling [15–18].

Mechanisms of Hypoxemia in Hepatopulmonary Syndrome

The three main mechanisms leading to hypoxemia in HPS are alveolar ventilation-perfusion imbalance, intrapulmonary shunt due to dilatation of pulmonary capillaries, and diffusion impairment to oxygen essentially due to a diffusion-perfusion defect [54].

Ventilation-perfusion imbalance is due to the coexistence of the lung region normally ventilated but overperfused. Overperfusion is the consequence of the hyperdynamic syndrome consecutive to the portal hypertension and increased volume of capillary bed due to neangiogenesis and vasodilatation. In many patients, hypoxemia resulting from a ventilation-perfusion imbalance is corrected by 100% oxygen test. Diffusion for oxygen is reduced because the distance between the alveoli and the red cells in the central stream of the dilated pulmonary microvessels is too great for complete equilibration of carbon monoxide with hemoglobin. This diffusion impairment to oxygen can be aggravated, in part, by a high cardiac output, resulting in a shorter transit time of the red blood cells and, hence, contributing to the development of a diffusion-perfusion imbalance [54].

Diagnosis of Hepatopulmonary Syndrome

Clinical Presentation

Although dyspnea is the most common symptom of hepatopulmonary syndrome, it is an entirely nonspecific and frequently reported symptom among those with chronic liver disease that is not complicated by intrinsic pulmonary disease. In addition, a high proportion of patients with HPS are likely to be asymptomatic. A characteristic of HPS is the typical complaint of platypnea (increased dyspnea from the supine-to-upright position) and the associated finding of orthodeoxia (decrease in PaO_2 >5% or >4 mm Hg from the supine-to-upright position). Spider naevi, digital clubbing, and cyanosis of the lips and nail beds are consistent findings in advanced HPS. Extrapulmonary complications of right-to-left pulmonary communications, such as the development of a brain abscess or intracranial hemorrhage, and hypoxemia-induced polycythemia, have been reported.

Gas Exchange Evaluation and Lung Function Test

Gas exchange evaluation is necessary to establish the diagnosis of HPS. Screening for HPS can be done by measuring transcutaneous oxygen saturation. If the saturation is less than 97%, there may be justification for further investigation by the completion of blood gas. Both forced spirometric results and static lung volumes are characteristically within normal limits in HPS in the absence of pulmonary comorbid conditions. A moderately to severely reduced DLCO, after adequate correction for anemia, appears to be a common functional marker of HPS.

Highlight of Intrapulmonary Shunt

Contrast-Enhanced Echocardiography. Transthoracic echocardiography with contrast enhancement (CE-TTE) is considered the gold standard for assessing intrapulmonary shunt, which is necessary for the diagnosis of HPS. It is commonly accomplished by hand agitation of 10 ml normal saline, resulting in microbubbles (<90 μm in diameter) which are injected into an upper-extremity vein. In the physiological condition, microbubbles are trapped in the pulmonary capillary bed, in which vascular diameter is <90 μm. In case of capillary dilatation, microbubbles can transit to pulmonary veins. Also, detection of microbubbles within the left atrium after three cardiac cycles is considered a positive contrast-enhanced echocardiography. Although positive CE-TTE results are found in 11–47% of patients with liver disease (with or without associated HPS), only 50% of these patients have arterial hypoxemia [55, 56]. The transesophageal echocardiography with contrast enhancement is probably more sensitive than CE-TTE, but is not routinely used because of the sedation necessity and risk of bleeding in esophageal varices [56].

Perfusion Lung Scanning. Whole-body 99mTcMAA scanning may be useful to detect intrapulmonary shunt in cases of cardiopulmonary disease, but this technique is less sensitive than contrast echocardiography and does not distinguish between an intracardiac and intrapulmonary shunt. The radionuclide approach allows the quantification of intrapulmonary vascular dilatations by assessment of systemic and pulmonary uptake. Finally, the combination of quantifying the severity of arterial deoxygenation and the degree of intrapulmonary shunting indices by 99mTcMAA can offer complementary information for the stratification of HPS patients at greater risk of OLT mortality [55, 57].

Pulmonary Angiography. Pulmonary angiography is not usually used to detect intrapulmonary shunt in patients with PoPH. Two angiographic patterns have been described in HPS. The first corresponds to the diffuse forms of vascular abnormalities with different degrees of severity. In the more advanced diffuse form, spongy or blotchy appearance can be observed. The second pattern, which is probably more rare, consists of focal arteriovenous communications similar to those seen in hereditary hemorrhagic telangiectasia [58, 59].

Management of Hepatopulmonary Syndrome

No medical treatment has demonstrated efficacy in the management of hepatopulmonary syndrome. Only OLT can lead to regression of this vascular condition. Therefore, it should be considered for severe forms of HPS.

Experiences with Medical Treatment. Many medical treatment targets for NO overproduction (methylene blue, L-NAME) or inflammation implicated in HPS pathophysiology (corticosteroid, nonsteroidal anti-inflammatory, pentoxifylline, norfloxacine) have been tried for this vascular condition. Some case reports have described improvement of gas exchange. However, no studies have demonstrated consistent improvement in oxygenation in a larger population of patients as all were of inadequate size to test efficacy. Only long-term oxygen therapy is available for symptomatic measures.

Liver Transplantation. Liver transplantation remains the best option to reverse HPS, unlike PoPH. Complete resolution of HPS following OLT has been observed in >80% of reported cases [58, 60–63]. As recommended by the United Network for Organ Sharing, the existence of a PaO_2 below 60 mm Hg due to HPS is a priority criterion for access to OLT, whatever the severity of the underlying liver disease. Considering transplantation for patients with severe HPS (PaO_2 <60 mm Hg) is justified by the excess mortality observed in this group of patients and the absence of alternative medical treatment demonstrating any efficacy in this pulmonary vascular condition [64]. If hypoxemia is mild-to-moderate ($PA\text{-}aO_2$ >15 mm Hg and/or PaO_2 60–80 mm Hg), periodic follow-up is recommended at least once a year, with assessment of lung function, including pulse oximetry and/or arterial blood gas levels if necessary. If hypoxemia progressively deteriorates in a symptomatic (breathless) patient, OLT can then be considered. If hypoxemia is severe (PaO_2 50–60 mm Hg), consideration of OLT is vital. If the hypoxemia is very severe or extreme (PaO_2 <50 mm Hg) and/or cardiopulmonary comorbid conditions exist, OLT needs to be considered on an individual basis after full assessment of the severity and prognosis of the associated extrahepatic disorders because excess postoperative mortality has been reported in these patients [54].

Conclusion

Pulmonary vascular disorders due to portal hypertension remain entities that are incompletely understood, difficult to treat, and often associated with a poor prognosis. The disorders should be systematically excluded in all OLT candidates or in symptomatic patients because of their impact on the management of the underlying liver disease. Recent reports have shown that treatment with PAH-specific agents may confer durable improvements in important clinical parameters for some patients with PoPH. However, the effectiveness of these agents has yet to be rigorously evaluated in randomized clinical studies. When PoPH is identified in patients otherwise deemed good candidates for OLT, therapeutic strategies should focus on improvements in pulmonary hemodynamics in order to optimize cardiac reserve during the peri- and postoperative periods and maximize the likelihood of a successful outcome. In contrast, no medical treatment has been shown to improve the HPS. OLT remains the only alternative therapeutic to reverse the more severe cases of HPS.

References

1 Rodriguez-Roisin R, Krowka MJ, Herve P, Fallon MB: Pulmonary-hepatic vascular disorders (PHD). Eur Respir J 2004;24:861–880.

2 Herve P, Lebrec D, Brenot F, Simonneau G, Humbert M, Sitbon O, Duroux P: Pulmonary vascular disorders in portal hypertension. Eur Respir J 1998;11:1153–1166.

3 Hadengue A, Benhayoun MK, Lebrec D, Benhamou JP: Pulmonary hypertension complicating portal hypertension: prevalence and relation to splanchnic hemodynamics. Gastroenterology 1991;100:520–528.

4 Colle IO, Moreau R, Godinho E, Belghiti J, Ettori F, Cohen-Solal A, Mal H, Bernuau J, Marty J, Lebrec D, et al: Diagnosis of portopulmonary hypertension in candidates for liver transplantation: a prospective study. Hepatology 2003;37:401–409.

5 Halank M, Ewert R, Seyfarth HJ, Hoeffken G: Portopulmonary hypertension. J Gastroenterol 2006;41:837–847.

6 Humbert M, Sitbon O, Chaouat A, Bertocchi M, Habib G, Gressin V, Yaici A, Weitzenblum E, Cordier JF, Chabot F et al: Pulmonary arterial hypertension in France: results from a national registry. Am J Respir Crit Care Med 2006;173:1023–1030.

7 Benza RL, Miller DP, Gomberg-Maitland M, Frantz RP, Foreman AJ, Coffey CS, Frost A, Barst RJ, Badesch DB, Elliott CG, et al: Predicting survival in pulmonary arterial hypertension: insights from the Registry to Evaluate Early and Long-Term Pulmonary Arterial Hypertension Disease Management (REVEAL). Circulation 2010;122:164–172.

8 Kawut SM, Krowka MJ, Trotter JF, Roberts KE, Benza RL, Badesch DB, Taichman DB, Horn EM, Zacks S, Kaplowitz N, et al: Clinical risk factors for portopulmonary hypertension. Hepatology 2008;48:196–203.

9 Roberts KE, Fallon MB, Krowka MJ, Brown RS, Trotter JF, Peter I, Tighiouart H, Knowles JA, Rabinowitz D, Benza RL, et al: Genetic risk factors for portopulmonary hypertension in patients with advanced liver disease. Am J Respir Crit Care Med 2009;179:835–842.

10 Le Pavec J, Souza R, Herve P, Lebrec D, Savale L, Tcherakian C, Jais X, Yaici A, Humbert M, Simonneau G, et al: Portopulmonary hypertension: survival and prognostic factors. Am J Respir Crit Care Med 2008;178:637–643.

11 Mandell MS, Groves BM: Pulmonary hypertension in chronic liver disease. Clin Chest Med 1996;17:17–33.

12 Roberts K, Fallon M, Krowka M, Brown R, Trotter J, Peter I, Tighiouart H, Knowles J, Rabinowitz D, Benza R, et al: Genetic risk factors for portopulmonary hypertension in patients with advanced liver disease. Am J Respir Crit Care Med 2009;179:835–842.

13 Provencher S, Herve P, Jais X, Lebrec D, Humbert M, Simonneau G, Sitbon O: Deleterious effects of beta-blockers on exercise capacity and hemodynamics in patients with portopulmonary hypertension. Gastroenterology 2006;130:120–126.

14 Van der Linden P, Le Moine O, Ghysels M, Ortinez M, Devière J: Pulmonary hypertension after transjugular intrahepatic portosystemic shunt: effects on right ventricular function. Hepatology 1996;23:982–987.

15 Benjaminov FS, Prentice M, Sniderman KW, Siu S, Liu P, Wong F: Portopulmonary hypertension in decompensated cirrhosis with refractory ascites. Gut 2003;52:1355–1362.

16 Chan C, Wang S, Lee F, Chang F, Lin H, Chu C, Chen C, Huang H, Lee S: Endothelin-1 induces vasoconstriction on portal-systemic collaterals of portal hypertensive rats. Hepatology 2001;33:816–820.

17 Kojima H, Sakurai S, Kuriyama S, Yoshiji H, Imazu H, Uemura M, Nakatani Y, Yamao J, Fukui H: Endothelin-1 plays a major role in portal hypertension of biliary cirrhotic rats through endothelin receptor subtype B together with subtype A in vivo. J Hepatol 2001;34:805–811.

18 Tièche S, De Gottardi A, Kappeler A, Shaw S, Sägesser H, Zimmermann A, Reichen J: Overexpression of endothelin-1 in bile duct ligated rats: correlation with activation of hepatic stellate cells and portal pressure. J Hepatol 2001;34:38–45.

19 O'Callaghan D, Gaine SP: Bosentan: a novel agent for the treatment of pulmonary arterial hypertension. Int J Clin Pract 2004;58:69–73.

20 Kuntzen C, Gülberg V, Gerbes A: Use of a mixed endothelin receptor antagonist in portopulmonary hypertension: a safe and effective therapy? Gastroenterology 2005;128:164–168.

21 Halank M, Miehlke S, Hoeffken G, Schmeisser A, Schulze M, Strasser R: Use of oral endothelin-receptor antagonist bosentan in the treatment of portopulmonary hypertension. Transplantation 2004;77:1775–1776.

22 Grander W, Eller P, Fuschelberger R, Tilg H: Bosentan treatment of portopulmonary hypertension related to liver cirrhosis owing to hepatitis C. Eur J Clin Invest 2006;36(suppl 3):67–70.

23 Stähler G, von Hunnius P: Successful treatment of portopulmonary hypertension with bosentan: case report. Eur J Clin Invest 2006;36(suppl 3):62–66.

24 Hoeper M, Halank M, Marx C, Hoeffken G, Seyfarth H, Schauer J, Niedermeyer J, Winkler J: Bosentan therapy for portopulmonary hypertension. Eur Respir J 2005;25:502–508.

25 Cartin-Ceba R, Swanson K, Iyer V, Wiesner R, Krowka M: Safety and efficacy of ambrisentan for the therapy of portopulmonary hypertension. Chest 2011;139:109–114.

26 van Giersbergen P, Popescu G, Bodin F, Dingemanse J: Influence of mild liver impairment on the pharmacokinetics and metabolism of bosentan, a dual endothelin receptor antagonist. J Clin Pharmacol 2003;43:15–22.

27 Galie N, Ghofrani HA, Torbicki A, Barst RJ, Rubin LJ, Badesch D, Fleming T, Parpia T, Burgess G, Branzi A, et al: Sildenafil citrate therapy for pulmonary arterial hypertension. N Engl J Med 2005;353:2148–2157.

28 Reichenberger F, Voswinckel R, Steveling E, Enke B, Kreckel A, Olschewski H, Grimminger F, Seeger W, Ghofrani HA: Sildenafil treatment for portopulmonary hypertension. Eur Respir J 2006;28:563–567.

29 Gough MS, White RJ: Sildenafil therapy is associated with improved hemodynamics in liver transplantation candidates with pulmonary arterial hypertension.
30 Hemnes AR, Robbins IM: Sildenafil monotherapy in portopulmonary hypertension can facilitate liver transplantation.
31 Krowka MJ, Swanson KL: How should we treat portopulmonary hypertension? Eur Respir J 2006;28:466–467.
32 Kuo P, Johnson L, Plotkin J, Howell C, Bartlett S, Rubin L: Continuous intravenous infusion of epoprostenol for the treatment of portopulmonary hypertension. Transplantation 1997;63:604–606.
33 Plotkin J, Kuo P, Rubin L, Gaine S, Howell C, Laurin J, Njoku M, Lim J, Johnson L: Successful use of chronic epoprostenol as a bridge to liver transplantation in severe portopulmonary hypertension. Transplantation 1998;65:457–459.
34 Krowka M, Frantz R, McGoon M, Severson C, Plevak D, Wiesner R: Improvement in pulmonary hemodynamics during intravenous epoprostenol (prostacyclin): a study of 15 patients with moderate to severe portopulmonary hypertension. Hepatology 1999;30:641–648.
35 O'Callaghan DS, Moutet A, Jais X, Yaici A, Savale L, Natali D, Parent F, Simonneau G, Humbert MJC, Doucet-Populaire F, et al: Catheter related-infections in pulmonary hypertension patients treated by continuous intravenous epoprostenol: experience of the French Referral Centre (abstract). Am J Respir Crit Care Med 2010;181:A3337.
36 Findlay JY, Plevak DJ, Krowka MJ, Sack EM, Porayko MK: Progressive splenomegaly after epoprostenol therapy in portopulmonary hypertension. Liver Transpl Surg 1999;5:362–365.
37 Minder S, Fischler M, Muellhaupt B, Zalunardo M, Jenni R, Clavien P, Speich R: Intravenous iloprost bridging to orthotopic liver transplantation in portopulmonary hypertension. Eur Respir J 2004;24:703–707.
38 Halank M, Marx C, Miehlke S, Hoeffken G: Use of aerosolized inhaled iloprost in the treatment of portopulmonary hypertension. J Gastroenterol 2004;39:1222–1223.
39 Hoeper MM, Seyfarth HJ, Hoeffken G, Wirtz H, Spiekerkoetter E, Pletz MW, Welte T, Halank M: Experience with inhaled iloprost and bosentan in portopulmonary hypertension. Eur Respir J 2007;30:1096–1102.
40 Melgosa M, Ricci G, García-Pagan J, Blanco I, Escribano P, Abraldes J, Roca J, Bosch J, Barberà J: Acute and long-term effects of inhaled iloprost in portopulmonary hypertension. Liver Transpl 2010;16:348–356.
41 Krowka M, Plevak D, Findlay J, Rosen C, Wiesner R, Krom R: Pulmonary hemodynamics and perioperative cardiopulmonary-related mortality in patients with portopulmonary hypertension undergoing liver transplantation. Liver Transpl 2000;6:443–450.
42 Rodríguez-Roisin R, Krowka M, Hervé P, Fallon M: Committee ETFP-HVDPS: Pulmonary-hepatic vascular disorders (PHD). Eur Respir J 2004; 24:861–880.
43 Swanson K, Wiesner R, Nyberg S, Rosen C, Krowka M: Survival in portopulmonary hypertension: Mayo Clinic experience categorized by treatment subgroups. Am J Transplant 2008;8: 2445–2453.
44 Fix O, Bass N, De Marco T, Merriman R: Long-term follow-up of portopulmonary hypertension: effect of treatment with epoprostenol. Liver Transpl 2007;13:875–885.
45 Savale L, Magnier R, Le Pavec J, O'Callaghan DS, Jais X, Natali D, Humbert MJC, Simonneau G, Sitbon O: Impact of pulmonary arterial hypertension specific therapy on portopulmonary hypertension (abstract). Am J Respir Crit Care Med 2010;181:A3339.
46 Kim BJ, Lee SC, Park SW, Choi MS, Koh KC, Paik SW, Lee SH, Hong KP, Park JE, Seo JD: Characteristics and prevalence of intrapulmonary shunt detected by contrast echocardiography with harmonic imaging in liver transplant candidates. Am J Cardiol 2004;94:525–528.
47 O'Callaghan D, Gaine SP: Hepatopulmonary syndromes: treatment of liver transplantation candidates. Curr Opin Organ Transplant 2002;7:107–113.
48 Berthelot P, Walker JG, Sherlock S, Reid L: Arterial changes in the lungs in cirrhosis of the liver – lung spider nevi. N Engl J Med 1966;274:291–298.
49 Jones F, Kuo P, Johnson L, Njoku M, Dixon-Ferguson M, Plotkin J: The coexistence of portopulmonary hypertension and hepatopulmonary syndrome. Anesthesiology 1999;90:626–629.
50 Nunes H, Lebrec D, Mazmanian M, Capron F, Heller J, Tazi KA, Zerbib E, Dulmet E, Moreau R, Dinh-Xuan AT, et al: Role of nitric oxide in hepatopulmonary syndrome in cirrhotic rats. Am J Respir Crit Care Med 2001;164:879–885.
51 Thenappan T, Goel A, Marsboom G, Fang YH, Toth PT, Zhang HJ, Kajimoto H, Hong Z, Paul J, Wietholt C, et al: A central role for CD68(+) macrophages in hepatopulmonary syndrome: reversal by macrophage depletion. Am J Respir Crit Care Med 2011;183:1080–1091.
52 Sztrymf B, Rabiller A, Nunes H, Savale L, Lebrec D, Le Pape A, de Montpreville V, Mazmanian M, Humbert M, Herve P: Prevention of hepatopulmonary syndrome and hyperdynamic state by pentoxifylline in cirrhotic rats. Eur Respir J 2004;23:752–758.
53 Tang L, Luo B, Patel RP, Ling Y, Zhang J, Fallon MB: Modulation of pulmonary endothelial endothelin B receptor expression and signaling: implications for experimental hepatopulmonary syndrome. Am J Physiol Lung Cell Mol Physiol 2007;292:L1467–L1472.
54 Rodriguez-Roisin R, Krowka MJ: Hepatopulmonary syndrome – a liver-induced lung vascular disorder. N Engl J Med 2008;358:2378–2387.
55 Krowka MJ, Wiseman GA, Burnett OL, Spivey JR, Therneau T, Porayko MK, Wiesner RH: Hepatopulmonary syndrome: a prospective study of relationships between severity of liver disease, PaO(2) response to 100% oxygen, and brain uptake after (99m)Tc MAA lung scanning. Chest 2000;118:615–624.
56 Aller R, Moya JL, Moreira V, Boixeda D, Cano A, Picher J, Garcia-Rull S, de Luis DA: Diagnosis of hepatopulmonary syndrome with contrast transesophageal echocardiography: advantages over contrast transthoracic echocardiography. Dig Dis Sci 1999;44:1243–1248.
57 Abrams GA, Jaffe CC, Hoffer PB, Binder HJ, Fallon MB: Diagnostic utility of contrast echocardiography and lung perfusion scan in patients with hepatopulmonary syndrome. Gastroenterology 1995;109:1283–1288.
58 Krowka M: Hepatopulmonary syndrome and liver transplantation. Liver Transpl 2000;6:113–115.
59 Krowka MJ, Dickson ER, Cortese DA: Hepatopulmonary syndrome. Clinical observations and lack of therapeutic response to somatostatin analogue. Chest 1993;104:515–521.
60 Krowka MJ: Hepatopulmonary syndrome versus portopulmonary hypertension: distinctions and dilemmas. Hepatology 1997;25:1282–1284.
61 Arguedas MR, Abrams GA, Krowka MJ, Fallon MB: Prospective evaluation of outcomes and predictors of mortality in patients with hepatopulmonary syndrome undergoing liver transplantation. Hepatology 2003;37:192–197.
62 Stavrou GA, Fruhauf NR, Lang H, Malago M, Saner F, Broelsch CE: Liver transplantation and severe hepatopulmonary syndrome. Transplantation 2003;76:746–747.
63 Taille C, Cadranel J, Bellocq A, Thabut G, Soubrane O, Durand F, Ichai P, Duvoux C, Belghiti J, Calmus Y, et al: Liver transplantation for hepatopulmonary syndrome: a ten-year experience in Paris, France. Transplantation 2003;75:1482–1489, discussion 1446–1447.
64 Schenk P, Schöniger-Hekele M, Fuhrmann V, Madl C, Silberhumer G, Müller C: Prognostic significance of the hepatopulmonary syndrome in patients with cirrhosis. Gastroenterology 2003;125:1042–1052.
65 Savale L, O'Callaghan DS, Magnier R, Le Pavec J, Herve P, Jais X, Seferian A, Humbert M, Simonneau G, Sitbon O: Current management approaches to portopulmonary hypertension. Int J Clin Pract Suppl 2011;169:11–18.

Dr. Laurent Savale, MD, PhD
Service de Pneumologie, Hôpital Antoine Béclère
157 rue de la Porte de Trivaux
FR–92140 Clamart (France)
Tel. +33 1 45 37 47 79, E-Mail laurent.savale@abc.aphp.fr

Humbert M, Souza R, Simonneau G (eds): Pulmonary Vascular Disorders.
Prog Respir Res. Basel, Karger, 2012, vol 41, pp 122–136

Pulmonary Hypertension in Congenital Heart Diseases

Cecile Tissot · Maurice Beghetti

Pediatric Cardiology Unit, The University Children's Hospital of Geneva, Geneva, Switzerland

Abstract

Pulmonary arterial hypertension (PAH) commonly arises in patients with congenital heart diseases (CHD), and is most often related with congenital shunt lesions. These patients initially exhibit a left-to-right (systemic-to-pulmonary) shunt, but as the disease progresses, vascular remodeling and dysfunction lead to an increase in pulmonary vascular resistance (PVR) with reversal of the shunt (right-to-left shunt or pulmonary-to-systemic) and finally Eisenmenger syndrome, the most advanced form of PAH. The pathological and structural abnormalities that occur within the pulmonary circulation of these patients are to some extent similar to those observed in other forms of PAH. Based on the physiopathological changes learned from other forms of PAH, the management of PAH associated with CHD has changed significantly over the past few years with the introduction of targeted therapies to address pulmonary vascular lesions. The best prevention of pulmonary vascular disease (PVD) in patients with CHD is early closure of the shunt. However, when a certain degree of PVD is present, there are no good preoperative parameters to indicate if surgical repair is safe and will be successful, even though hemodynamic assessment with pulmonary vasoreactivity testing remains the gold standard. Postoperative PAH, both in the immediate postsurgical period and in the long-term evolution, remains a challenge. The particular setting of single ventricle physiology and Fontan circulation is also a major concern as even a minimal increase in PVR may lead to failure of this circulation in the presence of pulmonary vascular lesions.

Pulmonary arterial hypertension (PAH) is a common complication in patients with congenital heart diseases (CHD), particularly in those with shunt lesions. Increased pulmonary blood flow or postcapillary pressure associated with CHD is well known to induce an increase in pulmonary pressure. Despite advances in the understanding of the pulmonary lesions leading to pulmonary vascular disease (PVD), surgical repair, and the discovery of targeted therapies in the pre- and postoperative period, pulmonary hypertension (PH) is still associated with significant mortality and morbidity rates in patients with CHD.

Based on hemodynamic definition of PAH [mean pulmonary artery pressure (PAP) >25 mm Hg] [1], almost all patients with a large unrestricted left-to-right shunt lesion present with PH. Nevertheless, the most important parameter to consider is the degree of PVD. Indeed, a patient with a left-to-right shunt, high pulmonary blood flow, and low pulmonary vascular resistance (PVR) will fulfill the requirements for a diagnosis of PAH, but will benefit from surgical closure of the shunt. In contrast, a patient with low pulmonary blood flow, high PVR, cyanosis secondary to reversal of the shunt, and Eisenmenger syndrome will not benefit from surgical closure of the shunt, but will potentially benefit from new targeted therapies for PAH.

The particular setting of single ventricle physiology and Fontan circulation is of particular interest as even a minimal increase in PVR may lead to failure of this circulation in the presence of pulmonary vascular lesions.

Pathophysiology

Increased PAP and/or pulmonary blood flow causes increased PVR related to active vasoconstriction and pathological remodeling of the pulmonary circulation consisting of decreased luminal area of the pulmonary arteries and/or diminished number of vessels. Increased wall stress and endothelial shear stress are thought to play a key role and serve as growth stimulus and increased matrix protein synthesis responsible for the remodeling lesions. In infants with CHD, vasoconstriction is predominant, but even older children and adults with markedly increased PVR may remain somewhat reactive to pulmonary vasodilatation. Because the normal physiologic response to increased flow is vasodilatation and decreased vascular resistance, the presence of increased PVR in the setting of increased pulmonary blood flow related to CHD suggests resting vasoconstriction and/or pulmonary vascular remodeling.

The pathophysiology of left-to-right congenital shunt lesions depends on the intracardiac level of shunting and also on other cardiovascular or extracardiac anomalies. Pretricuspid shunts are responsible for diastolic shunting, determined by the ventricular compliance, whereas posttricuspid shunts are responsible for systolic or systolodiastolic shunting, determined by the ratio of pulmonary to systemic vascular resistances (PVR/SVR). In posttricuspid shunts, the volume of shunt and pulmonary blood flow also depend on associated cardiovascular anomalies like left or right heart obstructive lesions and systolic ventricular function.

The distinction between reversible and irreversible PVD and the ability to predict whether the PVR will decrease following surgical correction of CHD is crucial. Indeed, in patients with Eisenmenger syndrome, closure of the pulmonary-to-systemic connection is associated with a worse clinical outcome than the natural history of the disease [2]. However, this is not so simple because even patients with Eisenmenger syndrome may show a small degree of vasodilatation in response to pulmonary vasodilator testing, providing rationale for therapy [3]. In small children (<2 years of age) with mildly elevated PVR, elimination of the shunt almost always results in normalization of PVR, whereas older patients with increased PAP and PVR may show progressive PVD even after surgical correction. It is generally assumed that medial hypertrophy regresses after removal of increased PAP and/or pulmonary blood flow.

Some variables have a major impact on the probability of reversal of PVD after surgical repair, i.e. type of CHD, patient age, and PVR at the time of surgical correction, and genetic and environmental factors can be responsible for considerable individual variability of the pulmonary vasculature to CHD. The rapidity of evolution of pulmonary vascular remodeling towards irreversible lesions depends whether the anatomical defect is associated with increased PAP, pulmonary blood flow, or both (fig. 1), and on individual and genetic predisposition [4]. For patients with a mild increase in pulmonary blood flow, such as an atrial septal defect (ASD), the risk of developing PVD is low <20 years. For children with a more pronounced increase in pulmonary blood flow and PAP, such as an isolated ventricular septal defect (VSD), closure performed in the first 6–12 months of life, even when PVR is elevated, reliably results in normalization of PVR, with a few exceptions, and the likelihood of favorable pulmonary vascular remodeling is even better when surgical closure is performed in the first year of life. CHD responsible for both an increase in PAP and pulmonary blood flow evolve more rapidly towards severe PVD compared to those with increased PAP or pulmonary blood flow alone. Complex cardiac lesions with increased PAP and pulmonary blood flow together with high pulmonary arterial oxygen saturation, low systemic arterial oxygen saturation, and polycythemia are at increased risk for the development of early PVD. For example, infants with unrepaired d-TGA and an intact ventricular septum may have increased pulmonary blood flow but normal PAP after the early neonatal period, and are at risk of developing increased PVR and PVD in the first year or two of life, which is more precocious compared to patients with an ASD. Infants with d-TGA and a VSD or patent ductus arteriosus have a predisposition to develop early severe PVD in the first year of life, and some patients may develop PVD despite neonatal arterial switch operation. Particular lesions prone to develop early PVD are common arterial trunk or aortic origin of a pulmonary artery. For the latter, pulmonary vascular changes may occur even in the protected lung supplied from the right ventricle, which emphasizes the role of other circulating vasoactive mediators besides increased PAP and pulmonary blood flow.

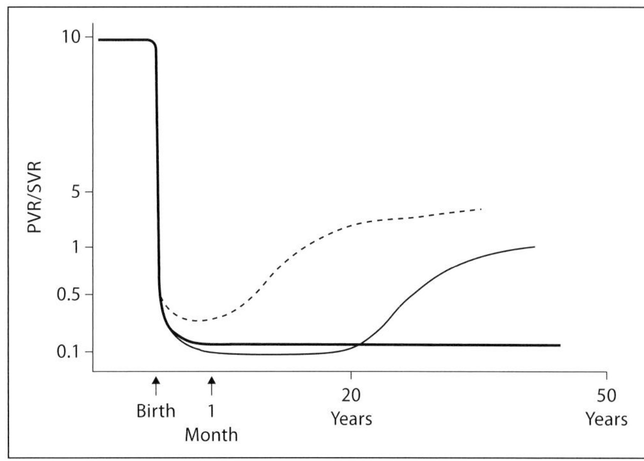

Fig. 1. Time course of change in the PVR/SVR ratio with normal pulmonary circulation with normal pattern of fall in pulmonary vascular resistance (thick line); high-pressure high-flow CHD, e.g. VSD (dotted line); and high-flow CHD, e.g. ASD (thin line) [53].

Table 1. Revised classification of pulmonary hypertension from Dana Point 2008 [5]

1	PAH
1.1	Idiopathic PAH
1.2	Heritable
1.2.1	BMPR2
1.2.2	ALK1, endoglin (with or without hereditary hemorrhagic telangiectasia)
1.2.3	Unknown
1.3	Drug- and toxin-induced
1.4	Associated with
1.4.1	Connective tissue diseases
1.4.2	HIV infection
1.4.3	Portal hypertension
1.4.4	CHD
1.4.5	Schistosomiasis
1.4.6	Chronic hemolytic anemia
1.5	Persistent PH of the newborn
1′	Pulmonary veno-occlusive disease and/or pulmonary capillary hemangiomatosis
2	PH owing to left heart disease
2.1	Systolic dysfunction
2.2	Diastolic dysfunction
2.3	Valvular disease
3	PH owing to lung diseases and/or hypoxia
3.1	Chronic obstructive pulmonary disease
3.2	Interstitial lung disease
3.3	Other pulmonary diseases with mixed restrictive and obstructive pattern
3.4	Sleep-disordered breathing
3.5	Alveolar hypoventilation disorders
3.6	Chronic exposure to high altitude
3.7	Developmental abnormalities
4	Chronic thromboembolic PH
5	PH with unclear multifactorial mechanisms
5.1	Hematologic disorders: myeloproliferative disorders, splenectomy
5.2	Systemic disorders: sarcoidosis, pulmonary Langerhans cell histiocytosis: lymphangioleiomyomatosis, neurofibromatosis, vasculitis
5.3	Metabolic disorders: glycogen storage disease, Gaucher's disease, thyroid disorders
5.4	Others: tumoral obstruction, fibrosing mediastinitis, chronic renal failure on dialysis

Table 2. PH related to CHD

Type of lesion	Lesion anatomy
Simple	ASD Sinus venosus defects VSD Patent ductus arteriosus (PDA) Aortopulmonary window Total or partial unobstructed anomalous pulmonary venous return
Combination	Combination of simple lesions
Complex	Atrioventricular septal defect Transposition of the great arteries with ventricular (VSD) or arterial shunt (PDA) Truncus arteriosus Single ventricle physiology with unobstructed pulmonary blood flow
Lesion dimensions	Small-to-moderate ASD ≤2 cm VSD and PDA ≤1 cm Large ASD >2 cm VSD and PDA >1 cm
Associated extracardiac anomalies	
Repair status	Unoperated Palliated Repaired

Definition and Classification

PAH is defined as a mean PAP ≥25 mm Hg at rest, with a normal pulmonary capillary wedge pressure (≤15 mm Hg) [1]. A revision of the classification including most of the forms of PH encountered in children was proposed at Dana Point in 2008 (table 1) [5]. Category 1 includes idiopathic and familial PAH as well as PAH associated with various diseases, including CHD. The rationale for the inclusion of PAH associated with CHD is that the histologies of Category 1 PAH diseases are indistinguishable from each other, with the plexiform lesion being the cornerstone of PVD. The most common form of associated PAH in children is related to CHD. In the new Dana Point classification, the denomination venous PH has been renamed to PH due to left heart disease and is now classified in Category 2. It is divided into PH related to left ventricular systolic dysfunction, left ventricular diastolic dysfunction, and left heart valvular diseases. Except for restrictive cardiomyopathy, PH secondary to left ventricular diastolic dysfunction is rare in children and the most common causes of PH related to left heart diseases in children are left-sided CHD and cardiomyopathies.

A classification of congenital shunt lesions associated with PAH has been proposed (table 2). In general, four clinical situations can be identified.

Eisenmenger Syndrome
Eisenmenger syndrome is a complication of left-to-right shunt lesions responsible for an increased PVR that becomes suprasystemic and is not reversible. This leads to inversion of the shunt, which becomes right-to-left with chronic cyanosis. The length of time required for evolution towards Eisenmenger syndrome depends on the level of the shunt, with more time needed in pretricuspid compared to posttricuspid shunt lesions. The risk of developing Eisenmenger syndrome also depends on the type of CHD, ranging from 10% for large ASD to 50% for VSD to almost 100% in common arterial trunk. Genetic predisposition also plays a role in the time needed to develop Eisenmenger syndrome for the same CHD, and it is well known that patients with Down syndrome are at increased risk for developing early PAH and Eisenmenger syndrome. In developed countries, early closure of the shunt has dramatically reduced the incidence of Eisenmenger syndrome, but it is still a major problem in developing countries.

Pulmonary Arterial Hypertension with Elevated Pulmonary Vascular Resisance Secondary to a Large Volume Left-to-Right Shunt
Patients with this condition have a large volume of left-to-right shunt (evaluated by the Qp/Qs) leading to increased pulmonary blood flow and increased PVR that is reversible. Indeed, it is crucial to ensure that closure of the shunt lesion and decrease in pulmonary blood flow will allow the PVR to normalize. In contrast, closure of the shunt in a patient with irreversible PVD and PVR will decrease his/her survival. This point is essential and there are currently no consensual criteria to predict which patient is at risk of keeping high PVR after surgical repair.

Pulmonary Arterial Hypertension Secondary to a Small Volume Left-to-Right Shunt
Such patients have a small volume of left-to-right shunt responsible for PAH and high PVR. In those patients, the evolution of PAH is similar to those with idiopathic PAH and cannot be totally explained by the shunt lesion, as the volume of shunting is disproportionate compared to the level of PAH. Some of those patients may have a genetic predisposition, although a clear mutation has not yet been found.

Pulmonary Arterial Hypertension after Surgical Repair of Congenital Heart Disease
These patients show persistent PAH in the postoperative period, whereas others may have reappearance of PAH months or years after initial successful surgical repair without residual shunt lesions. This is described more often in patients with associated left heart obstructive lesions, especially congenital mitral stenosis or pulmonary vein stenosis. For them, PAH was thought to be postcapillary in the preoperative period, but evolved towards PVD. Patients with d-TGA may also develop unexpected PAH in the postoperative period with a natural history mimicking idiopathic PAH.

Epidemiology and Genetics

In children, the predominant diagnoses of PAH are idiopathic and associated with CHD and shunt lesions [6]. Eisenmenger syndrome is rarely seen in developed countries nowadays because of early referral and surgical repair. Nevertheless, because of insufficient access to specialized care and late referral of patients in developing countries, CHD is still one of the most common etiologies of PAH worldwide. PAH appears to be a disease of ‘predisposed’ individuals in whom various stimuli may initiate the PVD process. A permissive genetic trait may account for the variability in expression of different degrees of PH to similar stimuli. A genetic mutation of the bone morphogenetic protein receptor type 2 on chromosome 2q33, a gene encoding a transforming growth factor-β receptor (the PPH1 gene), has been recognized in some patients with familial PAH (>50% of the patients), idiopathic PAH (approx. 20–25%), and sporadic cases of PAH (26%), and has been found in children [7, 8]. Mutation in the bone morphogenetic protein receptor type 2 is less common in PAH associated with CHD than in idiopathic PAH.

Assessment

Clinical History and Physical Exam
In children with congenital cardiac shunt lesions, feeding difficulties, poor weight gain, and recurrent respiratory tract infections are common signs of high pulmonary blood flow. The signs and symptoms of heart failure usually improve as PVR increases and the patient may be asymptomatic until reversal of shunt becomes obvious with arterial oxygen desaturation. In children with Eisenmenger syndrome, central cyanosis and digital clubbing is present. Those patients are at increased risk of developing hemoptysis in early adult life. The physical signs of PAH include a right ventricular lift and a loud second heart sound.

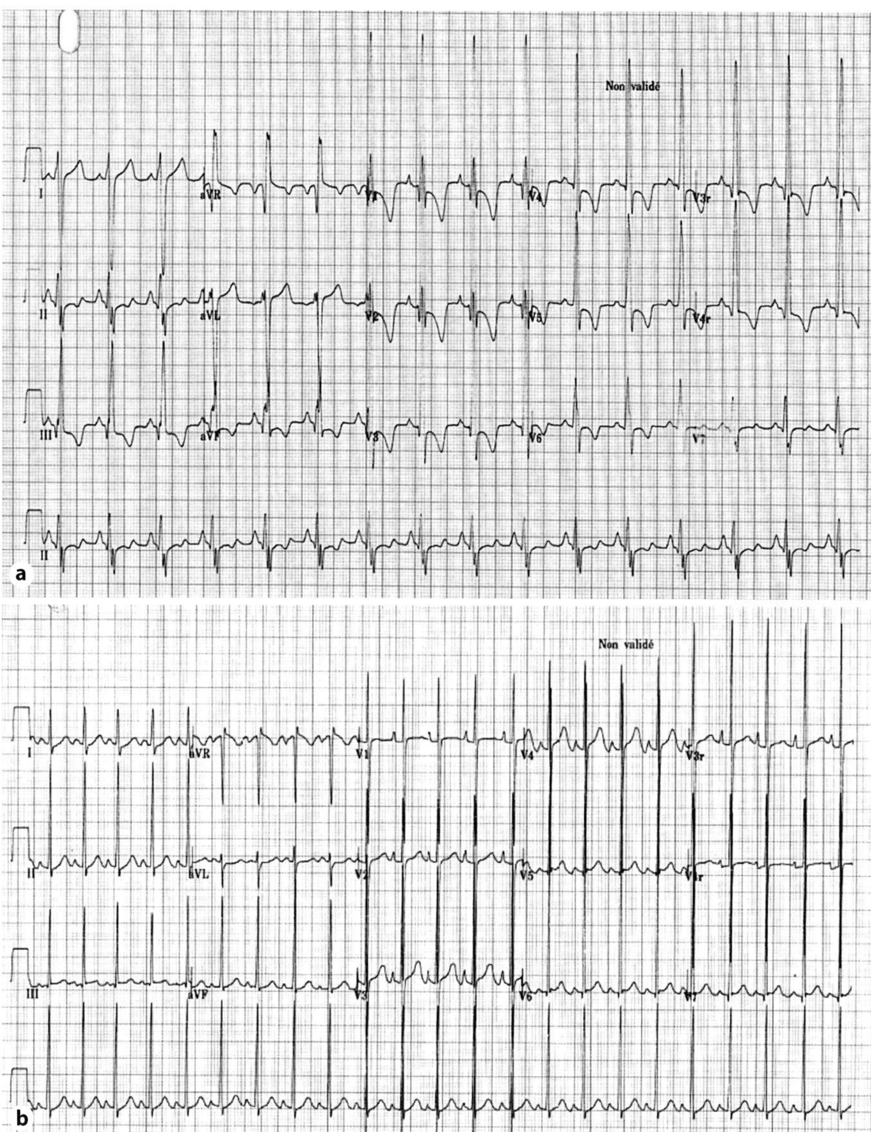

Fig. 2. Electrocardiogram of a child with idiopathic PAH (**a**) showing right ventricular hypertrophy and strain, right axis deviation, and incomplete right bundle branch block, and a child with truncus arteriosus and PAH (**b**), showing a normal QRS axis with biventricular hypertrophy.

Electrocardiogram

Electrocardiogram findings include right ventricular hypertrophy and strain, right atrial enlargement, and right axis deviation (fig. 2), which are superimposed on other Electrocardiogram abnormalities specific to each CHD.

Chest X-Ray

In children with PAH related to congenital shunt lesions, the chest X-ray is plethoric when the PVR is sufficiently low to allow high pulmonary blood flow and will show dilatation of the proximal vessels with peripheral hypoperfusion in cases of significant PAH (fig. 3). Cardiomegaly is a common finding in patients with shunt lesions and high pulmonary blood flow.

Echocardiography

Echocardiography is the key for the diagnosis of the CHD and allows hemodynamic assessment of pulmonary pressure, even though cardiac catheterization remains the gold standard. In children with congenital shunt lesions, systolic PAP can be estimated from the velocity of the shunt using the modified Bernoulli equation ($\Delta P = 4v^2$, where ΔP = pressure gradient and v = velocity). In cases of VSD or patent ductus arteriosus, right-to-left shunt or low-velocity left-to-right shunt may suggest the presence of elevated PAP (fig. 4).

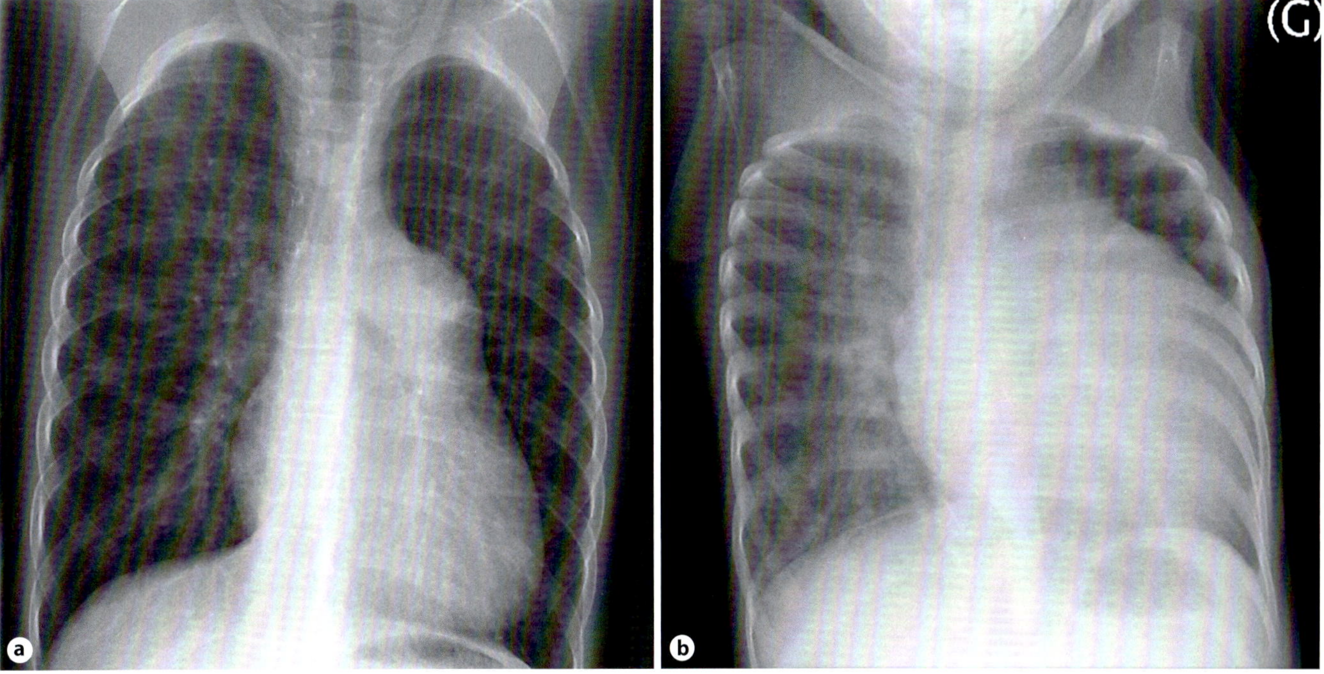

Fig. 3. Chest X-ray of a child with idiopathic PAH showing enlarged central pulmonary arteries and peripheral hypoperfusion (**a**), and of a child with a large patent ductus arteriosus and PAH showing cardiomegaly and increased pulmonary vascular markings (**b**).

In patients with tricuspid regurgitation and no pulmonary stenosis, echocardiography allows estimation of the systolic PAP by measuring the peak systolic pressure gradient from the right ventricle to the right atrium using the tricuspid regurgitation jet and the modified Bernoulli equation ($P = v^2$), and by adding the estimated right atrial pressure (fig. 5a). Echocardiography also allows estimation of end-diastolic and mean PAP from the pulmonary insufficiency flow velocity (fig. 5b).

Cardiac Catheterization

PAH must be confirmed by catheterization, and pulmonary vasoreactivity testing should be performed with inhaled nitric oxide (NO) [9, 10]. Protocols for pulmonary vasodilator testing are center-specific, but the use of 20 ppm NO with or without increased oxygen concentration for 10 min usually achieves sufficient pulmonary vasodilatation. In children with PAH related to CHD, calculation of pulmonary and systemic blood flow (Qp/Qs) and vascular resistance (PVR/SVR) using the Fick principle is essential. It is usually accepted that a baseline PVR index <6 WU × m^2 with a PVR/SVR ratio (PVR/SVR) <0.3 is indicative of a favorable outcome following surgical repair. In patients with a functional single ventricle, there is much debate but growing evidence that a mean PAP of >15 mm Hg may be associated with early and late mortality after the Fontan operation [11].

Exercise Capacity

In children aged ≥7–8 years, exercise capacity can be assessed with a 6-min walking test (6-MW test). The 6-MW test remains the standard tool for testing exercise capacity in most clinical trials in adults with PAH, but is difficult to standardize for children, even though recent publications of reference values in healthy children are now available [12]. As a result of the challenges involved in performing and interpreting the traditional treatment endpoints used in adults (primarily exercise capacity, but also functional capacity and quality of life), treatment response is difficult to quantify in children.

Brain Natriuretic Peptide

Brain natriuretic peptide is useful for assessing the progression of the disease, and change in brain natriuretic peptide measurements over time has been shown to significantly correlate with the change in the functional status, hemodynamics, echocardiographic parameters, and outcome in children with idiopathic PAH [13, 14]. Few data are available for children with PAH associated with CHD. One study showed that children and adolescents with

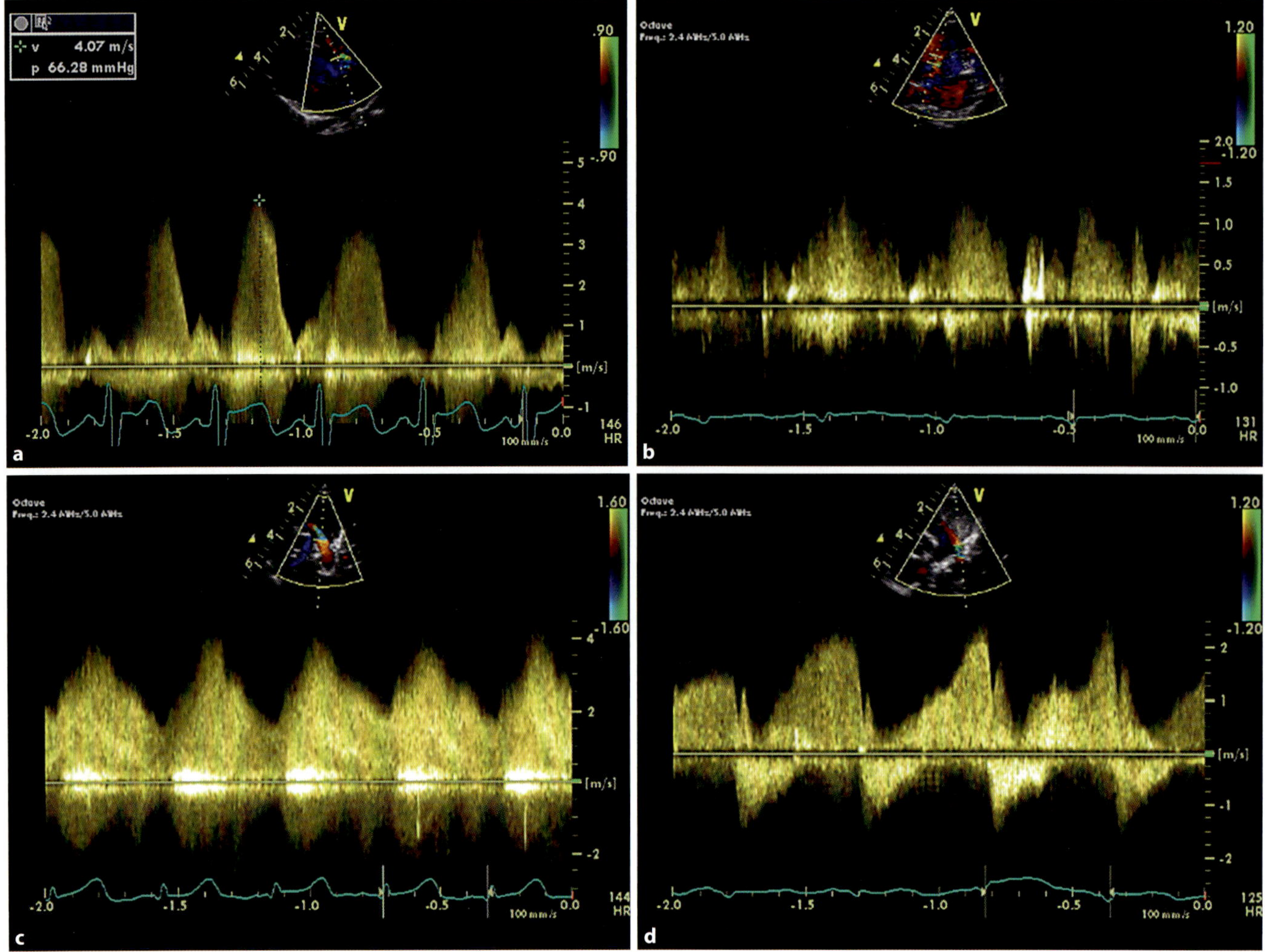

Fig. 4. Doppler echocardiography with high velocity left-to-right shunt (no PAH, **a**) and low velocity left-to-right shunt (infrasystemic PAH, **b**) across a VSD. Doppler echocardiography with high-velocity left-to-right shunt (no PAH, **c**) and low-velocity left-to-right shunt (infrasystemic PAH, **d**).

PAH related to congenital systemic-to-pulmonary shunts had enhanced systemic inflammation involving increased endothelial cell activation and platelet-mediated inflammation, and that N-terminal pro-brain natriuretic peptide levels correlated significantly with the level of C-reactive protein and von Willebrand factor [15].

Management of Pulmonary Arterial Hypertension Associated with Congenital Heart Disease

Patients with PAH associated with congenital shunt lesions which show acute response to vasodilator testing are considered candidates for surgical repair. Treatment for patients with CHD and nonreactive PAH (Eisenmenger syndrome) is based on the same selective pulmonary vasodilators as in idiopathic PAH, even if data are limited [16].

Operability

Most pulmonary vascular lesions related to CHD may be prevented by correction of the defect with closure of the shunt early enough to prevent permanent remodeling of the pulmonary vasculature and irreversible PVD. The window of opportunity for surgical correction and prevention of permanent PVD is wide and essentially lesion-specific, with posttricuspid shunt lesions prone to earlier PVD compared to pretricuspid shunt lesions. For a variable period of time after PVR starts to increase, changes in lung vasculature may

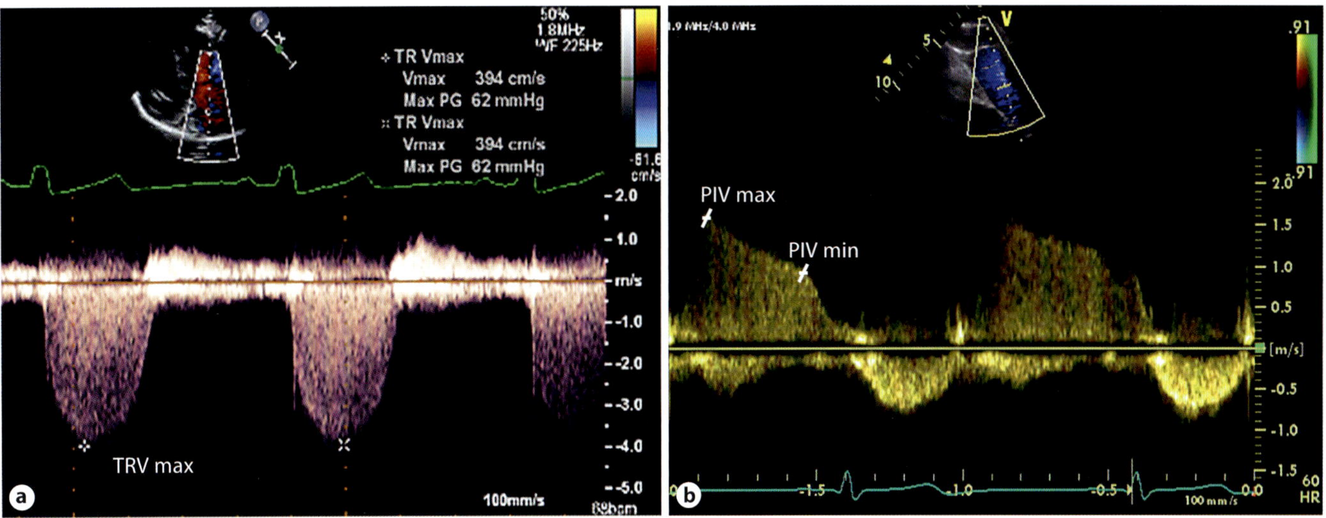

Fig. 5. Doppler echocardiography with high-velocity tricuspid regurgitation (**a**) allowing for estimation of right ventricular systolic pressure ($TRVmax^2$ + right atrial pressure), and with pulmonary insufficiency (**b**) allowing for estimation of end-diastolic pulmonary arterial pressure ($PIVmin^2$ + right atrial pressure) and mean pulmonary arterial pressure ($PIVmax^2$) using the modified Bernoulli equation.

still be reversible following correction of the CHD (operable situation). However, once irreversible PVD is established, closure of the shunt lesion may actually worsen the natural history (inoperable situation). The two main factors that affect patient outcome after surgical closure of shunt lesions have been identified as the age at repair and preoperative PVR. As mentioned previously, individual, environmental, and genetic susceptibilities also play a role and it is well known that patients with Down syndrome are prone to early and fixed pulmonary vascular remodeling, and have a more reactive pulmonary vascular bed in the postoperative period, prone to pulmonary hypertensive 'crisis'. There appears to be a spectrum in the development of pulmonary vascular lesions with a subset of patients with high PVR and advanced PVD in early infancy at one end and adults who remain operable with large left-to-right shunt lesions at the other.

It has been well described that higher preoperative pulmonary/systemic arterial pressure and resistance (PVR/SVR) ratios are associated with more advanced stages of PVD on lung biopsy and a higher incidence of early and late postoperative PH [17]. This relationship, however, is not constant and the degree of individual variability makes it difficult to apply a single cutoff value to determine operability. Nevertheless, risk stratification of patients with PAH and CHD is important [11, 18]. A baseline PVR index <6 WU × m^2 associated with a PVR/SVR ratio of <0.3 without a vasoreactivity test is interpreted as indicative of a favorable outcome following operations resulting in a biventricular circulation. Acute vasodilator challenge using NO and/or oxygen has been strongly encouraged if baseline PVR index is between 6 and 9 WU × m^2 in the presence of a PVR/SVR ratio of approx. 0.3–0.5. Although there is no absolute consensus, operability with a favorable outcome is considered likely if the following criteria are met: a decrease of 20% in the PVR index, a decrease of around 20% in the ratio of PVR/SVR, a final PVR index of <6 WU × m^2, and a final PVR/SVR ratio of <0.3.

These are very conservative numbers that may be adapted in the future. Technical difficulties leading to calculation errors (table 3) and other medical conditions need to be considered when undertaking vasodilator testing [19]. Another technique for assessing operability is to perform temporary balloon occlusion of the defect when feasible before deciding on suitability for closure of the shunt lesion. It remains unclear which preoperative hemodynamic parameter correlates best with the outcome and it can lead to difficulty in decision-making regarding operability of CHD, particularly in patients who present beyond infancy and early childhood.

It should be noted that the above criteria do not apply to patients with single ventricle physiology who are being assessed for a total cavopulmonary connection (Fontan procedure). In these patients, obtaining accurate hemodynamic measurements can be even more difficult. Ideally, they should have near normal levels of PVR and certainly ≤3 WU × m^2. A

Table 3. Sources of errors in flow and resistance calculation [19]

Sampling errors	Sampling obtained from different physiological states Streaming of blood Partial wedging of catheter (pulmonary artery) Nonrepresentative sampling (pulmonary vein)
Measurement errors	Diluted sample Air bubble Delay in sending/analyzing samples Nonstandardized equipment Failure to account for dissolved oxygen
Assumptions	Oxygen consumption Pulmonary venous saturation
Approximations	Mixed venous samples (using superior vena cava for mixed venous)
Associated medical conditions	Upper/lower airway obstruction Restrictive lung physiology Hypoventilation Parenchymal lung disease Reduced oxygen content in inhaled air (high altitude)

mean PAP of >15 mm Hg has been associated with both early and late mortality after the Fontan operation [11].

Pulmonary Artery Banding

There is clinical evidence that placing a restrictive band on the main pulmonary artery can reduce the PAP distal to the band and can reverse pathological pulmonary vascular remodeling. It has been described that high pulmonary blood flow results in impaired endothelium-mediated relaxation and increased vasomotor tone accompanied by histological changes in the vessel wall, which can potentially be reversed by reducing the pulmonary blood flow.

For neonates with a single ventricle physiology or complex CHD and unobstructed pulmonary blood flow (no pulmonary protection), the goal is to secure a normal PAP with pulmonary artery banding before proceeding to the cavopulmonary anastomosis.

Immediate Postoperative Care

It is in the immediate postoperative period that the child with PAH related to CHD is the most vulnerable. Postoperative pulmonary hypertensive 'crisis' is characterized by an acute and labile increase in PVR following cardiac surgery, related to heightened vascular reactivity secondary to vasospastic stimuli. Pulmonary hypertensive crisis leads to acute right heart failure, low cardiac output with systemic hypotension, and myocardial ischemia, and may be lethal. Patients with extracardiac syndromes (particularly Down syndrome) seem to be at increased risk. In general, early corrective surgery in the first 6 months of life decreases the risk of postoperative pulmonary hypertensive crisis, which is particularly true for atrioventricular septal defect and VSD. For high-risk cardiac lesions, like truncus arteriosus or d-TGA, surgical repair should be attempted even sooner [4]. Precipitating factors should be avoided, particularly stressful stimuli like tracheal suction, pain, and anxiety, as well as hypoxia, hypercapnia, acidosis, hyperthermia, or fluid overload. Adequate sedation, hyperventilation, and the use of sodium bicarbonate are useful strategies in the immediate postoperative care of such patients [20].

In general, there is no clear PAP indicating the need for postoperative specific pulmonary vasodilator therapy. However, patients with PH and signs of low cardiac output should be treated. Inhaled NO has become the accepted therapy because of its selective vasodilator effect on the pulmonary vascular bed. There is no optimal dosage, but there does not appear to be any benefit from doses exceeding 10–20 ppm [21]. Rebound PH is a common complication upon rapid withdrawal of NO [22] and can be minimized by slow weaning, particularly in the last 5 ppm, and adjunction of oral sildenafil.

Medical Therapy

PVD related to CHD may be prevented by early diagnosis and correction of the defect before permanent pulmonary vascular remodeling. Once the lesions are established and nonreactive to pulmonary vasodilator testing, therapy is supportive rather than designated to decrease PVR, even though patients with Eisenmenger syndrome may show some improvement with targeted therapies.

The main determinant of treatment is the response to vasodilator testing at cardiac catheterization. Acute responders with CHD-associated PAH are candidates for surgical repair with shunt closure, whereas nonresponders are candidates for targeted therapies. It is important to note that these therapies have not received approval for use in children, except for the pediatric formulation of bosentan which has been recently approved in Europe for the treatment of idiopathic PAH [23].

Patients with Eisenmenger syndrome are at particular risk during anesthesia and as a result of dehydration, chest infections, high altitude, and intravenous lines. It is also recommended to avoid strenuous exercise and not to participate in competitive sports.

Conventional Medical Therapy

Enhanced inspired oxygen is usually contraindicated in children with PAH associated with congenital shunt lesions and high pulmonary blood flow, but may be beneficial for those with concomitant hypoventilation or lung disease. Nevertheless, for those with right-to-left interatrial shunting, oxygen supplementation does not usually improve oxygen saturation. A controlled study in patients with Eisenmenger syndrome showed no benefit in survival or level of hemoglobin [24].

Anticoagulation is controversial because of the increased risk of hemoptysis and hemorrhage, but may be beneficial in patients with low cardiac output leading to sluggish blood flow through the pulmonary arteries or in those with hypercoagulable states at risk for thrombosis. The risk/benefit of anticoagulation should be carefully weighed. Low-dose warfarin is frequently used (INR of 1.5–2). For contraception, it is recommended to use oral contraceptive agents that have no estrogen content, so as to avoid the risk of a thromboembolic event.

NO is a potent vasodilator with a selective effect on pulmonary circulation. NO activates soluble guanylate cyclase in the pulmonary smooth muscle cells, which increases cGMP and decreases intracellular calcium concentration, leading to smooth muscle relaxation and vasodilation. NO is useful in all forms of PAH and has proven beneficial in the treatment of postoperative pulmonary hypertensive 'crisis' [25]. Rebound PAH is problematic and may prolong postoperative NO administration in some patients [22]. The delivery system is a major limitation.

Calcium channel blockers (CCB) inhibit calcium influx into cardiac and smooth muscle cells, causing pulmonary vasodilation. Chronic CCB are efficacious in patients with idiopathic PAH who demonstrate an acute response to vasodilator testing [6, 26]. Nevertheless, the efficacy of CCB in patients with Eisenmenger syndrome is not proven, as their use can result in an acute decrease in systemic arterial pressure and increased right-to-left shunting, which may lead to syncope and sudden death. Published experience with long-term CCB does not permit accurate assessment of their effects on PVR in patients with congenital cardiac lesions. For this reason, CCB is not indicated in PAH associated with CHD [1].

Targeted Pulmonary Arterial Hypertension Therapies

Treatment of patients with advanced PVD associated with CHD should be made in specialized centers. Based on known mechanisms of action and the endothelial dysfunction, three classes of drugs are commonly used for the treatment of children with PAH: prostacyclin analogues, endothelin receptor antagonists, and phosphodiesterase inhibitors.

Epoprostenol is a prostacyclin analogue with pulmonary and systemic vasodilatory properties mainly used by intravenous infusion. Epoprostenol has been shown to improve hemodynamics, quality of life, exercise capacity, and survival in adults and children with idiopathic PAH and associated PAH [26]. In adults and children with PAH associated with CHD, epoprostenol has been show to decrease PVR, improve oxygen delivery, and increase exercise capacity, with no demonstrated effect on survival [27, 28]. There are anecdotal reports of chronic infusion of epoprostenol permitting a sufficient decrease in PVR to permit closure of the shunt lesion in patients considered inoperable before therapy. The development of tolerance is possible and most children need periodic dose escalation. The optimal dose of intravenous epoprostenol shows significant patient variability, and should be titrated incrementally, with children usually needing much higher doses than adults. Epoprostenol has a short half-life (1–2 min) rendering a continuous intravenous infusion with a permanent central venous catheter necessary. Complications such as line sepsis, local infection, and catheter dislodgement are not unusual and can be responsible for life-threatening rebound PAH.

Iloprost is an inhaled prostacyclin analogue with a longer half-life. In children treated with iloprost, WHO functional class has been shown to be improved in 35%, remained unchanged in 50%, and decreased in 15% [29]. Lower-airway reactivity is a problem in some children, as well as poor compliance with the need for frequent aerosol administrations (6–8 times daily). The short- and long-term efficacy of inhaled iloprost is still controversial. In the critical care setting of CHD, inhaled iloprost has been shown to be as efficacious in lowering mean PVR and improve systemic oxygen saturation compared to NO [30]. Nevertheless, clinical deterioration, side effects, and poor compliance could limit its chronic administration in children [29]. Data on the use of chronic inhaled iloprost in CHD remains scarce.

Treprostinil is a prostacyclin analogue usually administered subcutaneously by continuous infusion. Unfortunately, when infused subcutaneously, discomfort at the infusion site is common and represents the most limiting factor. In a small series of children treated with subcutaneous treprostinil after failure of combined oral treatment or because of severe complications with intravenous epoprostenol, early significant improvement was noted in functional class, hemodynamics, and/or 6-minute walk distance in all patients [31]. Further studies in a larger number of patients are needed to confirm these encouraging findings.

Bosentan is an oral dual endothelin (ET-1) receptor antagonist acting on both the ET_A and ET_B receptors. In children with PAH, Barst et al. [32] demonstrated the beneficial effect of bosentan in lowering PAP and PVR. In an open uncontrolled study in children with PAH, bosentan was shown to lower mean PAP and PVR and improve WHO functional status and survival estimates at 1 and 2 years (98 and 91%, respectively) [33]. Nevertheless, in a study including both children and adults with PAH and systemic-to-pulmonary shunt, bosentan therapy was shown to produce only short-term improvement in WHO functional class and 6-MW test. There was a progressive decline in the beneficial effect of bosentan after 1 year, with a more pronounced decline in the children, who tended to have more severe disease at baseline [34]. In the first placebo-controlled trial in patients with Eisenmenger syndrome (BREATHE-5 study), bosentan was well tolerated and improved exercise capacity and hemodynamics without compromising peripheral oxygen saturation [35]. Longer follow-up data support the efficacy and safety profile reported in the preceding BREATHE-5 study, challenging the notion that PVD and severe functional impairment in these patients are not amenable to therapy [36]. Common side effects include dose-related hepatotoxicity, and liver function tests should be performed monthly. Beghetti et al. [37] recently reported on the safety of bosentan therapy in children with PAH. Elevated transaminase levels were reported in 2.7% of children compared with 7.8% of patients aged ≥12 years, and the overall discontinuation rate from bosentan was 14% in children compared with 28% in patients aged ≥12 years. Bosentan has been shown to be well tolerated with improved exercise capacity and hemodynamics without compromising peripheral oxygen saturation in a placebo-controlled trial in children with Eisenmenger syndrome [35]. A specific pediatric formulation has recently been approved in Europe [23].

Sitaxsentan and ambrisentan are oral selective ET_A receptor antagonists with a long half-life. They block the vasoconstrictor effect of ET_A receptors while maintaining the vasodilator effect and clearance function of ET_B receptors. Sitaxsentan has shown beneficial effects on exercise capacity and NYHA functional class in adult patients. Few data, however, are available in the CHD population, and the drug has recently been removed from the market. No data are available for ambrisentan.

Sildenafil is a phosphodiesterase inhibitor type 5 (PDE-5) that prevents the breakdown of cGMP resulting in pulmonary vasodilatation. PDE-5 is an acute pulmonary vasodilator as efficient as inhaled NO, and potentiates pulmonary vasodilatation when used together with NO. They may be particularly beneficial in situations where withdrawal of NO may lead to rebound PAH [38]. Sildenafil can be used orally or intravenous, but currently only oral sildenafil is available. Sildenafil has been approved for the treatment of WHO functional class II–IV PAH adult patients [39, 40], but the data in children remain limited. In a pilot study of 14 children with PAH [41], oral sildenafil significantly decreased PAP and PVR and improved the mean 6-MW test, but a plateau was reached between 6 and 12 months. In a small study of children with idiopathic PAH and PH associated with CHD, sildenafil was shown to be well tolerated and safe with improved oxyhemoglobin saturation and exercise capacity without significant side effects [42]. Recently, 3 months of sildenafil therapy in adults with Eisenmenger syndrome was shown to be tolerated and associated with significant improvement in quality of life, NYHA class, and exercise capacity [43]. Moreover, PDE-5 appears to be highly expressed in the hypertrophied human right ventricle and acute inhibition with oral sildenafil has been shown to improve right ventricular contractility. Preliminary safety and efficacy trials of oral sildenafil are underway in pediatric patients, in whom a significant number present CHD-PAH, and results are expected soon. Intravenous sildenafil has been shown to potentiate the increase in cGMP in response to NO in children with increased PVR related to CHD or postoperative state. Nevertheless, sildenafil infusion was associated with increased intrapulmonary shunting and augmentation of hypoxemia related to V/Q mismatch in the postoperative patient.

Combination therapy is an attractive option to simultaneously address the multiple pathophysiological pathways present in PAH. It is understandable that acting on the three different pathways of PAH may be more efficacious than acting on a single one in terms of additive or synergistic effects. Few data are available in children. In a pediatric study from Ivy et al. [44], bosentan was successfully used in children with idiopathic PAH on long-term epoprostenol therapy, and concomitant use of bosentan allowed for a decrease in epoprostenol dose and its associated side effects. In adult patients with Eisenmenger syndrome, treatment with bosentan significantly improved walking distance, pulmonary blood flow, and PVR; however, adding sildenafil to bosentan did not significantly improve walking distance, but did increase saturation at rest [45]. Whether combination therapy should be used as a first step by simultaneous initiation of two or more drugs or by addition of a second treatment to a previous therapy once insufficient is still not known; more studies are needed to help establish guidelines. Even if empiric combination of drugs is not uncommon in pediatric patients with PAH, there is a clear lack of studies in this area.

Medical Therapy in Special Conditions

Patients with nonoperable pre-Eisenmenger syndrome have a PVR considered too high for surgical repair, but they do not reach the diagnosis of Eisenmenger syndrome. So far, the therapeutic approach of this group is to watch and wait. However, with the upcoming new targeted therapies for treating PAH, the concept to treat and repair has emerged.

In PAH associated with CHD and large shunt lesions, it is thought that the pressure and/or volume load on the pulmonary vascular bed leads to pulmonary vascular remodeling and lesions. By reducing PVR, the possibility arises that pretreatment with vasodilators can be used to improve a patient's condition and an inoperable case could be considered operable; however, the pretreatment may not always be efficacious depending on the extensiveness and severity of the lesions. Although pretreatment may reduce PVR in these patients, PAH could remain postoperatively, resulting in a worse prognosis. Moreover, the reversal of vascular remodeling and lesion formation with pretreatment, leading to an initial decrease in PVR, could actually result in an increase in pulmonary blood flow, re-establishing the propensity towards pulmonary vascular damage and lesions later on.

There have been several case reports of pretreatment with prostacyclins or bosentan being used prior to CHD surgery to prepare borderline patients. These reports suggest some benefit to improve hemodynamics and make conditions more favorable for repair. Nevertheless, it is important to note that most patients had simple CHD like ASDs. A retrospective analysis of national registries on this type of data would be required in order to gain a complete picture.

Another special condition is persistent PH late after surgical repair. Series reflective of contemporary practice suggest that PH complicates 2% of patients undergoing CHD surgery. However, acute treatment and survival in the immediate postoperative period does not mean that PH resolves, and the patient may present persistent PAH after surgical repair with closed shunt. Literature on this subgroup of patients remains scarce, but the hemodynamics and prognosis appear very similar to idiopathic PAH [6]. This emphasizes the importance of an accurate decision for operability because survival may be better with a persistent shunt lesions and Eisenmenger syndrome than with a closed shunt and RV failure [2].

A further special condition is PH and the Fontan circulation. The Fontan procedure (total cavopulmonary connection) results in a pulmonary circulation very different from physiological conditions, and a small increase in PAP has a profound impact on the passive pulmonary blood flow. The process of ageing itself has potentially important effects, such as increasing PAP, and may lead to failure of the Fontan circulation over time. For this reason, the idea of treating failing Fontan patients with a therapy that lowers PVR has emerged [46]. Therapies approved for PAH may therefore provide benefits in this patient population, but few data have been reported in the literature thus far.

Inhaled NO has been shown to be predominantly effective in patients with central venous pressure ≥15 mm Hg and/or a transpulmonary pressure gradient ≥8 mm Hg. In the early postoperative period, inhaled NO and milrinone have been shown to be very effective in reducing the transpulmonary pressure gradient [47]. The use of prostacyclins, sildenafil, and bosentan in the perioperative course of Fontan or in late Fontan patients is seldom reported and limited to case reports. In adult patients with Fontan, oral administration of a single dose of sildenafil improves exercise capacity and hemodynamic response to exercise [48]. One study failed to show significant improvement after treatment with bosentan in a small group of patients with failing Fontan circulation, while some individuals did improve [49]. Given the important role of the pulmonary circulation in the Fontan physiology and the current lack of data, there is a need for clinical studies on the safety and efficacy of those potential therapies.

Interventional Treatment of Pulmonary Arterial Hypertension

Atrial septostomy with right-to-left shunting has been shown to be beneficial in patients with severe PAH and intractable right heart failure refractory to vasodilator treatment by maintaining cardiac output at the expense of increased hypoxemia [50]. This is used as a bridge to transplantation or in the absence of other therapeutic options in patients that are refractory to medical therapy. Atrial septostomy, blade balloon atrial septostomy, and graded balloon dilatation atrial septostomy are the different techniques used. This procedure should be performed in institutions with experience in performing atrial septostomy.

Surgical Treatment of Pulmonary Arterial Hypertension

In patients with severe PAH and high PVR, the congenital shunt lesion can be closed with left patent foramen ovale or creation of an ASD. Another alternative is to use partial

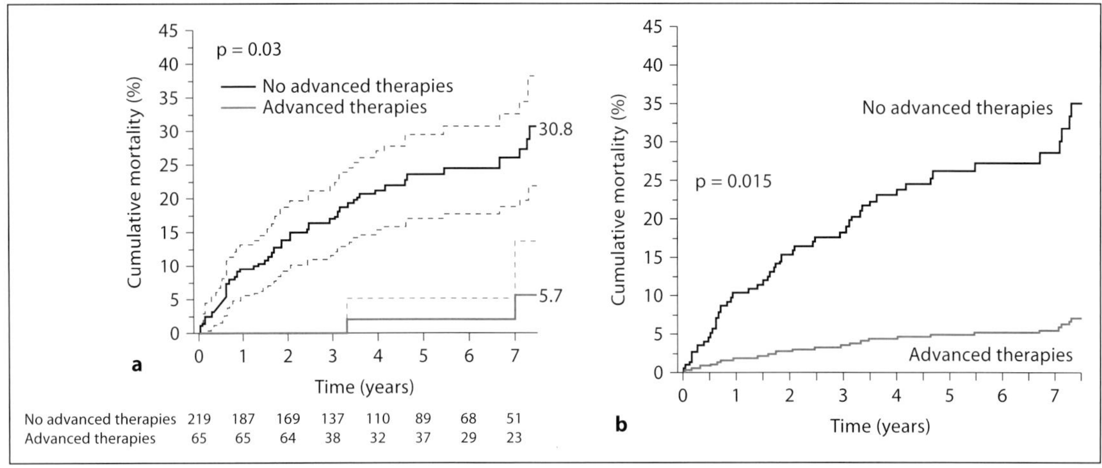

Fig. 6. Unadjusted (**a**) survival rate curves (with 95% CI) and adjusted (**b**) survival rate curves based on the propensity-score adjusted Cox model by treatment with advanced therapy (n = 287) [51].

closure of the shunt, allowing for some degree of right-to-left shunting. The use of a fenestrated VSD patch closure has been successfully reported with good outcome in children with high PVR. In patients with ASD or VSD, another technique is to apply 'flap-valve' closure of the shunt, allowing decompression of the right heart whenever the right ventricular pressure exceeds systemic levels, thus preventing right heart failure.

In patients with severe postoperative PAH in which atrial level shunting is not sufficient to alleviate right heart failure, creation of a Potts shunt (anastomosis between the left pulmonary artery and the descending aorta) may allow a decrease in right ventricular afterload with subsequent improvement in right ventricular function. Nevertheless, the high risk of the procedure makes it an experimental therapy that should be reserved for the treatment of children resistant to other forms of therapy.

Transplantation

Lung or heart-lung transplantation remains the only available treatment for patients not responding to vasodilator treatment or with certain lesions such as pulmonary vascular obstructive lesions, but is limited by the shortage of donors and the high incidence of bronchiolitis obliterans which limits the long-term survival after lung transplantation. Thus, transplantation should be reserved for children with PAH which has progressed despite optimal medical therapy, and children should be listed for transplantation when their probability of 2-year survival without transplantation is ≤50%.

Outcome

Patients with Eisenmenger syndrome are at high risk of death. In a 5-year retrospective study of children with PAH in the United Kingdom, the subpopulation with postoperative CHD-PAH fared far worse than those with PAH associated with complex (unoperated) CHD and Eisenmenger syndrome; almost one quarter of these children died [6]. Children with Eisenmenger syndrome had a greater cumulative survival time of 1.3 years, indicating that surgical repair is not necessarily always the best option. In a study of a contemporary cohort of adults with Eisenmenger syndrome, advanced therapy for PAH was associated with a lower risk of death (fig. 6) [51]. The mortality in Eisenmenger syndrome is related to the underlying cardiac defect and is worse in those with complex lesions. When compared with healthy individuals, median survival is reduced by approximately 20 years in Eisenmenger syndrome patients [52] (fig. 7).

Conclusion

Advances in the understanding of pulmonary vasculature have led to new therapeutic options for patients with CHD-PAH. In children with CHD, increased pulmonary blood flow is a potent stimulator to both active vasoconstriction and pathological remodeling of the pulmonary vascular bed leading to PVD and increased PVR. With the exception of a few high-risk congenital cardiac malformations or

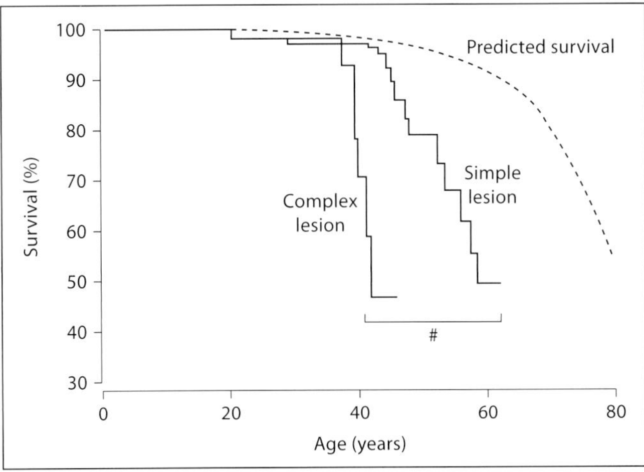

Fig. 7. Mortality in Eisenmenger syndrome is related to the underlying cardiac defect. # p = 0.02, comparison between Eisenmenger syndrome patients with simple and complex lesions [52].

predisposed individuals, irreversible PVD seldom occurs in the first 1–2 years of age. Timely diagnosis is crucial as early surgical repair of congenital shunt lesions and earlier treatment of PAH leads to improved outcome. Initial evaluation still includes acute vasodilator testing at cardiac catheterization, which helps determine operability of the CHD. The outcome of patients with Eisenmenger syndrome seems to be improved with careful follow-up and the use of targeted therapies. Several novel therapeutic agents are under investigation and evolving clinical research should better define the role of new treatments. Moreover, improved delivery of medical and surgical care in underprivileged areas should reduce PVD associated with CHD.

References

1 Task Force for Diagnosis and Treatment of Pulmonary Hypertension of European Society of Cardiology (ESC), European Respiratory Society (ERS), International Society of Heart and Lung Transplantation (ISHLT), Galiè N, Hoeper MM, Humbert M, et al: Guidelines for the diagnosis and treatment of pulmonary hypertension. Eur Heart J 2009;34:1219–1263.
2 Wood P: The Eisenmenger syndrome or pulmonary hypertension with reversed central shunt. I. Br Med J 1958;2:701–709.
3 Budts W, et al: Residual pulmonary vasoreactivity to inhaled nitric oxide in patients with severe obstructive pulmonary hypertension and Eisenmenger syndrome. Heart 2001;86:553–558.
4 Haworth SG: Pulmonary vascular disease in different types of congenital heart disease. Implications for interpretation of lung biopsy findings in early childhood. Br Heart J 1984;52:557–571.
5 Simonneau G, et al: Updated clinical classification of pulmonary hypertension. J Am Coll Cardiol 2009;54(1 suppl):S43–S54.
6 Haworth SG, Hislop AA: Treatment and survival in children with pulmonary arterial hypertension: the UK Pulmonary Hypertension Service for Children 2001–2006. Heart 2009;95:312–317.
7 Austin ED, Loyd JE, Phillips JA: 3rd Genetics of pulmonary arterial hypertension. Semin Respir Crit Care Med 2009;30:386–398.
8 Rosenzweig EB, et al: Clinical implications of determining BMPR2 mutation status in a large cohort of children and adults with pulmonary arterial hypertension. J Heart Lung Transplant 2008;27:668–674.
9 Berner M, et al: Inhaled nitric oxide to test the vasodilator capacity of the pulmonary vascular bed in children with long-standing pulmonary hypertension and congenital heart disease. Am J Cardiol 1996;77:532–535.
10 Balzer DT, et al: Inhaled nitric oxide as a preoperative test (INOP Test I): the INOP Test Study Group. Circulation 2002;106(12 suppl 1):I76–I81.
11 Giglia TM, Humpl T: Preoperative pulmonary hemodynamics and assessment of operability: is there a pulmonary vascular resistance that precludes cardiac operation? Pediatr Crit Care Med 2010;11(2 suppl):S57–S69.
12 Lammers AE, et al: The 6-minute walk test: normal values for children of 4–11 years of age. Arch Dis Child 2008;93:464–468.
13 Bernus A, et al: Brain natriuretic peptide levels in managing pediatric patients with pulmonary arterial hypertension. Chest 2009;135:745–751.
14 Van Albada ME, et al: Biological serum markers in the management of pediatric pulmonary arterial hypertension. Pediatr Res 2008;63:321–327.
15 Brun H, et al: Patients with pulmonary hypertension related to congenital systemic-to-pulmonary shunts are characterized by inflammation involving endothelial cell activation and platelet-mediated inflammation. Congenit Heart Dis 2009;4:153–159.
16 Beghetti M, Galie N: Eisenmenger syndrome a clinical perspective in a new therapeutic era of pulmonary arterial hypertension. J Am Coll Cardiol 2009;53:733–740.
17 Fried R, et al: Pulmonary arterial changes in patients with ventricular septal defects and severe pulmonary hypertension. Pediatr Cardiol 1986;7:147–154.
18 Feinstein JA: Evaluation, risk stratification, and management of pulmonary hypertension in patients with congenital heart disease. Semin Thorac Cardiovasc Surg Pediatr Card Surg Annu 2009;12:106–111.
19 Viswanathan S, Kumar RK: Assessment of operability of congenital cardiac shunts with increased pulmonary vascular resistance. Catheter Cardiovasc Interv 2008;71:665–670.
20 Adatia I, Beghetti M: Early postoperative care of patients with pulmonary hypertension associated with congenital cardiac disease. Cardiol Young 2009;19:315–319.
21 Beghetti M, et al: Continuous low dose inhaled nitric oxide for treatment of severe pulmonary hypertension after cardiac surgery in paediatric patients. Br Heart J 1995;73:65–68.
22 Atz AM, Adatia I, Wessel DL: Rebound pulmonary hypertension after inhalation of nitric oxide. Ann Thorac Surg 1996;62:1759–1764.
23 Beghetti M, et al: Pharmacokinetic and clinical profile of a novel formulation of bosentan in children with pulmonary arterial hypertension: the FUTURE-1 study. Br J Clin Pharmacol 2009;68:948–955.
24 Sandoval J, et al: Nocturnal oxygen therapy in patients with the Eisenmenger syndrome. Am J Respir Crit Care Med 2001;164:1682–1687.
25 Wessel DL: Inhaled nitric oxide for the treatment of pulmonary hypertension before and after cardiopulmonary bypass. Crit Care Med 1993;21(9 suppl):S344–S345.
26 Barst RJ, Maislin G, Fishman AP: Vasodilator therapy for primary pulmonary hypertension in children. Circulation 1999;99:1197–1208.

27 Fernandes SM, et al: Usefulness of epoprostenol therapy in the severely ill adolescent/adult with Eisenmenger physiology. Am J Cardiol 2003;91:632–635.

28 Rosenzweig EB, Kerstein D, Barst RJ: Long-term prostacyclin for pulmonary hypertension with associated congenital heart defects. Circulation 1999;99:1858–1865.

29 Ivy DD, et al: Short- and long-term effects of inhaled iloprost therapy in children with pulmonary arterial hypertension. J Am Coll Cardiol 2008;51:161–169.

30 Rimensberger PC, et al: Inhaled nitric oxide versus aerosolized iloprost in secondary pulmonary hypertension in children with congenital heart disease: vasodilator capacity and cellular mechanisms. Circulation 2001;103:544–548.

31 Ivy DD, Claussen L, Doran A: Transition of stable pediatric patients with pulmonary arterial hypertension from intravenous epoprostenol to intravenous treprostinil. Am J Cardiol 2007;99:696–698.

32 Barst RJ, et al: Pharmacokinetics, safety, and efficacy of bosentan in pediatric patients with pulmonary arterial hypertension. Clin Pharmacol Ther 2003;73:372–382.

33 Rosenzweig EB, et al: Effects of long-term bosentan in children with pulmonary arterial hypertension. J Am Coll Cardiol 2005;46:697–704.

34 van Loon RL, et al: Long-term effect of bosentan in adults versus children with pulmonary arterial hypertension associated with systemic-to-pulmonary shunt: does the beneficial effect persist? Am Heart J 2007;154:776–782.

35 Galie N, et al: Bosentan therapy in patients with Eisenmenger syndrome: a multicenter, double-blind, randomized, placebo-controlled study. Circulation 2006;114:48–54.

36 Gatzoulis MA, et al: Longer-term bosentan therapy improves functional capacity in Eisenmenger syndrome: results of the BREATHE-5 open-label extension study. Int J Cardiol 2008;127:27–32.

37 Beghetti M, et al: Safety experience with bosentan in 146 children 2–11 years old with pulmonary arterial hypertension: results from the European Postmarketing Surveillance program. Pediatr Res 2008;64:200–204.

38 Atz AM, Wessel DL: Sildenafil ameliorates effects of inhaled nitric oxide withdrawal. Anesthesiology 1999;91:307–310.

39 Galie N, et al: Sildenafil citrate therapy for pulmonary arterial hypertension. N Engl J Med 2005;353:2148–2157.

40 Michelakis ED, et al: Long-term treatment with oral sildenafil is safe and improves functional capacity and hemodynamics in patients with pulmonary arterial hypertension. Circulation 2003;108:2066–2069.

41 Humpl T, et al: Beneficial effect of oral sildenafil therapy on childhood pulmonary arterial hypertension: twelve-month clinical trial of a single-drug, open-label, pilot study. Circulation 2005;111:3274–3280.

42 Karatza AA, Bush A, Magee AG: Safety and efficacy of sildenafil therapy in children with pulmonary hypertension. Int J Cardiol 2005;100:267–273.

43 Tay EL, et al: Quality of life and functional capacity can be improved in patients with Eisenmenger syndrome with oral sildenafil therapy. Int J Cardiol 2011;149:372–376.

44 Ivy DD, et al: Weaning and discontinuation of epoprostenol in children with idiopathic pulmonary arterial hypertension receiving concomitant bosentan. Am J Cardiol 2004;93:943–946.

45 Iversen K, et al: Combination therapy with bosentan and sildenafil in Eisenmenger syndrome: a randomized, placebo-controlled, double-blinded trial. Eur Heart J 2010;31:1124–1131.

46 Beghetti, M: Fontan and the pulmonary circulation: a potential role for new pulmonary hypertension therapies. Heart 2010;96:911–916.

47 Cai J, et al: Nitric oxide and milrinone: combined effect on pulmonary circulation after Fontan-type procedure: a prospective, randomized study. Ann Thorac Surg 2008;86:882–888.

48 Giardini A, et al: Effect of sildenafil on haemodynamic response to exercise and exercise capacity in Fontan patients. Eur Heart J 2008;29:1681–1687.

49 Ovaert C, et al: The effect of bosentan in patients with a failing Fontan circulation. Cardiol Young 2009;19:331–339.

50 Sandoval J, et al: Graded balloon dilation atrial septostomy in severe primary pulmonary hypertension. A therapeutic alternative for patients nonresponsive to vasodilator treatment. J Am Coll Cardiol 1998;32:297–304.

51 Dimopoulos K, et al: Improved survival among patients with Eisenmenger syndrome receiving advanced therapy for pulmonary arterial hypertension. Circulation 2010;121:20–25.

52 Diller GP, et al: Long-term safety, tolerability and efficacy of bosentan in adults with pulmonary arterial hypertension associated with congenital heart disease. Heart 2007;93:974–976.

53 Kulik T, et al: Pulmonary arterial hypertension associated with congenital heart disease. Prog Pediatr Cardiol 2009;27:25–33.

Cecile Tissot
Pediatric Cardiology Unit, The University Children's Hospital of Geneva
6 rue Willy Donze
CH–1211 Geneva 14 (Switzerland)
Tel. +41 22 3824580, E-Mail cecile.tissot@hotmail.com

Chapter 14
Humbert M, Souza R, Simonneau G (eds): Pulmonary Vascular Disorders.
Prog Respir Res. Basel, Karger, 2012, vol 41, pp 137–142

Pulmonary Hypertension in Sickle Cell Disease

Florence Parent[a,b,c] · Laurent Savale[a,b,c] · Bernard Maitre[d,e] · Gérald Simonneau[a,b,c]

[a]Centre de Référence de l'Hypertension Pulmonaire Sévère, Service de Pneumologie et Réanimation Respiratoire, Hôpital Antoine Béclère (AP-HP), Clamart, [b]Université Paris-Sud, Faculté de Médecine, Kremlin-Bicêtre, [c]INSERM U999, Hypertension Artérielle Pulmonaire: Physiopathologie et Innovation Thérapeutique, Le Plessis Robinson, [d]Service de Pneumologie, hôpitaux intercommunal et H Mondor, Créteil, [e]Inserm U955 IMRB, Unité des Maladies Génétiques du Globule Rouge, hôpital H Mondor, Créteil, France

Abstract

Until recently, the prevalence and characteristics of pulmonary hypertension (PH) in adults with sickle cell disease (SCD) remained uncertain. During the past decade several studies have reported the prevalence of PH as defined by a tricuspid valve regurgitant jet velocity (TRJV) ≥2.5 m/s as high as 30%. However, in these studies the diagnosis of PH was not systematically confirmed on right heart catheterization (RHC), a procedure that is recommended in international guidelines. Most recent studies have reported that the prevalence of PH confirmed on RHC in the SCD population is lower than expected (6–10%). Moreover, postcapillary PH was the most frequent cause of PH. Actually, these two studies demonstrated that the positive predictive value of echocardiography for the detection of PH in this population was low (25–32%) when using a TRJV ≥2.5 m/s to define PH. Patients with SCD and precapillary PH have a distinct hemodynamic profile, with less marked increase in mean pulmonary artery pressure, higher cardiac output, and lower pulmonary vascular resistance than patients with idiopathic pulmonary arterial hypertension (PAH). However, PH confirmed by RHC confers an increased risk of death even when mild or moderate. None of the specific therapies approved for the treatment of PAH are currently approved for the treatment of PAH associated with SCD due to the lack of data in this specific population.

During the past decade, the prevalence of pulmonary hypertension (PH) in adults with sickle cell disease (SCD) has been reported to be as high as 30% [1–4]. In these studies, however, PH was defined by a tricuspid valve regurgitant jet velocity (TRJV) of at least 2.5 m/s and was not systematically confirmed on right heart catheterization (RHC). Moreover, in some of these studies, a TRJV of at least 2.5 m/s predicted an increased risk of death [1–3]. More recently, two studies reported that PH, confirmed on RHC, was less frequent than expected in adults with SCD, and that half of the patients at least had postcapillary PH [5, 6].

Thus, the true prevalence of PH in SCD remains controversial. Concerning physiopathology, some authors [7] recently suggested that hemolysis, which was believed to play a key role in the development of PH in SCD [8], could be less important than previously recognized.

SCD is a multisystem disease associated with episodes of acute illness and progressive organ damage, and is one of the most common severe monogenic disorders worldwide. SCD occurs in individuals who are homozygous for a GAG→GTG substitution in the β-globin chain of hemoglobin A, resulting in a hemoglobin called hemoglobin S which polymerizes on deoxygenation [9].

Hemoglobin polymerization, which leads to erythrocyte rigidity and vaso-occlusion, is central to the physiopathology of this disease, although the importance of chronic anemia, hemolysis, and vasculopathy has been established.

Recurrent episodes of vaso-occlusion and inflammation result in progressive damage to most organs, including the brain, kidneys, bones, and pulmonary and cardio-vascular system, and becomes apparent with increasing age. Among these complications, pulmonary involvement is common [acute chest syndrome (ACS), reactive airways disease, pulmonary fibrosis, PH] and a leading cause of mortality in SCD patients, especially ACS [10].

Epidemiology and Characteristics of Pulmonary Hypertension in Sickle Cell Disease

Epidemiology

For several years, retrospective studies have reported that 20–30% of adult patients with SCD have PH, and in some of these reports, patients with PH had a significantly increased mortality rate compared with patients without PH [11, 12]. In addition, autopsy studies have suggested that up to 75% of SCD patients have histological evidence of pulmonary arterial hypertension (PAH) at the time of death [13].

Gladwin et al. [1] have reported a PH screening study in 195 adult patients with SCD in stable condition. All of them were screened with transthoracic Doppler echocardiograms and PH was defined by a TRJV of at least 2.5 m/s. It was found in this study that 32% of patients with SCD had elevated pulmonary artery pressure (PAP; defined as a TRJV ≥2.5 m/s) and 9% had more severe elevated pressures defined as a TRJV ≥3 m/s. In this study, PH defined as a TRJV ≥2.5 m/s was associated with a significant increased risk of death when compared with a TRJV <2.5 m/s. The 18-month mortality rate was 16% for patients with a TRJV ≥2.5 m/s and <2% in patients with a TRJV <2.5 m/s. However, in this study, the diagnosis of PH was not systematically confirmed on RHC, a procedure that is recommended in international guidelines as the standard of care [14]. Moreover, in screening programs for PH in high-risk populations, the use of a definition of PH that is based on the results of echocardiography alone results in a substantial number of false positive diagnoses that are not confirmed on RHC [15–17].

Recently, two studies have been published [5, 6] and have addressed this issue using the same methodology. All patients with SCD underwent Doppler echocardiography with measurement of TRJV. RHC was performed in all patients in whom PH was suspected on the basis of a TRJV ≥2.5 m/s, and PH was defined according to international guidelines as a mean PAP of at least 25 mm Hg [14].

In the French study [5], 398 outpatients in stable condition were included at referral centers for SCD; the prevalence of a TRJV ≥2.5 m/s was 27%. In contrast, the prevalence of PH as confirmed on RHC was only 6.2%. Among the 24 patients with confirmed PH (mean PAP of at least 25 mm Hg), 13 had postcapillary PH, as defined by mean PAP ≥25 mm Hg and pulmonary-capillary wedge pressure ≥15 mm Hg, and the remaining 11 had precapillary PH, as defined by mean PAP ≥25 mm Hg and pulmonary-capillary wedge pressure <15 mm Hg.

In the Brazilian study [6], among the 80 adult patients included, 40% had a high TRJV ≥2.5 m/s on echocardiography and only 10% had mean PAP ≥25 mm Hg on RHC, including 6% of postcapillary PH.

Thus, the results of these two studies performed in France and Brazil [5, 6] are remarkably similar, showing a prevalence of PH of 6.2 and10%, respectively, which is lower than expected. Interestingly, postcapillary PH was the most frequent cause, with a prevalence of 3.3 and 6.2%, respectively, whereas the prevalence of precapillary PH was only 2.9 and 3.8%. In addition, these two studies clearly demonstrate that, when a threshold TRJV of 2.5 m/s was used to define PH, the predictive positive value of echocardiography for the detection of PH was only 25 and 32%, respectively.

Characteristics of Sickle Cell Disease Patients with Pulmonary Hypertension

In the US study by Gladwin et al. [1], all markers of hemolytic anemia, including low hemoglobin and hematocrit, high aspartate aminotransferase (but not alanine aminotransferase), high lactate dehydrogenase, and high direct bilirubin levels were all significant univariate predictors of a high TRJV ≥2.5 m/s. Multiple logistic regression analysis identified a history of renal or cardiovascular complications, elevated lactate dehydrogenase and alkaline phosphatase levels, and a history of priapism in men as independent predictors of high TRJV. These associated risk factors for high TRJV suggest that PH could be related to high rates of hemolysis in some SCD patients (see 'Physiopathology').

In the group of patients with confirmed PH, Fonseca et al. [6] observed a decrease in hemoglobin level and an increase in lactate dehydrogenase and aspartate aminotransferase levels when compared to patients without PH, also suggesting hyperhemolysis. However, other important markers of hemolysis, including reticulocyte count and unconjugated bilirubin level, were similar in the two groups. Moreover, lactate dehydrogenase and aspartate aminotransferase levels may be also influenced by liver dysfunction. In the study from Parent et al. [5], data regarding biological markers of hemolysis and the presence of PH are also discordant. Hemoglobin and indirect bilirubin levels were similar in patients with confirmed PH and in those without PH. In contrast, patients with confirmed PH had a significant increase in lactate dehydrogenase and aspartate aminotransferase levels, which may also have been influenced by liver dysfunction.

Interestingly, in all three studies, patients with a high TRJV or PH compared to other groups were older and had significantly higher creatinine levels [1, 5, 6]. The mean age of SCD patients with confirmed PH is 45 ±10 and 41 ±10 years in the French and Brazilian studies, respectively.

Table 1. Functional and hemodynamic profiles in SCD patients with confirmed PH

	Systolic PAP mm Hg	Diastolic PAP mm Hg	Mean PAP mm Hg	RAP mm Hg	PCWP mm Hg	Cardiac output or index	PVR dyn/s/cm^{-5}	NYHA FC III–IV %	6MWD m
Castro et al. [22] (n = 20)	54±12	25±8	36±8	–	16±6	8.6±1.8 l/min	184±26	–	–
Fonseca et al. [6] (n = 8)	48±13	–	31±9	–	16±6	4.9±1.7[1] l/min/m^2	176±120		460±152
Parent et al. [5] (n = 24)	44±7	19±6	30±6	10±6	16±7	8.7±1.9 l/min	138±58	38%	404±94

Results are means ± SD. PAP = Pulmonary artery pressure; RAP = right atrial pressure; PCWP = pulmonary capillary wedge pressure; PVR = pulmonary vascular resistance; NYHA FC = New York Heart Association functional class.
[1] Cardiac index (l/min/m^2).

Table 2. Hemodynamic profiles in SCD patients with precapillary PH

	Systolic PAP mm Hg	Diastolic PAP mm Hg	Mean PAP mm Hg	RAP mm Hg	PCWP mm Hg	Cardiac output or index	PVR dyn/s/cm^{-5}	NYHA FC III–IV %	6MWD m
Fonseca et al. [6] (n = 3)	52±18	–	33±9	–	10±3	5.1±1.3[1] l/min/m^2	240±152	–	419±246
Parent et al. [5] (n = 11)	43±7	15±5	28±4	5±2	10±3	8.2±1.6 l/min	178±55	45%	406±107

Results are means ± SD. PAP = Pulmonary artery pressure; RAP = right atrial pressure; PCWP = pulmonary capillary wedge pressure; PVR = pulmonary vascular resistance; NYHA FC = New York Heart Association functional class.
[1] Cardiac index (l/min/m^2).

Hemodynamic Characteristics of Sickle Cell Disease Patients with Pulmonary Hypertension and Survival

In all reports of hemodynamic results in SCD patients, half of the patients or more with confirmed PH had postcapillary PH suggesting a left-sided heart disease (table 1) [5, 6, 12, 18].

Patients with SCD and precapillary PH had a less marked increase in mean PAP, higher values of cardiac output, and lower levels of pulmonary vascular resistance than patients with idiopathic PAH (tables 1, 2) [5, 6, 12, 18]. Thus, in SCD patients, precapillary PH seems to be different than other forms of PAH. Moreover, despite having less severe hemodynamic impairment, these patients nonetheless had a clinically significant functional limitation, as assessed according to NYHA functional class, and a marked decrease in the 6-min walk distance (6MWD; tables 1, 2). This poor exercise tolerance, despite being only mild or moderate PH, is probably multifactorial. Anemia, intrinsic cardiac disease, and musculoskeletal problems may also contribute to worsening of functional status.

In some studies, including the one from Gladwin et al. [1], a TRJV ≥2.5 m/s independently predicted an increased risk of death in adult patients with SCD [2]; however, the proportion of these patients with confirmed PH with a mean PAP of at least 25 mm Hg on RHC is unknown. Fonseca et al. [6] reported only a trend for worse survival in patients with a TRJV of at least 2.5 m/s compared with patients with a TRJV <2.5 m/s. In contrast, what really makes the difference in terms of prognosis is to have confirmed PH on RHC. In the study by Fonseca et al. [6], these patients showed a worse survival compared with the remaining patients, regardless of the measured TRJV. Parent et al. [5] reported similar observations in the supplement to their publication, with mortality rates in patients with a TRJV <2.5 m/s, TRJV of at least 2.5 m/s without PH, and confirmed PH of 0.3, 1.4 and 12.5%, respectively. However, these results must be taken with caution due to the low rate of death.

Clinical Presentation and Screening of Pulmonary Hypertension in Sickle Cell Disease

Exertional dyspnea, the most typical sign of PH, is also very frequent in SCD patients due to chronic anemia. More specific symptoms, such as syncope and lower extremity edema are uncommon and usually associated with severe and advanced PH. Nowadays, because of the potential high mortality rate of PH in SCD, screening should be performed.

Doppler echocardiography is the essential first-line tool. It is important that such screening be performed in a steady state, as pulmonary pressures increase during vaso-occlusive crisis [19, 20]. In case of a high TRJV, RHC is mandatory to confirm PH according to the guidelines [14]. As described above, in the study from Parent et al. [5], when a threshold TRJV of 2.5 m/s was used to define PH, the positive predictive value of echocardiography was only 25%; if PH had been defined at a higher threshold, a TRJV of 2.9 m/s, the positive predictive value would have improved, but the sensitivity of the test would have decreased. Thus, the use of this single screening tool for the selection of SCD patients for RHC does not appear to be ideal, whatever threshold is selected. An alternative approach could be the use of the combination of TRJV, 6MWD and N-terminal pro-brain natriuretic peptide level to better select patients with a suspected PH requiring RHC, as reported in this study [5]. Actually, in several studies, the 6MWD is significantly lower in SCD patients with PH compared to patients without PH [5, 18]; in the same way, N-terminal pro-brain natriuretic peptide levels are significantly higher in patients with PH compared to patients without PH [5, 21]. Further studies are needed on this issue.

Acute Rises in Pulmonary Pressures during Vaso-Occlusive Crisis and during Acute Chest Syndrome

It has been reported that pulmonary pressures rise acutely during vaso-occlusive crisis and ACS [19, 20]. The study from Mekontso Dessap et al. [20] examined 84 consecutive SCD patients hospitalized for an ACS: 60% of the patients had a high TRJV on echocardiography (TRJV ≥2.5 m/s), and 13% of the patients manifested right heart failure. The patients with right heart failure had the higher rate of mortality. These data suggest that acute PH represents a major comorbidity during ACS.

ACS is a common complication of SCD and represents the leading cause of premature death in this patient population [22, 23]. During episodes of ACS, the marked increased of PAP may result in acute right heart failure and death in patients that otherwise have only mild PH when stable [19, 20].

Pathophysiology

The etiology of PAH in patients with SCD is probably multifactorial and several mechanisms can contribute to its development, especially intravascular hemolysis, chronic hypoxemia, in situ thrombosis, pulmonary embolism, and liver dysfunction with portal hypertension.

Hemolysis

Hemolysis is believed to play a key role in the development of PH in SCD patients. Several experimental and clinical studies have focused on the hypothesis that nitric oxide (NO) depletion by plasma hemoglobin in the microcirculation plays a central role in the pathogenesis of many manifestations of SCD, particularly PH [8]. In SCD, the release of hemoglobin into plasma during chronic intravascular hemolysis potently scavenges NO [24]. The half-life of NO in the vasculature is very short because of rapid reactions with red cell hemoglobin to form methemoglobin and nitrate [25]. Hemolysis also releases erythrocyte arginase into the plasma. Arginase metabolizes plasma arginine into ornithine, reducing the substrate for NO synthesis and participating in the reduction of NO bioavailability in SCD [26]. Accordingly, high arginase activity in plasma has been associated with a higher risk of PH and death in patients with SCD [26]. In addition, chronic hemolysis enhanced platelet activation and increased endothelin-1 release [8, 27].

NO is a critical signaling molecule produced by the endothelium that regulates basal vasodilator tone and inhibits platelet and hemostatic activation. All these mechanisms, described above, lead to decreased NO bioavailability and resistance to NO-dependent vasodilatation [8]. All of these events in turn lead to a vasculopathy characterized by endothelial dysfunction, increased vascular tone, inflammation and hypercoagulability, and finally to vascular remodeling, which potentially results in PH [8, 28].

In support of the role of hemolysis as an important mechanism in this disease, PH is also an increasingly recognized complication of other hemolytic anemias including thalassemia, spherocytosis, and stomatocytosis [28, 29]. However, this theory has recently been questioned by some authors [7], and further studies are needed to clarify the role of hemolysis in the pathogenesis of PH in patients with SCD.

Thrombosis
A hypercoagulable state is another mechanism in the development of PH in SCD. In SCD, several mechanisms lead to a hypercoagulable state. Depletion of NO, which is a potent inhibitor of platelet activation, leads to hypercoagulability [30]. Recent studies have suggested correlations between the rate of hemolysis and the levels of procoagulant factors in blood of SCD patients in a steady state (decrease of protein C and protein S level, increase of thrombin-antithrombin complex, tissue factor activation) [31–33]. Moreover, in patients with SCD, functional asplenia could also contribute to the development of PH. It has been reported that the loss of splenic function increases the circulation of platelet-derived mediators and that abnormal erythrocytes in the circulation induce platelet activation, promoting PH, microthrombosis, and red cell adhesion to the endothelium [32].

Thromboembolic complications have been reported in SCD patients, including pulmonary embolism and in situ thrombosis. Recently, in a study of 125 SCD patients presenting 144 ACS, a pulmonary embolism was diagnosed in 17% of the cases [34]. Some cases of patients with chronic thromboembolic PH have also been reported with pulmonary endarterectomy performed [35, 36].

Other Mechanisms
Iron overload, hepatitis C, or nodular regenerative hyperplasia produces liver dysfunction, which may lead to portopulmonary hypertension. Chronic anemia induces a high-output state which damages the pulmonary vasculature and, hence, contributes to the pathogenesis of PH. Recurrent ACS are not associated with PH in several studies [1–3, 19], although it is clearly demonstrated that pulmonary pressures may rise acutely during ACS and vaso-occlusive crisis [19, 20].

Therapeutic Considerations

There are no evidence-based guidelines for the management of PH in patients with SCD and there are limited data on this topic. As recommended for the work-up of any patient with PH, RHC is necessary to confirm the diagnosis and to categorize PH according to its cause (precapillary or postcapillary PH). In case of precapillary PH, a ventilation-perfusion lung scan must be performed to search for a chronic thromboembolic cause, which even in SCD patients is potentially curable [35, 36].

The treatment of PH in SCD patients requires a multidisciplinary approach that includes optimizing SCD therapy, treating chronic hypoxemia and thrombo-embolic disease, and identifying and treating comorbid cardiopulmonary conditions. The general approach usually includes optimizing SCD-specific therapy, with hydroxyurea and/or transfusion. Because hemolysis is a possible mechanism in the development of PH, it is likely that maximization of treatments to decrease the hemolytic rate would be beneficial, but data to confirm this hypothesis are lacking. Hydroxyurea has been shown to decrease the frequency of vaso-occlusive crisis and ACS, reduce the need for transfusions, and reduce mortality in SCD [37, 38]. Long-term transfusion therapy reduces the synthesis of sickle cells and decreases the incidence of stroke and pulmonary events [39]. Moreover, a higher hemoglobin level of 8–10 g/dl and a lower level of hemoglobin S might improve cardiopulmonary function and prevent the progression of PH.

Specific Therapy for Precapillary Pulmonary Hypertension
Specific therapies approved for the treatment of PAH include prostacyclin derivatives, endothelin receptor antagonists, and phosphodiesterase-5 inhibitors [40]. However, none of these agents are currently approved for the treatment of PAH associated with SCD due to the lack of data in this specific population. Recently, the effect of bosentan was assessed in a randomized, double-blind, placebo-controlled trial of patients with SCD and PH. Overall, bosentan appeared to be well tolerated, although the small sample size precluded an analysis of its efficacy [41]. Another randomized, double-blind, placebo-controlled study designed to evaluate the safety and efficacy of sildenafil was prematurely halted after interim analysis showed that sildenafil-treated patients were likely to have more acute sickle cell pain crisis (35%) compared to placebo-treated patients (14%) [42]. Furthermore, there was no evidence of treatment-related improvement at the time of study termination. Thus, the optimal management of this severe complication remains to be properly evaluated.

Conclusion

The prevalence of PH, confirmed on RHC, seems to be lower than initially reported (6–10%) in SCD patients in stable condition. Interestingly, postcapillary PH seems to be the most frequent cause of PH in these patients. Thus, precapillary PH associated with SCD is probably uncommon, and quite different from the other forms of PAH in terms of both its hemodynamic profile and response to specific PAH therapies.

References

1 Gladwin MT, Sachdev V, Jison ML, et al: Pulmonary hypertension as a risk factor for death in patients with sickle cell disease. N Engl J Med 2004;350:886–895.

2 Ataga KI, Moore CG, Jones S, et al: Pulmonary hypertension in patients with sickle cell disease: a longitudinal study. Br J Haematol 2006;134:109–115.

3 De Castro LM, Jonassaint JC, Graham FL, Ashley-Koch A, Telen MJ: Pulmonary hypertension associated with sickle cell disease: clinical and laboratory endpoints and disease outcomes. Am J Hematol 2008;83:19–25.

4 Gordeuk VR, Sachdev V, Taylor JG, Gladwin MT, Kato G, Castro OL: Relative systemic hypertension in patients with sickle cell disease is associated with risk of pulmonary hypertension and renal insufficiency. Am J Hematol 2008;83:15–18.

5 Parent F, Bachir D, Inamo J, et al: A hemodynamic study of pulmonary hypertension in sickle cell disease. N Engl J Med 2011;365:44–53.

6 Fonseca GH, Souza R, Salemi VM, Jardim CV, Gualandro SF: Pulmonary hypertension diagnosed by right heart catheterization in sickle cell disease. Eur Respir J 2011, E-pub ahead of print.

7 Bunn HF, Nathan DG, Dover GJ, et al: Pulmonary hypertension and nitric oxide depletion in sickle cell disease. Blood 2010;116:687–692.

8 Gladwin MT, Vichinsky E: Pulmonary complications of sickle cell disease. N Engl J Med 2008; 359:2254–2265.

9 Rees DC, Williams TN, Gladwin MT: Sickle-cell disease. Lancet 2010;376:2018–2031.

10 Vij R, Machado RF: Pulmonary complications of hemoglobinopathies. Chest 2010;138:973–983.

11 Sutton LL, Castro O, Cross DJ, Spencer JE, Lewis JF: Pulmonary hypertension in sickle cell disease. Am J Cardiol 1994;74:626–628.

12 Castro O, Hoque M, Brown BD: Pulmonary hypertension in sickle cell disease: cardiac catheterization results and survival. Blood 2003; 101:1257–1261.

13 Haque AK, Gokhale S, Rampy BA, Adegboyega P, Duarte A, Saldana MJ: Pulmonary hypertension in sickle cell hemoglobinopathy: a clinicopathologic study of 20 cases. Hum Pathol 2002; 33:1037–1043.

14 Galie N, Hoeper MM, Humbert M, et al: Guidelines for the diagnosis and treatment of pulmonary hypertension. Eur Respir J 2009;34:1219–1263.

15 Hachulla E, Gressin V, Guillevin L, et al: Early detection of pulmonary arterial hypertension in systemic sclerosis: a French nationwide prospective multicenter study. Arthritis Rheum 2005; 52:3792–3800.

16 Lapa M, Dias B, Jardim C, et al: Cardiopulmonary manifestations of hepatosplenic schistosomiasis. Circulation 2009;119:1518–1523.

17 Sitbon O, Lascoux-Combe C, Delfraissy JF, et al: Prevalence of HIV-related pulmonary arterial hypertension in the current antiretroviral therapy era. Am J Respir Crit Care Med 2008;177:108–113.

18 Anthi A, Machado RF, Jison ML, et al: Hemodynamic and functional assessment of patients with sickle cell disease and pulmonary hypertension. Am J Respir Crit Care Med 2007;175: 1272–1279.

19 Machado RF, Mack AK, Martyr S, et al: Severity of pulmonary hypertension during vaso-occlusive pain crisis and exercise in patients with sickle cell disease. Br J Haematol 2007;136:319–325.

20 Mekontso Dessap A, Leon R, Habibi A, et al: Pulmonary hypertension and cor pulmonale during severe acute chest syndrome in sickle cell disease. Am J Respir Crit Care Med 2008;177:646–653.

21 Machado RF, Anthi A, Steinberg MH, et al: N-terminal pro-brain natriuretic peptide levels and risk of death in sickle cell disease. JAMA 2006;296:310–318.

22 Castro O, Brambilla DJ, Thorington B, et al: The acute chest syndrome in sickle cell disease: incidence and risk factors. The Cooperative Study of Sickle Cell Disease. Blood 1994;84:643–649.

23 Vichinsky EP, Neumayr LD, Earles AN, et al: Causes and outcomes of the acute chest syndrome in sickle cell disease. National Acute Chest Syndrome Study Group. N Engl J Med 2000;342:1855–1865.

24 Reiter CD, Wang X, Tanus-Santos JE, et al: Cell-free hemoglobin limits nitric oxide bioavailability in sickle-cell disease. Nat Med 2002;8:1383–1389.

25 Graido-Gonzalez E, Doherty JC, Bergreen EW, Organ G, Telfer M, McMillen MA: Plasma endothelin-1, cytokine, and prostaglandin E2 levels in sickle cell disease and acute vaso-occlusive sickle crisis. Blood 1998;92:2551–2555.

26 Morris CR, Kato GJ, Poljakovic M, et al: Dysregulated arginine metabolism, hemolysis-associated pulmonary hypertension, and mortality in sickle cell disease. JAMA 2005;294:81–90.

27 Gladwin MT, Lancaster JR Jr, Freeman BA, Schechter AN: Nitric oxide's reactions with hemoglobin: a view through the SNO-storm. Nat Med 2003;9:496–500.

28 Farmakis D, Aessopos A: Pulmonary hypertension associated with hemoglobinopathies: prevalent but overlooked. Circulation 2011;123: 1227–1232.

29 Machado RF, Gladwin MT: Chronic sickle cell lung disease: new insights into the diagnosis, pathogenesis and treatment of pulmonary hypertension. Br J Haematol 2005;129:449–464.

30 Villagra J, Shiva S, Hunter LA, Machado RF, Gladwin MT, Kato GJ: Platelet activation in patients with sickle disease, hemolysis-associated pulmonary hypertension, and nitric oxide scavenging by cell-free hemoglobin. Blood 2007;110:2166–2172.

31 Ataga KI, Moore CG, Hillery CA, et al: Coagulation activation and inflammation in sickle cell disease-associated pulmonary hypertension. Haematologica 2008;93:20–26.

32 Westerman M, Pizzey A, Hirschman J, et al: Microvesicles in haemoglobinopathies offer insights into mechanisms of hypercoagulability, haemolysis and the effects of therapy. Br J Haematol 2008;142:126–135.

33 van Beers EJ, Spronk HM, Ten Cate H, et al: No association of the hypercoagulable state with sickle cell disease related pulmonary hypertension. Haematologica 2008;93:e42–e44.

34 Dessap AM, Deux JF, Abidi N, et al: Pulmonary artery thrombosis during acute chest syndrome in sickle cell disease. Am J Respir Crit Care Med 2011;184:1022–1029.

35 Yung GL, Channick RN, Fedullo PF, et al: Successful pulmonary thromboendarterectomy in two patients with sickle cell disease. Am J Respir Crit Care Med 1998;157:1690–1693.

36 Jerath A, Murphy P, Madonik M, Barth D, Granton J, de Perrot M: Pulmonary endarterectomy in sickle cell haemoglobin C disease. Eur Respir J 2011;38:735–737.

37 Charache S, Terrin ML, Moore RD, et al: Effect of hydroxyurea on the frequency of painful crises in sickle cell anemia. Investigators of the Multicenter Study of Hydroxyurea in Sickle Cell Anemia. N Engl J Med 1995;332:1317–1322.

38 Steinberg MH, Barton F, Castro O, et al: Effect of hydroxyurea on mortality and morbidity in adult sickle cell anemia: risks and benefits up to 9 years of treatment. JAMA 2003;289:1645–1651.

39 Adams RJ, McKie VC, Hsu L, et al: Prevention of a first stroke by transfusions in children with sickle cell anemia and abnormal results on transcranial Doppler ultrasonography. N Engl J Med 1998;339:5–11.

40 Humbert M, Sitbon O, Simonneau G: Treatment of pulmonary arterial hypertension. N Engl J Med 2004;351:1425–1436.

41 Barst RJ, Mubarak KK, Machado RF, et al: Exercise capacity and haemodynamics in patients with sickle cell disease with pulmonary hypertension treated with bosentan: results of the ASSET studies. Br J Haematol 2010;149:426–435.

42 Machado RF, Barst RJ, Yovetich NA, et al: Hospitalization for pain in patients with sickle cell disease treated with sildenafil for elevated TRV and low exercise capacity. Blood 2011;118:855–864.

Florence Parent, MD
Service de Pneumologie et réanimation respiratoire, Hôpital Antoine Béclère
157 rue de la Porte de Trivaux
FR–92140 Clamart (France)
Tel. +33 1 45 37 40 46, E-Mail florence.parent@abc.aphp.fr

Chapter 15

Humbert M, Souza R, Simonneau G (eds): Pulmonary Vascular Disorders.
Prog Respir Res. Basel, Karger, 2012, vol 41, pp 143–148

Schistosomiasis and Pulmonary Hypertension

Caio Julio Cesar Fernandes · Carlos Jardim · Andre Hovnanian · Susana Hoette · Luciana Kato Morinaga · Rogerio Souza

Pulmonary Department, Heart Institute, University of Sao Paulo Medical School, Sao Paulo, Brazil

Abstract

Schistosomiasis is the third leading parasitic disease in the world. It is present in 74 countries, infecting 200 million people. Each year 280,000 patients die because of the disease. One of its most severe complications is pulmonary arterial hypertension (PAH). Previous studies have shown that 5% of patients with hepatosplenic schistosomiasis develop PAH. It is believed today that the most prevalent cause worldwide of PAH is schistosomiasis. Specifics about schistosomiasis-associated PAH including epidemiological data, mechanisms of the disease, clinical and hemodynamic features, and modalities of treatment will be reviewed in this chapter.

Geographical and Epidemiological Aspects of Schistosomiasis and Schistosomiasis-Associated Pulmonary Hypertension

Schistosomiasis is one of the most prevalent chronic infectious diseases in the world, and is the third-leading endemic parasitic disease known following malaria and amebiasis [1]. According to the World Health Organization (WHO), there are 200 million patients infected worldwide, 120 million symptomatic patients, and 20 million with severe illness manifestations. The disease is responsible for 11,000 deaths and 1.7 million disability-adjusted life-years lost per year [2]. It is an infection highly related to poverty and lack of basic sanitation, and the main regions of the world afflicted by it are sub-Saharan Africa, China, Southeast Asia, and some areas of Latin America, particularly in Brazil). However, recent reports of schistosomiasis in nonendemic areas, basically due to migration and travel, have renewed the interest in the disease by the global medical community [3].

The global magnitude of schistosomiasis has led to several attempts of epidemic control worldwide, such as the Schistosomiasis Control Initiative. The Schistosomiasis Control Initiative, which has been implemented in some African countries, is a collaborative program focused on morbidity control that is supported by national health and education ministries and the Imperial College London [4]. Similar efforts are pursued by the Special Program for Research and Training in Tropical Diseases of the United Nations Development Program, the World Bank, and the WHO. These programs are of major importance in decreasing the morbidity and mortality associated with schistosomiasis [3].

The first description of the disease was in 1852 by Theodor Bilharz [5]. During an autopsy in Cairo, Egypt, he identified a unique worm in the mesenteric veins of a patient and first described it as bilharziasis, which would later be known as schistosomiasis. Despite the fact that the gastrointestinal and genitourinary tracts were the main systems afflicted, multiple organs have been described as targets of the disease since then. Specifically concerning the respiratory system, in 1932 S. Azmy Pasha [6] first described the most significant and severe form of pulmonary involvement: pulmonary hypertension associated with schistosomiasis (Sch-PH). He described 2 cases of patients with hepatosplenic schistosomiasis with secondary cor pulmonale, and found in the necropsy of these patients remarkable dilations in the pulmonary arteries. One of them also presented with schistosoma eggs in the pulmonary circulation and exuberant granulomatous formations and obliterative arteritis. As times goes by, the relevance of Sch-PH has been progressively acknowledged, mainly in the setting of pulmonary hypertension (PH) and its possible etiologies. It is believed that about 5% of patients diagnosed with hepatosplenic schistosomiasis mansoni may also present with PH [7], suggesting that Sch-PH is potentially the most prevalent cause of PH worldwide.

The importance of Sch-PH might be even greater in regions where schistosomiasis is endemic. Indeed, it is estimated that up to 30% of all PH patients followed at reference centers in Brazil have pulmonary arterial hypertension associated with schistosomiasis (Sch-PAH) [8]. In the updated classification of pulmonary arterial hypertension (PAH) [9], following better understanding of the mechanisms involved in Sch-PAH as well as its hemodynamic features, Sch-PAH has been reclassified within Group I (PAH), the one that raises the most interest in the area as well as the most researched of all five groups.

The Parasite Life-Cycle: Pathology and Immunology of the Infection

Schistosomiasis is caused by a group of parasite trematode worms of the Schistosomatidae family (derived from the Greek word for 'fissure' and named by Weinland due to the presence of the slit in the body of the female where the male is sheltered). Human infections are caused mainly by the *Schistosoma mansoni, Schistosoma haematobium,* and *Schistosoma japonicum,* respectively in their specific regions [3].

The life cycle of the parasite begins with the presence of its eggs in a fresh water reservoir. There they hatch and release the miracidium, the swimming larval form of the worm. The miracidium infects the intermediate host of the cycle: snails (*Biomphalaria* species to *S. mansoni, Bulinus* species to *S. haematobium,* and *Oncomelania* species to *S. japonicum*). Over 30 days they suffer morphologic modifications and are released again in the water in a caudate form named cercariae. The cercariae penetrate the skin of the definitive host, a human or other mammal, shed their tail becoming schistosomula, and reach the venous circulation en route to the lungs. In the pulmonary capillaries they perforate the alveolar-capillary barrier and go up the bronchial tree until the pharynx where they are swallowed. They reach the gut and migrate to the portal venous system where males and females mature and unite. Pairs of worms then migrate to the superior mesenteric veins (*S. mansoni*), the inferior mesenteric and superior hemorrhoidal veins (*S. japonicum*), or the vesical plexus (*S. haematobium*). Egg production begins 6 weeks after the primal infection and persists throughout the life of the worm, usually 3–5 years (there are, however, anecdotal reports of worms with 30 years of active life). The eggs then pass from the lumen of blood vessels into adjacent tissues, and many reach intestinal or bladder mucosa and are shed in the feces (*S. mansoni* and *S. japonicum*) or urine (*S. haematobium*). The life cycle is completed when the eggs reach a reservoir of fresh water reservoir [10].

About one third of the eggs produced by *S. mansoni* and *S. japonicum* do not follow the direction of the intestinal lumen and are deposited instead in the small veins of the liver as a natural consequence of the portal flow. During the late schistosomal infection, the immunologic response is mainly a CD4 lymphocyte T helper 2 one, with the mediation of IL-4 and IL-13, among other chemokines. The shift of response from T helper 1 to T helper 2 from the host is responsible for the formation of the granulomatous activity. The eggs therefore induce a presinusoidal granulomatous inflammatory response and periportal fibrosis with subsequent portal hypertension. In the presence of this condition, portacaval shunts open; in addition to the generation of pulmonary blood overflow, it enables the eggs to be carried to the lung capillaries where they lodge [11]. Most of the lesions associated with chronic schistosomiasis are not related to the worms, but to the released eggs and the secondary granulomatous inflammatory T helper 2 response. Some genetic factors of the definitive host are known to be related to the magnitude of this granulomatous response, particularly in the liver. Whether these factors are also co-related with the development of PH in the schistosomotic population remains to be studied.

Since the disease is mainly located in presinusoidal space, sparing the hepatocytes, liver failure is usually not a feature of schistosomiasis, even in the presence of advanced hepatosplenic disease and portal hypertension.

The Development of Pulmonary Hypertension in Schistosomiasis

In 1938 Shaw and Gareeb [12] published a case series of Sch-PH. Based on the presence of the eggs in the pulmonary vessels, they believed that the eggs had a mechanical effect and induced PH by physical vascular obstruction, basically due to the embolic mechanism, inducing secondary right ventricular insufficiency, and suggested the first proposed mechanism of the genesis of PH in schistosomiasis.

Ever since the 1960s, this hypothesis was contested. Pathologic studies of this period indeed identified the presence of eggs in the vessels of Sch-PH patients. Nevertheless, it was found in both frequency and magnitude to be clearly insufficient to generate PH merely by physical vascular

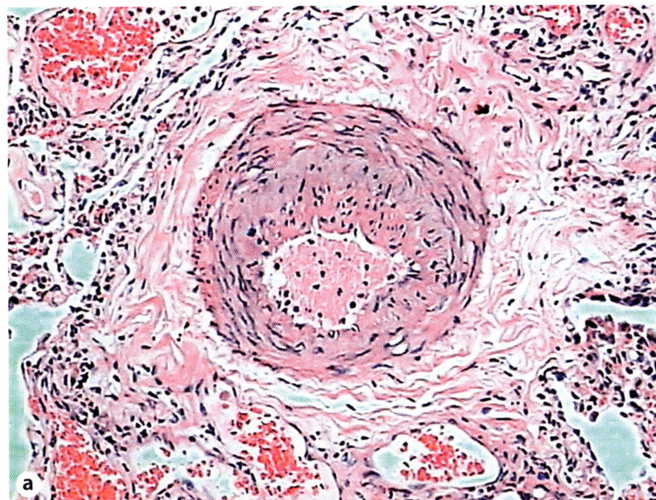

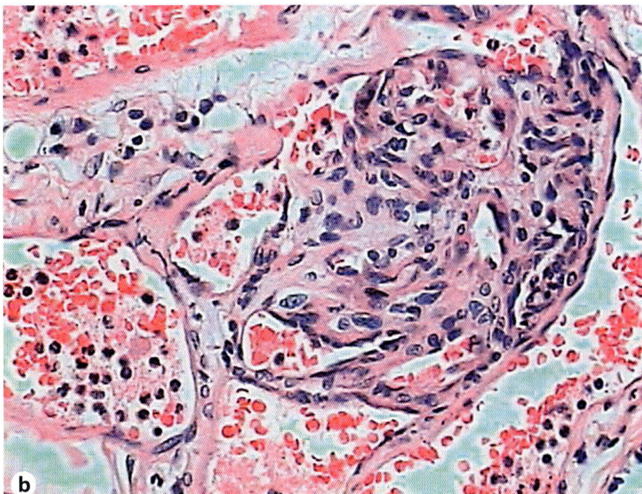

Fig. 1. Hematoxylin and eosin-stained lung biopsy of a patient with Sch-PAH. Despite the eventual presence of perivascular granulomatous lesions and mechanical vascular obstruction by the schistosoma egg (**a**), the vascular plexiform lesions unrelated to the eggs (**b**) were far more frequent and very similar to the ones found in IPAH.

obstruction. Some authors then hypothesized that the presence or maybe just the passage of the eggs or the worm during its life cycle induces nongranulomatous inflammatory endothelitis in the pulmonary circulation of genetically susceptible patients, and the abnormal healing process would be responsible by the PH genesis. Chaves [13, 14], among others, did not identify marked pathologic differences in the plexiform lesions of Sch-PH and primary PH [nowadays idiopathic PAH (IPAH)] patients. Besides, the plexiform lesions of Sch-PH did not present any relation to the angiomatoid lesions characteristically related to the schistosoma egg when these were found [13–14]. These data were re-evaluated and confirmed in a case series that also supported the existence of a spectrum of vascular lesions not related to the presence of eggs or granuloma [15] (fig. 1).

Recently, an experimental study in mice identified a direct relation between the quantity of schistosoma eggs in the pulmonary circulation and the induced granulomatous response with the degree of right ventricle remodeling. It is possible then to speculate that the inflammatory response may be proportional to the quantity of antigen released in the lung tissue, reinforcing the possibility of this so-called 'inflammatory' mechanism of disease. Different cytokines have been implicated with the immunological processes that modulate chronic host response to schistosoma infection (mainly in the setting of hepatosplenic disease), as IL-13, interferon-γ, TNF, and IL-5. Nevertheless, their specific role in each phase of human schistosomiasis is still to be determined [16].

Nevertheless, it is quite evident that not just the exposition to the schistosoma egg is enough to induce PH in schistosomotic patients. The low relative prevalence of PAH in schistosomiasis (4.6%) is evidence that other factors may intervene in the PH genesis [7], otherwise all schistosomotic patients would develop PH. In light of this information, some authors have hypothesized that Sch-PH may not be related to the egg presence at all and may be just another form of portopulmonary hypertension, where, in patients with portal hypertension, the opening of portacaval shunts would generate blood overflow in the pulmonary circulation and subsequently endothelial dysfunction and PH [17]. In fact, Sch-PH shares with portopulmonary hypertension many clinical features (e.g. the better hemodynamic profile at diagnosis and the lack of acute response to vasodilator challenge) [18]. Again, however, the prevalence of Sch-PH leaves some doubt about this theory. While just 1–2% of patients with portal hypertension develop PH [19], more than the double of this prevalence is found in Sch-PH, meaning at least that the schistosomotic patient is more susceptible to pulmonary blood overflow than the ordinary patient with portal hypertension. This is possibly due to the presence or passage of the egg in the lung vessel and may be secondary to the inflammatory response induced by it. Today it is believed that, besides an individual predisposition, Sch-PH may be related to multiple hit mechanisms, including mechanical impaction of *S. mansoni* eggs within the pulmonary vessels, the consequent inflammatory process in the lung vasculature, and the higher blood flow that occurs in portal hypertension because of arteriovenous shunts.

The classification of schistosomiasis in the setting of PAH follows the timeline of it becoming better understood. In 1988, the Evian classification of PH put schistosomiasis in the inflammatory group along with sarcoidosis, which could have had incorrect implications in terms of treatment [20]. The revised classification, from the international symposium held in Venice in 2003 [21], relocated schistosomiasis in the nonthrombotic embolic group, emphasizing the mechanical effect of egg obstruction in the lung vasculature. In 2008 at the last international symposium held in Dana Point, schistosomiasis was reclassified as a form of PAH (Group I), reflecting recent findings regarding pathology and hemodynamic presentation [9].

Clinical Features of Pulmonary Hypertension Associated with Schistosomiasis

Clinical presentation of Sch-PH is very similar to that of IPAH [7]. The symptoms of progressive dyspnea, chest pain, dry cough, lower-extremity edema, and eventually syncope may be present, which worsens progressively over years at a rate slower than the progression of IPAH. Recent data show other similarities among these two entities concerning clinical aspects, such as mean age at diagnosis (roughly the third to fifth decade of life), functional class at diagnosis, and baseline 6-min walk time [18].

It is known that the initial contact with the parasite might happen many years before the onset of PH symptoms and still be schistosomiasis that is responsible for the disease since it is the consequence of the egg position which is responsible for the genesis of PH and not necessarily active schistosomiasis. In other words, a patient exposed to the worm in childhood, even if adequately treated ensuring the elimination of the parasite, may develop PH in his 40s or 50s, depending on the time of the exposure and the individual predisposition [13]. Therefore, the epidemiologic information about schistosomiasis always needs to be researched, even in nonendemic areas, since the patient may originally be from a high prevalence region of the disease.

Remarkably, most Sch-PH patients do not present with severe symptoms of portal hypertension and the diagnosis of schistosomiasis is usually given much later than the diagnosis of PH. Considering these data, it is possible to imagine that schistosomotic patients that evolve to PH may be the ones in whom the portacaval shunts are more effective, sparing somehow the portal circulation after the beginning of the process.

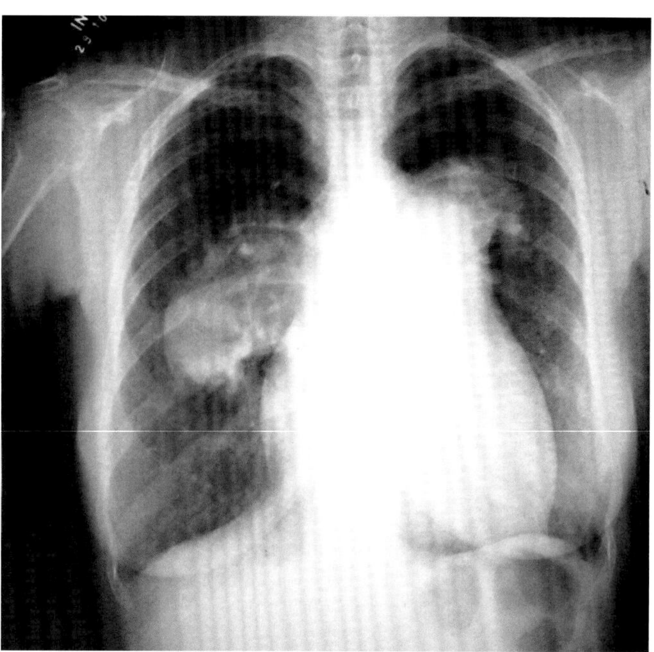

Fig. 2. Chest X-ray of a patient with Sch-PAH displaying the enlargement of the main pulmonary arteries.

The radiological features somehow reinforce this hypothesis since they suggest an insidious process with remarkable vascular dilatations [22]. The main pulmonary artery enlargement is more pronounced when compared with IPAH, even considering the severity of the hemodynamic profile, and are similar to the ones found in congenital heart disease-associated PH, suggesting a slower rate of progression and greater compliance of the pulmonary arteries (fig. 2).

Diagnostic Strategy

The diagnosis of schistosomiasis is based mainly on environmental exposure to the parasite and identification of the parasite eggs in stool examination or rectal biopsy [10]. Abdominal ultrasonographic findings such as enlargement of the left lobe of the liver or periportal fibrosis may suggest schistosomiasis and have a high positive predictive value in prevalent areas [23]. These hepatosplenic abnormalities may support the association of schistosomiasis with PAH; however, schistosomiasis may also cause PAH in the absence of portal abnormalities. Serologies, by means of ELISA technique, may identify previous contact with multiple forms of *Schistosoma*, but utility is mainly in patients from nonendemic areas since the massive population exposure lowers the value of serologies as a disease marker [24].

The cardiovascular investigation of Sch-PH follows the same algorithm suggested for other etiologies of PH. After clinical suspicion, an echocardiogram is performed; when signs of PH are present, right heart catheterization is mandatory to confirm elevated pulmonary artery pressure and determine the main vascular territory implicated (pre- or postcapillary) [25]. A recent study comparing consecutive newly diagnosed patients with schistosomiasis-related PAH and IPAH from the same period of time showed that schistosomiasis patients displayed a more preserved hemodynamic profile at diagnosis. Furthermore, none of the schistosomiasis patients displayed acute vasodilation in response to nitric oxide challenge as compared with an approximate 15% response in the idiopathic [18].

The prognosis of Sch-PH also seems to be better than IPAH. Recent data demonstrated that independently of hemodynamic severity at baseline, Sch-PH patients had a better 3-year survival than what would be expected for patients with IPAH, suggesting a more benign course of the disease (86 vs. 52%, respectively) [18]. These findings are similar to what is believed for portopulmonary hypertension, as recently demonstrated by Le Pavec et al. [26], mainly if the subgroup of patients without liver cirrhosis is considered, which is another similarity between these two conditions.

Therapy of Pulmonary Hypertension Associated with Schistosomiasis

Conventional therapy for PAH such as diuretics and oxygen should be implemented as needed to all patients with Sch-PH. Particularities in the conventional therapy for PAH to this population of patients includes caution in the implementation of anticoagulation since there is a risk of life-threatening bleeding due to the presence of esophageal varices. The use of high-dosage calcium channel blockers is not advised because of the presence of portal hypertension in virtually all cases, and absence of response to the vasodilator test.

The response of schistosomiasis-associated PAH to specific PH therapy requires further study. Preliminary reports noted improvement in right ventricular function with sildenafil (assessed by MRI) [27]. There is a theoretical benefit in the use of endothelin receptor antagonists or prostanoids, but hard data is lacking. Unpublished data from our group demonstrated a statistically significant improvement of baseline hemodynamics and clinical parameters (6-min walk test and functional class) with specific PH treatment available (sildenafil and bosentan), but further studies addressing endpoints such as mortality or time to clinical worsening with specific PH therapy are still needed.

The effect of antiparasitic treatment in the course of Sch-PH is questionable. In theory, it would be interesting to decrease the rate of egg position and, consequently, the time and quantity of antigen exposure, decreasing the secondary inflammatory response. Nevertheless, a great number of Sch-PH patients do not carry the viable worm at the time of diagnosis. In the hepatosplenic disease, response to antiparasitic treatment varies greatly, ranging from no effect to resolution of periportal fibrosis [28]. Antiparasitic treatment is not believed to have a significant effect on the pulmonary circulation, but at least one case report cited significant improvement in hemodynamics after treatment [29]. However, as the treatment of the parasite requires one-day treatment with praziquantel, a drug with few side effects, it is reasonable to treat all diagnosed patients even in the absence of viable worms or eggs.

Conclusion

Schistosomiasis is one of the most prevalent chronic infectious diseases in the world. One of its most severe complications is PH, which may occur in up to 5% of patients with hepatosplenic schistosomiasis. The prevalence of schistosomiasis is so overwhelming that Sch-PH may be the most prevalent cause of PH around the world. Nevertheless, despite its epidemiologic importance, much still remains to be understood about this disease. Multiple pathways have been described as potential mechanisms of diseases of Sch-PH, such as egg embolism in a physical manner, egg-triggered inflammatory disease, or pulmonary blood overflow due to the opening of portacaval shunts in a similar way to portopulmonary hypertension; it is quite possible that each one of these has a role.

The clinical features of Sch-PH are very similar to the ones of IPAH, but less severe and with a longer evolution. The natural history of the disease was described, with a 3-year rate of survival of 86%. Nevertheless, the experience in providing health care to these patients shows that Sch-PH patients may take longer to deteriorate, but when they do they follow the same path downstream, such as IPAH.

The response to specific PH treatment still needs to be addressed, but small studies suggest a significant benefit with the use endothelin antagonist receptors and inhibitors of phosphodiesterase 5, concerning clinical and hemodynamic parameters. To date, there is no data available on mortality and specific PH treatment in Sch-PH.

References

1 Salanitri J, Stanley P, Hennessy O: Acute pulmonary schistosomiasis. Australas Radiol 2002;46:435–437.

2 Vennervald B, Dunne D: Morbidity in schistosomiasis: an update. Curr Opin Infect Dis 2004;17:439–447.

3 Ross AG BP, Sleigh AC, Olds GR, Li Y, Williams GM, McManus DP: Schistosomiasis. N Engl J Med 2002;346:1212–1220.

4 World Health Organization: Schistosomiasis and soil transmitted helminth infections. Fifty-fourth World Health Assembly, resolution WHA54.19. World Health Organization, Geneva, 2001.

5 Bilharz T: Further observations concerning Distonum Haematobium, from a letter to C. T. von Siebald. Z Wissensch Zool 1853;4:454–456.

6 Azmy S, Effat S: Pulmonary arteriosclerosis of a bilharzial nature. J Egypt Med Assoc 1932;15:87.

7 Lapa M DB, Jardim C, Fernandes CJ, Dourado PM, Figueiredo M, Farias A, Tsutsui J, Terra-Filho M, Humbert M, Souza R: Cardio-pulmonary manifestations of hepatosplenic schistosomiasis. Circulation 2009;119:1518–1523.

8 Lapa MS FE, Jardim C, Martins Bdo C, Arakaki JS, Souza R: Clinical characteristics of pulmonary hypertension patients in two reference centers in the city of Sao Paulo (in Portuguese). Rev Assoc Med Bras 2006;52:139–143.

9 Simonneau G, Robbins IM, Beghetti M, Channick RN, Delcroix M, Denton CP, Elliott CG, Gaine SP, Gladwin MT, Jing ZC, Krowka MJ, Langleben D, Nakanishi N, Souza R: Updated clinical classification of pulmonary hypertension. J Am Coll Cardiol 2009;54:43–54.

10 Prata A: Esquistossomose Mansônica; in Veronessi R, Foccacia R, Dietze R (eds): Doenças Infecciosas e Parasitárias, ed 8. Rio de Janeiro, Guanabara Koogan, 1991, pp 838–855.

11 Meira J: Esquistossomose Mansônica; in Meira D (ed): Clínica de Doenças Tropicais e Infecciosas. Rio de Janeiro, Interlivros Edições, 1991, pp 401–450.

12 Shaw A, Ghareeb A: Pathogenesis of the pulmonary schistossomiasis in Egypt with special reference to Ayerza's disease. J Pathol Bacteriol 1938;46:401–429.

13 Chaves E: The pathology of the arterial pulmonary vasculature in Manson's schistosomiasis. Dis Chest 1966;50:72–77.

14 Chaves E: Plexiform lesions in chronic cor pulmonale in schistosomiasis (in Portuguese). Hospital (Rio J) 1965;68:635–645.

15 Pozzan G, Souza R, Jardim C, Dolhnikoff M, Mello G, Canzian M, Bernardi F, Mauad T, Grunberg K: Histopathological features of pulmonary vascular disease in chronic *Schistosomia mansoni* infection are not different from those in idiopathic pulmonary hypertension. Am J Respir Crit Care Med 2008;177:A443.

16 Crosby A, Jones FM, Southwood M, Stewart S, Schermuly R, Butrous G, Dunne DW, Morrell NW: Pulmonary vascular remodeling correlates with lung eggs and cytokines in murine schistosomiasis. Am J Respir Crit Care Med 2010;181: 279–288.

17 Pereira GJ, Bestetti R, Leite M, Santos R, Ramos S, Lucchesi F, et al: Portopulmonary hypertension syndrome in schistosomiasis mansoni. Trans R Soc Trop Med Hyg 2002;96:427–428.

18 Fernandes C, Jardim C, Hovnanian A, Hoette S, Dias B, Souza S, et al: Survival in schistosomiasis-associated pulmonary arterial hypertension. J Am Coll Cardiol 2010;56:715–720.

19 Hadengue A BM, Lebrec D, Benhamou JP: Pulmonary hypertension complicating portal hypertension: prevalence and relation to splanchnic hemodynamics. Gastroenterology 1991;100: 520–528.

20 Rich S, Rubin L, L Abenhail, et al: Executive summary from the World Symposium on Primary Pulmonary Hypertension (Evian, France, September 6–10, 1998). World Health Organization, 1998. http://wwwwhoint/ncd/cvd/pphhtml.

21 Simmoneau G, Galiè N, Rubin L, Langleben D, Seeger W, Domenighetti G, Gibbs S, Lebrec D, Speich R, Beghetti M, Rich S, Fishman A: Clinical classification of pulmonary hypertension. J Am Coll Cardiol 2004;43:5S–12S.

22 Figueiredo C, Souza R, Ota J: Pulmonary hypertension in schistosomiasis: a chest CT study. Am J Respir Crit Care Med 2004;169:A174.

23 Hatz C, Jenkins J, Ali Q, Abdel-Wahab M, Cerri G, Tanner M: A review of the literature on the use of ultrasonography in schistosomiasis with special reference to its use in field studies. 2. *Schistosoma mansoni*. Acta Trop 1992;51: 15–28.

24 Igreja RP MJ, Goncalves MM, Barreto MM, Peralta JM: *Schistosoma mansoni*-related morbidity in a low-prevalence area of Brazil: a comparison between egg excretors and seropositive non-excretors. Ann Trop Med Parasitol 2007;101:575–584.

25 Galiè N, Hoeper M, Humbert M, Torbicki A, Vachiery J, Barbera J, et al: Guidelines for the diagnosis and treatment of pulmonary hypertension. Task Force for Diagnosis and Treatment of Pulmonary Hypertension of European Society of Cardiology (ESC); European Respiratory Society (ERS); International Society of Heart and Lung Transplantation (ISHLT). Eur Respir J 2009;34: 1219–1263.

26 Le Pavec J, Souza R, Herve P, Lebrec D, Savale L, Tcherakian C, Jais X, Yaici A, Humbert M, Simonneau G, Sitbon O: Portopulmonary hypertension: survival and prognostic factors. Am J Respir Crit Care Med 2008;178:637–643.

27 Loureiro R, Mendes A, Bandeira A, Cartaxo H, Sa D: Oral sildenafil improves functional status and cardiopulmonary hemodynamics in patients with severe pulmonary hypertension secondary to chronic pulmonary schistosomiasis: a cardiac magnetic resonance study. American Heart Association, New Orleans, 2004.

28 Richter J: Evolution of schistosomiasis-induced pathology after therapy and interruption of exposure to schistosomes: a review of ultrasonographic studies. Acta Trop 2000;77:111–131.

29 Bouree P, Piveteau J, Gerbal, JL, Halpen G: Pulmonary arterial hypertension due to bilharziasis. Apropos of a case due to Schistosoma haematobium having been cured by praziquantel (in French). Bull Soc Pathol Exot 1990;83:66–71.

Rogerio Souza, MD, PhD
Pulmonary Circulation Unit
Pulmonary Department, Heart Institute, University of Sao Paulo Medical School
Av. Dr. Eneas de Carvalho Aguiar, 44
Sao Paulo, 05403-000 (Brazil)
Tel. +55 11 26 61 56 95, E-Mail rogerio.souza@incor.usp.br

Chapter 16

Humbert M, Souza R, Simonneau G (eds): Pulmonary Vascular Disorders.
Prog Respir Res. Basel, Karger, 2012, vol 41, pp 149–160

Pulmonary Veno-Occlusive Disease

David Montani[a–c] · Alice Huertas[a–c] · Peter Dorfmüller[a–c] · Marc Humbert[a–c]

[a]Université Paris-Sud, Faculté de Médecine, Kremlin-Bicêtre, [b]AP-HP, Centre National de Référence de l'Hypertension Pulmonaire Sévère, Service de Pneumologie et Réanimation Respiratoire, Hôpital Antoine Béclère, Clamart, [c]INSERM U999, Hypertension Artérielle Pulmonaire: Physiopathologie et Innovation Thérapeutique, LabEx LERMIT, Centre Chirurgical Marie-Lannelongue, Le Plessis-Robinson, France

Abstract
Pulmonary veno-occlusive disease (PVOD) is a rare disorder that can be misdiagnosed as idiopathic pulmonary arterial hypertension (PAH) and accounts for 5–10% of cases initially considered as idiopathic PAH. PVOD and idiopathic PAH share a similar clinical presentation, genetic background, and hemodynamic profile. Chest high-resolution computed tomography (HRCT) may be suggestive, but definitive diagnosis necessitates a surgical lung biopsy. However, this procedure presents high risks in these patients and is generally not recommended. Therefore, a noninvasive diagnostic approach using chest HRCT, arterial blood gas analysis, pulmonary function tests, and bronchoalveolar lavage may be helpful to detect PVOD. PVOD is characterized by a poor prognosis and the possibility of developing severe pulmonary edema with specific PAH therapy. Lung transplantation remains the treatment of choice.

Pulmonary veno-occlusive disease (PVOD) is a rare disorder classified as a subgroup of pulmonary arterial hypertension (PAH) [1]. PAH is a heterogeneous group of diseases, defined as an increase in resting mean pulmonary arterial pressure ≥25 mm Hg, which can lead to right heart failure and death [1, 2]. PVOD and idiopathic PAH share several characteristics, from risk factors to clinical presentation, which can easily lead to misdiagnosis between these two conditions. Both PVOD and PAH are severe and have clinical and hemodynamic similarities (table 1). These two conditions can only be distinguished by the PVOD histopathological hallmark, which is represented by a widespread fibrous intimal proliferation that predominantly involves the pulmonary venules and small veins [3, 4], while idiopathic PAH is characterized by a major remodeling of small precapillary pulmonary arteries with frequent plexiform and possible thrombotic lesions. Histological proof is required for a definitive diagnosis of PVOD. Since surgical lung biopsy is a high-risk procedure in these patients, the differential diagnosis between PVOD and PAH is often challenging.

The importance of establishing a correct and early diagnosis is justified by the worse prognosis in PVOD patients compared to idiopathic PAH patients, and by the risk of developing severe pulmonary edema with specific PAH therapy by PVOD patients [5]. Another important clinical hallmark of PVOD is that patients exposed to novel PAH-specific treatments may experience an abrupt and potentially life-threatening deterioration [6]. Clinical worsening as a result of disease progression is almost universal and few patients are alive more than 2 years after diagnosis. It has been hypothesized that idiopathic PAH and PVOD may represent two parts of the same disease spectrum, with lesions preferentially affecting precapillary vessels in PAH and postcapillary vessels in PVOD. Because of the differences in pathological assessment, response to specific PAH therapy, and prognosis, PVOD is now more clearly identified as a unique subgroup of PAH (revised classification of the 4th World Symposium on Pulmonary Hypertension) [1]. PVOD remains a challenging entity from both a diagnostic and therapeutic point of view. This review aims to provide current knowledge of PVOD.

Epidemiology and Risk Factors

As PVOD is a difficult-to-diagnose subgroup of a rare disease, the prevalence and incidence are difficult to evaluate. PVOD, without any associated conditions, is an infrequent subgroup of a rare disease and is usually considered to

Table 1. Characteristics of idiopathic PAH and idiopathic PVOD

	IPAH	PVOD
Genetic mutations	*BMPR2* mutations in 10–40% of cases	cases of *BMPR2* mutation
Epidemiology/risk factors		
Female predominance	yes (F/M ratio = 2)	no (F/M ratio = 1)
Tobacco exposure	unrelated	more frequent and higher exposure than in IPAH
Chemotherapy	case reports	case reports
Clinical exam		
Auscultatory crackles	no	possible
Clubbing	possible	possible
Hemoptysis	possible	possible
Pulmonary function tests		
FEV_1, FVC, TLC	normal (possible mild restrictive pattern)	normal (possible mild restrictive pattern)
DLCO and DLCO/VA	often reduced	lower than IPAH
PaO_2 at rest	often reduced	lower than IPAH
Chest HRCT	mild abnormalities	frequent association of abnormalities including centrilobular ground-glass opacities, septal lines, and lymph node enlargement
Bronchoalveolar lavage	normal	possible occult alveolar hemorrhage
Management		
Acute NO testing	when positive, it is predictive of long-term CCB response and better prognosis	not a predictor of CCB response (risk of pulmonary edema after initiation of CCB)
Response to PAH therapy	improve hemodynamics, functional status and outcome	may deteriorate PVOD with a risk of pulmonary edema; cases of transient stabilization (bridge therapy to LTx)

IPAH = Idiopathic PAH; VA = alveolar volume; LTx = lung transplantation; CCB = calcium channel blocker; FEV_1 = forced expiratory volume in 1 s; FVC = forced vital capacity ratio; TLC = total lung capacity; HRCT = high-resolution computed tomography.

represent about 5–10% of histological cases where patients were initially diagnosed as 'idiopathic' PAH [7]. As observed in idiopathic PAH, PVOD has been diagnosed throughout a very wide age range, from the first weeks of life to the seventh decade [7]. With regard to sex distribution, PVOD occurs equally in men and women, whereas idiopathic PAH has a clear female predominance [2, 8–10].

As previously described in idiopathic PAH, we have shown that even in the absence of a diagnosed autoimmune disorder, PVOD shares a similar autoimmune background with idiopathic PAH: autoantibodies (antinuclear, antiphospholipid, or thyroid antibodies) were found in 30 and 33% in PVOD and idiopathic PAH, respectively [8]. PVOD can also occur in conditions usually associated with pulmonary hypertension, including connective tissue diseases [11–13], sarcoidosis [14], pulmonary Langerhans' cell histiocytosis [7, 15, 16], and, more rarely, HIV infection [17–19].

There is a clear and significant risk of developing PAH after anorexigen (fenfluramine derivatives) exposure, and it has been clearly demonstrated that PAH associated with anorexigens shares a similar presentation and evolution as idiopathic PAH [20–24]. We have recently reported a case of a PVOD in a patient with a history of fenfluramine exposure, thus suggesting a possible association between anorexigen exposure and PVOD [8].

PVOD has been reported in association with various chemotherapy regimens, including bleomycin, BCNU, and mitomycin [25–28], and after bone marrow transplantation [29–36]. Chemical exposure has been suggested to influence the development of PVOD, while it is not considered as a risk factor of PAH. This association has been reported in isolated case reports; however, the two largest series of PVOD found no significant association with chemical exposure, but did not include specific exposure history elicited by questionnaire [8, 9]. In a recent series, we reported higher tobacco exposure and an increased proportion of smokers in PVOD as compared to idiopathic PAH [8]. Even if it has been previously demonstrated that tobacco exposure may contribute to pulmonary vascular injury [37, 38], it is not clear why tobacco exposure would be a specific risk factor for PVOD and not for PAH [21].

In idiopathic PAH, germline mutations in the bone morphogenetic protein receptor 2 *(BMPR2)* gene are detected in about 75% of familial cases and in 10–40% of apparently idiopathic PAH [39–41]. The distinction between idiopathic and familial *BMPR2* mutation carriers may in fact be artificial because all these cases are a genetic form of PAH. Therefore, recent expert discussion pleads in favor of the term 'heritable' PAH [1]. Interestingly, PVOD could appear in a familial context and some patients with a definite diagnosis of PVOD have been reported to carry a *BMPR2* mutation. These observations suggest the existence of a genetic risk factor in the development of PVOD [8, 42–46]. The involvement of *BMPR2* mutation in the development of PVOD emphasizes once more the similarities between PVOD and PAH. As in heritable PAH, heritable PVOD may occur in the absence of *BMPR2* mutation, suggesting that other genetic risk factors may also be contributing to the disease process. These results support systematic screening for a possible familial history of pulmonary vascular disease and similar genetic counseling in both PAH and PVOD patients.

Clinical Presentation

Idiopathic PAH and PVOD have very similar clinical presentations; therefore, the differentiation between these two entities is difficult and the clinical exam is most often unhelpful. As in PAH, progressive dyspnea on exertion is the main symptom in PVOD, although often neglected by patients, leading to the frequent diagnostic delay. In PVOD, most of the patients have severe exertional dyspnea with a New York Heart Association (NYHA) functional class III or IV at the time of the diagnosis [8, 9]. We found no difference in NYHA functional class at diagnosis between patients displaying PVOD as compared to idiopathic PAH. Right-sided cardiac dysfunction and right ventricular failure, due to the sustained pressure overload, often complicate the more advanced stages of the disease. Signs of right heart failure are frequently elicited on clinical examination. Cardiac auscultation reveals a prominent pulmonic component of the second heart sound and a systolic murmur of tricuspid regurgitation [9]. Respiratory auscultatory crackles may occur in PVOD patients with predominant pulmonary infiltrates, but the precise prevalence is unknown [7, 9]. Pleural effusions have been suggested to be more frequent in PVOD; however, studies focused on radiography with high-resolution computed tomography (HRCT) of the chest show a similar proportion of pleural effusions in both diseases [8, 9, 47, 48]. Hemoptysis has been described in PVOD; however, in a recent study, we reported that hemoptysis was observed infrequently and equally in both idiopathic PAH and PVOD, confirming that alveolar hemorrhage in PVOD is generally occult [8, 49]. Clubbing and Raynaud's phenomenon have been reported as clinical signs in PVOD, but this was not reproduced in our recent series, as these signs remain rare and can also occur in idiopathic PAH [8].

Diagnosis

Histopathological Assessment

In idiopathic PAH, the characteristic pathological abnormalities are represented by fibrotic and proliferative changes located in muscular arteries less than 500 μm in diameter. Different compartments of the vessel may contribute to the thickening of the arterial wall, and, hence, various histological patterns may occur [3]. They include isolated medial hypertrophy, concentric and eccentric nonlaminar intimal fibrosis, concentric laminar intimal fibrosis (also known as 'onion-skin' lesions), and complex lesions [3]. Thrombotic lesions, also known as in situ thrombosis, are a frequent pattern in different PAH subgroups. A peculiar entity within the pathological classification of vasculopathies in pulmonary hypertension is referred to as the complex lesions [3], associating plexiform lesions with dilation lesions. The former represents the most illustrious form of vascular change in PAH and was considered for a long time as a pathognomonic feature of idiopathic PAH [50]. However, this presumption has been revised and it has been reported that plexiform lesions may occur in PAH associated with other conditions [3]. Dilation lesions are usually found distally to plexiform lesions and correspond to thin-walled and congestive precapillary pulmonary vessels. Arteritis, including transmural inflammation and fibrinoid necrosis, may be sporadically present in severe pulmonary hypertension, whereas perivascular inflammatory infiltrate is frequently encountered in the range of diseased vessels. In PVOD, the observed postcapillary lesions affect septal veins and

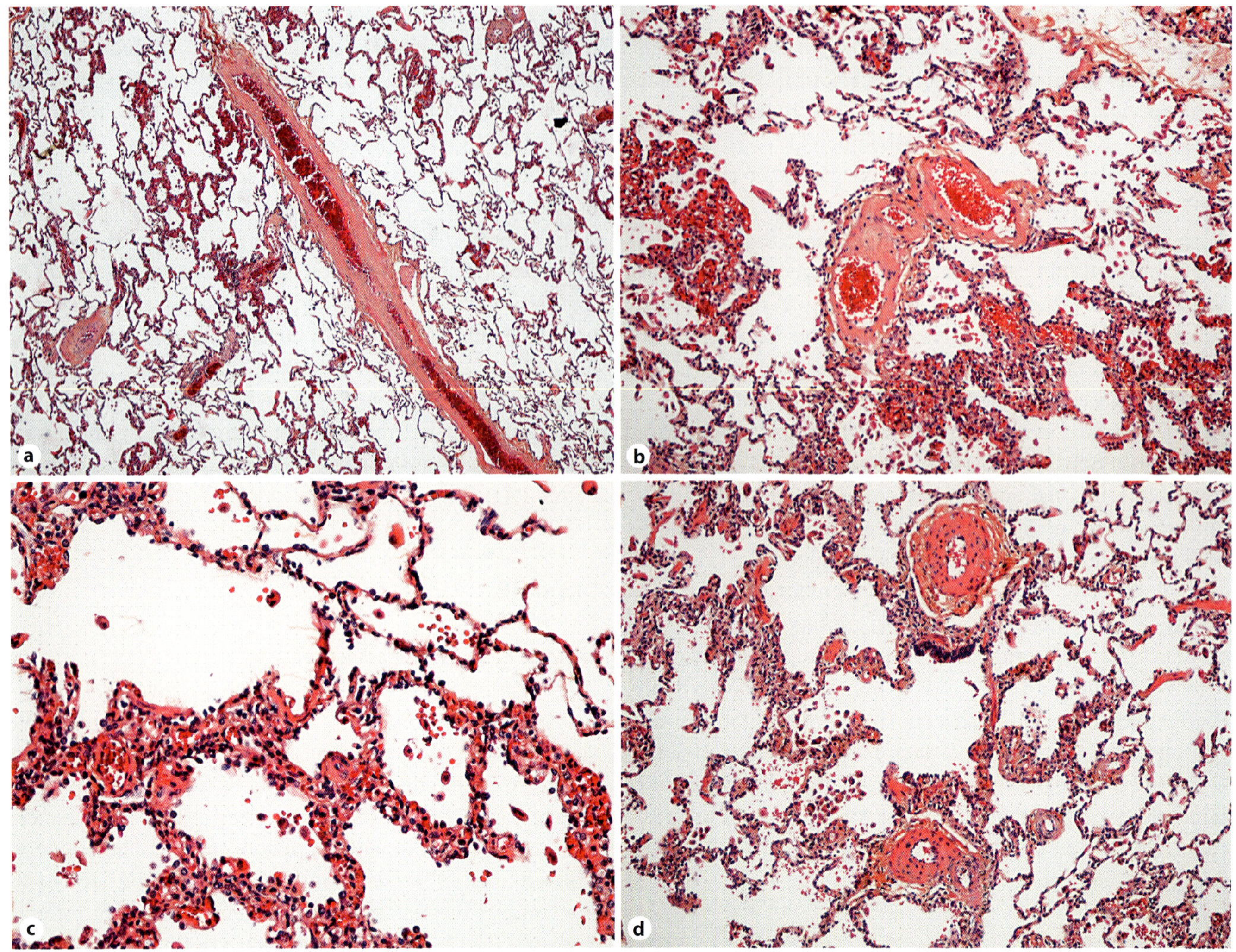

Fig. 1. Pulmonary vascular lesions in a patient suffering from PVOD (hematoxylin-eosin staining). **a** Septal vein displaying fibrosis with cushion-like narrowing of the native lumen. **b** Preseptal venules with occlusive intimal fibrosis. **c** Thickening of alveolar septa due to focal multiplication of alveolar capillaries. **d** Associated precapillary remodeling in the same patient with typical muscular hyperplasia of small arterioles.

preseptal venules, and consist of fibrous remodeling of the intima, which may occlude the lumen of pulmonary veins (fig. 1). Occult alveolar hemorrhage in bronchoalveolar lavage fluid may be evaluated using the Golde score. It frequently occurs in patients displaying PVOD contrarily to idiopathic PAH where alveolar hemorrhage is classically absent [49]. Interestingly, venous lesions and postcapillary obstruction in PVOD are commonly associated with capillary remodeling, including angiectasia and even capillary angioproliferation (fig. 1). A doubling or tripling of the alveolar septal capillary layers may focally be observed. Despite the constant occurrence of arterial lesions in the lungs of PVOD patients, complex lesions, as defined here above, do usually not occur in the context of PVOD [3].

Hemodynamic Evaluation

Pulmonary Capillary Wedge Pressure

As for all patients with suspected PAH, hemodynamic evaluation is required in PVOD to confirm the diagnosis. Both idiopathic PAH and PVOD patients have evidence of severe precapillary PAH with an elevated resting mean pulmonary arterial pressure equal to or greater than 25 mm Hg with a pulmonary capillary wedge pressure (PCWP) equal to or less than 15 mm Hg [1, 5, 51–53]. When biopsy-proven idiopathic PAH patients were compared with a group with biopsy-proven PVOD in a recent large series, similar hemodynamic characteristics were observed with the exception of right atrial pressure, which was lower in PVOD [8].

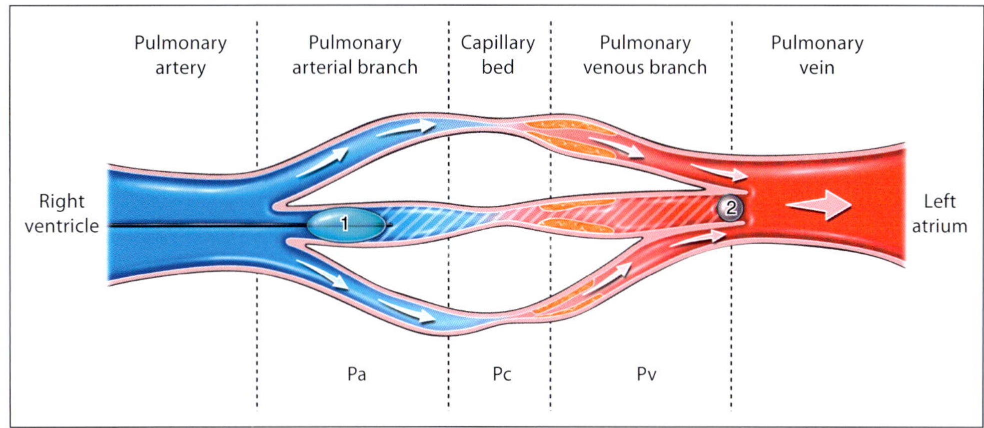

Fig. 2. Measurement of PCWP in PVOD (Reprinted with permission from Montani D et al. [5]). Diagram explaining why PCWP is usually normal in PVOD. PVOD mostly affects small pulmonary veins, leading to an elevation of pressure in this region (Pv) as well as to an elevation in true pulmonary capillary pressure (Pc) and precapillary pulmonary arterial pressure (Pa). Larger pulmonary veins are usually not affected by PVOD, and it is in fact the pressure here that is reflected by PCWP: the static column of blood (hatched) occluded by pulmonary arterial catheter wedging or balloon inflation of a pulmonary arterial branch (balloon 1) reflects the pressure in a vein of similar diameter (balloon 2), usually of a larger size than those vessels affected by PVOD. Therefore, this measurement technique does not reflect the important elevation of pressure in the smaller diameter vessels associated with PVOD. Pv = pressure in small pulmonary veins; Pc = true pulmonary capillary pressure; Pa = pulmonary artery pressure.

Case reports [54] and case series [8, 9, 49] demonstrated that PCWP is usually normal (<15 mm Hg) in PVOD patients. The difference between PVOD and idiopathic PAH is at the level of obstruction to blood flow, noted in precapillary vessels in PAH and in capillary as well as postcapillary vessels in PVOD. By definition, true capillary pressure and measured PCWP are normal (<15 mm Hg) in idiopathic PAH. By contrast, in PVOD, the postcapillary obstruction leads to an elevated true capillary pressure [55, 56], although not of PCWP. During hemodynamic evaluation, the measured PCWP is reflective of the pressure in the column of blood distal to the inflated balloon (fig. 2). Then, PCWP reflects the pressure in a pulmonary vein of similar diameter to the occluded pulmonary arterial branch, which is larger than the small veins affected by PVOD, explaining the normal PCWP usually obtained in PVOD patients [3, 5, 8] (fig. 2). In conclusion, because PCWP does not reflect true capillary pressure but reflects the pressure in large veins, PCWP is not helpful to discriminate idiopathic PAH and PVOD. Measurement of the true capillary pressure may theoretically be useful in PVOD; the principle of true capillary pressure measurement is extrapolated from a canine model whereby the pressure decay following balloon occlusion is mathematically analyzed to represent the emptying of the capillary compartment [57]. Interestingly, Fesler et al. [58] showed that patients displaying PVOD may have higher true capillary pressure than PAH patients using this method [59].

Acute Vasodilator Testing

In idiopathic PAH, acute vasoreactivity testing is predictive of long-term responsiveness to calcium channel blockers [53, 60]. There are clear differences in the long-term prognosis in the group of idiopathic PAH patients who have a positive response to this challenge when compared to non-responders [53, 60]. There is a recent report of one patient with PVOD who responded to nitric oxide (NO); however, within 48 h after initiation of calcium channel blocker therapy, severe pulmonary edema developed [8]. This suggests that an acute vasodilator response in PVOD is not predictive of a better prognosis and that calcium channel blockers should be avoided in PVOD, even in the context of a positive acute test. The main concern in PVOD is the risk of pulmonary edema with pulmonary vasodilators such as continuous intravenous epoprostenol and other specific PAH therapies [6, 8, 9]. Pulmonary edema has been described following vasodilator testing [6, 9]; however, in a recent series of 24 histologically confirmed PVOD patients, inhalation of 10 ppm NO for a short period (5–10 min) was used to test acute vasoreactivity. In this study, none of the patients developed pulmonary edema acutely [8]. This regimen of NO administration seems to be safe in patients with suspected PVOD. However, in this series, acute vasoreactivity testing was unable to predict those patients who later developed pulmonary edema following initiation of a PAH-specific therapy. It appears that acute vasoreactivity testing is probably not helpful in the management of PVOD patients, as calcium channel blocker responders have not been described. Furthermore, acute vasoreactivity testing is not predictive of those patients at risk of developing pulmonary edema with specific PAH therapy. Given these important observations, there may be little merit of systemically performing vasodilator studies in patients with a strong clinical suspicion of PVOD since the hemodynamic findings are unlikely to have an impact on therapeutic decisions.

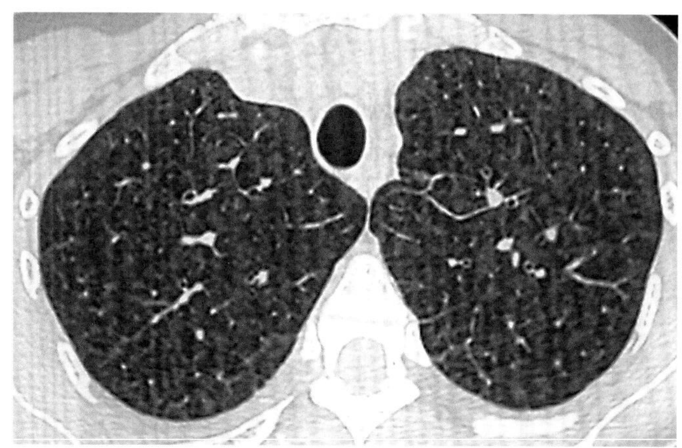

Fig. 3. HRCT of the chest in PVOD, showing marked ground-glass opacities with centrilobular pattern, ground-glass opacities with poorly defined nodular opacities, and septal lines.

Noninvasive Tools

The gold standard for a definite diagnosis of PVOD requires histological analysis of a lung sample. As this patient population often presents with more advanced disease, surgical lung biopsy is invasive and quite risky. Therefore, there is a need to use less invasive tools to aid in the diagnosis of suspected PVOD. Recent data have shown that HRCT of the chest, arterial blood gases, pulmonary function tests, and bronchoalveolar lavage could be helpful to define a subgroup of PAH with a high probability of PVOD.

Transthoracic Echocardiography

Transthoracic echocardiography is an important initial noninvasive diagnostic tool in the evaluation of all patients in whom pulmonary hypertension is suspected [61]. A systolic pulmonary artery pressure cutoff greater than 40 mm Hg, as estimated by the velocity of the regurgitating flow through the tricuspid valve, is a sensitive but unspecific diagnostic threshold. False positives using this value are common and formal diagnosis of pulmonary hypertension requires confirmation by right heart catheterization. Furthermore, there are no distinct echocardiographic features that help distinguish PVOD from other forms of pulmonary hypertension. Nonetheless, echocardiography is useful to exclude the presence of associated left ventricular, valvular, or pericardial abnormalities [62].

High-Resolution Computed Tomography of the Chest

In idiopathic PAH, the radiographic findings are generally limited to enlargement of the right and left pulmonary arteries without evidence of pulmonary parenchymal abnormalities. In contrast, the chest radiograph in PVOD may show significant abnormalities with Kerley B lines or signs of pulmonary edema, most frequently occurring after initiation of pulmonary vasodilator therapy [6, 8, 9, 47, 63]. HRCT of the chest may also help to discriminate PVOD and PAH in less acute situations [8, 9, 47, 48]. It has been clearly demonstrated that HRCT in PVOD was characterized by a higher frequency of centrilobular ground-glass opacities, septal lines (fig. 3), and mediastinal lymph node enlargement as compared to idiopathic PAH [48]. Pleural effusion and other abnormal parenchymal findings were not significantly associated with PVOD [48]. We have reported that the presence of two or three radiological abnormalities (including lymph node enlargement, septal lines, and centrilobular ground-glass opacities) were present in 75% of HRCT from patients displaying histologically proven PVOD [8]. However, this means that one quarter of histologically proven PVOD patients had only one or no radiological abnormalities on HRCT; inversely, 15% of patients with confirmed idiopathic PAH had two or three abnormalities [8]. These findings suggest that HRCT was a useful tool to discriminate PVOD, but normal HCRT could not rule out the diagnosis of PVOD, and should be included in a multifactorial noninvasive approach.

Pulmonary Function Testing and Oxygen Parameters

Results of previous reports have suggested that PVOD patients may have mild obstructive or restrictive patterns noted on pulmonary function testing [9]. However, a large series of 'idiopathic' PVOD patients showed that these patients had normal mean values of forced expiratory volume in 1 s, forced expiratory volume in 1 s/forced vital capacity ratio, and total lung capacity. Indeed, no difference was observed in pulmonary function tests analyzed during spirometry and plethysmography as compared to idiopathic PAH [8]. A decrease in diffusing lung capacity of carbon monoxide (DLCO) has been well established in patients displaying idiopathic PAH and PVOD [9, 64]. However, we compared DLCO and DLCO/alveolar volume between PVOD and PAH patients, and the results indicated that both these parameters were more significantly reduced in PVOD as compared to idiopathic PAH [8]. PVOD patients usually had a very low DLCO and in this series, half of the histologically confirmed PVOD patients had a mean DLCO of 52 ± 19% as compared to 71 ± 15% in idiopathic PAH patients [8].

Hypoxemia has been reported in patients displaying PVOD or idiopathic PAH [9, 53]. Our recent report showed that the baseline partial pressure of arterial oxygen (PaO_2) at rest is significantly lower in PVOD patients than in idiopathic PAH patients (61 ± 17 and 75 ± 14, respectively) [8]. This study also evaluated the partial pressure of arterial carbon dioxide which was decreased in a similar pattern in both PVOD and PAH patients. Many factors likely contribute to the pathophysiological mechanisms of exaggerated hypoxemia in PVOD patients in comparison to patients with idiopathic PAH. These include a probable combination of more extensive obliteration of the pulmonary vascular bed, a diffusion limitation, possible alveolar hemorrhage, and pulmonary edema in the most severe cases.

The 6-minute walk distance (6MWD) has been found to correlate with functional status and survival in idiopathic PAH. Additionally, it is used as a measure of baseline severity and a surrogate marker of response to treatment in idiopathic PAH. Only a few studies have evaluated this parameter in PVOD. A series comparing idiopathic PAH and PVOD patients demonstrated a significantly lower 6MWD in the PVOD group [49]. Our recent case series showed that PVOD patients had a similar 6MWD compared to the PAH patients; however, the PVOD patients had lower nadir pulse oxygen saturation during the test [8].

Bronchoalveolar Lavage

In patients undergoing an evaluation for PAH, bronchoscopy is rarely performed as a routine investigation. However, in the context of possible PVOD, a bronchoscopic evaluation with bronchoalveolar lavage may be helpful [49]. In PVOD, it has been suggested that hyperemia of the lobar and segmental bronchi may be observed on bronchoscopic airway inspection as it was described in mitral stenosis, where chronic pulmonary venous hypertension leads to engorgement and dilatation of the bronchial venous plexus and veins [65, 66]. Of note, bronchial biopsies are not informative of PVOD and transbronchial biopsies are contraindicated in patients with pulmonary hypertension due to the risk of life-threatening hemoptysis [67]. When comparing the bronchoalveolar lavage results of 8 PVOD patients and 11 idiopathic PAH patients, Rabiller et al. [49] showed a significantly elevated percentage of hemosiderin-laden macrophages and a higher Golde score, demonstrating that PVOD may be associated with occult alveolar hemorrhage. The absence of alveolar hemorrhage could not exclude the diagnosis of PVOD; however, confirmation of alveolar hemorrhage is highly subjective of PVOD. As histological diagnosis is difficult to obtain in this patient population, the role of bronchoscopy to detect occult alveolar hemorrhage as part of the diagnostic work-up for suspected PVOD is somewhat attractive.

Prognosis

Historically, the prognosis has been poor in idiopathic PAH and, unfortunately, the survival in PVOD seems to be even more dismal than for idiopathic PAH. Data suggest that the 1-year mortality rate may be as high as 72% in PVOD [9], and the most recent series of a group of 24 histologically confirmed severe PVOD patients found a mean time from first symptoms (or diagnosis confirmed by right heart catheterization) to death or lung transplantation of 24.4 ± 22.2 months (or 11.8 ± 16.4, respectively), which is significantly lower in PVOD when compared to 57.9 ± 38.2 months (or 42.3 ± 29.9, respectively) for patients with idiopathic PAH [8]. In this series, even if baseline parameters including NYHA functional class, 6MWD, and baseline hemodynamics are similar between the idiopathic PAH and the PVOD groups, PVOD patients seem to have a poorer prognosis, suggesting that these parameters might be less accurate for predicting the evolution of PVOD than they are in idiopathic PAH. Unfortunately, treatment options are very limited in PVOD. Therefore, early diagnosis and referral for lung transplantation in appropriate patients are critical in PVOD.

Therapy

Conventional Therapy

A significant aggravating factor in PAH is hypoxic vasoconstriction. Therefore, oxygen therapy should be considered and initiated in hypoxemic patients with both idiopathic PAH and PVOD [53]. It has been noted that PVOD patients have a lower PaO_2 at rest than idiopathic PAH patients, suggesting that PVOD patients may require oxygen therapy earlier than other PAH patients [8]. In appropriate patients with resting or exercise-induced hypoxemia, oxygen therapy may provide symptomatic benefit as well as avoid PAH deterioration [53].

Patients with idiopathic PAH have improved outcomes with the initiation of warfarin therapy. Although there are no specific data pertaining to PVOD, the rationale is similar and related to reducing organized thrombi [68] and subsequent in situ thrombosis, which are manifest in both conditions [69]. The current recommendations suggest warfarin therapy with an international normalized ratio to be maintained between 1.5 and 2.5 in idiopathic PAH [53]. This recommendation has been generalized to all PAH patients without contraindications, despite the fact that the evidence was obtained only in the idiopathic PAH group. In PVOD, one could suggest that caution should be taken in the application of anticoagulation because of the frequent association with occult alveolar hemorrhage. However, we reported the same proportion of hemoptysis in idiopathic PAH and PVOD, even with the use of anticoagulation. As in idiopathic PAH, no data support the role of immunosuppressive therapy in 'idiopathic' PVOD, but it may be of interest in PAH or PVOD associated with other inflammatory conditions, including sarcoidosis, mixed connective tissue disease, and systemic lupus erythematosus, but not in scleroderma-associated PAH [14, 70, 71].

A number of additional measures are routinely advised for PVOD patients, although these are mostly based on expert consensus, often with extrapolation from historical studies in other diseases. Empiric evidence from well-designed prospective clinical trials to support the use of most of these 'conventional' therapies is lacking as published studies are mostly of a retrospective or uncontrolled retrospective nature. Indeed, some of these interventions likely offer only symptomatic benefits without necessarily impacting on prognosis. Nevertheless, their application is biologically plausible and thus broadly advocated [72].

General recommendations include limiting of physical activity to tolerance and avoidance of concomitant medications that can potentially aggravate pulmonary hypertension (such as β-adrenergic receptor blockers) or interfere with the metabolism of vitamin K antagonist anticoagulation therapy. Vaccinations to prevent pneumococcal pneumonia and influenza are advised. Given a possible etiological link between tobacco exposure and PVOD, smoking cessation advice and appropriate pharmacotherapy is particularly important and should routinely be offered to cigarette smokers. Diuretics offer symptomatic benefit in those with right ventricular volume overload that is not controlled by dietary measures alone. The effect of diuretics on mortality in PVOD has not been systemically examined.

The additional hemodynamic stresses of pregnancy and delivery are poorly tolerated in PVOD patients, being associated with increased rate of deterioration and very high mortality rates. Moreover, commonly prescribed treatments (e.g. warfarin and bosentan) are known teratogens. Female patients of child-bearing potential should therefore be counseled on effective contraception measures.

Specific Pulmonary Arterial Hypertension Therapies

Presently, the evidence for specific vasodilator therapies is strong in idiopathic PAH [52–54, 73–75], but is modest and conflicting in PVOD, and the primary concern remains the risk of pulmonary edema. Recent reports have illustrated the occurrence of pulmonary edema with different specific PAH therapies (prostacyclins, endothelin receptor antagonists, phosphodiesterase type 5 inhibitors, calcium channel blockers) highlighting that pulmonary edema is not limited to a single therapeutic class and can occur with all specific PAH therapies [5, 8]. One of the suspected mechanisms is a relative vasodilatation of the precapillary resistance vessels greater than the pulmonary capillaries and veins, associated with increased blood flow that leads to an increase of transcapillary hydrostatic pressure and transudation of fluid into the pulmonary interstitium and alveoli. Furthermore, lymphatic involvement is frequently observed in PVOD and may participate in the mechanism of pulmonary edema by a decrease in fluid reabsorption. In our recent cohort of histologically confirmed PVOD patients, 7 of 16 patients who received specific PAH developed pulmonary edema. However, none of these patients developed pulmonary edema during acute testing with NO, nor were any of the clinical, functional, or hemodynamic characteristics predictive of the onset of this complication after initiation of specific PAH therapy [8]. In selected cases, mild clinical improvement or stabilization with continuous intravenous epoprostenol [9, 76–79], and iloprost therapy [80, 81], oral sildenafil [82, 83] has been reported. In contrast with idiopathic PAH, the benefits of specific PAH treatments in patients with PVOD remain unclear.

Immunomodulatory Agents

The basis for the use of immunosuppressive agents in some selected PAH patients was initially anecdotal with rare reports of clinical and hemodynamic improvements in PAH and PVOD patients, suggesting the use of corticosteroids, cyclophosphamide, and azathioprine [17, 29, 70, 71, 84, 85].

PVOD is also thought to be present in some cases of pulmonary hypertension patients displaying sarcoidosis. However, in these patients, the pulmonary vascular component may be less responsive to treatment with glucocorticoids than the parenchymal lung disease [14]. There is mounting evidence that PAH is a significant inflammatory component [86], and that PAH in some connective tissue diseases responds well to immunosuppressive therapy [71, 76, 85]. Specific patients who may improve with immunosuppression include those with mixed connective tissue disease and systemic lupus erythematosus, but not in scleroderma-associated PAH [71, 85]. A full histopathological assessment has shown that severe connective tissue disease-associated PAH has a major venous pathological component in 75% of cases [11]. In cases where such venous occlusion was observed, the postcapillary arterial involvement was important, and there was also an association with local inflammatory infiltrates [11]. The reason why this subset of connective tissue disease-associated PAH patients do not improve with pulmonary vasodilator therapy might be due at least in part to venous involvement. More studies are needed to understand whether PVOD, either idiopathic or associated with other conditions such as connective-tissue diseases, is responsive to immunosuppressive therapies. Currently, corticosteroids or immunosuppressive therapy should only be considered in the context of sarcoidosis or connective tissue disease (except scleroderma).

Lung Transplantation

Lung transplantation is the only curative intervention of PAH and historically it was the only form of treatment for severe PAH. However, with the advent of specific PAH therapy, transplantation is now considered in idiopathic PAH when the disease progresses despite optimal medical management [51–53, 87, 88]. As the prognosis in PVOD patients is worse than in idiopathic PAH and because of limited medical therapy, lung transplantation should be considered and discussed early in the course of PVOD. In these patients, PAH-specific therapies may serve as a bridge to lung transplantation [79]. No specific data is available on survival of PVOD patients after transplantation, but it has been suggested to be broadly similar to that in idiopathic PAH.

Conclusion

PVOD is a rare subgroup of PAH characterized by specific pathological changes of postcapillary venous pulmonary vessels. PVOD shares a broadly similar clinical presentation with idiopathic PAH (table 1), making this diagnosis much more challenging to the clinician. In contrast with idiopathic PAH, patients with PVOD have a poorer prognosis and are at risk of developing pulmonary edema with specific PAH therapy. Hemodynamic parameters do not help discriminate between these two diseases, and even if PVOD is defined by involvement of postcapillary and capillary vessels, PCWP is normal (<15 mm Hg) in both groups. However, there are some features that may help to discriminate between the two entities in order to prevent risky histological confirmation. These include and may identify a higher probability of PVOD: history of tobacco exposure, oxygen parameters (low PaO_2 at rest, low SpO_2 during 6-min walk test), pulmonary functional tests (low DLCO), HRCT of the chest (centrilobular ground-glass opacities, septal lines, lymph node enlargement), and occult alveolar hemorrhage on bronchoalveolar lavage when feasible. In PVOD, cautious initiation of specific PAH therapy may be considered, but should not delay consideration and referral for lung transplantation, which remains the best treatment. Further studies are needed to understand the pathophysiology of this subgroup of PAH, the role of specific PAH therapies, and whether new therapeutic approaches with antiproliferative therapies might be helpful.

Expert Commentary

There is now a wealth of accumulated clinical experience with strategies employing combinations of PAH-specific drugs in order to target the multifarious aberrant molecular pathways characteristic of the disorder and thereby theoretically to enhance therapeutic gain. Indeed, this approach is routinely pursued in many expert centers, despite a lack of robust evidence demonstrating additional clinical benefit. Theoretically, the risk of pulmonary edema developing in the context of PVOD might be further increased by using a regimen involving more than one pulmonary vasodilator. However, in patients with severe disease and poor expected survival time, cautious introduction of additional treatments has been attempted in the hope of slowing clinical deterioration. Nonetheless, experience is extremely limited to date and this approach is not recommended outside of expert centers due to the risk of severe pulmonary edema.

5-Year View

In recent years, remarkable advances in the pharmacologic options available to clinicians treating PAH patients have been made. Regulatory approval has now been granted for a number of drug therapies that manifest pulmonary-specific vasodilatory and antiproliferative effects, resulting in meaningful and sustained improvements in relevant clinical parameters. As our understanding of the pathophysiology of PVOD and PAH increases, so does the identification of possible therapeutic targets and potential novel treatments. In 5 years' time, further studies will be needed in order to refine the understanding of the molecular characteristics of PVOD and PAH. The discovery of agents that modify these aberrant pathways will determine whether new therapeutic approaches with antiproliferative therapies might have any role in the PVOD.

Key Issues

- PVOD is a rare form of PAH with several similarities but worse prognosis.
- PVOD has been described as idiopathic, heritable, or complicating other conditions, such as connective tissue diseases, HIV infection, chronic respiratory disease, malignancy, or bone marrow transplantation, among others.
- The PVOD histopathological hallmark is represented by a widespread fibrous intimal proliferation that predominantly affects the postcapillary venous pulmonary vessels, venules, and small veins.
- Compared to PAH, PVOD is characterized by a higher male/female ratio, higher tobacco exposure, lower arterial oxygen tension at rest, lower diffusing capacity of the lung for carbon monoxide, and lower oxygen saturation nadir during the 6-min walk test.
- Surgical lung biopsy is considered the definitive diagnostic test, but is associated with significant risk and is not recommended.
- A noninvasive approach using HRCT of the chest, arterial blood gas analyses, pulmonary function tests, and bronchoalveolar lavage could be helpful for the detection of PVOD.
- Treatment of PVOD is challenging as exposure to pulmonary vasodilators and PAH-specific therapies may precipitate acute pulmonary edema.
- Lung transplantation is the treatment of choice.

References

1 Simonneau G, Robbins IM, Beghetti M, et al: Updated clinical classification of pulmonary hypertension. J Am Coll Cardiol 2009;54(1 Suppl): S43–S54.
2 Rubin LJ: Primary pulmonary hypertension. N Engl J Med 1997;336:111–117.
3 Pietra GG, Capron F, Stewart S, et al: Pathologic assessment of vasculopathies in pulmonary hypertension. J Am Coll Cardiol 2004;43(12 Suppl S):25S–32S.
4 Lantuejoul S, Sheppard MN, Corrin B, Burke MM, Nicholson AG: Pulmonary veno-occlusive disease and pulmonary capillary hemangiomatosis: a clinicopathologic study of 35 cases. Am J Surg Pathol 2006;30:850–857.
5 Montani D, Price LC, Dorfmuller P, et al: Pulmonary veno-occlusive disease. Eur Respir J 2009; 33:189–200.
6 Palmer SM, Robinson LJ, Wang A, Gossage JR, Bashore T, Tapson VF: Massive pulmonary edema and death after prostacyclin infusion in a patient with pulmonary veno-occlusive disease. Chest 1998;113:237–240.
7 Mandel J, Mark EJ, Hales CA: Pulmonary veno-occlusive disease. Am J Respir Crit Care Med 2000;162:1964–1973.
8 Montani D, Achouh L, Dorfmuller P, et al: Pulmonary veno-occlusive disease: clinical, functional, radiologic, and hemodynamic characteristics and outcome of 24 cases confirmed by histology. Medicine (Baltimore) 2008;87:220–233.
9 Holcomb BW Jr, Loyd JE, Ely EW, Johnson J, Robbins IM: Pulmonary veno-occlusive disease: a case series and new observations. Chest 2000;118:1671–1679.
10 Humbert M, Sitbon O, Chaouat A, et al: Pulmonary arterial hypertension in France: results from a national registry. Am J Respir Crit Care Med 2006;173:1023–1030.
11 Dorfmüller P, Humbert M, Perros F, et al: Fibrous remodeling of the pulmonary venous system in pulmonary arterial hypertension associated with connective tissue diseases. Hum Pathol 2007;38:893–902.
12 Zhang L, Visscher D, Rihal C, Aubry MC: Pulmonary veno-occlusive disease as a primary cause of pulmonary hypertension in a patient with mixed connective tissue disease. Rheumatol Int 2007;27:1163–1165.
13 Johnson SR, Patsios D, Hwang DM, Granton JT: Pulmonary veno-occlusive disease and scleroderma associated pulmonary hypertension. J Rheumatol 2006;33:2347–2350.
14 Nunes H, Humbert M, Capron F, et al: Pulmonary hypertension associated with sarcoidosis: mechanisms, haemodynamics and prognosis. Thorax 2006;61:68–74.
15 Fartoukh M, Humbert M, Capron F, et al: Severe pulmonary hypertension in histiocytosis X. Am J Respir Crit Care Med 2000;161:216–223.
16 Hamada K, Teramoto S, Narita N, Yamada E, Teramoto K, Kobzik L: Pulmonary veno-occlusive disease in pulmonary Langerhans' cell granulomatosis. Eur Respir J 2000;15:421–423.
17 Escamilla R, Hermant C, Berjaud J, Mazerolles C, Daussy X: Pulmonary veno-occlusive disease in a HIV-infected intravenous drug abuser. Eur Respir J 1995;8:1982–1984.
18 Hourseau M, Capron F, Nunes H, Godmer P, Martin A, Kambouchner M: Pulmonary veno-occlusive disease in a patient with HIV infection. A case report with autopsy findings (in French). Ann Pathol 2002;22:472–475.
19 Ruchelli ED, Nojadera G, Rutstein RM, Rudy B: Pulmonary veno-occlusive disease. Another vascular disorder associated with human immunodeficiency virus infection? Arch Pathol Lab Med 1994;118:664–666.
20 Humbert M, Nunes H, Sitbon O, Parent F, Hervé P, Simonneau G: Risk factors for pulmonary arterial hypertension. Clin Chest Med 2001;22:459–475.
21 Abenhaim L, Moride Y, Brenot F, et al: Appetite-suppressant drugs and the risk of primary pulmonary hypertension. International Primary Pulmonary Hypertension Study Group. N Engl J Med 1996;335:609–616.
22 Souza R, Humbert M, Sztrymf B, et al: Pulmonary arterial hypertension associated with fenfluramine exposure: report of 109 cases. Eur Respir J 2008;31:343–348.
23 Douglas JG, Munro JF, Kitchin AH, Muir AL, Proudfoot AT: Pulmonary hypertension and fenfluramine. Br Med J (Clin Res Ed) 1981;283: 881–883.
24 Gurtner HP: Aminorex and pulmonary hypertension. A review. Cor Vasa 1985;27:160–171.
25 Joselson R, Warnock M: Pulmonary veno-occlusive disease after chemotherapy. Hum Pathol 1983;14:88–91.
26 Knight BK, Rose AG: Pulmonary veno-occlusive disease after chemotherapy. Thorax 1985;40: 874–875.

27 Swift GL, Gibbs A, Campbell IA, Wagenvoort CA, Tuthill D: Pulmonary veno-occlusive disease and Hodgkin's lymphoma. Eur Respir J 1993;6:596–598.

28 Waldhorn RE, Tsou E, Smith FP, Kerwin DM: Pulmonary veno-occlusive disease associated with microangiopathic hemolytic anemia and chemotherapy of gastric adenocarcinoma. Med Pediatr Oncol 1984;12:394–396.

29 Hackman RC, Madtes DK, Petersen FB, Clark JG: Pulmonary venoocclusive disease following bone marrow transplantation. Transplantation 1989;47:989–992.

30 Williams LM, Fussell S, Veith RW, Nelson S, Mason CM: Pulmonary veno-occlusive disease in an adult following bone marrow transplantation. Case report and review of the literature. Chest 1996;109:1388–1391.

31 Kuga T, Kohda K, Hirayama Y, et al: Pulmonary veno-occlusive disease accompanied by microangiopathic hemolytic anemia 1 year after a second bone marrow transplantation for acute lymphoblastic leukemia. Int J Hematol 1996;64:143–150.

32 Troussard X, Bernaudin JF, Cordonnier C, et al: Pulmonary veno-occlusive disease after bone marrow transplantation. Thorax 1984;39:956–957.

33 Salzman D, Adkins DR, Craig F, Freytes C, LeMaistre CF: Malignancy-associated pulmonary veno-occlusive disease: report of a case following autologous bone marrow transplantation and review. Bone Marrow Transplant 1996;18:755–760.

34 Seguchi M, Hirabayashi N, Fujii Y, et al: Pulmonary hypertension associated with pulmonary occlusive vasculopathy after allogeneic bone marrow transplantation. Transplantation 2000;69:177–179.

35 Trobaugh-Lotrario AD, Greffe B, Deterding R, Deutsch G, Quinones R: Pulmonary veno-occlusive disease after autologous bone marrow transplant in a child with stage IV neuroblastoma: case report and literature review. J Pediatr Hematol Oncol 2003;25:405–409.

36 Bunte MC, Patnaik MM, Pritzker MR, Burns LJ: Pulmonary veno-occlusive disease following hematopoietic stem cell transplantation: a rare model of endothelial dysfunction. Bone Marrow Transplant 2008;41:677–686.

37 Wright JL, Tai H, Churg A: Cigarette smoke induces persisting increases of vasoactive mediators in pulmonary arteries. Am J Respir Cell Mol Biol 2004;31:501–509.

38 Wright JL, Tai H, Churg A: Vasoactive mediators and pulmonary hypertension after cigarette smoke exposure in the guinea pig. J Appl Physiol 2006;100:672–678.

39 Rosenzweig EB, Morse JH, Knowles JA, et al: Clinical implications of determining BMPR2 mutation status in a large cohort of children and adults with pulmonary arterial hypertension. J Heart Lung Transplant 2008;27:668–674.

40 Sztrymf B, Coulet F, Girerd B, et al: Clinical outcomes of pulmonary arterial hypertension in carriers of BMPR2 mutation. Am J Respir Crit Care Med 2008;177:1377–1383.

41 Humbert M: Update in pulmonary hypertension 2008. Am J Respir Crit Care Med 2009;179:650–656.

42 Runo JR, Vnencak-Jones CL, Prince M, et al: Pulmonary veno-occlusive disease caused by an inherited mutation in bone morphogenetic protein receptor II. Am J Respir Crit Care Med 2003;167:889–894.

43 Machado RD, Aldred MA, James V, et al: Mutations of the TGF-beta type II receptor BMPR2 in pulmonary arterial hypertension. Hum Mutat 2006;27:121–132.

44 Aldred MA, Vijayakrishnan J, James V, et al: BMPR2 gene rearrangements account for a significant proportion of mutations in familial and idiopathic pulmonary arterial hypertension. Hum Mutat 2006;27:212–213.

45 Davies P, Reid L: Pulmonary veno-occlusive disease in siblings: case reports and morphometric study. Hum Pathol 1982;13:911–915.

46 Voordes CG, Kuipers JR, Elema JD: Familial pulmonary veno-occlusive disease: a case report. Thorax 1977;32:763–766.

47 Dufour B, Maitre S, Humbert M, Capron F, Simonneau G, Musset D: High-resolution CT of the chest in four patients with pulmonary capillary hemangiomatosis or pulmonary venoocclusive disease. AJR Am J Roentgenol 1998;171:1321–1324.

48 Resten A, Maitre S, Humbert M, et al: Pulmonary hypertension: CT of the chest in pulmonary venoocclusive disease. AJR Am J Roentgenol 2004;183:65–70.

49 Rabiller A, Jais X, Hamid A, et al: Occult alveolar haemorrhage in pulmonary veno-occlusive disease. Eur Respir J 2006;27:108–113.

50 Wagenvoort CA: The pathology of primary pulmonary hypertension. J Pathol 1970;101:Pi.

51 Galie N, Hoeper MM, Humbert M, et al: Guidelines for the diagnosis and treatment of pulmonary hypertension. Eur Respir J 2009;34:1219–1263.

52 Galie N, Hoeper MM, Humbert M, et al: Guidelines for the diagnosis and treatment of pulmonary hypertension: the Task Force for the Diagnosis and Treatment of Pulmonary Hypertension of the European Society of Cardiology (ESC) and the European Respiratory Society (ERS), endorsed by the International Society of Heart and Lung Transplantation (ISHLT). Eur Heart J 2009;30:2493–2537.

53 Humbert M, Sitbon O, Simonneau G: Treatment of pulmonary arterial hypertension. N Engl J Med 2004;351:1425–1436.

54 Rambihar VS, Fallen EL, Cairns JA: Pulmonary veno-occlusive disease: antemortem diagnosis from roentgenographic and hemodynamic findings. Can Med Assoc J 1979;120:1519–1522.

55 Gaar KA Jr, Taylor AE, Owens LJ, Guyton AC: Pulmonary capillary pressure and filtration coefficient in the isolated perfused lung. Am J Physiol 1967;213:910–914.

56 Grimbert FA: Effective pulmonary capillary pressure. Eur Respir J 1988;1:297–301.

57 Cope DK, Allison RC, Parmentier JL, Miller JN, Taylor AE: Measurement of effective pulmonary capillary pressure using the pressure profile after pulmonary artery occlusion. Crit Care Med 1986;14:16–22.

58 Fesler P, Pagnamenta A, Vachiery JL, et al: Single arterial occlusion to locate resistance in patients with pulmonary hypertension. Eur Respir J 2003;21:31–36.

59 Souza R, Amato MB, Demarzo SE, et al: Pulmonary capillary pressure in pulmonary hypertension. Crit Care 2005;9:R132–R138.

60 Sitbon O, Humbert M, Jais X, et al: Long-term response to calcium channel blockers in idiopathic pulmonary arterial hypertension. Circulation 2005;111:3105–3111.

61 McLaughlin VV, Archer SL, Badesch DB, et al: ACCF/AHA 2009 expert consensus document on pulmonary hypertension a report of the American College of Cardiology Foundation Task Force on Expert Consensus Documents and the American Heart Association developed in collaboration with the American College of Chest Physicians; American Thoracic Society, Inc.; and the Pulmonary Hypertension Association. J Am Coll Cardiol 2009;53:1573–1619.

62 Rubin LJ: American College of Chest Physicians: Diagnosis and management of pulmonary arterial hypertension: ACCP evidence-based clinical practice guidelines. Chest 2004;126(1 Suppl):7S–10S.

63 Swensen SJ, Tashjian JH, Myers JL, et al: Pulmonary venoocclusive disease: CT findings in eight patients. AJR Am J Roentgenol 1996;167:937–940.

64 Elliott CG, Colby TV, Hill T, Crapo RO: Pulmonary veno-occlusive disease associated with severe reduction of single-breath carbon monoxide diffusing capacity. Respiration 1988;53:262–266.

65 Matthews AW, Buchanan R: A case of pulmonary veno-occlusive disease and a new bronchoscopic sign. Respir Med 1990;84:503–505.

66 Ohmichi M, Tagaki S, Nomura N, Tsunematsu K, Suzuki A: Endobronchial changes in chronic pulmonary venous hypertension. Chest 1988;94:1127–1132.

67 Wahidi MM, Rocha AT, Hollingsworth JW, Govert JA, Feller-Kopman D, Ernst A: Contraindications and safety of transbronchial lung biopsy via flexible bronchoscopy. A survey of pulmonologists and review of the literature. Respiration 2005;72:285–295.

68 Wagenvoort CA, Wagenvoort N: The pathology of pulmonary veno-occlusive disease. Virchows Arch A Pathol Anat Histol 1974;364:69–79.

69 Chazova I, Robbins I, Loyd J, et al: Venous and arterial changes in pulmonary veno-occlusive disease, mitral stenosis and fibrosing mediastinitis. Eur Respir J 2000;15:116–122.

70 Jais X, Launay D, Yaici A, et al: Management of lupus and mixed connective tissue disease-associated pulmonary arterial hypertension. Arthritis Rheum 2008;58:521–531.

71 Sanchez O, Sitbon O, Jais X, Simonneau G, Humbert M: Immunosuppressive therapy in connective tissue diseases-associated pulmonary arterial hypertension. Chest 2006;130:182–189.
72 Alam S, Palevsky HI: Standard therapies for pulmonary arterial hypertension. Clin Chest Med 2007;28:91–115, viii.
73 Barst RJ, Rubin LJ, Long WA, et al: A comparison of continuous intravenous epoprostenol (prostacyclin) with conventional therapy for primary pulmonary hypertension. The Primary Pulmonary Hypertension Study Group. N Engl J Med 1996;334:296–302.
74 Sitbon O, Humbert M, Nunes H, et al: Long-term intravenous epoprostenol infusion in primary pulmonary hypertension: prognostic factors and survival. J Am Coll Cardiol 2002;40:780–788.
75 Montani D, O'Callaghan D, Jaïs X, et al: Implementing the ESC/ERS pulmonary hypertension guidelines: real-life cases from a national referral centre. Eur Respir Rev 2009;18:231–249.
76 Okumura H, Nagaya N, Kyotani S, et al: Effects of continuous IV prostacyclin in a patient with pulmonary veno-occlusive disease. Chest 2002;122:1096–1098.
77 Resten A, Maitre S, Humbert M, et al: Pulmonary arterial hypertension: thin-section CT predictors of epoprostenol therapy failure. Radiology 2002;222:782–788.
78 Davis LL, deBoisblanc BP, Glynn CE, Ramirez C, Summer WR: Effect of prostacyclin on microvascular pressures in a patient with pulmonary veno-occlusive disease. Chest 1995;108:1754–1756.
79 Montani D, Jaïs X, Price LC, et al: Cautious epoprostenol therapy is a safe bridge to lung transplantation in pulmonary veno-occlusive disease. Eur Respir J 2009;34:1348–1356.
80 Shackelford GD, Sacks EJ, Mullins JD, McAlister WH: Pulmonary venoocclusive disease: case report and review of the literature. AJR Am J Roentgenol 1977;128:643–648.
81 Hoeper MM, Eschenbruch C, Zink-Wohlfart C, et al: Effects of inhaled nitric oxide and aerosolized iloprost in pulmonary veno-occlusive disease. Respir Med 1999;93:62–64.
82 Kuroda T, Hirota H, Masaki M, et al: Sildenafil as adjunct therapy to high-dose epoprostenol in a patient with pulmonary veno-occlusive disease. Heart Lung Circ 2006;15:139–142.
83 Barreto AC, Franchi SM, Castro CR, Lopes AA: One-year follow-up of the effects of sildenafil on pulmonary arterial hypertension and veno-occlusive disease. Braz J Med Biol Res 2005;38:185–195.
84 Gilroy RJ Jr, Teague MW, Loyd JE: Pulmonary veno-occlusive disease. Fatal progression of pulmonary hypertension despite steroid-induced remission of interstitial pneumonitis. Am Rev Respir Dis 1991;143:1130–1133.
85 Dorfmüller P, Perros F, Balabanian K, Humbert M: Inflammation in pulmonary arterial hypertension. Eur Respir J 2003;22:358–363.
86 Sanchez O, Humbert M, Sitbon O, Simonneau G: Treatment of pulmonary hypertension secondary to connective tissue diseases. Thorax 1999;54:273–277.
87 Sitbon O, Humbert M, Simonneau G: Primary pulmonary hypertension: current therapy. Prog Cardiovasc Dis 2002;45:115–128.
88 Cassart M, Gevenois PA, Kramer M, et al: Pulmonary venoocclusive disease: CT findings before and after single-lung transplantation. AJR Am J Roentgenol 1993;160:759–760.

David Montani, MD, PhD
Centre National de Référence de l'Hypertension Pulmonaire Sévère
Service de Pneumologie, Hôpital Antoine Béclère
Assistance Publique – Hôpitaux de Paris, Université Paris-Sud
157 rue de la Porte de Trivaux
FR–92140 Clamart (France)
Tel. +33 1 45 37 47 72, E-Mail david.montani@abc.aphp.fr

Chapter 17

Humbert M, Souza R, Simonneau G (eds): Pulmonary Vascular Disorders.
Prog Respir Res. Basel, Karger, 2012, vol 41, pp 161–168

Pulmonary Hypertension and Left Heart Disease

Yochai Adir[a] · Nazzareno Galiè[b]

[a]Pulmonary Division, Carmel Medical Center, Faculty of Medicine, Technion, Institute of Technology, Haifa, Israel;
[b]Institute of Cardiology, University of Bologna, Bologna, Italy

Abstract

Pulmonary arterial hypertension (PAH) is defined as a group of rare diseases characterized by a progressive increase of pulmonary vascular resistance (PVR) leading to right ventricular failure and premature death. A more frequent scenario is the patient with pulmonary hypertension (PH) in the setting of left heart disease (PH-LHD, Group 2) with elevated left-sided cardiac filling pressures. PH-LHD can result from any of a number of pathological or functional abnormalities. In the past, rheumatic mitral stenosis was the most common cause of this entity; however, today PH-LHD most commonly results from heart failure (HF) related to systolic and/or diastolic dysfunction of the left ventricle. Such patients require optimization of therapies for LHD. However, it is not uncommon that in a subset of patients, even with such optimization, clinically meaningful PH remains and for some of them PH is 'out of proportion' to their underlying disease state. In this setting, there are no evidence-based data to support the use of PAH-specific therapies. This chapter reviews the epidemiology, pathophysiology, risk factors, and treatment controversies concerning PH related to HF with reduced left ventricular ejection fraction, preserved left ventricle ejection fraction, and mitral and aortic valve disease.

Pulmonary hypertension (PH) is defined as mean pulmonary artery pressure (PAP) >25 mm Hg at rest and pulmonary vascular resistance (PVR) >3 Wood units in the presence of normal pulmonary capillary wedge pressure (PCWP) measured during right heart catheterization (RHC) [1]. The clinical classification of PH comprises heterogeneous conditions with different clinical presentations, pathophysiology, and management. The first category of the clinical classification termed 'pulmonary arterial hypertension' (PAH) is defined as a group of rare diseases characterized by a progressive increase of PVR leading to right ventricular failure and premature death. PAH includes idiopathic PAH (IPAH), heritable PAH, and PAH related to risk factors or associated conditions such as connective tissue diseases, congenital heart disease, HIV infection, chronic hemolytic anemia, and portal hypertension [1]. As Group 1 PAH is a rare disease, the more frequent scenario is the patient with PH in the setting of left heart disease (PH-LHD, Group 2) with elevated left-sided cardiac filling pressures as assessed by PCWP or left ventricular end-diastolic pressure. PH-LHD can result from any of a number of pathological or functional abnormalities. In the past, rheumatic mitral stenosis (MS) was the most common cause of this condition; however, today PH-LHD most commonly results from heart failure (HF) related to systolic and/or diastolic dysfunction of the left ventricle [2, 3].

It is well known that elevation of left-sided filing pressures can generate PH by passive or reactive mechanisms; however, it is still unclear what risk factors are involved, how to predict which patient will develop PH, and to what degree.

Most patients will have a passive increase in PAP due to the backward transmission of the elevation of the left atrial pressures. In this case, at the RHC an elevated PCWP and mean PAP will be found together with a normal transpulmonary pressure gradient (TPG; defined as mean PAP minus PCWP, normal values <12 mm Hg) and usually a normal PVR. Interventions which normalize the PCWP, such as diuretic therapy, would also be expected to normalize PAP [3].

In a second, smaller group of patients, a component of the PH is a result of functional and/or structural abnormalities of the distal pulmonary arteries caused by the chronically elevated pressures. These patients will have an increase of mean

PAP with increased TPG (>12 mm Hg) and PVR (>3 Wood units); as opposed to the 'passive' form, lowering the PCWP to normal may not normalize the TPG [2]. These patients can develop severe PH which is also defined as 'reactive' or 'out of proportion'. Pathological changes in this group are characterized by enlarged and thickened pulmonary veins, pulmonary capillary dilatation, interstitial edema, alveolar hemorrhage, and lymphatic vessel and lymph node enlargement. Distal pulmonary arteries may be affected by medial hypertrophy and intimal fibrosis, explaining the 'fixed' component of the elevated PAP [4].

Heart Failure with Reduced Left Ventricular Ejection Fraction

PH is present in about two thirds of the patients with severe HF with reduced left ventricular ejection fraction (LVEF), commonly associated with right ventricular dysfunction [5]. Elevated PAP and abnormal right ventricular function are important determinants of exercise capacity and prognosis in patients with HF and reduced LVEF. When right ventricular failure complicates the course of HF and reduced LVEF, a cardiorenal syndrome with progressive renal insufficiency, hyponatremia, and diuretic resistance may develop. In the advanced stages, patients have severe tricuspid regurgitation due to tricuspid annulus dilatation, with increased jugular venous pressure, chronic liver congestion, ascites, and peripheral edema. Ghio et al. [5] followed 377 patients with moderate-to-severe HF (LVEF <35%) for a median of 17 months after performing RHC. They found that patients with PH and reduced right ventricular function had the worse prognosis and survival among patients with advanced HF and reduced LVEF. The prognosis in patients with normal right ventricular function and PH was similar to that of patients with normal PAP. In contrast, when PAP was normal, reduced right ventricular function did not carry an additional risk. However, a previous study found that right ventricular dysfunction is more common in patients with dilated cardiomyopathy as compared to patients with ischemic cardiomyopathy (65 vs. 16%), although the mean PAP was the same in both groups, suggesting that the impact of PH per se on the prognosis may be difficult to assess.

Reactive and fixed PH is considered to be a contraindication to orthotopic heart transplantation since the right ventricle of the implanted organ will fail acutely due to the high PVR, resulting in allograft failure and death. The risk is directly proportional to both PVR and TPG.

Butler et al. [6] studied 182 patients with baseline normal pulmonary pressures or reversible PH, defined as a decrease in PVR ≤2.5 Wood units, who underwent heart transplantation. Patients with PASP >50 mm Hg and TPG ≥16 had a higher mortality rate, suggesting that pretransplant PH, even when reversible to a PVR ≤2.5 Wood units, is associated with a higher posttransplant mortality rate. Specific values of PVR and TPG have been proposed as risk predictors. HF patients with a TPG <12mm Hg or PVR <3 Wood units are considered suitable with an acceptable risk in most transplant centers, whereas patients with a TPG ≥15 mm Hg or PVR ≥5 Wood units, despite acute reversibility testing, are not considered appropriate candidates. Following a successful transplantation in patients with mild-to-moderate PH, the PAP values tend to normalize over a period of 6–12 months; however, the greater the PH level prior to surgery, the longer the time to resolution. In some patients an incomplete resolution may be observed, with residual elevations in PAP and PVR.

In patients with HF, reduced LVEF, and PH, the traditional therapy for HF, such as diuretics, angiotensin-converting enzyme inhibitors, angiotensin II receptor antagonists, and β-adrenergic blocking agents, may result in the reduction of PH. However, if the patient remains significantly symptomatic despite these measures and moderate-to-severe PH persists, RHC may be indicated in order to clarify the hemodynamic details. Also, a search for other causes of PH should be undertaken such as lung function tests, ventilation-perfusion scanning, and polysomnography.

In case of 'out of proportion' PH despite optimization of the traditional therapy for HF, there are no clear indications for additional measures. In fact, there is no evidence that the drugs approved for PAH are effective and safe in this setting. The main concern is that by decreasing PVR, the consequent increase in venous return to the left ventricle may increase left heart filling pressures, resulting in deterioration rather than improvement.

Early experiences evaluating PAH-specific treatments in the setting of left ventricular failure were disappointing. Sueta et al. [7] studied the efficacy of acute and prolonged effects (12 weeks) of continuous intravenous epoprostenol on 33 patients with severe HF. Epoprostenol administration resulted in significant reductions in mean PAP, PVR, and PCWP, and a marked increase in cardiac output. These beneficial hemodynamic effects persisted with long-term infusions. Based on this and other studies suggesting clinical benefit of intravenous epoprostenol, a large randomized controlled study [Flolan International Randomized Survival Trial (FIRST)] was initiated [8]. The FIRST study randomized 471 patients with advanced HF to receive continuous epoprostenol infusion plus standard care or standard care alone. Although hemodynamic improvement was seen acutely among patients receiving epoprostenol with an increase in cardiac index and a decrease in PCWP and PVR, the study was terminated prematurely due to a strong trend toward increased mortality rates in patients receiving epoprostenol. Based on the findings of this study, chronic use of epoprostenol in patients with HF is considered contraindicated.

Explanations for the increased mortality rates include sympathetic stimulation due to systemic vasodilatory effects and/or unknown detrimental effects of prostanoids in this setting. The more recent data on the inhaled prostacyclin analogue iloprost which apparently show short-term beneficial effects in patients undergoing assessment for heart transplantation, with improvements recorded in mean PAP, PVR, and PCWP during vasoreactivity testing, has to be considered with caution.

Endothelin plasma levels have been shown to be elevated in HF and to correlate with severity. Endothelin plasma levels may contribute to the excessive systemic and pulmonary vasoconstriction that is present in HF. In animal models of HF, treatment with both selective and nonselective endothelin receptor antagonists (ERAs) prevented left ventricular remodeling and improved exercise capacity.

Studies investigating the short-term hemodynamic effect of ERAs in patients with chronic HF were initially encouraging. A randomized placebo-controlled study evaluated the hemodynamic effects of 6-hour infusions of tezosentan compared with placebo in 61 patients with New York Heart Association class III–IV HF. This trial demonstrated increased cardiac index with reduction in PCWP, PVR, and SVR. A short-term study evaluating a 2-week therapy with the nonselective ERA bosentan in 36 patients with symptomatic HF despite treatment with standard regimen resulted in a reduction of both systemic and pulmonary pressures and an increase in cardiac output. These initial encouraging results prompted long-term randomized trials. In the REACH-1 (Research on Endothelin Antagonists in Chronic Heart Failure) study, 370 patients with advanced HF (NYHA functional class IIIB/IV) received bosentan or placebo and were followed-up for 26 weeks. The target dose of bosentan was 500 mg twice a day, much higher than the current recommended dose for PAH. The trial was stopped prematurely due to safety issues, namely elevated liver transaminases, but the question of possible long-term benefit using lower doses was raised based on a trend towards reduction in morbidity and mortality [9]. A larger study, the ENABLE (Endothelin Antagonist Bosentan for Lowering Cardiac Events in Heart Failure) trial evaluated the effects of low-dose bosentan in patients with severe HF (LVEF <35%, NYHA class IIIb/IV). A total of 1,613 patients were randomized to receive either bosentan (125 mg twice a day) or placebo. However, no improvement in outcome was demonstrated between patients treated with bosentan and conventional treatment versus conventional treatment alone. There was an increased risk of early HF exacerbations due to fluid retention in patients treated with bosentan.

The reasons for the lack of efficacy of ERA treatment in HF are unclear and may include the small relevance of the endothelin system activation in patients already treated with the approved drugs for HF. Previous studies in animal models and in humans suggest that endothelial dysfunction is present in HF with a relative deficiency in nitric oxide production. Inhaled nitric oxide administered to patients with HF lowers PVR, increases cardiac index, and improves exercise capacity without altering systemic arterial pressure, suggesting that phosphodiesterase type 5 (PDE5) inhibition may reduce PVR and improve cardiac performance. Furthermore, recent studies reported that PDE5 is also present within cardiac myocytes and PDE5 inhibition resulted in antihypertrophic, antiapoptotic, and ischemic preconditioning effects. Preliminary clinical studies tested the effects of acute administration of sildenafil in patients with PH secondary to systolic HF, and reported that sildenafil improves exercise capacity, gas exchange, and pulmonary hemodynamics in a dose-dependent manner. The hemodynamic benefits are specific to the pulmonary circulation and are most dramatic in patients with severe PH.

Lewis et al. [10] examined the outcomes of 34 patients with symptomatic left ventricular systolic dysfunction and associated PH before and after randomization to either sildenafil or placebo for 12 weeks. Sildenafil improved peak oxygen consumption, PVR, and cardiac output with exercise. There was also improvement in exercise capacity and quality of life [10]. The dose of sildenafil was 50 mg three times daily at completion of the study, which was higher than the dose approved for PAH (20 mg three times a day). We can speculate that higher doses may offer additional benefits, particularly over longer durations of treatment.

A recent study reported 6 patients with severe HF excluded from heart transplantation due to severe PH. The patients were treated with sildenafil 50 mg b.i.d. for 1 month. Five patients had significant reductions in PVR and TPG. However, since no patient had undergone heart transplantation at the time of publication, the clinical relevance of the hemodynamic improvement is unclear. PDE5 inhibitors are the only class of PAH-approved drugs without a formal multicenter randomized trial in HF patients. Therefore, the favorable results observed in small single-center studies are to be considered with extreme caution as similar results were also observed after epoprostenol and ERAs (and contradicted by large clinical trials).

Long-term use of PDE5 inhibitors in HF patients has not been investigated to date and there are concerns that long-term PDE5 inhibition might produce adverse events, such as an increase in mortality rates as seen with milrinone, a PDE3 inhibitor.

Heart Failure with Preserved Left Ventricle Ejection Fraction (Diastolic Heart Failure) and Pulmonary Hypertension

HF with preserved LVEF is a clinical syndrome characterized by the same symptoms and signs of HF with reduced LVEF, and it is usually due to left ventricular diastolic dysfunction [11]. From a conceptual perspective, HF with preserved LVEF occurs when the left ventricle is unable to accommodate an adequate volume of blood during diastole at normal diastolic pressures and maintain an appropriate stroke volume. These abnormalities are caused by a decrease in ventricular relaxation and/or an increase in ventricular stiffness. The prevalence of HF with preserved LVEF increases with age, approaching 50% in HF patients >70 years of age. It is more common among women and major risk factors include systemic hypertension, ischemic heart disease, diabetes, and obesity. The clinical manifestations of HF with preserved LVEF may not differ from those of PAH and are characterized by dyspnea on exercise and eventually overt right ventricular failure and peripheral edema. However, important and distinctive symptoms are orthopnea and paroxysmal nocturnal dyspnea, both of which are not features of PAH.

The prevalence and severity of PH in patients with HF with preserved LVEF is poorly defined. Klapholz et al. [12] reported a mean systolic PAP of 47 ± 17 mm Hg in 44% of 272 patients hospitalized for exacerbation of HF with normal LVEF on echocardiography. A community-based study of 244 patients with HF with preserved LVEF (age 76 ± 13 years; 45% males) reported that PH was highly prevalent (83%), often severe (median PSAP was 48 mm Hg, measured by echocardiography), and strongly predictive of mortality. The development of PH was related to the extent of pulmonary venous hypertension as estimated by Doppler indexes. However, after accounting for this passive component of PH, the severity of PH suggests that some cases may have been affected by 'out of proportion' PH. A retrospective analysis of 477 consecutive echocardiographic studies in subjects with HF with preserved LVEF demonstrated an association between the severity and grade of diastolic dysfunction and estimated PAP.

Echocardiography may provide a broad estimation of the left ventricular diastolic dysfunction; however, in patients with chronic atrial fibrillation, the assessment of left ventricular diastolic function is difficult.

Interestingly, 'borderline' PCWP at rest may be found on RHC in patients with HF with preserved LVEF and PH, particularly if diuretics are used. In this scenario, an exercise test or fluid challenge at the time of RHC may induce an increase of PCWP. However, there is no consensus on specific protocols for both exercise and fluid challenge, and age-related PCWP normal values are not available in these settings.

The relationship of the metabolic syndrome to HF with preserved LVEF is increasingly recognized. Compared with patients with HF and reduced LVEF, individuals with HF with preserved LVEF are typically older and more likely to be women, with a higher likelihood of having hypertension (prevalence up to 88%), obesity (prevalence of BMI >30 approx. 40%), and atrial fibrillation [13]. In conjunction, the prevalence of diabetes (about 30%) and coronary artery disease (40–50% of patients with HF with preserved LVEF) are substantial, being similar to that in patients with HF and reduced LVEF [14]. Individuals with the metabolic syndrome and normal left ventricular systolic function frequently show abnormalities in left ventricular diastolic function (i.e. impaired relaxation). These findings are also evident in subjects with only one or two metabolic syndrome criteria (or premetabolic syndrome), and components of the metabolic syndrome such as hypertension and obesity are independent predictors for the development of HF with preserved LVEF. Whether the presence of the metabolic syndrome also confers increased risk for PH is unknown, although it might be a plausible hypothesis. A recent study reported 17 patients (77% females) with diastolic dysfunction and pulmonary venous hypertension which were characterized by two or more features of the metabolic syndrome [14]. The majority of patients reported to have 'out of proportion' PH associated with HF with preserved LVEF were obese postmenopausal women. The decrease of estrogens in the postmenopausal period may alter endothelial homeostasis. The effects of estrogen on the pulmonary vasculature are complex and not fully understood. Estrogens increase prostacyclin release and enhance the production of nitric oxide.

Additionally, estrogens downregulate the gene expression of endothelin. In animal models, estrogens or hormone replacement therapy have been shown to attenuate the severity of PH and increase survival. Studies in scleroderma patients suggest that estrogen replacement therapy may prevent the development of PH. On the other hand, it is known that adipose tissue is a storage site for estrogens and that obesity is a high-leptin state; both factors are considered to be angoigenic. In postmenopausal women, plasma leptin levels fall but hormone replacement therapy causes an increase in leptin production and in VEGF serum levels. A previous study [15] reported that 47.6% of 467 women with severe PH (defined as mean PAP >45 mm Hg by RHC) were obese (BMI >30) and 43% received estrogen replacement therapy. One additional study collected information from 88 women with severe PH: 46% of them met the criteria for obesity, 81% reported prior use of replacement hormone therapy, and 70% reported treatment lasting longer than 10 years.

Obesity is considered to be a risk factor for the development of PH and has been shown to increase right ventricular wall thickness and volume [16]. Furthermore, recent studies have shown a correlation between right heart dysfunction and increased weight. Obstructive sleep apnea is common in obese patients and increased BMI is associated with worsening degrees of obstructive sleep apnea. Severe obstructive sleep apnea was found to be independently associated with PH and directly related to the severity of disease and presence of diastolic dysfunction. During sleep, repetitive chronic upper airway collapse and oxygen desaturation can lead to hypoxic pulmonary vasoconstriction that eventually can result in PH. However, it is not known to what degree obstructive sleep apnea, independent of coexisting pulmonary or heart disease, contributes to sustain daytime PH. Furthermore, it is unclear whether obesity by itself has a role in the development of PH. An epidemiological study reported that the prevalence of PH in obstructive sleep apnea syndrome patients ranges from 17 to 52%, with most patients suffering from relatively mild disease. Treatment of obstructive sleep apnea with continuous positive airway pressure can lower daytime PAP, which suggests that it is plausible that obstructive sleep apnea may be an independent cause of PH [17].

Diabetes as a predictor of subsequent HF was first described in the Framingham Heart Study. Recently, the association between diabetes or impaired glucose regulation and altered left ventricular function has been reported. Insulin may act as a growth factor in the myocardium and sustained hyperinsulinemia has been shown to increase myocardial mass and decrease cardiac output in rats. A recent study reported that insulin resistance increased the stimulating effects of angiotensin II on cellular hypertrophy and collagen production in individuals with hypertension, leading to myocardial hypertrophy and fibrosis and diastolic HF. Furthermore, insulin resistance was related to advanced HF with poor prognosis.

Insulin resistance may also be linked to PH. Reduced pulmonary mRNA expression of peroxisome proliferator-activated receptor-γ (PPAR-γ), a ligand-activated nuclear receptor and transcription factor that regulates adipogenesis and glucose metabolism was found in patients with PAH [18]. Furthermore, reduced pulmonary mRNA expression of apolipoprotein E (apoE), a protective factor known to reduce circulating oxidized low-density lipoprotein and atherogenesis in the vessel wall was also reported. Deficiency of both PPAR-γ and apoE has been linked to insulin resistance and the metabolic syndrome. A recent study reported that insulin resistance, low plasma adiponectin levels, and deficiency of apoE may be risk factors for PAH and that PPAR-γ activation can reverse PH in an animal model.

Systemic hypertension and peripheral vascular stiffness are known as an independent risk factor for the development of HF with preserved LVEF. Furthermore, recent studies have demonstrated that the metabolic syndrome amplifies the age-associated increases in vascular thickness and stiffness. Vascular stiffness, in turn, may contribute not only to the development of HF with preserved LVEF, but may also involve directly the pulmonary vasculature leading to increased PVR and PAP.

Since the mechanisms underlying HF with preserved LVEF are still under debate, it is not surprising that there is no evidence-based treatment for patients with HF with preserved LVEF, and obviously there are no data on the treatment approach to patients complicated by PH. Treatment of HF with preserved LVEF is primarily linked to the underlying etiology. Aggressive management of systemic hypertension should be instituted, especially in patients with left ventricular hypertrophy and diabetes mellitus. Sodium restriction and judicious use of diuretics and nitrates to relieve symptoms of congestion along with drugs that slow the heart rate and improve diastolic filling time, such as β-blockers and the calcium channel blockers. Recently, several studies have demonstrated that angiotensin II receptor antagonist drugs improve exercise tolerance in this setting. The CHARM (Candesartan in Heart Failure: Assessment of Reduction in Mortality and Morbidity)-Preserved trial suggested that treatment with candesartan reduces hospitalization related to diastolic HF, although there were no effects on mortality [19].

Apparently, despite the normalization of the left atrial pressures, a proportion of these patients are still left with significant PH. Whether modification of the metabolic syndrome features such as dietary control, weight reduction, and blood pressure control would result in an improvement of symptoms and PAP in patients with HF with preserved LVEF is still an open question and worth investigation.

An additional question is whether PAH-specific therapy may be beneficial or detrimental in patients with 'out of proportion' PH and HF with preserved LVEF. The evolving data on the possible advantages of PDE5 inhibition, discussed above, promoted the initiation of the RELAX trial, which is trying to address the effectiveness of sildenafil in patients with a clinical diagnosis of HF and LVEF ≥50%, focusing on exercise capacity as the primary endpoint.

Mitral and Aortic Valve Disease and Pulmonary Hypertension

Development of PH in association with mitral valve disease has been shown to be a marker of severity. PH frequently complicates MS and may significantly influence long-term prognosis [20]. The increase in PAP may be out of proportion to the degree of left atrial pressure increase, reflecting an increase in PVR. Elevation of PVR is an important pathophysiological event in MS, and the level of PAP is an indicator of surgical risk. Interestingly, there is a subset of mildly symptomatic patients with severe MS and severe PH who are usually young and have preserved sinus rhythm.

Several clinical studies have shown that removing the mitral valve gradient, either surgically or with percutaneous balloon valvuloplasty, will result in an immediate fall in PAP. The degree of the fall, however, can be quite variable, with some patients achieving normal hemodynamics immediately following the procedure while others require many months to improve. Fawzy et al. [21] reported that in patients with MS and severe PH, the pulmonary pressure regressed to normal levels over 6–12 months after successful mitral balloon valvuloplasty. The magnitude and rate of regression may be related to the severity of the pulmonary vascular disease which in turn may be related to the duration of PH and to constitutional factors. These may either induce more severe vascular disease or slow the reverse remodeling of the obstructive changes in the distal pulmonary arteries.

PH can also occur in patients with mitral regurgitation (MR). The presence of PH in patients with MR may be associated with decreased cardiac output and it conveys a poor prognosis. Rosenhek et al. [22] evaluated the outcome of a watchful waiting strategy in patients with asymptomatic severe MR until they were referred to surgery when symptoms occurred or when asymptomatic patients developed left ventricular dilatation, left ventricular dysfunction, PH, or recurrent atrial fibrillation. Only 5 of 132 patients, followed for a median of 62 months, developed new onset of atrial fibrillation or PH. These findings are in correlation with the ACC/AHA guidelines for the management of patients with valvular heart disease [23], which recommend mitral valve surgery for asymptomatic patients with chronic severe MR, preserved left ventricular function, and PH (pulmonary artery systolic pressure >50 mm Hg at rest or >60 mm Hg with exercise).

PH frequently complicates the perioperative management of patients undergoing mitral valve surgery and may be aggravated by the endothelial dysfunction due to the cardiopulmonary bypass procedure. Exacerbation of PH may result in acute right ventricular failure, which is associated with high morbidity and mortality. A recent study randomized 20 patients with chronic PH undergoing mitral valve repair to receive inhaled iloprost or intravenous nitroglycerine. The drugs were administered during the weaning from cardiopulmonary bypass. Inhaled iloprost selectively decreased PVR index and TPG with an associated improvement in indices of right ventricular function and was apparently more pulmonary-selective than intravenous nitrogylycerine. However, the real clinical benefit of these effects is not clear.

PH in the setting of aortic valve stenosis and/or regurgitation is less common than in mitral valve diseases. Silver et al. [24] performed RHCs in 45 patients with aortic stenosis. In 13 patients (29%), PH, defined as pulmonary artery systolic pressure >50 mm Hg, was found. Patients with aortic stenosis and PH had a higher incidence of congestive HF, a lower LVEF and cardiac index, and more MR as compared with patients with aortic stenosis and normal PAP. Eight of the 13 patients had a TPG ≥10 mm Hg, suggesting a reactive component of the elevated PAP.

Malouf et al. [25] analyzed the clinical characteristics and outcomes of 47 patients (mean age: 78 years) with severe PH and severe aortic stenosis. Aortic valve replacement was performed in 37 patients (79%) and 10 patients (21%) were treated conservatively. Fifteen patients died (32%) in the group that underwent aortic valve replacement, whereas mortality was much higher in the conservatively treated group – 80% on follow-up. Severe PH as opposed to the severity of left ventricular systolic dysfunction or concomitant coronary artery bypass grafting was an independent predictor of perioperative mortality. However, it seems that the prognosis for patients with aortic stenosis and severe PH treated conservatively without aortic valve replacement is dismal. Although aortic valve replacement is associated with higher mortality in presence of PH, the potential benefits outweigh the risk of surgery.

The incidence of PH (pulmonary artery systolic pressure ≥60 mm Hg) in 139 patients with severe aortic regurgitation was reported to be 24%. All patients had high left-sided filling pressures, suggesting that PH was a consequence of severe long-standing regurgitation with ventricular dysfunction. Aortic valve replacement in the patients with severe aortic regurgitation and PH resulted in decreased PVR and normalization of the PAP in most patients with no increased mortality compared to patients with no PH.

Conclusion

LHD is the most common cause of PH and is usually linked to HF either with impaired or preserved LVEF as well as mitral and aortic valve disease. The presence of PH in patients who have LHD predicts a poor outcome. In a subgroup of patients, the elevation of PAP appears to be out of proportion to the elevated left-sided filling pressures. The exact mechanisms for this phenomenon are currently unknown.

The optimal treatment of the underlying LHD is recommended in patients with PH due to LHD. Patients with 'out of proportion' PH due to LHD should follow the same indication. In this setting, only appropriately sized and long-term randomized controlled studies may define the safety and efficacy of PAH-approved drugs.

References

1 Galiè N, Hoeper MM, Humbert M, Torbicki A, Vachiery JL, Barbera JA, Beghetti M, Corris P, Gaine S, Gibbs JS, Gomez-Sanchez MA, Jondeau G, Klepetko W, Opitz C, Peacock A, Rubin L, Zellweger M, Simonneau G, ESC Committee for Practice Guidelines (CPG): Guidelines for the diagnosis and treatment of pulmonary hypertension: the Task Force for the Diagnosis and Treatment of Pulmonary Hypertension of the European Society of Cardiology (ESC) and the European Respiratory Society (ERS), endorsed by the International Society of Heart and Lung Transplantation (ISHLT). Eur Heart J 2009;30:2493–2537.

2 Oudiz RJ: Pulmonary hypertension associated with left-sided heart disease. Clin Chest Med 2007;28:233–241.

3 Rich S, Rabinovitch M: Diagnosis and treatment of secondary (non-category 1) pulmonary hypertension. Circulation 2008;118:2190–2199.

4 Pietra GG CF, Stewart S, Leone O, Humbert M, Robbins IM, Reid LM, Tuder RM: Pathologic assessment of vasculopathies in pulmonary hypertensio. J Am Coll Cardiol 2004;43:25S–32S.

5 Ghio S, Gavazzi A, Campana C, Inserra C, Klersy C, Sebastiani R, Arbustini E, Recusani F, Tavazzi L: Independent and additive prognostic value of right ventricular systolic function and pulmonary artery pressure in patients with chronic heart failure. J Am Coll Cardiol 2001;37:183–188.

6 Butler J, Stankewicz MA, Wu J, Chomsky DB, Howser RL, Khadim G, Davis SF, Pierson RN 3rd, Wilson JR: Pre-transplant reversible pulmonary hypertension predicts higher risk for mortality after cardiac transplantation. J Heart Lung Transplant 2005;24:170–177.

7 Sueta CA, Gheorghiade M, Adams K, Bourge RC, Murali S, Uretsky BF, Pritzker MR, McGoon MD, Butman SM, Grossman SH: Safety and efficacy of epoprostenol in patients with severe congestive heart failure. Am J Cardiol 1995;75:34A-43A.

8 Califf RM, Adams KA, McKenna WJ, Gheorghiade M, Uretsky BF, McNulty SE, Darius H, Schulman K, Zannad F, Handberg-Thurmond E, Harrell FE Jr, Wheeler W, Soler-Soler J, Swedberg K: A randomized controlled trial of epoprostenol therapy for severe congestive heart failure: the Flolan International Randomized Survival Trial (FIRST). Am Heart J 1997;134:44–54.

9 Mylona P, Cleland JG: Update of REACH-1 and MERIT-HF clinical trials in heart failure. Cardio net Editorial Team. Eur J Heart Fail 1999;1:197–200.

10 Lewis GD, Shah R, Shahzad K, Camuso JM, Pappagianopoulos PP, Hung J, Tawakol A, Gerszten RE, Systrom DM, Bloch KD, Semigran MJ: Sildenafi l improves exercise capacity and quality of life in patients with systolic heart failure and secondary pulmonary hypertension. Circulation 2007;116:1555–1562.

11 Paulus WJ, Tschope C, Sanderson JE, Rusconi C, Flachskampf FA, Rademakers FE, Marino P, Smiseth OA, De Keulenaer G, Leite-Moreira AF, Borbély A, Edes I, Handoko ML, Heymans S, Pezzali N, Pieske B, Dickstein K, Fraser AG, Brutsaert DL: How to diagnose diastolic heart failure: a consensus statement on the diagnosis of heart failure with a normal ejection fraction by the Heart Failure and Echocardiography Associations of the European Society of cardiology. Eur Heart J 2007;28:2539–2550.

12 Klapholz M, Maurer M, Lowe AM, Messineo F, Meisner JS, Mitchell J, Kalman J, Phillips RA, Steingart R, Brown EJ Jr, Berkowitz R, Moskowitz R, Soni A, Mancini D, Bijou R, Sehhat K, Varshneya N, Kukin M, Katz SD, Sleeper LA, Le Jemtel TH, New York Heart Failure Consortium: Hospitalization for heart failure in the presence of a normal left ventricular ejection fraction: results of the New York Heart Failure Registry. J Am Coll Cardiol 2004;43:1432–1438.

13 Hogg K, Swedberg K, McMurray J: Heart failure with preserved left ventricular systolic function; epidemiology, clinical characteristics, and prognosis. J Am Coll Cardiol 2004;43:317–327.

14 Robbins IM, Newman JH, Johnson RF, Hemnes AR, Fremont RD, Piana RN, Zhao DX, Byrne DW: Association of the metabolic syndrome with pulmonary venous hypertension. Chest 2009;136:31–36.

15 Taraseviciute A, Voelkel NF: Severe pulmonary hypertension in postmenopausal obese women. Eur J Med Res 2006;11:198–202.

16 Amad K, Brennan J, Alexander J: The cardiac pathology of chronic exogenous obesity. Circulation 1965;32:740–745.

17 Arias M, García-Río F, Alonso-Fernández A, Martínez I, Villamor J: Pulmonary hypertension in obstructive sleep apnoea: effects of continuous positive airway pressure: a randomized, controlled cross-over study. Eur Heart J 2006;27:1106–1113.

18 Ameshima S, Golpon H, Cool CD, Chan D, Vandivier RW, Gardai SJ,Wick M, Nemenoff RA, Geraci MW, Voelkel NF: Peroxisome proliferator-activated receptor gamma (PPARgamma) expression is decreased in pulmonary hypertension and affects endothelial cell growth. Circ Res 2003;92:1162–1169.

19 Yusuf S, Pfeffer MA, Swedberg K, Granger CB, Held P, McMurray JJ, Michelson EL, Olofsson B, Ostergren J: CHARM Investigators and Committees. Effects of candesartan in patients with chronic heart failure and preserved left-ventricular ejection fraction: the CHARM-Preserved trial. Lancet 2003;362:777–781.

20 Walston A, Peter RH, Morris JJ, Kong Y, Behar VS: Clinical implications of pulmonary hypertension in mitral stenosis. Am J Cardiol 1973;32:650–655.

21 Fawzy ME, Hassan W, Stefadouros M, Moursi M, El Shaer F, Chaudhary MA: Prevalence and fate of severe pulmonary hypertension in 559 consecutive patients with severe rheumatic mitral stenosis undergoing mitral balloon valvotomy. J Heart Valve Dis 2004;13:942–947.

22 Rosenhek R, Rader F, Klaar U, Gabriel H, Krejc M, Kalbeck D, Schemper M, Maurer G, Baumgartner H: Outcome of watchful waiting in asymptomatic severe mitral regurgitation. Circulation 2006;113:2238–2244.

23 Bonow RO, Carabello BA, Chatterjee K, de Leon AC Jr, Faxon DP, Freed MD, Gaasch WH, Lytle BW, Nishimura RA, O'Gara PT, O'Rourke RA, Otto CM, Shah PM, Shanewise JS, Smith SC Jr, Jacobs AK, Adams CD, Anderson JL, Antman EM, Fuster V, Halperin JL, Hiratzka LF, Hunt SA, Lytle BW, Nishimura R, Page RL, Riegel B: ACC/AHA 2006 guidelines for the management of patients with valvular heart disease: a report of the American College of Cardiology/American Heart Association Task Force on Practice Guidelines (Writing Committee to Revise the 1998 Guidelines for the Management of Patients with Valvular Heart Disease) developed in collaboration with the Society of Cardiovascular Anesthesiologists endorsed by the Society for Cardiovascular Angiography and Interventions and the Society of Thoracic Surgeons. J Am Coll Cardiol 2006;48:1–149.

24 Silver K, Aurigemma G, Krendel S, Barry N, Ockene I, Alpert J: Pulmonary artery hypertension in severe aortic stenosis: incidence and mechanism. Am Heart J 1993;125:146–150.

25 Malouf JF, Enriquez-Sarano M, Pellikka PA, Oh JK, Bailey KR, Chandrasekaran K, Mullany CJ, Tajik AJ: Severe pulmonary hypertension in patients with severe aortic valve stenosis: clinical profile and prognostic implications. J Am Coll Cardiol 2002;40:789–795.

Yochai Adir, MD
Pulmonary Divison, Carmel Medical Center
7 Michal St., Haifa (Israel)
Tel. +972 4 825 8342, E-Mail adir-sh@zahav.net.il

Chapter 18
Humbert M, Souza R, Simonneau G (eds): Pulmonary Vascular Disorders.
Prog Respir Res. Basel, Karger, 2012, vol 41, pp 169–177

Pulmonary Hypertension in Chronic Obstructive Pulmonary Disease

Emmanuel Weitzenblum[a] · Ari Chaouat[b] · Matthieu Canuet[a] · Alain Ducoloné[a] · Romain Kessler[a]

[a]Department of Pulmonology, Nouvel Hôpital Civil, Strasbourg, [b]Department of Respiratory Diseases and Respiratory Intensive Care, CHU de Nancy, Vandoeuvre les Nancy, Nancy, France

Abstract

Pulmonary hypertension (PH) is a common complication of advanced chronic obstructive pulmonary disease (COPD) and its presence is associated with decreased survival. Owing to its frequency, COPD is by far the most common cause of PH. PH is consecutive to the elevation of pulmonary vascular resistance which is due to functional and morphological factors (chronic alveolar hypoxia is the most important). PH is generally mild to moderate, with mean pulmonary artery pressure (PAP) usually ranging between 20 and 35 mm Hg at rest in a stable state of the disease. A small proportion of COPD patients may present a severe or 'disproportionate' PH with a resting PAP >35–40 mm Hg. The prognosis is poor in these patients; PH usually worsens during exercise, sleep, and severe exacerbations of the disease. These acute increases in afterload may favor the development of right heart failure. The diagnosis of PH relies on Doppler echocardiography, and right heart catheterization is needed in a minority of patients. Treatment of PH in COPD relies on long-term oxygen therapy (≥16 h/day), which generally stabilizes, or at least attenuates, and sometimes reverses the progression of PH. 'New' vasodilator drugs have rarely been used in COPD. Patients with severe PH should be referred to a specialist PH center where the possibility of inclusion in controlled clinical trials should be considered.

Chronic obstructive pulmonary disease (COPD) is a major cause of morbidity and mortality with an increasing prevalence during the past decades [1]. One established complication of advanced COPD is the development of pulmonary hypertension (PH). Typically, PH appears when airflow limitation is severe and is associated with chronic alveolar hypoxia.

In the present classification of PH, Group 3 is entitled 'Pulmonary Hypertension Associated with Lung Diseases and/or Hypoxemia' [2]. That group includes COPD, interstitial lung diseases, alveolar hypoventilation disorders, and other less frequent causes of PH. Owing to its frequency, COPD is by far the most common cause of PH.

With time, PH may lead to the development of right ventricular enlargement which may result in right ventricular failure, but it should be emphasized that PH is only one among several complications of advanced COPD and that the prognosis of COPD is linked to the severity of respiratory insufficiency rather than the occurrence of PH, which is essentially a 'marker' of long-standing hypoxemia [3].

This chapter is devoted to PH resulting from COPD with the aim to cover all aspects of PH in COPD, from epidemiology to therapy.

Definitions

The current definition of PH is resting mean pulmonary artery pressure (PAP) ≥25 mm Hg [2, 4]. It is accepted that normal mean PAP is between 8 and 20 mm Hg [2, 4–6]. In the past, PH complicating chronic respiratory disease was generally defined by resting PAP >20 mm Hg [7], which is slightly different from the present definition of PH [2, 4] and is explained by the fact that a resting PAP >20 mm Hg was considered as being abnormal, even in elderly subjects. These various definitions should be kept in mind when comparing studies, particularly in terms of prevalence of PH in COPD [8].

Severe PH in COPD could be defined by PAP >35 or >40 mm Hg in patients investigated at rest during a stable state of the disease, but there is in fact no consensual definition of severe PH in COPD [8].

In the 'natural history' of COPD, PH is often preceded by an abnormally large increase in PAP during exercise, defined by a mean pressure >30 mm Hg for a mild level of exercise [9]. The term 'exercising pulmonary hypertension' has been used, but the term 'pulmonary hypertension' should be reserved for resting PH [10].

Prevalence of Pulmonary Hypertension in Chronic Obstructive Pulmonary Disease

Determination of prevalence of PH in COPD has been impeded by difficulties in obtaining valid data from an adequate sample of COPD. The main reason is that right heart catheterization (RHC), the gold standard for the diagnosis of PH, cannot be performed on a large scale in COPD patients for ethical reasons, and Doppler echocardiography, which is the best noninvasive method [11], is often inaccurate in COPD patients [12].

Studies from hospital-based samples are available, but they have no real epidemiological value. The prevalence of PH defined by PAP >20 mm Hg ranges from 35 to more than 90% [13–17]. In the studies conducted by Scharf et al. [15], Thabut et al. [16], and Chaouat et al. [17], 5, 13.5, and 5.8% of the COPD patients had severe PH (PAP >35 mm Hg), respectively.

The study by Williams and Nicholl [18] aimed to determine the prevalence of subjects at risk of developing PH (markedly hypoxemic COPD) in the general population (of Sheffield, UK). They estimated that 0.3% of adults aged ≥45 years were at risk. Extrapolating for England and Wales, this would represent 60,000 subjects. However, these data were obtained more than 20 years ago, whereas the incidence and prevalence of COPD have markedly increased in recent years. The prevalence of COPD is estimated to be approximately 5% in the adult population in most European countries [19] and 6% of COPD patients have severe or very severe disease and are at risk of PH [8] (this would represent approx. 1.5 million patients for Europe).

Pathology

The structural basis of PH in COPD includes three potential mechanisms: remodeling, reduction in the total number of pulmonary vessels, and pulmonary thrombosis. However, the only demonstrated morphological basis is the remodeling of pulmonary arteries and arterioles. Remodeling includes muscularization of pulmonary arterioles (<80 μm), which can extend to the periphery in precapillary vessels (20 μm), and changes in the intima: intimal thickening is observed in muscular pulmonary arteries and in pulmonary arterioles [20, 21]. These intimal lesions are characterized by the development of longitudinal muscle and fibrosis. The other component of intimal thickness is the occurrence of inner muscular tubes, i.e. a new layer of circular smooth muscle sandwiched between internal and external lamina in pulmonary arterioles [20].

It has been known for many years that pulmonary vascular remodeling is present not only in end-stage COPD, but also in patients with mild COPD [21–23]. It has been shown in recent years that smokers with normal lung function may also develop intimal thickening in pulmonary muscular arteries [24]. These structural abnormalities could be the consequence of endothelial dysfunction of pulmonary arteries, probably induced by cigarette smoke [24]. However, the clinical relevance of these early abnormalities is presently unknown and it should be emphasized that they have been observed in mild COPD patients and in smokers not exhibiting PH.

Pathophysiology

Three variables can contribute to the elevation of PAP: pulmonary artery 'capillary' pressure (PCP; also known as wedge pressure or occlusion pressure), cardiac output, and pulmonary vascular resistance (PVR).

The role of an elevated cardiac output is in COPD almost negligible. An abnormally elevated PCP at rest has been observed by some authors in a relatively high percentage of COPD patients [15, 25]. However, many of these patients had associated left heart disease [25]. One hypothesis is that the increase in intrathoracic pressure in emphysematous patients may induce an increase in PCP. This has been frequently observed during exercise [26] and has been attributed to dynamic hyperinflation [27]. Actually, at rest and during a steady state of the disease, PCP is most often normal in COPD patients not exhibiting associated significant left heart disease. Thus, PH is precapillary, almost exclusively accounted for by the increased PVR [10, 28].

The factors leading to an increased PVR in COPD are listed in table 1. These factors are numerous, but alveolar hypoxia is predominant. Two distinct mechanisms of action of alveolar hypoxia must be considered: acute alveolar hypoxia causes pulmonary vasoconstriction, and chronic

Table 1. Factors leading to increased PVR in COPD

Factors	Consequences on pulmonary hemodynamics and pulmonary vascular bed
Emphysema	reduction (destruction) of the pulmonary vascular bed
Airway obstruction	increased intrathoracic (and intravascular) pressure during expiration
Acute alveolar hypoxia[1]	pulmonary vasoconstriction
Chronic alveolar hypoxia[1]	pulmonary vascular remodeling
Polycythemia	hyperviscosity
Lung and systemic inflammation	pulmonary vascular remodeling (including pulmonary arterial fibrosis)

[1] Most important factor.

hypoxia induces with time structural changes in the pulmonary vascular bed, i.e. remodeling of the pulmonary vasculature [29].

Acute hypoxia induces in humans, as well as in almost all species of mammals, a rise of PVR and PAP that is accounted for by hypoxic pulmonary vasoconstriction [30, 31]. Hypoxic pulmonary vasoconstriction is observed in normal subjects [31] as well as in patients with chronic respiratory disease [32]. This vasoconstriction is localized in the resistance pulmonary arteries (<500 μm) and its precise mechanism has recently been better identified [33]. There has been a marked improvement of the knowledge of the smooth muscle cell potassium channels involved in the regulation of the pulmonary vasomotor tone [33] and of the endothelium-derived mediators [34]. In normal humans, the reactivity of the pulmonary circulation to acute hypoxia varies from one individual to another and this interindividual variability is also found in COPD patients [35], but the potential clinical consequences of this variability are presently unknown. The situations which bear the closest analogy with acute hypoxic challenges are severe exacerbations of COPD leading to acute respiratory failure and the sleep-related episodes of worsening hypoxemia.

PH is generally observed in COPD patients exhibiting pronounced chronic hypoxemia [arterial oxygen tension (PaO_2) <55–60 mm Hg). There is some degree of similarity between the structural changes observed in COPD patients exhibiting PH ('remodeling' of the pulmonary vascular bed) and those present in healthy people living at altitudes >3,500 m [36], which suggests that alveolar hypoxia is the main cause of the pulmonary vascular remodeling in COPD even though this concept has been challenged by the results of one morphological study [20].

Chronic alveolar hypoxia is not the only factor leading to elevated PVR. Patients with advanced COPD have marked morphological changes of the lung (including loss of capillaries and reduction of the pulmonary vascular bed), particularly when emphysema is severe, and these changes could partly account for the increased PVR [15, 20].

It has been hypothesized that inflammation of the pulmonary arteries could contribute to pulmonary vascular remodeling in COPD and to the elevation of PVR [37]. However, few studies have confirmed this hypothesis [38]. It has also been recently shown that systemic inflammation increases the risk of developing PH in COPD [39, 40]. The issue of the role of inflammation in PH complicating COPD remains controversial [41].

Finally, the occurrence and the degree of severity of PH in COPD could be modulated by genetic factors as suggested by recent studies [42, 43]. Much more studies are needed in this field.

Diagnosis of Pulmonary Hypertension in Chronic Obstructive Pulmonary Disease

Symptoms and physical signs are of little help in the diagnosis of PH. Dyspnea is present in advanced COPD patients with and without PH. Dyspnea is the consequence of airflow limitation and pulmonary hyperinflation rather than PH.

Physical signs occur late, being observed at an advanced stage of the disease far after the development of PH. Peripheral (ankle) edema is the best sign of right heart failure (RHF), but it is not specific and can arise from other causes (in some patients with PH it does not occur at all). A murmur of tricuspid regurgitation, suggesting right ventricular dilatation, is rarely present in COPD patients, which can be explained by the mild-to-moderate degree of PH in COPD.

The detection of right ventricular hypertrophy by electrocardiography has high specificity but low sensitivity. A normal ECG does not exclude the presence of PH in COPD patients [44]. Similarly the radiological signs of PH lack both sensitivity and specificity [44].

Magnetic resonance imaging is probably the best method for the measurement of right ventricular ejection fraction [45], right ventricular mass, and the diameter of the pulmonary artery, but its role in the diagnosis strategy of PH in COPD is not well established. Doppler echocardiography is by far the best method for a noninvasive diagnosis of PH [11]. The maximum velocity of the tricuspid regurgitation jet allows the calculation of the right ventricular-to-right atrial gradient according to the Bernoulli equation. The gradient is added to right atrial pressure (5 or 10 mm Hg) to give an estimated value of right ventricular systolic pressure that is equal to pulmonary artery systolic pressure. With the same technique (continuous wave Doppler echocardiography), it is possible in case of pulmonary regurgitation to estimate the pulmonary artery diastolic pressure.

However, in COPD the chance of obtaining tricuspid regurgitation signals of sufficient quality is generally low [46]. In the large series (n = 374) of candidates for lung transplantation (most of them being COPD) investigated by Arcasoy et al. [12], the estimation of systolic PAP was possible in only 44% of the patients, and 52% of pressure estimations were found to be inaccurate when compared with pressures measured during RHC (>10 mm Hg difference). In a recent study [47], the bias of Doppler echocardiography in the measurement of systolic PAP compared with RHC was 2.8 mm Hg (95% CI: 18.7–24.0), which is high when one takes into account the modest level of PH (PAP <35 mm Hg in most COPD patients).

PAP can also be estimated from Doppler pulmonary flow velocity curves since the correlations between PAP and the time to peak pulmonary blood velocity (acceleration time measured by pulsed Doppler echocardiography) are strong [48]. To our knowledge the evaluation of right ventricular dysfunction with the Tei index and the tricuspid annular displacement has not been performed in COPD patients [8]. Plasma brain natriuretic peptide could be a biomarker of PH in chronic lung diseases [49], but studies are needed to determine whether it is a useful diagnostic tool in COPD patients.

RHC continues to be the gold standard for the diagnosis of PH [10, 28]. It allows the direct measurement of PAP, PCP, right heart filling pressures, and cardiac output. Measurements can be repeated after therapeutic interventions (oxygen, vasodilators). The major drawback of RHC is indeed its invasive nature. Furthermore, there is no evidence-based study demonstrating its clinical value in advanced COPD. Therefore RHC cannot be used routinely.

In COPD patients, Doppler echocardiography must be performed when PH is suspected (patients with chronic hypoxemia, severe and very severe COPD, i.e. stages 3 and 4 of the GOLD classification). The indications for RHC should be limited to the cases where there is a suspicion of severe PH (systolic pressure estimated from Doppler echocardiography >50–60 mm Hg. RHC can help to differentiate diastolic left heart failure from severe precapillary PH in COPD. Accordingly, RHC may be useful for prescribing the most appropriate treatment.

Table 2. Comparison of PH in COPD, IPAH, and CTEPH from three studies

	COPD	IPAH	CTEPH
Study	[14]	[50]	[51]
Patients, n	62	259	500
Age, years	55 ± 8	50	–
FEV_1, ml	1,170 ± 390	–	–
FEV_1, % predicted	–	>70	–
PaO_2, mm Hg	60	–	–
$PaCO_2$, mm Hg	45	–	–
PAP, mm Hg	26 ± 6	56	46
PCP, mm Hg	8 ± 2	8	8
Cardiac output, l/min/m^2	3.8 ± 1.1	2.3	2.2

Values are means ± SD. FEV_1 = Forced expiratory volume in 1 s; $PaCO_2$ = arterial carbon dioxide tension.

Main features of Pulmonary Hypertension in Chronic Obstructive Pulmonary Disease

The main characteristic of PH in COPD is probably its mild-to-moderate degree, with resting PAP in a stable state of the disease usually ranging between 20 and 35 mm Hg. This modest degree of PH, well recognized in COPD [14], is very different from other causes of PH such as chronic thromboembolic PH (CTEPH) and idiopathic pulmonary arterial hypertension (IPAH), where PAP is usually >40–50 mm Hg. Table 2 compares the pulmonary hemodynamic data of COPD patients exhibiting PH [14, 17], a series of patients from the French Registry of Pulmonary Hypertension [50] and a series of CTEPH from San Diego (Calif., USA) [51]. It can be seen that PH is severe in IPAH (mean PAP of 56 mm Hg) and CTEPH (46 mm Hg), but is rather mild in COPD (26 and 25 mm Hg, respectively). In COPD, when PH occurs, PVR is moderately increased and cardiac output is in the normal range, contrasting with IPAH and CTEPH (table 2). A PAP >40 mm Hg is unusual in COPD patients, except when they are investigated during an acute exacerbation [10] or when there is an associated cardiopulmonary disease [8]. The consequences of the modest level of PH include the absence or late occurrence of RHF. However, PH, even if mild at baseline, may

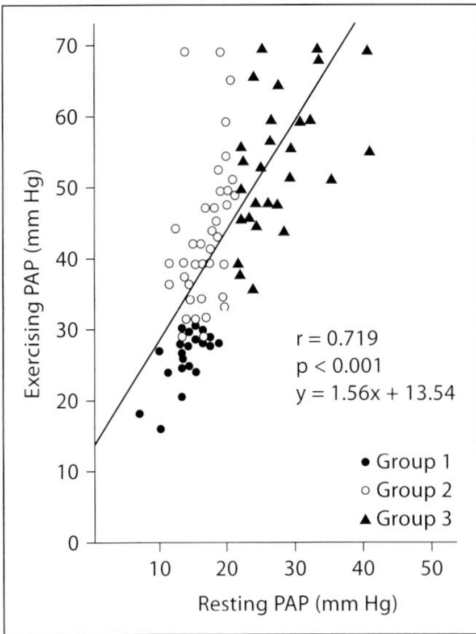

Fig. 1. Resting and exercising mean PAP in a large series of COPD patients. Group 1: resting PAP <20 mm Hg and exercising PAP <30 mm Hg. Group 2: resting PAP <20 mm Hg and exercising PAP >30 mm Hg. Group 3: resting PAP >20 mm Hg (PH; personal data).

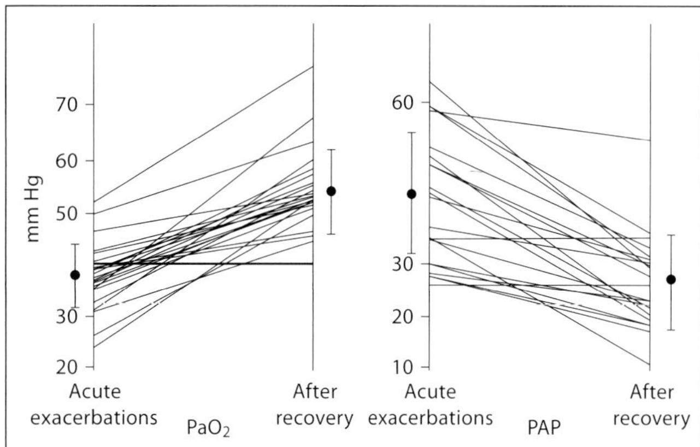

Fig. 2. Evolution of PaO_2 and mean PAP in a series of COPD patients investigated during acute exacerbations and after recovery. The pronounced improvement in PaO_2 (from a mean of 38 mm Hg to 53 mm Hg) is accompanied by a profound decrease in PAP (from a mean of 44 to 27 mm Hg; personal data).

worsen during exercise, sleep, and acute exacerbations of the disease [10].

PAP increases during steady state exercise notably in advanced COPD patients with resting PH [13, 52], as illustrated in figure 1 which shows that in these patients (Group 3) PAP rises from a mean of 27 to 55 mm Hg during a 30- to 40-Watt exercise of 7–10 min duration. This is explained by the fact that PVR does not decrease during exercise in these patients, whereas it does in healthy subjects. This means that daily activities such as climbing stairs or even walking can induce marked PH.

Acute increases of PAP during sleep have been observed in COPD patients with respiratory failure [53]. They are principally observed in REM sleep during which dips in oxygen saturation are more severe. These episodes of sleep-related desaturation are not caused by apneas, except if COPD is associated with a sleep apnea syndrome, but by alveolar hypoventilation and/or ventilation-perfusion mismatching [53]. The more profound the dips of hypoxemia, the more severe the peaks of PH (PAP can increase by >10 mm Hg from its baseline value).

In patients with advanced COPD, severe exacerbations can lead to acute respiratory failure, characterized by a worsening of hypoxemia and hypercapnia. In patients exhibiting PH, there is a simultaneous increase of PAP from its baseline value [54]. PAP may increase by as much as 20 mm Hg, but usually returns to its baseline after recovery, as shown in figure 2. The striking parallel between changes in PaO_2 and PAP suggests the presence of hypoxic pulmonary vasoconstriction.

Thus, even though PH is usually mild to moderate in COPD patients, it may increase markedly during exercise, sleep, and exacerbations of the disease; these acute increases of afterload, especially during exacerbations, can favor the development of RHF [55].

Severe and 'Out of Proportion' Pulmonary Hypertension

As mentioned earlier, in most COPD patients, PH (when present) is mild to moderate with a resting PAP ranging between 20 and 35 mm Hg. A minority of COPD patients exhibit severe PH which can be defined by resting PAP >35 mm Hg [15, 16] or >40 mm Hg [17]. This level of PH is considered to be 'out of proportion' in COPD patients investigated during a stable state of the disease.

Chaouat et al. [17] found that of 998 COPD patients investigated, when clinically stable, with RHC, only 27 had resting PAP ≥40 mm Hg. Among them, 16 had an associated disease explaining in part the severity of PH: left heart disease in 2 patients, CTEPH in 2 patients, and associated restrictive lung disease in 6 patients (mainly severe obesity plus obstructive sleep apneas). It is recommended that the presence of an associated cardiac or pulmonary disease should be

Table 3. Severe ('disproportionate') PH in COPD

	Severe PH (PAP> 40 mm Hg) without associated cardiopulmonary disease (n = 11)	'Usual' PH (PAP = 20–40 mm Hg) (n = 16)	Control group without PH (PAP <20 mm Hg) (n = 14)
Age, years	67	66	62
FEV_1, % of predicted	50	27	35
FEV_1/VC, %	49	34	39
DLCO, ml/min/mm Hg	4.6	10.3	13
PaO_2, mm Hg	46	56	72
$PaCO_2$, mm Hg	32	47	40
$AaDO_2$, mm Hg	56	30	28
PAP, mm Hg	48	25	16
PCP, mm Hg	6	7	7.5
Cardiac output, l/min/m^2	2.3	2.8	3.3
TPR, IU/m^2	21.3	9.0	4.0

Comparison of a group with severe PH to a group with 'usual' PH and a group without PH [17]. Values are means ± SD. VC = Vital capacity. DLCO = transfer factor of carbon monoxide; $AaDO_2$ = alveolar-arterial difference of PO_2; TPR = total pulmonary resistance.

investigated in COPD patients with severe PH [17]. Finally, only 11 patients (1.1%) had COPD as the only cause of severe PH, which underlines the fact that severe PH is uncommon in COPD [17]. These patients exhibit a distinctive pattern with less severe airflow limitation, but more severe hypoxemia, hypocapnia, and markedly decreased DLCO [17], as illustrated in table 3. Using statistical analysis, Thabut et al. [16] identified a similar subgroup of 16 patients with severe PH and observed identical results (table 3).

Patients of Thabut et al. [16] and Chaouat et al. [17] with severe PH represent a subset of COPD patients in whom pulmonary vascular disease is predominant. Actually, some characteristics of the COPD subgroup with severe PH (low cardiac output, hypocapnia, low DLCO) are similar to those observed in IPAH. Due to the severity and the scattered number of COPD patients with severe (or 'out of proportion') PH, these patients should be referred to an expert center of pulmonary vascular diseases so that RHC can be performed and they should be included in registries and clinical trials [2].

Evolution and Prognosis of Pulmonary Hypertension in Chronic Obstructive Pulmonary Disease

The 'natural history' of PH in COPD is not fully understood [9], but several studies have shown that the progression of PH is generally slow and that PAP may remain stable over periods of 2–5 years [56, 57]. In a study in which 93 patients were followed for 5–12 years, the changes in PAP were rather small: +0.5 mm Hg/year for the group as a whole [58]. The evolution of PAP was identical in patients with and without initial PH. A study on the 'natural history' of pulmonary hemodynamics in COPD patients with an initial PAP <20 mm Hg showed that only 33 of 121 developed PH (PAP >20 mm Hg) after a mean interval of 6.8 ± 2.9 years [9].

Nevertheless, a minority of advanced COPD patients exhibit a marked worsening of PAP during follow-up [58]. These patients do not differ from the others at the onset, but are characterized by a progressive deterioration of PaO_2 and $PaCO_2$ during the evolution [57, 58] and there is a significant correlation between the changes in PaO_2 and PAP [58]. The longitudinal evolution of PH is favorably influenced by long-term oxygen therapy (LTOT; see below).

Does PH lead with time to RHF? The classic view of the development of RHF in COPD patients is as follows [59]: PH increases the work of the right ventricle, which leads to right ventricle enlargement (hypertrophy plus dilatation), which can result in right ventricle dysfunction (systolic, diastolic). Later, RHF can be observed in some COPD patients. There is a relationship between the severity of PH and the development of RHF.

Peripheral edema is frequently observed in advanced COPD patients and is considered to reflect RHF, but the possible occurrence of RHF in these patients has been questioned [60], particularly because the degree of PH is most often mild in COPD. Peripheral edema may simply indicate the presence of secondary hyperaldosteronism induced by functional renal insufficiency, and is not synonymous with heart failure [59, 60].

The role of pressure overload in the development of RHF in these patients has been debated. It has been denied by MacNee et al. [61], but another study from our group [55] has led to different conclusions: in 9 of 16 patients with marked peripheral edema during an exacerbation of COPD, hemodynamic signs of RHF were present during the episode of edema and were probably accounted for by a significant worsening of PH (from 27 ± 5 to 40 ± 6 mm Hg, $p < 0.001$), which in turn was explained by a worsening of hypoxemia. Thus, many patients with advanced COPD will never develop RHF; however, some patients will experience episodes of 'true' RHF during exacerbations of the disease accompanied by a worsening of PH [55].

The level of PAP is a good indicator of prognosis [14, 62] in COPD. The prognosis is worse in patients with PH compared with patients without PH and is particularly poor for patients with a severe degree of PH (>35–40 mm Hg) [62], including patients with disproportionate PH [17]. The 5-year survival rate of COPD patients with PH (PAP >20 mm Hg) is about 50% [14, 62], but these results were obtained before the era of LTOT, which significantly improves the prognosis of markedly hypoxemic patients (most of them exhibiting PH) [63, 64]. Of interest, PAP is still an excellent prognosis indicator in COPD patients treated with LTOT [3].

Treatment of Pulmonary Hypertension in Chronic Obstructive Pulmonary Disease

The treatment of PH in COPD is based on oxygen therapy (LTOT). This raises the important question as to whether it is necessary to treat PH in COPD with methods other than LTOT? PH, even if modest in most patients, may worsen during acute exacerbations and these acute increases in PAP may contribute to the development of RHF [57]. This could represent an argument for the treatment of PH which must be also considered in all cases of severe PH (PAP >35–40 mm Hg).

Long-Term Oxygen Therapy
Alveolar hypoxia is considered the major cause of the elevation of PVR and PAP in COPD. Accordingly, LTOT is a logical treatment of PH in COPD. The well-known Nocturnal Oxygen Therapy Trial (NOTT) [63] and Medical Research Council (MRC) Study [64] were not principally devoted to pulmonary hemodynamics, but RHC was performed at the onset in all patients and follow-up data were available in a relatively high number of patients. In the MRC study [64], LTOT patients had a stable PAP after 1 year, whereas control patients had a significant increase in PAP. In the NOTT [63], continuous LTOT (≥18 h/day) slightly but significantly decreased resting and exercising PAP after 6 months, whereas nocturnal LTOT (10–12 h/day) did not.

These pivotal studies were confirmed by further studies more specifically devoted to pulmonary hemodynamic evolution under LTOT [65, 66], which showed either a tendency to the reversal of the progression of PH [65] or a stabilization of PH under LTOT [66] over periods of 2–6 years. PAP seldom returns to normal. The best hemodynamic results have been obtained in the studies in which the daily duration of LTOT was the longest (>16–18 h/day) [63, 65]. Accordingly, one should recommend continuous oxygen therapy.

Vasodilator Drugs
Experience with vasodilators (prostanoids, endothelin receptor antagonists, phosphodiesterase 5 inhibitors) has come from the treatment of IPAH. It is tempting to use these drugs in cases of PH complicating COPD, particularly in the (rare) cases of severe ('disproportionate') PH. Unfortunately, there have been very few studies in this field. To our knowledge, there has only been one controlled study in which COPD patients with mild resting PH or no resting PH at all received bosentan or placebo; however, the results were disappointing and included a worsening of gas exchange abnormalities [67], which is a well-known deleterious effect of vasodilators in COPD.

Nitric oxide is a selective and potent pulmonary vasodilator. One long-term study (3 months) in 40 patients already on LTOT showed that the addition of nitric oxide produced a significant improvement in PAP, PVR, and cardiac output [68]. However, inhaled NO is far from being routinely used in stable COPD patients at the present time.

It is currently recommended not to treat COPD patients with drugs dedicated to IPAH outside of trials and to refer patients with severe PH to a regional specialist PH center [2].

References

1 Celli BR, MacNee W: Standards for the diagnosis and treatment of patients with COPD: a summary of the ATS/ERS position paper. Eur Respir J 2004;23:932–946.

2 Galié N, Hoeper MM, Humbert M, et al: Guidelines for the diagnosis and treatment of pulmonary hypertension. Eur Respir J 2009;34:1219–1263.

3 Oswald-Mammosser M, Weitzenblum E, Quoix E, et al: Prognostic factors in COPD patients receiving long-term oxygen therapy. Chest 1995;107:1193–1198.

4 Badesch DB, Champion HC, Sanchez MA, et al: Diagnosis and assessment of pulmonary arterial hypertension. J Am Coll Cardiol 2009;54:S55–S66.

5 Tartulier M, Bourret M, Deyrieux F: Les pressions artérielles pulmonaires chez l'homme normal. Effets de l'âge et de l'exercice musculaire. Bull Physiopathol Respir 1972;8:1295–1321.

6 Naeije R: Pulmonary vascular function; in Peacock AJ, Rubin LJ (eds): Pulmonary Circulation: Diseases and Their Treatment. London, Arnold, 2004, pp 3–13.

7 Bishop JM: Cardiovascular complications of chronic bronchitis and emphysema. Med Clin North Am 1973;57:771–780

8 Chaouat A, Naeije R, Weitzenblum E: Pulmonary hypertension in COPD. Eur Respir J 2008;32:1371–1385

9 Kessler R, Faller M, Weitzenblum E, et al: 'Natural history' of pulmonary hypertension in a series of 131 patients with chronic obstructive lung disease. Am J Respir Crit Care Med 2001;164:219–222.

10 Weitzenblum E: Chronic cor pulmonale. Heart 2003;89:225–230.

11 Naeije R, Torbicki A: More on the non invasive diagnosis of pulmonary hypertension: Doppler echocardiography revisited. Eur Respir J 1995;8: 1445–1449.

12 Arcasoy SM, Christie JD, Ferrari VA, et al: Echocardiographic assessment of pulmonary hypertension in patients with advanced lung disease. Am J Respir Crit Care Med 2003;167: 735–740.

13 Burrows B, Kettel LJ, Niden AH, et al: Patterns of cardiovascular dysfunction in chronic obstructive lung disease. N Engl J Med 1972;286:912–918.

14 Weitzenblum E, Hirth C, Ducolone A, et al: Prognostic value of pulmonary artery pressure in chronic obstructive pulmonary disease. Thorax 1981;36:752–758.

15 Scharf S, Igbal M, Keller C, et al: Hemodynamic characterization of patients with severe emphysema. Am J Respir Crit Care Med 2002;166:314–322.

16 Thabut G, Dauriat G, Stern JB, et al: Pulmonary hemodynamics in advanced COPD candidates for lung volume reduction surgery or lung transplantation. Chest 2005;127:1531–1536.

17 Chaouat A, Bugnet AS, Kadaoui N, et al: Severe pulmonary hypertension and chronic obstructive pulmonary disease. Am J Respir Crit Care Med 2005;172:189–194.

18 Williams BT, Nicholl JP: Prevalence of hypoxaemic chronic obstructive lung disease with reference to long-term oxygen therapy. Lancet 1985;2: 369–372.

19 Boutin-Forzano S, Moreau D, Kalaboka S, et al: Reported prevalence and co-morbidity of asthma, chronic bronchitis and emphysema: a pan-European estimation. Int J Tuberc Lung Dis 2007;11:695–702.

20 Wilkinson M, Langhorne CA, Heath D, et al: A pathophysiological study of 10 cases of hypoxic cor pulmonale. Q J Med 1988;66:65–85.

21 Magee F, Wright JL, Wiggs BR, et al: Pulmonary vascular structure and function in chronic obstructive pulmonary disease. Thorax 1988;43: 183–189.

22 Hale KA, Niewoehner DE, Cosio MG: Morphologic changes in the muscular pulmonary arteries: relationship to cigarette smoking, airway disease, and emphysema. Am Rev Respir Dis 1980;122:273–278.

23 Wright JL, Lawson L, Pare PD, et al: The structure and function of the pulmonary vasculature in mild chronic obstructive pulmonary disease. The effect of oxygen and exercise. Am Rev Respir Dis 1983;128:702–707.

24 Santos S, Peinado VI, Ramirez J, et al: Characterization of pulmonary vascular remodelling in smokers and patients with mild COPD. Eur Respir J 2002;19:632–638.

25 Chabot F, Schrijen F, Poincelot F, et al: Interpretation of high wedge pressure on exercise in patients with chronic obstructive pulmonary disease. Cardiology 2001;95:139–145.

26 Lockhart A, Tzareva M, Nader F, et al: Elevated pulmonary artery wedge pressure at rest and during exercise in chronic bronchitis: fact or fancy. Clin Sci 1969;37:503–517.

27 Butler J, Schrijen F, Henriquez A, et al: Cause of the raised wedge pressure on exercise in chronic obstructive pulmonary disease. Am Rev Respir Dis 1988;138:350–354.

28 Barbera JA, Peinado VI, Santos S: Pulmonary hypertension in chronic obstructive pulmonary disease. Eur Respir J 2003;21:892–905.

29 Heath D: Remodeling of the pulmonary vasculature in hypoxic lung disease; in Peacock AJ (ed): Pulmonary Circulation. London, Chapman & Hall, 1996, pp 71–79.

30 Von Euler US, Liljestrand G: Observation of the pulmonary arterial blood pressure in the cat. Acta Physiol Scand 1946;12:301–320.

31 Motley HL, Cournand A, Werko L, et al: The influence of short periods of induced acute hypoxia upon pulmonary artery pressure in man. Am J Physiol 1947;150:315–320.

32 Fishman AP, McClement J, Himmelstein A, et al: Effects of acute anoxia on the circulation and respiration in patients with chronic pulmonary disease studied during the steady state. J Clin Invest 1952;31:770–781.

33 Archer S, Michelakis E: The mechanism(s) of hypoxic pulmonary vasoconstriction: potassium channels, redox 02 sensors, and controversies. News Physiol Sci 2002;17:131–137.

34 Faller DV: Endothelial cell responses to hypoxic stress. Clin Exp Pharmacol Physiol 1999;26:74–84.

35 Weitzenblum E, Schrijen F, Mohan-Kumar T, et al: Variability of the pulmonary vascular response to acute hypoxia in chronic bronchitis. Chest 1988;94:772–778.

36 Penaloza D, Sime F, Banchero N, et al: Pulmonary hypertension in healthy men born and living at high altitude. Med Thorac 1962;19:449–460.

37 Wright JL, Levy RD, Churg A: Pulmonary hypertension in chronic obstructive pulmonary disease: current theories of pathogenesis and their implications for treatment. Thorax 2005;60:605–609.

38 Peinado VI, Barbera JA, Abate P, et al: Inflammatory reaction in pulmonary muscular arteries of patients with mild chronic obstructive pulmonary disease. Am J Respir Crit Care Med 1999;159:1605–1611.

39 Joppa P, Petrasova D, Stancak B, et al: Systemic inflammation in patients with COPD and pulmonary hypertension. Chest 2006;130:326–333.

40 Eddahibi S, Chaouat A, Tu L, et al: Interleukin-6 gene polymorphism confers susceptibility to pulmonary hypertension in chronic obstructive pulmonary disease. Proc Am Thorac Soc 2006;3: 475–476.

41 Hoeper MM, Welte T: Systemic inflammation, COPD, and pulmonary hypertension. Chest 2007; 131:634–635.

42 Eddahibi S, Chaouat A, Morrell N, et al: Polymorphism of the serotonin transporter gene and pulmonary hypertension in chronic obstructive pulmonary disease. Circulation 2003;108:1839–1844.

43 Chaouat A, Savale L, Chouaid C, et al: Role for interleukin-6 in COPD-related pulmonary hypertension. Chest 2009;136:678–687.

44 Oswald-Mammosser M, Oswald T, Nyankiye E, et al: Non-invasive diagnosis of pulmonary hypertension in chronic obstructive pulmonary disease. Comparison of ECG, radiological measurements, echocardiography and myocardial scintigraphy. Eur J Respir Dis 1987;71:419–429.

45 Vonk-Noordegraaf A, Marcus JT, Holverda S, et al: Early changes of cardiac structure and function in COPD patients with mild hypoxemia. Chest 2005;127:1898–1903.

46 Tramarin R, Torbicki A, Marchandise B, et al: Doppler echocardiographic evaluation of pulmonary artery pressure in chronic obstructive pulmonary disease. A European multicentre study. Eur Heart J 1991;12:103–111.

47 Fisher MR, Criner GJ, Fishman AP, et al: Estimating pulmonary artery pressures by echocardiography in patients with emphysema. Eur Respir J 2007;30:914–921.
48 Torbicki A, Skwarski K, Hawvrylkiewicz I, et al: Attempts at measuring pulmonary arterial pressure by means of Doppler echocardiography in patients with chronic lung disease. Eur Respir J 1989;2:856–860.
49 Leuchte HH, Baumgartner RA, Nounou ME, et al: Brain natriuretic peptide is a prognostic parameter in chronic lung disease. Am J Respir Crit Care Med 2006;173:744–750.
50 Humbert M, Sitbon O, Chaouat A, et al: Pulmonary arterial hypertension in France: results from a national registry. Am J Respir Crit Care Med 2006;173:1023–1030.
51 Jamieson SW, Kapelanski DP, Sakakibara N, et al: Pulmonary endarterectomy: experience and lessons learned in 1,500 cases. Ann Thorac Surg 2003;76:1457–1462.
52 Horsfield K, Segel N, Bishop JM: The pulmonary circulation in chronic bronchitis at rest and during exercise breathing air and 80% oxygen. Clin Sci 1968;43:473–483.
53 Fletcher EC, Levin DC: Cardiopulmonary hemodynamics during sleep in subjects with chronic obstructive pulmonary disease: the effect of short and long-term oxygen. Chest 1984;85:6–14.
54 Abraham AS, Cole RB, Green ID, et al: Factors contributing to the reversible pulmonary hypertension of patients with acute respiratory failure studied by serial observations during recovery. Circ Res 1969;24:51–60.
55 Weitzenblum E, Apprill A, Oswald M, et al: Pulmonary hemodynamics in patients with chronic obstructive pulmonary disease before and during an episode of peripheral edema. Chest 1994; 105:1377–1382.
56 Schrijen F, Uffholtz H, Polu JM, et al: Pulmonary and systemic hemodynamic evolution in chronic bronchitis. Am Rev Respir Dis 1978;117:25–31.
57 Weitzenblum E, Loiseau A, Hirth C, et al: Course of pulmonary hemodynamics in patients with chronic obstructive pulmonary disease. Chest 1979;75:656–662.
58 Weitzenblum E, Sautegeau A, Ehrhart M, et al: Long-term course of pulmonary arterial pressure in chronic obstructive pulmonary disease. Am Rev Respir Dis 1984;130:993–998.
59 MacNee W: Pathophysiology of cor pulmonale in chronic obstructive pulmonary disease. Am J Respir Crit Care Med 1994;150:833–852,1158–1168.
60 Richens JM, Howard P: Oedema in cor pulmonale. Clin Sci (Lond)1982;62:255–259.
61 MacNee W, Wathen C, Flenley DC, et al: The effects of controlled oxygen therapy on ventricular function in patients with stable and decompensated cor pulmonale. Am Rev Respir Dis 1988;137:1289–1295.
62 Bishop JM, Cross KW: Physiological variables and mortality in patients with various categories of chronic respiratory disease. Bull Eur Physiopathol Respir 1984;20:495–500.
63 Continuous or nocturnal oxygen therapy in hypoxemic chronic obstructive lung disease: a clinical trial. Nocturnal Oxygen Therapy Trial Group. Ann Intern Med 1980;93:391–398.
64 Long-term domiciliary oxygen therapy in chronic hypoxic cor pulmonale complicating chronic bronchitis and emphysema. Report of the Medical Research Council Working Party. Lancet 1981;1:681–686.
65 Weitzenblum E, Sautegeau A, Ehrhart M, et al: Long term oxygen therapy can reverse the progression of pulmonary hypertension in patients with chronic obstructive pulmonary disease. Am Rev Respir Dis 1985;131:493–498.
66 Zielinski J, Tobiasz M, Hawrylkiewicz I, et al: Effects of long-term oxygen therapy on pulmonary hemodynamics in COPD patients. A 6-year prospective study. Chest 1998;113:65–70.
67 Stolz D, Rasch H, Linka A, et al: A randomised controlled trial of bosentan in severe COPD. Eur Respir J 2008;32:619–628.
68 Vonbank K, Ziesche R, Higenbottam TW, et al: Controlled prospective randomised trial on the effects on pulmonary haemodynamics of the ambulatory long-term use of nitric oxide and oxygen in patients with severe COPD. Thorax 2003;58:289–293.

Emmanuel Weitzenblum
Department of Pulmonology
Nouvel Hôpital Civil
FR–67091 Strasbourg (France)
E-Mail emmanuel.weitzenblum@chru-strasbourg.fr

Chapter 19

Humbert M, Souza R, Simonneau G (eds): Pulmonary Vascular Disorders.
Prog Respir Res. Basel, Karger, 2012, vol 41, pp 178–198

Pulmonary Hypertension Complicating Interstitial and Granulomatous Lung Diseases

Hilario Nunes[a] · Yurdagul Uzunhan[a] · Thomas Gille[a] · Gaelle Dauriat[d] · Michel Brauner[b] · Marianne Kambouchner[c] · Dominique Valeyre[a]

University Paris 13, UPRES EA 2363, Assistance Publique Hôpitaux de Paris, Avicenne Hospital and Departments of [a]Pneumology, [b]Radiology and [c]Pathology, Bobigny, and [d]Assistance Publique Hôpitaux de Paris, Bichat Hospital, Departement of Pneumology, Paris, France

Abstract

Pulmonary hypertension (PH) carries a poor prognosis in interstitial lung diseases (ILDs). Its prevalence depends on the underlying condition, the most common being idiopathic pulmonary fibrosis, connective tissue disease-related ILD, sarcoidosis, and pulmonary Langerhans cell histiocytosis (PLCH). Although hypoxic vasoconstriction and loss of pulmonary capillaries are important in the pathogenesis of ILD-associated PH, other mechanisms may play a role, including the release of diverse cytokines and growth factors during fibrogenesis which induce vascular remodeling. This intrinsic vasculopathy may prevail in the venous side in sarcoidosis and PLCH. As a result, a small proportion of ILD patients may exhibit 'out of proportion' PH, i.e. more severe than expected from functional impairment (mean pulmonary artery pressure >35–40 mm Hg). The accuracy of echocardiography for the detection of PH is weak in ILDs. Management of ILD-associated PH mainly relies on supplemental oxygen and lung transplantation in otherwise eligible patients. Treatments targeted to the underlying ILD do not usually affect the course of PH, with the exception of rare cases of nonfibrotic sarcoidosis responding to corticosteroids. Data on the efficacy and safety of pulmonary arterial hypertension-specific agents are lacking. Further controlled trials are warranted and should integrate the concept of disproportionate PH in their design.

Pulmonary hypertension (PH) is a serious complication of interstitial lung diseases (ILDs). Its frequency is extremely variable and largely depends on the underlying ILD and stage of severity, with sarcoidosis, pulmonary Langerhans cell histiocytosis (PLCH), connective tissue diseases (CTDs), and idiopathic pulmonary fibrosis (IPF) being the most commonly associated with PH. PH results in substantial morbidity and adversely impacts the survival of affected patients. Since the advent of new therapeutic strategies for pulmonary arterial hypertension (PAH), there has been a dramatic resurgence of interest in ILD-associated PH.

This review examines the current literature regarding the prevalence, pathogenesis, prognosis, and therapeutic management of ILD-associated PH with a focus on the most recent knowledge.

General Considerations

Before describing the features of PH in each ILD, it is necessary to review briefly the classification of ILDs and that of PH as well as consider the principles that apply to the general assessment of patients with ILD-associated PH.

Classification of Interstitial Lung Diseases

ILDs encompass a heterogeneous group of disorders of known or unknown origin that are characterized by diffuse opacities on chest radiography. The lung interstitium is the primary site of injury for ILDs, resulting in various combinations of inflammation and fibrosis [1]. However, ILDs frequently involve not only the interstitium, but also the airspaces, peripheral airways, and vessels. ILDs are separated into four categories (fig. 1): (1) ILDs of known cause, such as those related to occupational or environmental exposures, drugs, CTDs, or vasculitis; (2) idiopathic interstitial pneumonias (IIPs); (3) granulomatous lung disorders; and (4) rare forms of ILDs with distinctive and well-defined

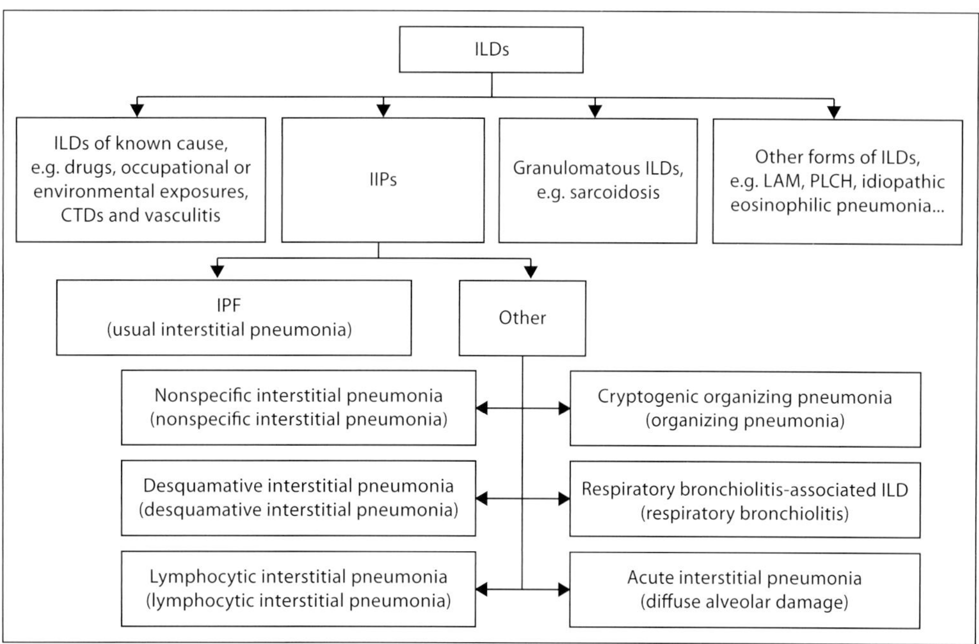

Fig. 1. Classification of ILDs. ILDs are separated into four categories: (1) ILDs of known cause, such as those in relation with occupational or environmental exposures, drugs, CTDs, or vasculitis; (2) IIPs; (3) granulomatous lung disorders, e.g. sarcoidosis; and (4) rare forms of ILDs with distinctive and well-defined clinicopathological features such as PLCH, LAM, and chronic idiopathic eosinophilic pneumonia. IIPs include seven clinico-radiological-pathological entities to which a histologic pattern, indicated in parenthesis, corresponds. Because its prognosis is much more severe, it is important to distinguish IPF from the other IIPs.

clinicopathological features, such as PLCH, lymphangioleiomyomatosis (LAM), chronic idiopathic eosinophilic pneumonia, pulmonary alveolar proteinosis, etc. [1].

The granulomatous lung disorder category usually designates sarcoidosis, which has the hallmark of discrete well-formed immune granuloma [1]. The international consensus statement adopted by the ATS and ERS in 2002 provides a standardized classification and nomenclature of the IIPs as well as uniform diagnostic criteria based on seven clinico-radiological-pathological entities [1]. Because its prognosis is devastating, the most important distinction among the IIPs is that between IPF and the other IIPs, in particular nonspecific interstitial pneumonia with which differential diagnosis may be confusing.

Classification of Pulmonary Hypertension

PH is defined as an increase in mean pulmonary arterial pressure (mPAP) ≥25 mm Hg at rest on right heart catheterization (RHC). In an attempt to assist physicians in their clinical practice, an updated clinical classification of PH derived from the Dana Point meeting was published in 2009 [2]. Group 3 refers to 'PH due to lung diseases and/or hypoxia' including ILDs. Group 5 was created for 'PH with unclear and/or multifactorial mechanisms' where several ILDs including sarcoidosis, PLCH, LAM, neurofibromatosis, and vasculitis have been placed. This distinction from Group 3 seems relevant as the pathogenesis of PH for these disorders is much more complex than merely parenchymal involvement and/or hypoxia. Another important point of the new classification is that pulmonary veno-occlusive disease (PVOD) is distinguished but not completely separated from PAH in Group 1' [2]. However, several authors continue to consider PVOD as a syndrome rather than a disease entity.

New Concept of 'Out of Proportion' Pulmonary Hypertension

Classically, morphologic changes characterizing PH due to ILDs include medial hypertrophy and intimal obstructive proliferation of the distal pulmonary arteries (PA) with a variable degree of destruction of the vascular bed in fibrotic zones. In this setting, PH has long been believed to result exclusively from hypoxic vasoconstriction and loss of capillaries, and mPAP rarely exceeds 35–40 mm Hg [2, 3].

This postulation has recently been questioned. Indeed, mPAP does not correlate well with the degree of restrictive physiology and PaO_2 in ILDs. Also, patients sometimes display 'out of proportion' PH, i.e. mPAP >40 mm Hg, which seems insufficiently explained by lung mechanical disturbances and raises the possibility of an intrinsic vasculopathy. 'Out of proportion' PH has been a matter of growing attention, chiefly in sarcoidosis and PLCH. Accordingly, the role of endothelial dysfunction and vasoconstrictor/proliferative-vasodilator/antiproliferative imbalance which promotes vascular remodeling has been emphasized in ILD-associated PH. Thereby, primary vascular changes are observed in areas unaffected by parenchymal involvement [4–7] and veins are sometimes predominantly concerned [6, 7]. The interrelationship of pulmonary fibrogenesis and vascular remodeling is detailed in the section on IPF, but may have implications for other forms of fibrotic ILDs. Besides these unifying mechanisms, others may be unique to sarcoidosis and PLCH, as discussed in the dedicated sections.

Diagnosis Challenges in Interstitial Lung Disease-Associated Pulmonary Hypertension

As PH bears a severe prognosis in ILDs, early diagnosis and consideration of treatment options may be keys to improving patient outcome. The clinical picture of underlying respiratory disorder can mask PH and delay its recognition. Several symptoms should, however, prompt diagnostic intervention: dyspnea more severe than one would expect from functional impairment, chest pain, palpitations, and near syncope on exertion. Physical signs include a loud P2 component to the second heart sound, a fixed, split S2, a holosystolic murmur of tricuspid regurgitation, and a diastolic murmur of pulmonic regurgitation. Signs of right-sided heart insufficiency are generally late findings. ECG may demonstrate signs of right ventricule strain and chest radiography may show right cardiomegaly and PA enlargement.

Transthoracic Doppler Echocardiography

Transthoracic Doppler echocardiography (TTE) is not perfect, but remains the most appropriate modality for the noninvasive assessment of PH in ILDs [8]. The peak velocity of the tricuspid regurgitation jet is measurable in only 44–54% of patients with ILDs, and even if available, estimation of the systolic PAP (sPAP) is often inaccurate [9–11]. Furthermore, there is no validated threshold of sPAP with a reasonable sensitivity and specificity in such a context [10]. Arcasoy et al. [9] examined the performance of TTE in 106 patients with diverse forms of ILDs referred for lung transplantation, using RHC as the gold standard. The estimation of sPAP was achieved only in 54%. Despite the significantly higher likelihood of obtaining an estimation of sPAP in ILDs, the accuracy of TTE was much worse than in obstructive lung diseases. There was a good correlation between sPAP estimated on TTE and measured on RHC, but the values were within 10 mm Hg in only 37% of the patients with ILDs. When considering estimated sPAP in excess of 45 mm Hg as a determinant of PH, the sensitivity, specificity, and positive and negative predictive values of TTE were 85, 17, 60, and 44%, respectively. When right ventricular abnormalities were used as a surrogate diagnostic marker of PH, the sensitivity, specificity, and positive and negative predictive values of TTE were 76, 53, 57, and 74% respectively [9]. Similar results have been found in restricted populations of IPF patients [10, 11]. Thus, the absence of increased sPAP appears to be suboptimal for excluding significant PH and does not obviate the need for RHC in selected patients. Right ventricular abnormalities are valuable additional parameters to reinforce suspicion of PH, independent of tricuspid regurgitation velocity [9].

Right Heart Catheterization

Although definite diagnosis relies on invasive measurements, not all patients with ILDs and suspected PH should undergo confirmatory RHC. The Task Force guidelines for the diagnosis and treatment of PH assert the following indications for RHC: (1) proper diagnosis of PH in candidates for transplantation, (2) suspected 'out of proportion' PH potentially amenable to be enrolled in a clinical trial with specific PAH drug therapy, (3) frequent episodes of right heart failure, and (4) inconclusive echocardiographic study in cases with a high index of clinical suspicion [3]. We would add the situation of persistent uncertainty with left heart disease and particularly diastolic dysfunction which is not uncommon in patients with ILDs [12–18] and frequently underscored by TTE [13, 14]. A diagnosis algorithm is proposed in figure 2.

RHC also allows the assessment of the severity of hemodynamic impairment, providing significant information on prognosis [14, 19, 20]. As therapy with high doses of calcium channel blockers currently has no role in Group 3 PH, acute vasodilator challenge is not recommended in the majority of patients with ILDs, but may still be useful for some patients in Group 5. Once PH is confirmed,

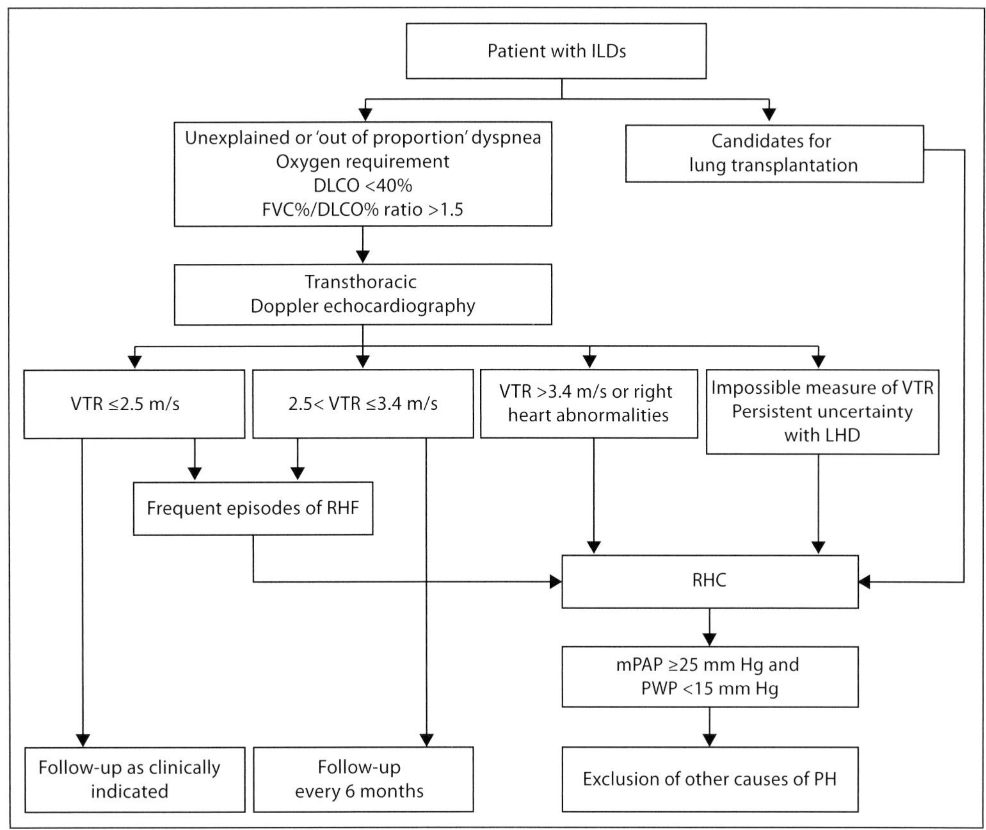

Fig. 2. Proposed algorithm for the diagnosis of ILD-associated PH. Several parameters should prompt the search for PH in patients with ILDs: unexplained or 'out of proportion' dyspnea, i.e. more severe than expected on the basis of functional impairment, oxygen requirement, DLCO <40% of predicted value, and FVC%/DLCO% ratio >1.5. Although imperfect, TTE remains the most appropriate test for the detection of PH by means of the measure of the peak velocity of tricuspid regurgitation jet (VTR) and the presence of morphologic abnormalities of the right heart. A proper diagnosis of PH relies on invasive measurements, but not all patients should undergo confirmatory RHC. This should be performed in candidates for transplantation; in suspected 'out of proportion' PH potentially amenable to specific PAH drug therapy, i.e. with a VTR >3.4 m/s (estimated sPAP >55–60 mm Hg); in cases with frequent episodes of right heart failure (RHF) or with persistent uncertainty with left heart disease (LHD); and particularly diastolic dysfunction. Precapillary PH is defined as an increase in mPAP ≥25 mm Hg with normal pulmonary wedge pressure (PWP). Other causes of PH should be excluded carefully.

a comprehensive workup is intended to scrupulously rule out the other classical causes of PH, in particular pulmonary embolism, unrecognized CTDs, or obstructive sleep apnea.

Other Screening Tools

Several other screening tools have been evaluated to detect PH in patients with ILDs.

High-Resolution CT. High-resolution CT (HRCT) can show an increased caliber of PA (widest diameter of the main PA >29 mm or superior to that of the ascending aorta). Even so, the PA diameter and PA/aorta ratio failed to predict the presence of PH in two studies on IPF [21] or various other fibrotic ILDs [22]. PA dilatation may occur even in the absence of significant PH, possibly because the restrictive lung physiology may result in a traction effect on the mediastinal vascular structures, distending the PA independently of the underlying PAP.

Natriuretic Peptides. Brain natriuretic peptide (BNP) or N-terminal pro-BNP may be helpful biomarkers for the detection of PH in patients with ILDs. In the study by Leuchte et al. [23] on patients with diverse fibrotic ILDs, elevated plasma BNP levels were predictive of moderate-to-severe PH, as defined by mPAP >35 mm Hg on RHC, with

100% sensitivity and 89% specificity. BNP is also independently associated with a higher risk of mortality in ILDs [24–26].

Pulmonary Function Tests and 6-Min Walk Test. Several studies have aimed to detect PH with pulmonary function tests in patients with ILDs, but in general, their contribution is modest. Hypoxemia, the need for supplemental oxygen, and/or a low DLCO are the parameters that most consistently identify patients with PH in ILDs [12, 16, 17, 19, 21, 27–32]. For instance, it has been demonstrated that oxygen requirement together with a DLCO <40% is specific but poorly sensitive for detecting PH in IPF patients [27]. In ILDs, however, the reduction of DLCO may be due to both interstitial and vascular involvement as well as emphysema, which are occasionally combined. For this reason several authors have postulated that a high FVC%/DLCO% ratio, reflecting a disproportionately reduced DLCO for the degree of restriction, may better gauge vascular involvement [16, 30–33]. In the study by Steen et al. [31] on systemic scleroderma (SSc), PH was strongly associated with an initial DLCO <55% and FVC%/DLCO% ratio >1.4. Among all patients in whom this ratio was >1.4, 22% developed PH, compared with only 2% of those whose ratio was inferior [31]. Nathan et al. [16] showed that the FVC%/DLCO% ratio performed just slightly better than DLCO separately and was still unsatisfactory in IPF patients. A cut point of 1.5 was associated with an almost twofold-higher risk of associated PH (43.1 vs. 27.0%) [16].

Zisman et al. [11] applied a multivariable linear regression model combining the FVC%/DLCO% ratio and resting SpO_2 at room air in a retrospective study of IPF patients with available RHC. The equation generated by the model showed a sensitivity of 71%, specificity of 81%, positive predictive value of 71%, and negative predictive value of 81% for the diagnosis of PH. Interestingly, the predictive ability of the model was substantially better than TTE [11]. The advantage of this approach is that it can be used for almost every IPF patient, while echocardiographic estimation of sPAP is possible in only half of the cases. The prediction formula has been further validated in an independent external cohort [34].

The measure of membrane and capillary blood components is theoretically capable of discriminating the respective part of interstitial and vascular involvement in the reduction of DLCO, but its role for the detection of ILD-associated PH has never been evaluated. The 6-min walk test (6MWT) alone is inadequate to predict PH in patients with ILDs, but exercise desaturation may improve the accuracy of detection yielded by TTE [8, 10, 29].

Treatment Challenges in Interstitial Lung Disease-Associated Pulmonary Hypertension

Because of limited publications, no recommendation can be drawn on the optimal management strategy for ILD-associated PH. The reports regarding the effects of treatment directed to the underlying ILD, including immunosuppressive therapy, are contradictory and may depend on the nature of ILD and causal mechanisms of PH. Supportive therapy includes supplemental oxygen and diuretics as needed. Long-term oxygen administration has been shown to prevent the progression of PH in patients with chronic obstructive pulmonary disease. By extension and despite less clear publications, the same is accepted for patients with ILDs. It is speculated that the benefit of oral anticoagulants in idiopathic PAH is explained by the role of in situ thrombosis [3]. Abnormalities in coagulation and fibrinolytic pathways have also been described in ILDs, in particular IPF. This, together with the possible presence of nonspecific risk factors for venous thromboembolism, including heart failure and immobility, represents the rationale for anticoagulation in ILD-associated PH. Unfortunately, no data exists in such a context; therefore, the benefit/risk balance has to be weighed and openly discussed with the patients.

Considering the pathogenetic links between ILDs and PH on the one hand, and some similar structural abnormalities of pulmonary vessels between ILDs-associated PH and PAH on the other, the use of PAH-specific agents is appealing. There are four classes of PAH specific agents: (1) calcium channel blockers, which are reserved for a small subset of patients with positive acute vasoreactivity testing; (2) prostacyclin analogues; (3) endothelin-1 (ET-1) receptor antagonists; and (4) phosphodiesterase-5 inhibitors [3]. Published experience on the efficacy and safety of PAH therapy in ILD-associated PH is scarce and mainly consists of the assessment of acute hemodynamic effects and case reports or uncontrolled small series. There has long been concern over systemic pulmonary vasodilators leading to an aggravation of hypoxemia because of the inhibition of hypoxic pulmonary vasoconstriction with subsequent increased ventilation/perfusion mismatch and shunting. Because of this, delivery of these medications to well-ventilated lung units via inhalation, including nitric oxide or prostanoids, has been preferred [35]. Yet, while decreased arterial oxygenation is actually observed with calcium channel blockers and intravenous epoprostenol [35, 36], it is not with oral sildenafil, a phosphodiesterase-5 inhibitor [36] or bosentan, the dual ET-1 receptor A and B antagonist [37].

In summary, long-term oxygen is the cornerstone of patients with ILD-associated PH who are hypoxemic on rest or during exercise. According to the Task Force guidelines, the use of PAH-targeted therapy is discouraged when mPAP <40 mm Hg [3]. It may be proposed to patients with 'out of proportion' PH in expert centers, ideally as part of a randomized controlled trial [3], even if the feasibility of a clinical trial is difficult in such uncommon conditions. Given the risk of pulmonary edema, these drugs should be used with caution in patients with suspected PVOD, as reported in sarcoidosis or PLCH. In patients with end-stage ILDs, the indication of lung transplantation, when otherwise appropriate, should be strengthened by the presence of PH.

Idiopathic Pulmonary Fibrosis

IPF is a distinctive type of chronic fibrosing interstitial pneumonia of unknown cause limited to the lung and associated with a pathological appearance of usual interstitial pneumonia. A set of criteria have been established for a definite diagnosis of IPF in the absence of surgical lung biopsy [38]. Although its precise frequency remains unclear, IPF is the most frequent IIP with a prevalence of approximately 20.2 and 13.2 cases per 100,000 for males and females, respectively. The prognosis is poor with a mean survival ranging from 2 to 4 years and no treatment with unequivocally proven efficacy. IPF progresses in a relentless and often gradual manner, but the course may also be a step-like process, with periods of relative steadiness punctuated by episodes of acute exacerbations, i.e. acute respiratory decompensations with no identifiable cause [38].

Frequency
Several studies have estimated the frequency of PH in patients with IPF, employing various methods to diagnose and criteria to define PH (table 1). In the prospective study of King et al. [39] on 238 unselected IPF patients, 20% had enlarged PA indicative of PH on chest radiography. Nadrous et al. [28] retrospectively reviewed 88 patients who underwent TTE at their initial visit and showed that PH, as defined by sPAP >35 mm Hg, was present in 84%. However, there is probably an overestimation with this study, as evaluation was not systematic but left to the discretion of the investigators. Most studies on IPF-associated PH have been conducted in patients referred for lung transplantation as they routinely undergo RHC, which creates obvious selection biases. In this setting, reported rates of prevalence range from 31.6 to 46.1% [16, 17, 27, 40] and increase from 39% at the time of listing for lung transplantation to 78% at the time of transplantation [41].

Table 1. Main studies on the prevalence of PH in patients with IPF

Population	Method	Definition	Prevalence, %	Reference
Prospective; initial evaluation, n = 238[1]	Chest X-ray	Enlarged PA	20	[39]
Retrospective; initial evaluation, n = 88[1]	TTE	sPAP > 35 mm Hg	84.1	[28]
Retrospective; transplant evaluation				
n = 79[1]	RHC	mPAP ≥25 mm Hg (mPAP >40 mm Hg)	31.6 (2)	[27]
n = 118[1, 2]	RHC	mPAP ≥25 mm Hg	40.7	[16]
n = 2,525[3]	RHC	mPAP ≥25 mm Hg (mPAP >40 mm Hg)	46.1 (9.1)	[17]
n = 376[3]	RHC	mPAP ≥25 mm Hg	36	[40]

[1] In these studies, the ATS/ERS criteria for IPF were verified.
[2] The study of Nathan et al. [16] is an update of the initial cohort of Lettieri et al. [27].
[3] In these studies, patients were identified from the registry maintained by the United Network for Organ Sharing and the Organ Procurement and Transplant Network of the United States. The diagnosis of 'IPF' was based on the reports of the referring transplant center.

Pathogenesis
The pathobiology of PH in IPF is incompletely understood and the complexity of pathobiologic paradigms that characterize IPF might also apply to PH complicating this condition. The old hypothesis explaining the mechanisms for the development of PH in IPF was based on hypoxic vasoconstriction and pulmonary capillary loss following scar tissue accumulation. However, PH can be seen in the absence of hypoxemia, irrespective of its severity, and lung volumes are neither closely linked with mPAP [16, 17, 19, 21, 27, 28], nor extent and severity of fibrosis on HRCT [21]. Actually, it seems that vessel abnormalities in IPF involve all sections of the vascular bed. The pathologic features in pulmonary vessels of IPF lungs show spatially and temporally heterogeneous changes with a broad range of structural alterations,

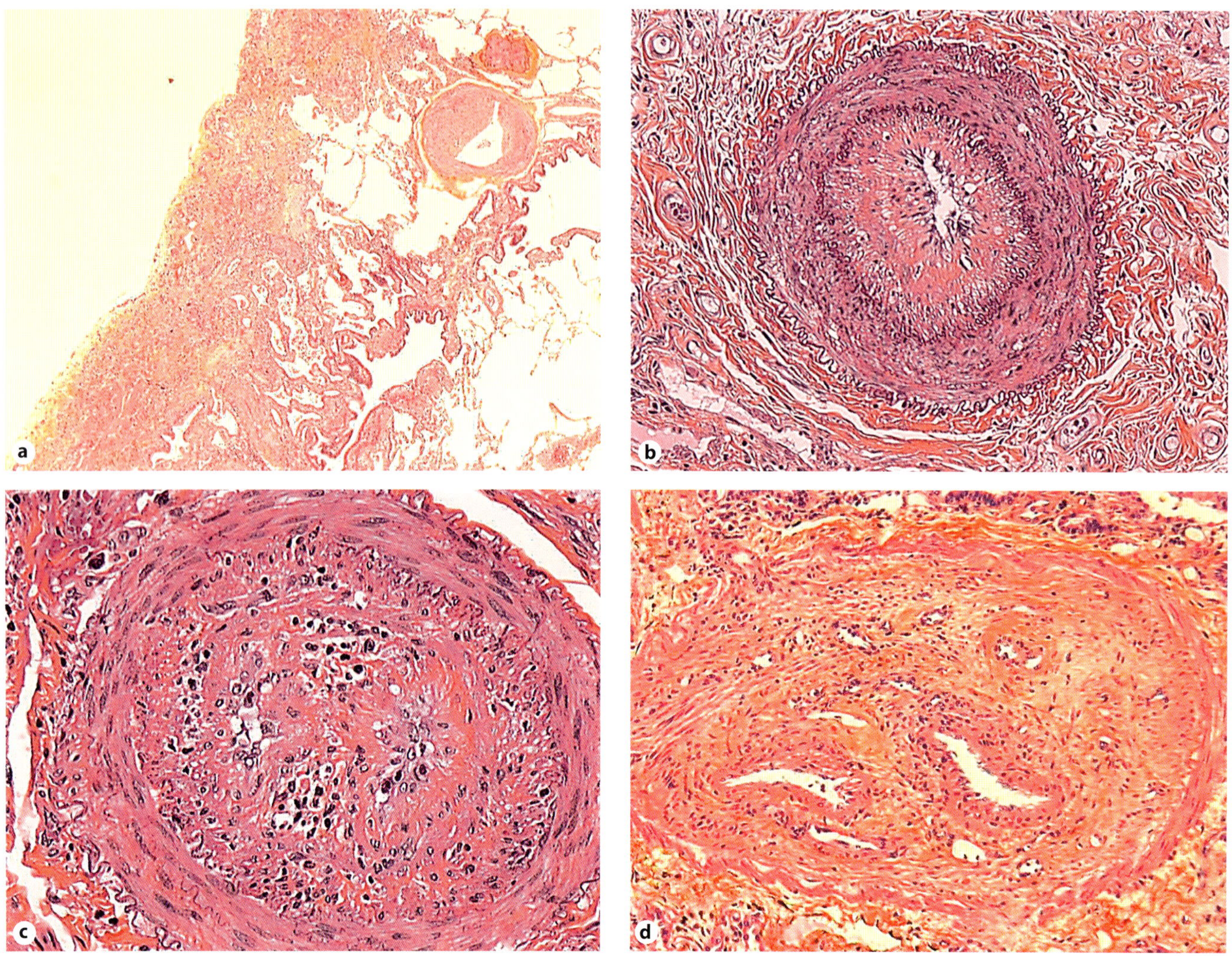

Fig. 3. Pulmonary artery changes in a patient with IPF-associated PH. The figure shows a pattern of usual interstitial pneumonia with arterial changes consisting of severe medial hypertrophy and intimal fibrosis (**a**, **b**) near an area of subpleural lung fibrosis (**a**). Some of the PA show evidence of plexiform lesions with early (**c**) or advanced recanalization (**d**).

from isolated thickening of the smooth muscle layer and proliferative intima lesions, to complete occlusion of the distal PA by scar tissue and plexiform lesions (fig. 3). Vascular density decreases with rising severity of pulmonary fibrosis, but increases in unaffected regions [42, 43]. Vessel ablation has been shown to occur particularly within fibroblastic foci and in areas of honeycombing [42]. In nonfibrotic zones, occlusion of venules has been observed as well as increased alveolar capillary density, hemosiderin deposition, and muscularized arterioles [4, 5]. Additionally, the presence of iron deposition and alveolar capillary density in the lung biopsy of patients with IPF appears to be predictive of PH [5].

The pathogenetic concepts of PH share mechanisms implicated in the development of pulmonary fibrosis (fig. 4). Structural and cellular lesions may result from an abnormal wound healing process. A repetitive injury provokes the damage of alveolar epithelial cells and basement membranes, followed by exudation of fibrin. The dialogue between fibroblasts and alveolar epithelial cells is then disrupted leading to an excess of alveolar epithelial cell apoptosis and an accumulation of myofibroblasts with increased deposition of extracellular matrix. Many mediators, including cytokines and growth factors, are produced in this context, such as transforming growth factor (TGF)-β, platelet-derived growth factor, connective tissue growth factor, ET-1, and angiotensin II [44, 45]. With decreased production of vascular endothelial growth factor, this environment may induce endothelial cell (EC) apoptosis and/

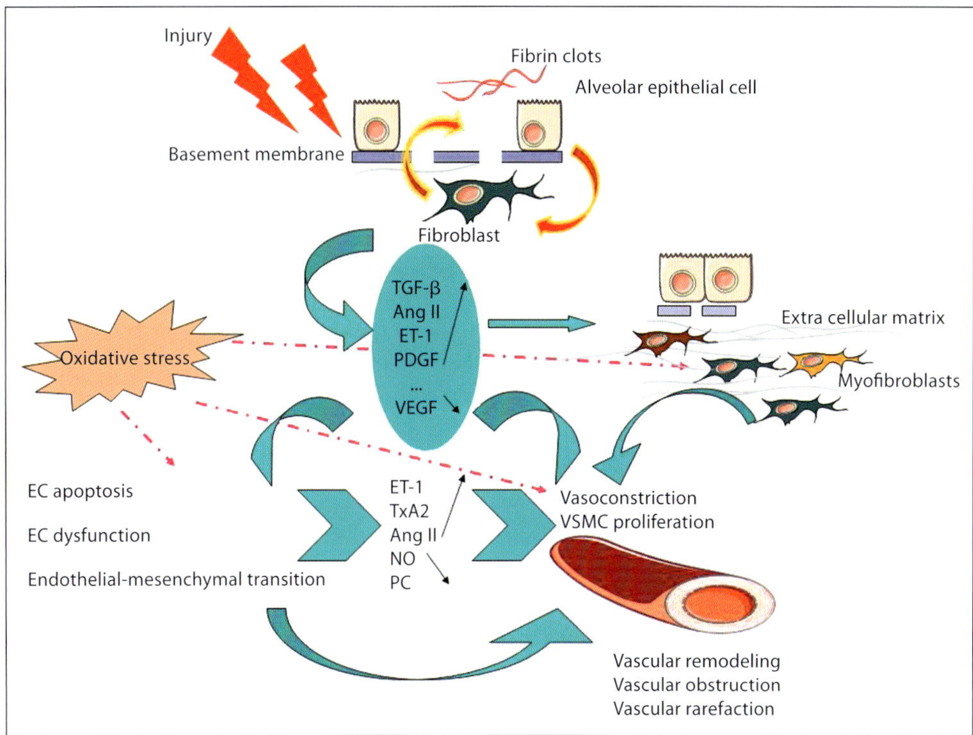

Fig. 4. Shared pathogenetic mechanisms between IPF and PAH. TxA2 = thromboxane; Ang II = angiotensin II; NO = nitric oxide; PC = prostacyclin; PDGF = platelet-derived growth factor; VEGF = vascular endothelial growth factor; VSMC = vascular smooth muscle cell.

or EC dysfunction [46]. The latter condition, a key event in this situation, leads to a decreased production of vasodilators like nitric oxide and prostacyclin, and increased release of angiotensin II, thromboxane A2, and ET-1, favoring vasoconstriction and vascular smooth muscle cell proliferation. Furthermore, TGF-β and ET-1 independently promote fibroblast resistance to apoptosis, proliferation, and activation [47]. The available evidence strongly supports increased oxidative stress in the pathogenesis of both fibrogenesis and PH through myofibroblast accumulation, vasoconstriction, vascular smooth muscle cell proliferation, and EC modifications. Another relevant setting is the reduction in cross-sectional vascular area through thrombotic obstruction of vessels. Indeed, a procoagulant state is generated. The alveolar fibrin clots due to impaired intra-alveolar fibrinolysis may provide a lead structure for fibroblast chemotactic migration and proliferation as well as for neovascularization. In addition to EC apoptosis or dysfunction, a transdifferentiation of these cells to mesenchymal cells is described and may contribute to both vascular remodeling and lung fibrogenesis [48]. These pathogenetic concepts, schematized on figure 4, primarily relate to IPF-associated PH, but may also have implications for other forms of fibrotic ILDs, including CTDs and granulomatous diseases such as sarcoidosis.

Diagnosis

A screening algorithm is proposed in figure 2. Several potential causes of PH need to be carefully searched in IPF patients because the following comorbidities are frequently associated: left heart dysfunction [15–18], in particular coronary artery disease [49], thrombo-embolic disease [49, 50], and obstructive sleep apnea [51]. IPF-associated PH is usually mild to moderate, with only 2–9.1% of transplantation candidates having a mPAP >40 mm Hg [17, 27]. However, PH progresses rapidly as demonstrated on serial RHC data where the rate of change of the mPAP is 3.8 mm Hg/month [41].

Clinical Impact and Prognosis

PH has an influence on functional status, quality of life, and ultimately survival of IPF patients. Patients with PH are more dyspneic than those without PH, as expressed by the Borg scale [52]. They are more likely to require some or total assistance for activities of daily living and are more frequently hospitalized [17]. PH also appears to pose an additional burden on exercise capacity of IPF patients, with a shorter distance walked and/or a greater desaturation on the 6MWT [8, 10, 23, 27, 40], a lower peak Vo_2, and a more pronounced ventilatory inefficiency on cardiopulmonary exercise testing as compared with those without PH [52].

Most importantly, there is a clearly documented association between PH and the risk of death in IPF independently of functional parameters and whatever the method of diagnosis, i.e. RHC [19, 27], TTE [26, 28], or even chest radiography [39]. In the IPF transplant cohort of Lettieri et al. [27], the overall mortality rates were 60 vs. 29.9% (OR: 2.6) and the 1-year mortality rates were 28 vs. 5.5% in patients with and without PH, respectively. There was also a linear correlation between mPAP and outcomes with higher pressures associated with a greater risk of mortality. Interestingly, even a mild increase in mPAP may have prognosis implications in IPF. Hamada et al. [19] demonstrated that a subset of patients with normal PAP comprised between 17 and 25 mm Hg experienced worse survival rates. Lastly, in an autopsy study on 42 consecutive IPF patients, PH or cor pulmonale was the immediate cause of death in 2 subjects, but was a contributing factor for mortality in 40% [53].

Treatment

There is no expectancy that regimens currently used in IPF have an effect on PH, as none of them has proven efficacy in IPF itself. One study suggested that anticoagulant therapy may improve survival in IPF probably by decreasing the mortality related to acute exacerbations [54]. These pilot results have encouraged clinicians to prescribe anticoagulants in IPF-associated PH. However, there was no mention about the potential link between the observed effect and the presence of PH, and this nonrandomized trial had major deficiencies which preclude any firm conclusion. Patients with IPF-associated PH should be considered for lung transplantation without delay [55]. The choice of transplantation procedure should always be based on the patient, but double-lung transplantation is the favored surgical approach in patients with severe PH [55]. Whether preoperative hemodynamics affect the outcome of IPF patients who undergo lung transplantation is a matter of debate. A recent large cohort of 195 patients who received double-lung transplantation for IPF revealed that preoperative mPAP >35 mm Hg was associated with a higher risk of death at 3 months posttransplantation [56].

To date, not much has been written about the benefits of PAH-targeted therapy. Acute aerosolization of prostacyclin or iloprost markedly decreases PAP with the advantage of not worsening gas exchange [35]. However, its chronic effect has not been evaluated. Sildenafil may selectively block phosphodiesterase-5 in well-ventilated regions of the lung and therefore improve gas exchange [36]. A placebo-controlled trial found a small but significant difference in arterial oxygenation, DLCO, degree of dyspnea, and quality of life favoring sildenafil in a population with advanced IPF defined as DLCO <35%. However, the study was not designed to determine whether the benefits of sildenafil were driven by the subgroup of patients with PH [57]. Collard et al. [58] reported an open-label 3-month study of sildenafil in 14 patients with IPF-associated PH. Among the 11 patients who completed serial 6MWTs, 57% improved their walk distance by more than 20% and overall mean amelioration was 49 m. Despite the rationale for ET-1 blockade in IPF-associated PH, the only available study with bosentan in IPF excluded patients with PH [59]. In the retrospective series of Minai et al. [60] on 19 patients with PH complicating various fibrotic ILDs, the benefit of PAH drugs was less likely to occur and appeared to be less sustained in IPF. Among the 8 patients with IPF-associated PH, 5 were initially treated with bosentan and 3 with intravenous epoprostenol. Six patients were considered responders, as defined by an increase in 6MWT distance >50 m at 3 or 6 months, but 2 of them had deteriorated significantly at the 1-year follow-up either on 6MWT, WHO class, or estimated sPAP. Further investigation of PAH agents in the treatment of IPF-associated PH is ongoing with several clinical trials underway (www.clinicaltrials.gov).

Combined Pulmonary Fibrosis and Emphysema Syndrome

Combined pulmonary fibrosis and emphysema (CPFE) syndrome has recently been individualized as a discrete entity rather than a particular phenotype of IPF (fig. 5). Hence, CPFE is characterized by the association of distinct features, including intense tobacco smoking, male predominance, severe dyspnea, unexpected subnormal spirometric findings, severely impaired DLCO, profound hypoxemia at exercise, high frequency of PH, and dismal prognosis [61]. The prevalence of echocardiographic PH was 47% in the series of 61 patients studied by Cottin et al. [61] and 90% in that of Mejia et al. [62] on 29 patients, as defined by an estimated sPAP >45 and 50 mm Hg, respectively. In the Mexican study, patients with CPFE syndrome had a 19-fold increase in the risk of developing PH in comparison with those with IPF without emphysema [62]. Likewise, there were positive correlations between hemodynamics and the extent of emphysema on HRCT, but not with lung volumes and DLCO [62].

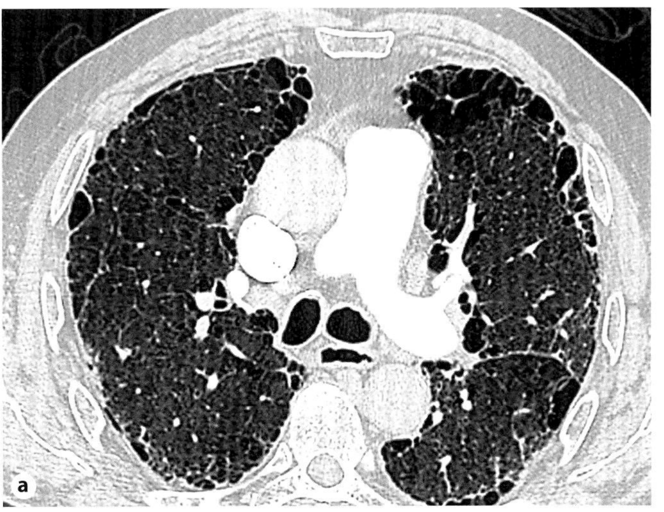
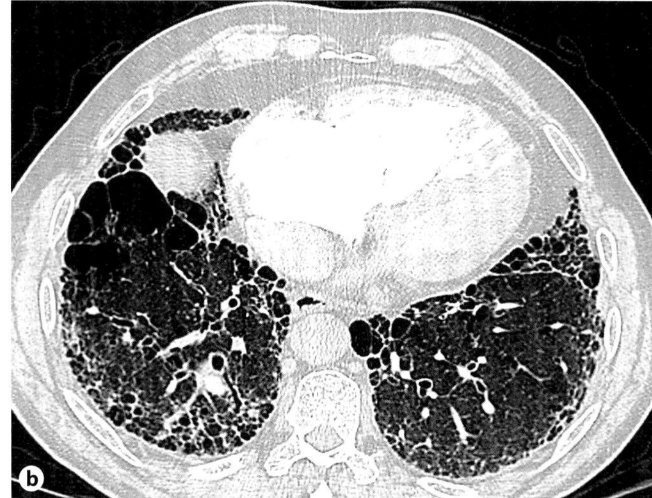

Fig. 5. Patient with PH complicating combined pulmonary fibrosis and emphysema. The scan shows emphysema predominating in the upper lobes (**a**) and basal subpleural honeycombing (**b**). Note the enlargement of right heart cavities (**b**).

PH complicating CPFE syndrome is severe. On RHC, mPAP is >35 mm Hg in 68% of cases and >40 mm Hg in 48% [63]. The survival of patients with CPFE syndrome is worse than that of patients with IPF alone, this pejorative outcome being at least partially determined by PH per se independently of emphysema. Indeed, in the study by Mejia et al. [62], the two strongest variables that predicted time to death in the whole population with IPF were FVC <50% and severe PH (estimated sPAP >75 mm Hg). The presence of emphysema as a significant predictor of survival was lost in the stratified analysis because of the strong association with severe PH. In the study by Cottin et al. [61], the only significant difference in survival in CPFE syndrome was found between patients with or without PH at diagnosis, with a 5-year survival rate of 25 vs. 75%, respectively.

In the French series enrolling 40 patients with CPFE syndrome and PH confirmed by RHC, 24 received first-line treatment with bosentan, sildenafil, or inhaled iloprost. No significant effect was observed regarding NHYA class, 6MWT, or estimated sPAP after 3–6 months, and treatment was not associated with a better survival [63].

Connective Tissue Disease-Related Interstitial Lung Disease

ILD and PH are the two most frequent and serious complications of CTDs, and can occur either separately or in association [64]. The histologic pattern of ILD in the context of CTDs is usually, although not universally, nonspecific interstitial pneumonia. CTD-associated PH may result from a primary pulmonary arteriopathy (Group 1 of the PH classification), ILD (Group 3), or occasionally left heart disease (Group 2) [2, 3]. The pathological picture of CTD-associated PAH is generally indistinguishable from that of classical idiopathic PAH, although pulmonary venous involvement may be more frequent [2, 3]. PAH occurs principally in SSc, systemic lupus erythematosus, and mixed CTD; to a lesser extent it occurs in rheumatoid arthritis, inflammatory myopathies, and Sjögren's syndrome. SSc is the CTD where the issue of ILD and PH association is the most relevant.

Frequency

In a recent cohort of 619 patients with SSc, 22.5% had evidence of isolated restrictive lung physiology suggestive of ILD, 19.2% had PAH alone (assessed by TTE), and 18.1% had combined restrictive ventilatory deficit along with PH [30]. Launay et al. [65] retrospectively studied 197 consecutive patients with SSc and found that PH was present in 21.8% of the 110 patients with ILD.

Pathogenesis

The prevalence of PH may be significantly higher in patients with CTD-related ILD than in those with IIPs [66]. In patients with SSc-related ILD, there is no correlation between lung volumes and PH [32, 65]. In the study of Launay et al. [65] the prevalence and severity of PH did not differ between ILD patients with or without significant reduction in lung volumes. A lower PaO_2 appeared as the unique independent factor significantly associated with PH, regardless of the extent of fibrosis. Lastly, PH was out of proportion to the degree of fibrosis in 33.3% of cases, suggesting a superimposed vasculopathy. The mechanisms of PH can be intricate. Thus, the presence of pulmonary fibrosis on chest radiography is an independent factor significantly associated with left ventricular dysfunction in patients with SSc [67].

Diagnosis

Classically, ILD is prone to develop in patients with diffuse cutaneous SSc and/or antitopoisomerase I antibody, while isolated PAH is more frequent in patients with the limited cutaneous form of disease and/or anticentromere antibody. According to Steen et al. [68] there is a subset of patients with antinucleolar antibody that have a unique mixture of both pulmonary fibrosis and authentic PAH, this latter being often severe.

A screening algorithm is proposed in figure 2. It has been suggested that the presence of pericardial abnormalities, including pericardial effusion, thickness of the anterior pericardial recess, and pericardial thickening, is a good indicator of echocardiographic PH in patients with ILD complicating SSc [69].

Clinical Impact and Prognosis

Survival of patients with SSc and ILD-associated PH is particularly grim. In fact, Trad et al. [32] demonstrated that echocardiographic PH was, together with age, the sole predictor of mortality in 52 patients with ILD among a retrospective cohort of diffuse cutaneous SSc, with a 5.07-fold increase in risk of death. In another study by Mathai et al. [70] on 59 consecutive patients with SSc and PAH or ILD-associated PH confirmed by RHC, survival was significantly worse in those with ILD-associated PH, with 1-, 2-, and 3-year survival rates of 82, 46, and 39%.

Treatment

Combining corticosteroids and cyclophosphamide has proven efficacy in SSc-related ILD, but is inefficient on SSc-PAH (contrary to other CTDs such as systemic lupus erythematosus or mixed CTD). Very little is known about the effect of immunosuppressive therapy in ILD-associated PH. Eight patients of the cohort of Trad et al. [32] received at least 6 monthly pulses of intravenous cyclophosphamide. sPAP increased significantly during this regimen while TLC and DLCO remained stable during the same period.

Patients with SSc-PAH have been included in most of the major clinical trials for regulatory approval of PAH medications. Treatment of SSc-PAH follows the same strategy as in idiopathic PAH, although the magnitude of the response is lower, possibly because of a more frequent involvement of pulmonary veins [2, 3]. The effect of vasomodulating therapy in PH complicating SSc-related ILD is not well understood. The only available randomized-controlled trial with bosentan in SSc-related ILD excluded patients with PH. In the retrospective series of Minai et al. [60] on 19 patients with PH and various fibrotic ILDs, 5 patients had CTDs. Four of them were initially given intravenous epoprostenol and 1 was given bosentan. All were considered responders, as defined by an increase in 6MWT distance >50 m at 3 or 6 months, but 2 had deteriorated significantly at 1-year follow-up on 6MWT, dyspnea, or estimated sPAP.

Lung transplantation may represent a viable therapeutic option to consider for patients with end-stage lung disease [71].

Sarcoidosis

Sarcoidosis is a multisystemic disorder of unknown etiology characterized by the formation of immune granulomas in affected tissues, particularly the lung and the lymphatic system. The disease has an estimated prevalence of 1–40/100,000 and mainly affects 25- to 40-year-old people with a predilection for women and Blacks. Multiple phenotypes are seen according to presentation, involved organs, disease duration, and severity [72]. While spontaneous remissions occur in nearly two thirds of the patients within 2–3 years, therapy is required and/or the course is chronic in a third of the patients.

Frequency

The exact prevalence of PH complicating sarcoidosis remains to be established. The wide distribution in published rates is most likely due to the use of different measurement techniques, selection of diverse patient populations, or various stages of disease. PH affects 1–6% of unselected patients with sarcoidosis [73–77], but it is much more frequent in advanced lung disease [12] or symptomatic patients [13].

The only available prospective study was conducted by Handa et al. [75]. They evaluated 212 consecutive outpatients with sarcoidosis by TTE and found that an estimated sPAP >40 mm Hg was present in 5.7%. Unfortunately, RHC

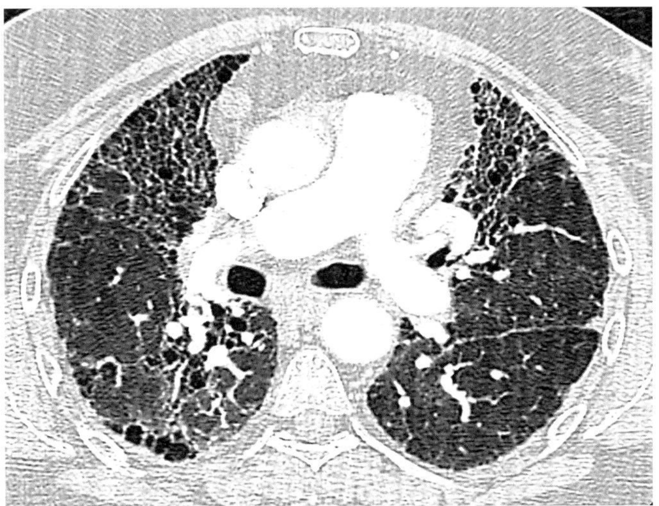

Fig. 6. Patient with PH complicating stage IV sarcoidosis. The scan shows pulmonary fibrosis with honeycombing and bronchial distortion and a significantly increased caliber of the main PA as compared with aorta.

was not performed to confirm the diagnosis of PH [75]. Shorr et al. [12] retrospectively reviewed a US cohort of 363 sarcoid patients listed for lung transplantation who had completed RHC. PH was identified in 73.8% of cases and mPAP was >40 mm Hg in 36.1%. Lastly, in the retrospective study by Baughman et al. [14], 130 patients with persistent dyspnea despite systemic therapy for their sarcoidosis were systematically explored with RHC; 38.5% had evidence of PH.

No difference has been observed in terms of sarcoidosis phenotype or demographic characteristics between patients with or without PH with the exception of possible male gender predominance [75].

Pathogenesis

Sarcoidosis-associated PH may fit into all five categories of PH classification. However, as its pathophysiology is complex, it has been classified under category 5 [2, 3].

Destruction of the Distal Capillary Bed and/or Hypoxemia

The majority of sarcoid patients with PH have evidence of stage IV on chest radiography [7, 29, 33, 75], and they are more hypoxemic and/or require supplemental oxygen more frequently than those without PH [7, 12, 29, 33, 75] (fig. 6). However, 31.8–40% of patients develop PH in the absence of patent pulmonary fibrosis [7, 33] and a small subset of cases have no apparent underlying lung disease (stage 0 and I) [7, 33, 75, 78]. Moreover, hemodynamic measurements do not correlate well with spirometric parameters and PaO_2 [7, 13, 75, 79], and mPAP is significantly higher in sarcoidosis than in IPF for equivalent respiratory impairment [80]. Finally, the degree of PH is sometimes disproportionate to functional abnormalities [7, 12, 81] and PH may even be more severe when it occurs in patients without fibrotic disease [7]. Taken together, these findings support the idea that mechanisms other than the destruction of the distal capillary bed and hypoxemia may play a role in the development of sarcoidosis-associated PH. These include specific vasculopathy, local increased vasoreactivity, extrinsic compression of pulmonary vessels, myocardial dysfunction, and portal hypertension.

Specific Vasculopathy

Vascular involvement is very common in pulmonary sarcoidosis, reaching 69–100% of cases according to pathological studies [82, 83]. Changes consist of occlusive or destructive lesions due to the invasion of vessel walls by granulomas or perivascular fibrosis [82, 83] (fig. 7). Vascular involvement can be observed at all levels, from large branches of PA to small veins, but it prevails in the venous side, reflecting the lymphatic predilection of sarcoidosis [82, 83] (fig. 7). Despite frequent vascular involvement, clinically significant PH is rare.

A type of PVOD-like disease is now a well-recognized cause of sarcoidosis-associated PH [7, 84, 85]. The occlusive narrowing of interlobular veins by granuloma can mimic PVOD and result in PH. This mechanical granulomatous PVOD has been pathologically authenticated in few cases with nonfibrotic sarcoidosis [84, 85]. Additionally, Nunes et al. [7] described an intrinsic occlusive venopathy in explanted lungs from 5 patients with sarcoidosis-associated PH. This venopathy was characterized by marked intimal fibrosis and recanalization of the interlobular septal veins associated with chronic hemosiderosis. Conversely, arterial changes were minor with no evidence of plexiform or thrombotic lesions. Scattered granuloma were present in veins in 4 of 5 cases, whereas arterial granulomas were seen in only 2 cases and neither venous nor arterial granulomas could be found in 1 patient.

Local Increased Vasoreactivity

The potential role of heightened reactivity of the pulmonary vasculature to vasoactive mediators has been raised because a number of patients with sarcoidosis-associated PH have shown a reduction in mPAP and/or pulmonary vascular resistance to acute vasodilator challenge with

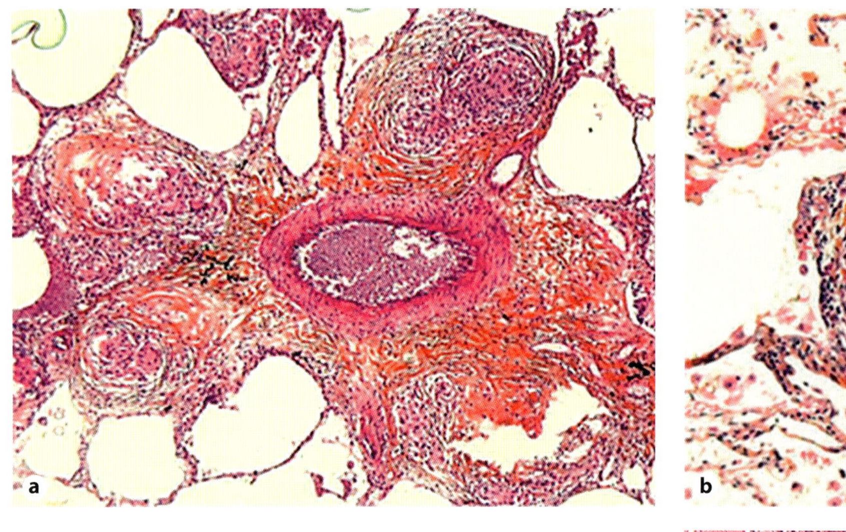

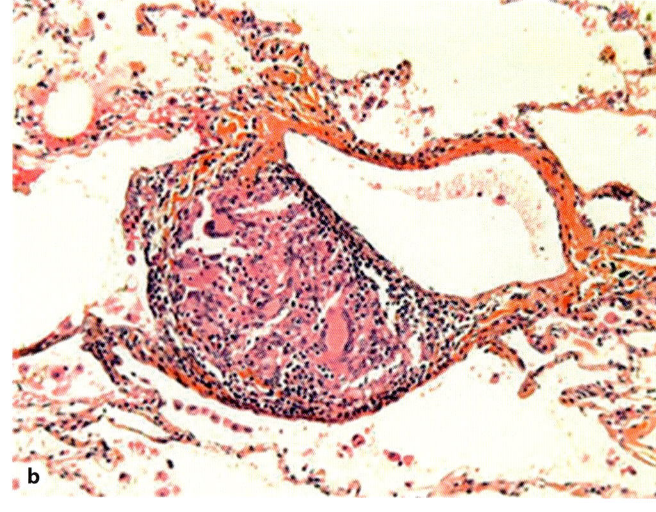

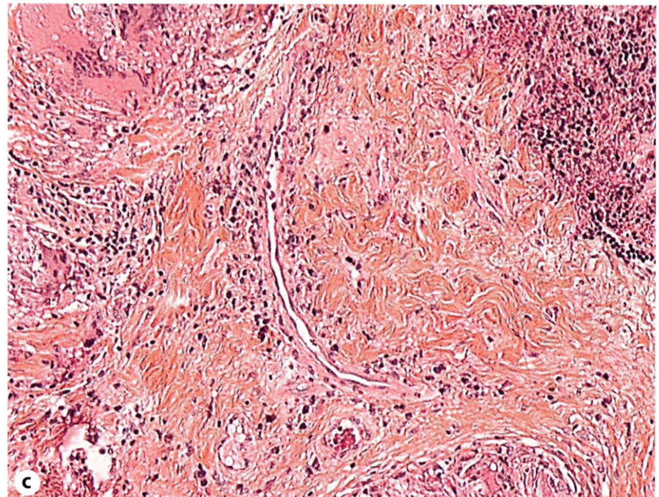

Fig. 7. Patient with pulmonary sarcoidosis. The figure shows several nonnecrotizing granulomas surrounding PA (**a**) and invading the wall of interlobular veins (**b**). The venular lumen is completely narrowed by granuloma simulating PVOD (**c**).

inhaled nitric oxide or prostacyclin [81, 86, 87]. It has been shown that levels of ET-1 in plasma [88] and BAL fluid [89, 90] are elevated in some, albeit not all, patients with sarcoidosis as compared with controls. Unfortunately, data are currently limited and none has correlated ET-1 with clinical phenotype of sarcoidosis, in particular the presence of PH.

Extrinsic Compression of Pulmonary Vessels

Sarcoidosis-associated PH may be caused by extrinsic compression of the proximal PA by enlarged lymph nodes or fibrosing mediastinitis [7, 91, 92] (fig. 8). Compression of the large pulmonary veins is much rarer and can result in localized edema. Although occasionally described in early stages of sarcoidosis, PA compression is much more frequent in patients with long-standing disease. This mechanism was demonstrated in 21.4% of patients with PH and radiographic stage IV in the study by Nunes et al. [7].

Left Heart Dysfunction

Myocardial involvement is not rare in sarcoidosis and may lead to left ventricular systolic or diastolic dysfunction. When sarcoid patients with persistent dyspnea are thoroughly investigated by RHC, left ventricular dysfunction as defined by an elevated PWP >15 mm Hg is revealed in 11.3–15.4% [13, 14], which represents 28.6% of all cases with PH [14]. In sarcoid patients awaiting lung transplantation, although within normal values for the vast majority of cases, PWP is on average significantly higher in the presence of PH. It is also independently associated with PH, which indicates that subtle impairment in cardiac performance may

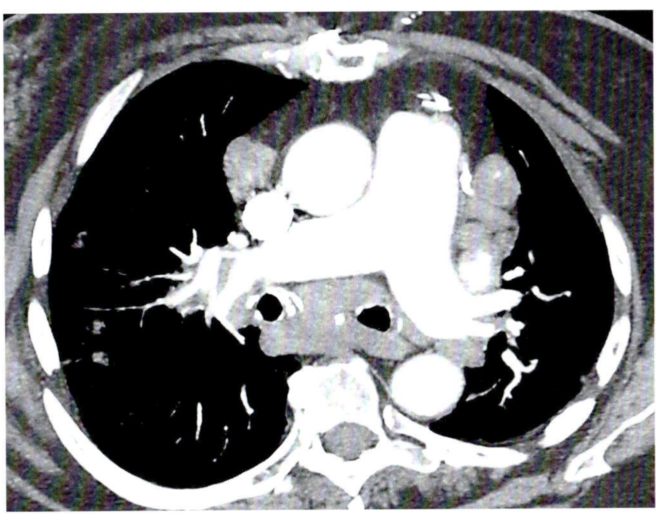

Fig. 8. Patient with sarcoidosis-associated PH. The scan shows multiple calcified lymph nodes with a bilateral extrinsic compression of large PA.

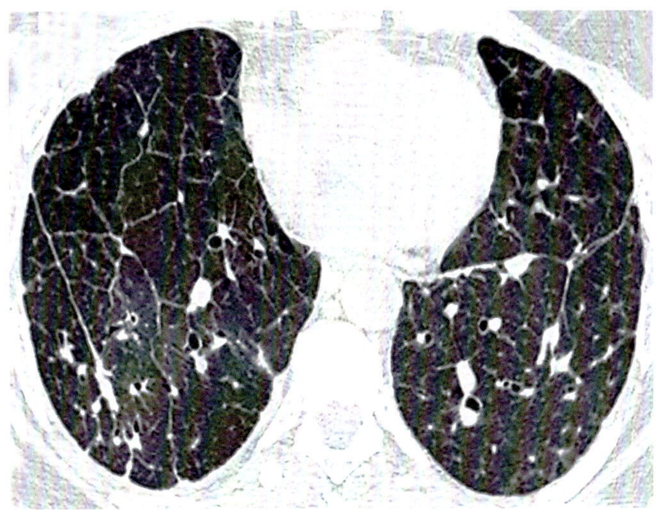

Fig. 9. Patient with sarcoidosis-associated PH. The scan shows a network of septal lines and ground-glass opacities suggestive of PVOD.

nonetheless exist and reflects left ventricular diastolic dysfunction [12].

Portal Hypertension
PH may also be the consequence of hepatic sarcoidosis which can lead, albeit rarely, to cirrhosis and portal hypertension [93].

Diagnosis
A screening algorithm is proposed in figure 2. Raynaud's phenomenon is occasionally noted in sarcoidosis-associated PH as in idiopathic PAH [7]. The severity of sarcoidosis-associated PH is extremely variable. About one quarter of the patients present with signs of right-sided heart failure [7, 33]. PH seems more severe in patients without than with pulmonary fibrosis [7], with 85.4% [7] and 36.1–53.3% [7, 12] having levels of mPAP >35–40 mm Hg, respectively.

Once PH is confirmed, it is imperative to delineate which mechanism is operative since this dictates therapeutic options. For that purpose, contrast-enhanced HRCT is crucial. First, it allows for the diagnosis of extrinsic vascular compression (fig. 8). Second, several findings may hint to PVOD, such as extensive ground-glass opacities and/or thickened interlobular septa (fig. 9). Although these signs may be related solely to sarcoidosis, Nunes et al. [7] showed that patients with sarcoidosis-associated PH had a significantly higher frequency of ground-glass attenuation and septal lines as compared to sarcoid controls without PH. It is sometimes tricky to differentiate extrinsic vascular compression from pulmonary embolism, which sometimes requires pulmonary angiography. Hepatic ultrasound is necessary to exclude portopulmonary hypertension. In cases with suspected myocardial involvement, several cardiac tests complement RHC.

Clinical Impact and Prognosis
PH accounts for refractory dyspnea [13] and reduced exercise capacity [94] in sarcoid patients. Furthermore, PH is well-known to portend a poor outcome [7, 14, 78, 80, 95, 96]. In transplantation candidates, mPAP is an independent predictor of death together with oxygen requirement [95, 96]. In a cohort of stage IV patients originating from a non-transplant center, the development of PH was also independently associated with mortality, and intractable right heart failure was the first cause of death.

In the retrospective series by Nunes et al. [7] on 22 patients with sarcoidosis-associated PH, the 5-year survival rate was 59%, which was significantly worse than for controls without PH. In the study by Baughman et al. [14], the relative risk of death in the presence of PH without left ventricular dysfunction versus no PH was 10.39 and 3.14 when comparing PH without or with left ventricular dysfunction.

Treatment
Therapy for sarcoidosis-associated PH should take into account the prominent underlying mechanism of PH. With respect to corticosteroids, published results are somewhat discrepant. PH can worsen despite corticosteroids [97–101] as

well as dramatically improve [102, 103]. In the study of Nunes et al. [7], 10 patients with sarcoidosis-associated PH received high doses of oral prednisone. There was no treatment effect in the 5 patients with stage IV, but a sustained improvement was obtained in 3 of the 5 cases without pulmonary fibrosis.

There have been several recent publications of case reports or uncontrolled small series on long-term responses to PAH therapy for sarcoidosis-associated PH with variable results, as summarized in table 2 [13, 60, 78, 81, 87, 104–106]. These conflicting results are confusing for clinicians and spark the need for prospective randomized placebo-controlled trials. Obviously, successful reports are more likely to be published, which produces a bias. Moreover, a more rational approach is critical to define which patients to treat (according to radiographic stage, lung function and/or mPAP), which drug to use, and whether it should be used after immunosuppressive therapy or in association. Lastly, one case of sudden death and one case of acute pulmonary edema have been described following intravenous epoprostenol, probably because of PVOD [87]. Clinical trials are underway to determine the efficiency and safety of PAH therapy in sarcoidosis-associated PH (www.clinicaltrials.gov).

Considering the high mortality rate of patients with sarcoidosis-associated PH, evaluation for lung transplantation should be discussed early. Interestingly, angioplasty and stenting of the PA with sustained hemodynamic and functional improvement has been reported in 2 sarcoid patients with extrinsic compression from mediastinal fibrosis [91].

Pulmonary Langerhans Cell Histiocytosis

In adults, PLCH is a smoking-related ILD characterized pathologically by bronchiolocentric stellate nodules composed of large numbers of Langerhans cells admixed with other inflammatory cells, often organized as loosely formed granulomas [107]. PLCH is very rare and predominantly affects adults aged 20–40 years. The disease is commonly associated with irreversible airflow obstruction and highly variable clinical outcomes. It may regress either spontaneously or after smoking cessation. In a minority of patients, however, PLCH may progress to pulmonary fibrosis and honeycomb lung with obstructive, restrictive, or mixed patterns of lung mechanics [107].

Frequency
Although the occurrence of PH is exceptional in patients with early PLCH, severe PH may be a common event in the course of advanced lung disease. In the study by Fartoukh et al. [6], all the 21 patients with PLCH referred for lung transplantation had evidence of PH on RHC. Dauriat et al. [108] set up a study in eleven French transplant centers. PH was present in 91.7% of the 36 transplanted patients who underwent RHC and mPAP was >35 mm Hg in 72.5% of cases. In the retrospective cohort of Chaowalit et al. [109] on 123 patients with PLCH, TTE was carried out in 17 cases because of suspected PH, shortness of breath, cor pulmonale, or palpitations. Of them, 13 had an estimated sPAP >35 mm Hg with no other identifiable cause of PH, which represented 2.4% of the whole population and 76.5% of symptomatic patients. Regrettably, only 4 patients underwent RHC confirming PH in all cases.

Pathogenesis
As sarcoidosis, PLCH is now classified under Group 5 of the PH classification [2, 3]. The degree of PH complicating PLCH is not related to the measures of pulmonary function or PaO_2 [6, 109–111], and mPAP is significantly higher in patients with PLCH than those with IPF [6, 110], LAM [110, 111], or other chronic obstructive pulmonary diseases [6] for similar alteration in pulmonary function. Additionally, in the majority of cases, PLCH-associated PH is severe and of much greater magnitude than would be anticipated on the basis of lung physiology only [6, 108, 111]. Taken together, these findings suggest that other mechanisms than the destruction of vascular bed and hypoxemia may be at play.

Several authors have alluded to the importance of vascular involvement in PLCH. Crausman et al. [112] elegantly demonstrated that indices reflecting pulmonary vascular dysfunction (DLCO, baseline VD/VT, and exercise VD/VT) are abnormal in patients with early PLCH, which may pave the way for the subsequent development of PH. These indices are strongly correlated with exercise limitation, whereas ventilatory function and gas exchanges are not [112]. Pathologically, vascular involvement is not uncommon in PLCH [113–115], though in general mild [114]. Vascular changes are usually within regions of prominent PLCH inflammation with an extension to the walls of small-to-medium-sized PA adjacent to bronchioles in the center of pulmonary lobules (fig. 10). Despite the bronchiolocentric distribution of PLCH lesions, interlobular septal veins may also be affected [113–115].

The development of PH has been ascribed to the presence of intense and widespread vasculopathy [6, 109, 111, 116]. Fartoukh et al. [6] analyzed the lung samples from 12 patients with PLCH-associated PH and found that all of them exhibited changes affecting both small-to-medium-sized intralobular PA and interlobular septal veins, with

Table 2. Main series on long-term PAH-targeted therapy for sarcoidosis-associated PH[1]

Patients characteristics	Agent	Effect	Outcomes	Reference
n = 7 Stage III: n = 1; IV: n = 6 Baseline mPAP = 55 ± 4 mm Hg Baseline PVR = 896 ± 200 dyne•s•cm^{-5}	iNO: n = 4 iNO + EPO : n = 1 CCB: n = 2	Patients treated with iNO: improvement in the 6MWT distance for 5/5 and in NYHA for 3/5; worsening in hemodynamics in 3/3 tested patients Patients treated with CCB: worsening in 2/2	6 patients died 2 patients alive under iNO for 1.5 and 2 years awaiting transplantation	[81]
n = 15/22 (7 patients could not complete 16 weeks of therapy for several reasons) Stage 0: n = 1; I: n = 1; II: n = 1; III: n = 1; IV: n = 11 Baseline mPAP = 36 (20–62) mm Hg and PVR = 488 (157–1,304) dyne•s•cm^{-5}	iloprost	Patients were followed prospectively At 16 weeks therapy, 8/15 patients were considered responders as defined as either an increase in 6MWT distance ≥30 m or a decrease in the PVR ≥20% Globally, the SGRQ activity score decreased significantly	NA	[104]
n = 5 Stage I: n = 1; III: n = 1; IV: n = 3 Baseline mPAP = 58 ± 7 mm Hg Baseline PVR = 1,142±568 dyne•s•cm^{-5}	IV EPO	Improvement in NYHA for all patients	4 patients alive and 1 transplanted after an average of 29 months therapy	[87]
n = 6	IV EPO: n=3 Bosentan: n=3	4 initial responders (increase in 6MWD >50 m at 3-6 months therapy): 2 with EPO and 2 with bosentan; only 1 responder at 12 months' therapy	NA	[60]
n = 7 Baseline mPAP = 53.4 ± 13.4 mm Hg	Bosentan: n = 4 Bosentan + EPO: n = 1 EPO: n = 1 CCB: n = 1	Significant improvement in hemodynamics in 4/5 tested patients (bosentan: n = 2; EPO: n = 1; CCB: n = 1) and stability in 1/5 (CCB)	Follow-up between 4 and 8 months; 2 patients died	[13]
n = 12 Patients with end-stage disease referred for lung transplantation Baseline mPAP = 48 ± 15 mm Hg and PVR: 856 ± 384 dyne•s•cm^{-5}	Sildenafil	Treatment was given for a median duration of 4 (1–12) months Significant improvement in hemodynamics in 9 tested patients (mPAP: –8 mmHg, PVR: –392 dyne•s•cm^{-5}) with a decrease in PVR ≥20% in 6/9 No significant change in the 6MWT distance	NA	[105]
n = 22 Stage 0: n = 3; II: n = 3; III: n = 1; IV: n = 15 Baseline mPAP = 46.1 ± 2.7 mm Hg Baseline PVR = 810 ± 89.1 dyne•s•cm^{-5}	Initial monotherapy: bosentan: n = 12 sildenafil: n = 9 EPO: n = 1 Various combination therapies (inadequate response to initial monotherapy): n = 8	Improvement in NYHA in 9 patients, significant increase in 6MWT distance in 18 tested patients (+59 m), significant improvement in hemodynamics in 12 tested patients (mPAP: –9.1 mm Hg, PVR: –350 dyne•s•cm^{-5}) Patients with a higher FVC had a greater increment in exercise capacity	Median of 11 months of follow-up; 1- and 3-year transplant-free survival rates: 90 and 74%	[78]

All studies were retrospective and uncontrolled. PVR = Pulmonary vascular resistance; iNO = inhaled nitric oxide; IV = intravenous; EPO = epoprostenol; CCB = calcium channel blockers; SGRQ = St. George's Respiratory Questionnaire; NA = not available.

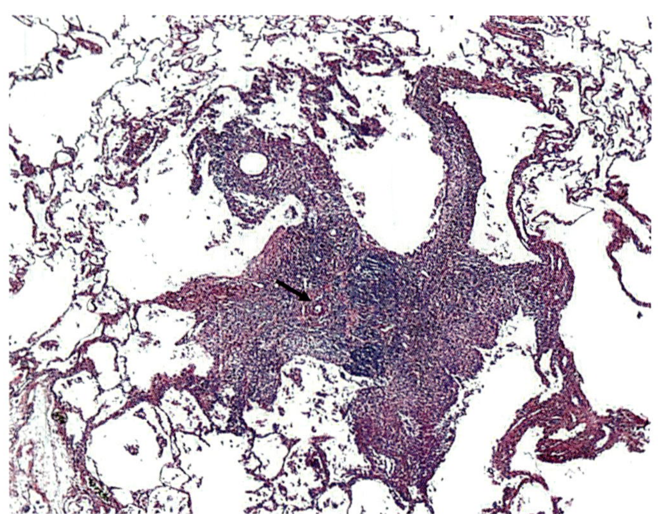

Fig. 10. Patient with PLCH. The figure shows concentric thickening of the arterial wall (arrow) within a florid pulmonary Langerhans cell granuloma.

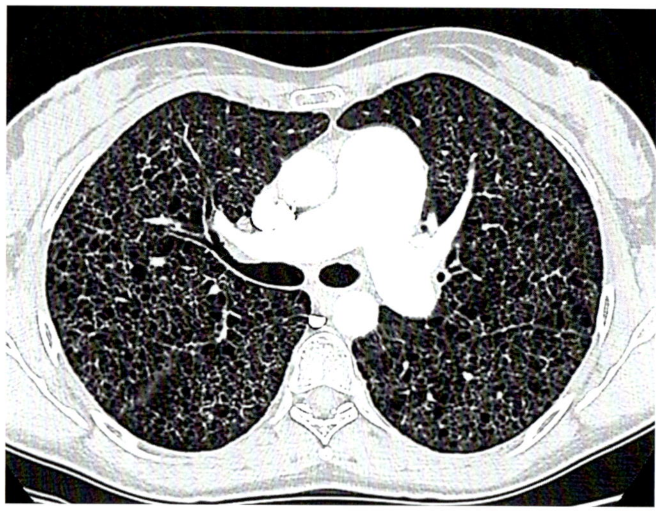

Fig. 11. Patient with PLCH-associated PH. The scan shows extensive cysts and a significantly increased caliber of the main PA as compared with aorta.

prominent venous participation. Involvement of the PA consisted of proliferative arteriopathy with intimal fibrosis and medial hypertrophy, leading to arterial obliteration in 60% of cases. There was no evidence of plexiform or thrombotic lesions. Involvement of the veins consisted of intimal fibrosis, medial hypertrophy, and obliteration in 75%. Aspects of PVOD with venular obliteration, hemosiderosis, and capillary dilatation were detected in one third of the patients. On the other hand, Langerhans cell infiltration of a vessel was observed in only one case and vascular abnormalities were noted in areas remote from histiocytosis X nodules in half of the patients [6]. It is fascinating that the vasculopathy worsened in the 6 patients from whom two subsequent lung samples (before and after the occurrence of PH) were available, whereas parenchymal and bronchiolar lesions remained relatively steady, suggesting that its progression was independent [6].

It is intriguing that, in contrast to sarcoidosis, PLCH-associated PH has almost not been reported in the absence of long-standing lung disease, which is probably due to the different distribution of granuloma between the two disorders (primarily bronchiolocentric vs. lymphatic). Instead, the venopathy observed in PLCH-associated PH resembles that of fibrotic sarcoidosis, and may share similar pathophysiology. Granuloma may have an indirect role through the production of various cytokines and growth factors implicated in vascular remodeling. For example, a number of these mediators can be released by granulomas of PLCH such as platelet-derived growth factor, TGF-β, and IL1 [117, 118].

Diagnosis

A screening algorithm is proposed in figure 2. Raynaud's phenomenon is occasionally noted in PLCH-associated PH as in idiopathic PAH [6]. PLCH-associated PH is generally severe, with HRCT showing extensive lesions (fig. 11). The majority of patients present with already important dyspnea, NYHA III or IV, and signs of right heart failure [6, 109]. At RHC, mPAP ranges from 43.6 to 59 mm Hg, the level of mPAP being over 45–50 mm Hg in about half to two thirds of the cases [6, 108, 111]. Acute vasodilator trial was positive in 31% of cases in a series [6].

Clinical Impact and Prognosis

In the retrospective cohort of patients with PLCH of Chaowalit et al. [109], 38.5% of the 13 subjects with echocardiographic PH died during the 55.5-month follow-up. The causes of death were related to the underlying lung disease and the median survival after PH diagnosis was 7.6 months. PH augmented the risk of mortality by 22.8. Interestingly, patients affected with PLCH referred for lung transplantation, even with higher degrees of PH, have a much better survival rate compared with those with IPF [110].

Treatment

Very little information is available on the treatment of PLCH-associated PH. One case was reported, which improved with corticosteroids [119]. In this observation, open lung biopsy showed evidence of medial hypertrophy of PA in areas of pulmonary fibrosis, but no vascular granulomas. Surprisingly, venous involvement was not mentioned. The patient stopped smoking and was given high doses of prednisone. mPAP and pulmonary vascular resistance diminished, with mPAP passing from 35 to 26 mm Hg at 9 months on RHC while pulmonary function tests and blood gases remained unchanged [119]. Conversely, another case deteriorated rapidly and died despite corticosteroids. Autopsy revealed a pattern of PVOD [116].

Because of the prominent venous involvement, intravenous epoprostenol may be hazardous in patients with PLCH-associated PH. Of note, Fartoukh et al. [6] reported 2 patients with severe PLCH-associated PH who experienced acute pulmonary edema on epoprostenol. Concerning other specific PAH agents, only one case has been reported with bosentan [120]. The patient was referred for lung transplantation because of end-stage PLCH and was diagnosed with severe PH. He was then started on diuretics, warfarin and bosentan, which was followed by improved dyspnea, 6MWT distance, and hemodynamics. Benefit was maintained for a total of 7 years, with mPAP passing from 41 to 30 mm Hg, so that inscription on the transplant list was postponed [120].

Lung transplantation is the therapy of choice for PLCH-associated PH. Despite a recurrence rate of the disease of approximately 20% after lung transplantation, postransplant results are good and very close to those obtained for other disorders [108].

Other Interstitial Lung Diseases

PH has been described in many other ILDs as a consequence of lung disease and/or hypoxia. The prevalence of PH in idiopathic nonspecific interstitial pneumonia is unknown and its presence should raise the possibility of forme fruste CTD. The echocardiographic prevalence of PH (sPAP >35 mm Hg) has been estimated at 6.7% in a cohort of 120 unselected patients with LAM [121].

Conclusion

While its prevalence is variable according to underlying ILD, PH signifies a grave outcome whatever ILD. There are recent shreds of evidence suggesting that PH may be more complex than just the result of parenchymal lung disease and hypoxemia. Intrinsic vasculopathy may play an important role, in particular in sarcoidosis and PLCH. Therapeutic intervention with PAH-targeted therapy may be helpful in ILD-associated PH, but the lack of specific studies leaves many uncertainties in this area. Although difficult in such rare and life-threatening conditions, prospective randomized-controlled trials are warranted and it is essential that their design distinguish patients with 'out of proportion' PH. Finally, a great effort should be put in the constitution of international registries to obtain data from patients with ILD-associated PH.

References

1 American Thoracic Society, European Respiratory Society: American Thoracic Society/European Respiratory Society International Multidisciplinary Consensus Classification of the Idiopathic Interstitial Pneumonias. This joint statement of the American Thoracic Society (ATS), and the European Respiratory Society (ERS) was adopted by the ATS board of directors, June 2001 and by the ERS Executive Committee, June 2001. Am J Respir Crit Care Med 2002;165: 277–304.

2 Simonneau G, Robbins IM, Beghetti M, et al: Updated clinical classification of pulmonary hypertension. J Am Coll Cardiol 2009;54:S43–S54.

3 Galie N, Hoeper MM, Humbert M, et al: Guidelines for the diagnosis and treatment of pulmonary hypertension. Eur Respir J 2009;34:1219–1263.

4 Colombat M, Mal H, Groussard O, et al: Pulmonary vascular lesions in end-stage idiopathic pulmonary fibrosis: histopathologic study on lung explant specimens and correlations with pulmonary hemodynamics. Hum Pathol 2007; 38:60–65.

5 Kim KH, Maldonado F, Ryu JH, et al: Iron deposition and increased alveolar septal capillary density in nonfibrotic lung tissue are associated with pulmonary hypertension in idiopathic pulmonary fibrosis. Respir Res 2010;11:37.

6 Fartoukh M, Humbert M, Capron F, et al: Severe pulmonary hypertension in histiocytosis X. Am J Respir Crit Care Med 2000;161:216–223.

7 Nunes H, Humbert M, Capron F, et al: Pulmonary hypertension associated with sarcoidosis: mechanisms, haemodynamics and prognosis. Thorax 2006;61:68–74.

8 Modrykamien AM, Gudavalli R, McCarthy K, Parambil J: Echocardiography, 6-minute walk distance, and distance-saturation product as predictors of pulmonary arterial hypertension in idiopathic pulmonary fibrosis. Respir Care 2010; 55:584–588.

9 Arcasoy SM, Christie JD, Ferrari VA, et al: Echocardiographic assessment of pulmonary hypertension in patients with advanced lung disease. Am J Respir Crit Care Med 2003;167: 735–740.

10 Nathan SD, Shlobin OA, Barnett SD, et al: Right ventricular systolic pressure by echocardiography as a predictor of pulmonary hypertension in idiopathic pulmonary fibrosis. Respir Med 2008; 102:1305–1310.

11 Zisman DA, Ross DJ, Belperio JA, et al: Prediction of pulmonary hypertension in idiopathic pulmonary fibrosis. Respir Med 2007;101:2153–2159.

12 Shorr AF, Helman DL, Davies DB, Nathan SD: Pulmonary hypertension in advanced sarcoidosis: epidemiology and clinical characteristics. Eur Respir J 2005;25:783–788.
13 Baughman RP, Engel PJ, Meyer CA, Barrett AB, Lower EE: Pulmonary hypertension in sarcoidosis. Sarcoidosis Vasc Diffuse Lung Dis 2006;23: 108–116.
14 Baughman RP, Engel PJ, Taylor L, Lower EE: Survival in sarcoidosis associated pulmonary hypertension: the importance of hemodynamic evaluation. Chest 2010;138:1078–1085.
15 Papadopoulos CE, Pitsiou G, Karamitsos TD, et al: Left ventricular diastolic dysfunction in idiopathic pulmonary fibrosis: a tissue Doppler echocardiographic (corrected) study. Eur Respir J 2008;31:701–706.
16 Nathan SD, Shlobin OA, Ahmad S, Urbanek S, Barnett SD: Pulmonary hypertension and pulmonary function testing in idiopathic pulmonary fibrosis. Chest 2007;131:657–663.
17 Shorr AF, Wainright JL, Cors CS, Lettieri CJ, Nathan SD: Pulmonary hypertension in patients with pulmonary fibrosis awaiting lung transplant. Eur Respir J 2007;30:715–721.
18 Jastrzebski D, Nowak J, Ziora D, et al: Left ventricular dysfunction in patients with interstitial lung diseases. Eur Respir J 2009;33:702–703, author reply 3–4.
19 Hamada K, Nagai S, Tanaka S, et al: Significance of pulmonary arterial pressure and diffusion capacity of the lung as prognosticator in patients with idiopathic pulmonary fibrosis. Chest 2007;131:650–656.
20 Corte TJ, Wort SJ, Gatzoulis MA, Macdonald P, Hansell DM, Wells AU: Pulmonary vascular resistance predicts early mortality in patients with diffuse fibrotic lung disease and suspected pulmonary hypertension. Thorax 2009;64:883–888.
21 Zisman DA, Karlamangla AS, Ross DJ, et al: High-resolution chest CT findings do not predict the presence of pulmonary hypertension in advanced idiopathic pulmonary fibrosis. Chest 2007;132:773–779.
22 Devaraj A, Wells AU, Meister MG, Corte TJ, Hansell DM: The effect of diffuse pulmonary fibrosis on the reliability of CT signs of pulmonary hypertension. Radiology 2008;249:1042–1049.
23 Leuchte HH, Neurohr C, Baumgartner R, et al: Brain natriuretic peptide and exercise capacity in lung fibrosis and pulmonary hypertension. Am J Respir Crit Care Med 2004;170:360–365.
24 Leuchte HH, Baumgartner RA, Nounou ME, et al: Brain natriuretic peptide is a prognostic parameter in chronic lung disease. Am J Respir Crit Care Med 2006;173:744–750.
25 Corte TJ, Wort SJ, Gatzoulis MA, et al: Elevated brain natriuretic peptide predicts mortality in interstitial lung disease. Eur Respir J 2010;36: 819–825.
26 Song JW, Song JK, Kim DS: Echocardiography and brain natriuretic peptide as prognostic indicators in idiopathic pulmonary fibrosis. Respir Med 2009;103:180–186.
27 Lettieri CJ, Nathan SD, Barnett SD, Ahmad S, Shorr AF: Prevalence and outcomes of pulmonary arterial hypertension in advanced idiopathic pulmonary fibrosis. Chest 2006;129:746–752.
28 Nadrous HF, Pellikka PA, Krowka MJ, et al: Pulmonary hypertension in patients with idiopathic pulmonary fibrosis. Chest 2005;128:2393–2399.
29 Bourbonnais JM, Samavati L: Clinical predictors of pulmonary hypertension in sarcoidosis. Eur Respir J 2008;32:296–302.
30 Chang B, Wigley FM, White B, Wise RA: Scleroderma patients with combined pulmonary hypertension and interstitial lung disease. J Rheumatol 2003;30:2398–2405.
31 Steen VD, Graham G, Conte C, Owens G, Medsger TA Jr: Isolated diffusing capacity reduction in systemic sclerosis. Arthritis Rheum 1992;35:765–770.
32 Trad S, Amoura Z, Beigelman C, et al: Pulmonary arterial hypertension is a major mortality factor in diffuse systemic sclerosis, independent of interstitial lung disease. Arthritis Rheum 2006;54:184–191.
33 Sulica R, Teirstein AS, Kakarla S, Nemani N, Behnegar A, Padilla ML: Distinctive clinical, radiographic, and functional characteristics of patients with sarcoidosis-related pulmonary hypertension. Chest 2005;128:1483–1489.
34 Zisman DA, Karlamangla AS, Kawut SM, et al: Validation of a method to screen for pulmonary hypertension in advanced idiopathic pulmonary fibrosis. Chest 2008;133:640–645.
35 Olschewski H, Ghofrani HA, Walmrath D, et al: Inhaled prostacyclin and iloprost in severe pulmonary hypertension secondary to lung fibrosis. Am J Respir Crit Care Med 1999;160:600–607.
36 Ghofrani HA, Wiedemann R, Rose F, et al: Sildenafil for treatment of lung fibrosis and pulmonary hypertension: a randomised controlled trial. Lancet 2002;360:895–900.
37 Gunther A, Enke B, Markart P, et al: Safety and tolerability of bosentan in idiopathic pulmonary fibrosis: an open label study. Eur Respir J 2007; 29:713–719.
38 American Thoracic Society: Idiopathic pulmonary fibrosis: diagnosis and treatment. International consensus statement. American Thoracic Society (ATS), and the European Respiratory Society (ERS). Am J Respir Crit Care Med 2000; 161:646–664.
39 King TE Jr, Tooze JA, Schwarz MI, Brown KR, Cherniack RM: Predicting survival in idiopathic pulmonary fibrosis: scoring system and survival model. Am J Respir Crit Care Med 2001;164: 1171–1181.
40 Lederer DJ, Arcasoy SM, Wilt JS, D'Ovidio F, Sonett JR, Kawut SM: Six-minute-walk distance predicts waiting list survival in idiopathic pulmonary fibrosis. Am J Respir Crit Care Med 2006;174:659–664.
41 Nathan SD, Shlobin OA, Ahmad S, et al: Serial development of pulmonary hypertension in patients with idiopathic pulmonary fibrosis. Respiration 2008;76:288–294.
42 Renzoni EA, Walsh DA, Salmon M, et al: Interstitial vascularity in fibrosing alveolitis. Am J Respir Crit Care Med 2003;167:438–443.
43 Ebina M, Shimizukawa M, Shibata N, et al: Heterogeneous increase in CD34-positive alveolar capillaries in idiopathic pulmonary fibrosis. Am J Respir Crit Care Med 2004;169:1203–1208.
44 Richter A, Yeager ME, Zaiman A, Cool CD, Voelkel NF, Tuder RM: Impaired transforming growth factor-beta signaling in idiopathic pulmonary arterial hypertension. Am J Respir Crit Care Med 2004;170:1340–1348.
45 Schermuly RT, Dony E, Ghofrani HA, et al: Reversal of experimental pulmonary hypertension by PDGF inhibition. J Clin Invest 2005;115:2811–2821.
46 Farkas L, Farkas D, Ask K, et al: VEGF ameliorates pulmonary hypertension through inhibition of endothelial apoptosis in experimental lung fibrosis in rats. J Clin Invest 2009;119:1298–1311.
47 Kulasekaran P, Scavone CA, Rogers DS, Arenberg DA, Thannickal VJ, Horowitz JC: Endothelin-1 and transforming growth factor-beta1 independently induce fibroblast resistance to apoptosis via AKT activation. Am J Respir Cell Mol Biol 2009;41:484–493.
48 Hashimoto N, Phan SH, Imaizumi K, et al: Endothelial-mesenchymal transition in bleomycin-induced pulmonary fibrosis. Am J Respir Cell Mol Biol 43:161–172.
49 Hubbard RB, Smith C, Le Jeune I, Gribbin J, Fogarty AW: The association between idiopathic pulmonary fibrosis and vascular disease: a population-based study. Am J Respir Crit Care Med 2008;178:1257–1261.
50 Sode BF, Dahl M, Nielsen SF, Nordestgaard BG: Venous thromboembolism and risk of idiopathic interstitial pneumonia: a nationwide study. Am J Respir Crit Care Med 181:1085–1092.
51 Lancaster LH, Mason WR, Parnell JA, et al: Obstructive sleep apnea is common in idiopathic pulmonary fibrosis. Chest 2009;136:772–778.
52 Glaser S, Noga O, Koch B, et al: Impact of pulmonary hypertension on gas exchange and exercise capacity in patients with pulmonary fibrosis. Respir Med 2009;103:317–324.
53 Daniels CE, Yi ES, Ryu JH: Autopsy findings in 42 consecutive patients with idiopathic pulmonary fibrosis. Eur Respir J 2008;32:170–174.
54 Kubo H, Nakayama K, Yanai M, et al: Anticoagulant therapy for idiopathic pulmonary fibrosis. Chest 2005;128:1475–1482.
55 Trulock EP, Edwards LB, Taylor DO, Boucek MM, Keck BM, Hertz MI: Registry of the International Society for Heart and Lung Transplantation: twenty-third official adult lung and heart-lung transplantation report–2006. J Heart Lung Transplant 2006;25:880–892.
56 Whelan TP, Dunitz JM, Kelly RF, et al: Effect of preoperative pulmonary artery pressure on early survival after lung transplantation for idiopathic pulmonary fibrosis. J Heart Lung Transplant 2005;24:1269–1274.

57 Zisman DA, Schwarz M, Anstrom KJ, Collard HR, Flaherty KR, Hunninghake GW: A controlled trial of sildenafil in advanced idiopathic pulmonary fibrosis. N Engl J Med 2010;363:620–628.

58 Collard HR, Anstrom KJ, Schwarz MI, Zisman DA: Sildenafil improves walk distance in idiopathic pulmonary fibrosis. Chest 2007;131:897–899.

59 King TE Jr, Behr J, Brown KK, et al: BUILD-1: a randomized placebo-controlled trial of bosentan in idiopathic pulmonary fibrosis. Am J Respir Crit Care Med 2008;177:75–81.

60 Minai OA, Sahoo D, Chapman JT, Mehta AC: Vaso-active therapy can improve 6-min walk distance in patients with pulmonary hypertension and fibrotic interstitial lung disease. Respir Med 2008;102:1015–1020.

61 Cottin V, Nunes H, Brillet PY, et al: Combined pulmonary fibrosis and emphysema: a distinct underrecognised entity. Eur Respir J 2005;26: 586–593.

62 Mejia M, Carrillo G, Rojas-Serrano J, et al: Idiopathic pulmonary fibrosis and emphysema: decreased survival associated with severe pulmonary arterial hypertension. Chest 2009;136: 10–15.

63 Cottin V, Le Pavec J, Prevot G, et al: Pulmonary hypertension in patients with combined pulmonary fibrosis and emphysema syndrome. Eur Respir J 2010;35:105–111.

64 Tyndall AJ, Bannert B, Vonk M, et al: Causes and risk factors for death in systemic sclerosis: a study from the EULAR Scleroderma Trials and Research (EUSTAR) database. Ann Rheum Dis 2010;69:1809–1815.

65 Launay D, Mouthon L, Hachulla E, et al: Prevalence and characteristics of moderate to severe pulmonary hypertension in systemic sclerosis with and without interstitial lung disease. J Rheumatol 2007;34:1005–1011.

66 Todd NW, Lavania S, Park MH, et al: Variable prevalence of pulmonary hypertension in patients with advanced interstitial pneumonia. J Heart Lung Transplant 2010;29:188–194.

67 Allanore Y, Meune C, Vonk MC, et al: Prevalence and factors associated with left ventricular dysfunction in the EULAR Scleroderma Trial and Research group (EUSTAR) database of patients with systemic sclerosis. Ann Rheum Dis 2010;69:218–221.

68 Steen VD, Lucas M, Fertig N, Medsger TA Jr: Pulmonary arterial hypertension and severe pulmonary fibrosis in systemic sclerosis patients with a nucleolar antibody. J Rheumatol 2007;34:2230–2235.

69 Fischer A, Misumi S, Curran-Everett D, et al: Pericardial abnormalities predict the presence of echocardiographically defined pulmonary arterial hypertension in systemic sclerosis-related interstitial lung disease. Chest 2007;131:988–992.

70 Mathai SC, Hummers LK, Champion HC, et al: Survival in pulmonary hypertension associated with the scleroderma spectrum of diseases: impact of interstitial lung disease. Arthritis Rheum 2009;60:569–577.

71 Schachna L, Medsger TA Jr, Dauber JH, et al: Lung transplantation in scleroderma compared with idiopathic pulmonary fibrosis and idiopathic pulmonary arterial hypertension. Arthritis Rheum 2006;54:3954–3961.

72 Statement on sarcoidosis. Joint Statement of the American Thoracic Society (ATS), the European Respiratory Society (ERS) and the World Association of Sarcoidosis and Other Granulomatous Disorders (WASOG) adopted by the ATS Board of Directors and by the ERS Executive Committee, February 1999. Am J Respir Crit Care Med 1999; 160:736–755.

73 Battesti JP, Georges R, Basset F, Saumon G: Chronic cor pulmonale in pulmonary sarcoidosis. Thorax 1978;33:76–84.

74 Gluskowski J, Hawrylkiewicz I, Zych D, Wojtczak A, Zielinski J: Pulmonary haemodynamics at rest and during exercise in patients with sarcoidosis. Respiration 1984;46:26–32.

75 Handa T, Nagai S, Miki S, et al: Incidence of pulmonary hypertension and its clinical relevance in patients with sarcoidosis. Chest 2006;129: 1246–1252.

76 Mayock RL, Bertrand P, Morrison CE, Scott JH: Manifestations of sarcoidosis. Analysis of 145 patients, with a review of nine series selected from the literature. Am J Med 1963;35:67–89.

77 Rizzato G, Pezzano A, Sala G, et al: Right heart impairment in sarcoidosis: haemodynamic and echocardiographic study. Eur J Respir Dis 1983; 64:121–128.

78 Barnett CF, Bonura EJ, Nathan SD, et al: Treatment of sarcoidosis-associated pulmonary hypertension. A two-center experience. Chest 2009; 135:1455–1461.

79 Emirgil C, Sobol BJ, Herbert WH, Trout K: The lesser circulation in pulmonary fibrosis secondary to sarcoidosis and its relationship to respiratory function. Chest 1971;60:371–378.

80 Shorr AF, Davies DB, Nathan SD: Outcomes for patients with sarcoidosis awaiting lung transplantation. Chest 2002;122:233–238.

81 Preston IR, Klinger JR, Landzberg MJ, Houtchens J, Nelson D, Hill NS: Vasoresponsiveness of sarcoidosis-associated pulmonary hypertension. Chest 2001;120:866–872.

82 Rosen Y, Moon S, Huang CT, Gourin A, Lyons HA: Granulomatous pulmonary angiitis in sarcoidosis. Arch Pathol Lab Med 1977;101:170–174.

83 Takemura T, Matsui Y, Saiki S, Mikami R: Pulmonary vascular involvement in sarcoidosis: a report of 40 autopsy cases. Hum Pathol 1992;23: 1216–1223.

84 Hoffstein V, Ranganathan N, Mullen JB: Sarcoidosis simulating pulmonary veno-occlusive disease. Am Rev Respir Dis 1986;134:809–811.

85 Jones RM, Dawson A, Jenkins GH, Nicholson AG, Hansell DM, Harrison NK: Sarcoidosis-related pulmonary veno-occlusive disease presenting with recurrent haemoptysis. Eur Respir J 2009; 34:517–520.

86 Milman N, Svendsen CB, Iversen M, Videbaek R, Carlsen J: Sarcoidosis-associated pulmonary hypertension: acute vasoresponsiveness to inhaled nitric oxide and the relation to long-term effect of sildenafil. Clin Respir J 2009;3:207–213.

87 Fisher KA, Serlin DM, Wilson KC, Walter RE, Berman JS, Farber HW: Sarcoidosis-associated pulmonary hypertension: outcome with long-term epoprostenol treatment. Chest 2006;130: 1481–1488.

88 Letizia C, Danese A, Reale MG, et al: Plasma levels of endothelin-1 increase in patients with sarcoidosis and fall after disease remission. Panminerva Med 2001;43:257–261.

89 Reichenberger F, Schauer J, Kellner K, Sack U, Stiehl P, Winkler J: Different expression of endothelin in the bronchoalveolar lavage in patients with pulmonary diseases. Lung 2001;179: 163–174.

90 Terashita K, Kato S, Sata M, Inoue S, Nakamura H, Tomoike H: Increased endothelin-1 levels of BAL fluid in patients with pulmonary sarcoidosis. Respirology 2006;11:145–151.

91 Hamilton-Craig CR, Slaughter R, McNeil K, Kermeen F, Walters DL: Improvement after angioplasty and stenting of pulmonary arteries due to sarcoid mediastinal fibrosis. Heart Lung Circ 2009;18:222–225.

92 Toonkel RL, Borczuk AC, Pearson GD, Horn EM, Thomashow BM: Sarcoidosis-associated fibrosing mediastinitis with resultant pulmonary hypertension: a case report and review of the literature. Respiration 2010;79:341–345.

93 Salazar A, Mana J, Sala J, Landoni BR, Manresa F: Combined portal and pulmonary hypertension in sarcoidosis. Respiration 1994;61:117–119.

94 Baughman RP, Sparkman BK, Lower EE: Six-minute walk test and health status assessment in sarcoidosis. Chest 2007;132:207–213.

95 Arcasoy SM, Christie JD, Pochettino A, et al: Characteristics and outcomes of patients with sarcoidosis listed for lung transplantation. Chest 2001;120:873–880.

96 Shorr AF, Davies DB, Nathan SD: Predicting mortality in patients with sarcoidosis awaiting lung transplantation. Chest 2003;124:922–928.

97 Barst RJ, Ratner SJ: Sarcoidosis and reactive pulmonary hypertension. Arch Intern Med 1985;145:2112–2114.

98 Damuth TE, Bower JS, Cho K, Dantzker DR: Major pulmonary artery stenosis causing pulmonary hypertension in sarcoidosis. Chest 1980;78: 888–891.

99 Portier F, Lerebours-Pigeonniere G, Thiberville L, et al: Sarcoidosis simulating a pulmonary veno-occlusive disease (in French). Rev Mal Respir 1991;8:101–102.

100 Smith LJ, Lawrence JB, Katzenstein AA: Vascular sarcoidosis: a rare cause of pulmonary hypertension. Am J Med Sci 1983;285:38–44.

101 Gluskowski J, Hawrylkiewicz I, Zych D, Zielinski J: Effects of corticosteroid treatment on pulmonary haemodynamics in patients with sarcoidosis. Eur Respir J 1990;3:403–407.

102 Davies J, Nellen M, Goodwin JF: Reversible pulmonary hypertension in sarcoidosis. Postgrad Med J 1982;58:282–285.

103 Rodman DM, Lindenfeld J: Successful treatment of sarcoidosis-associated pulmonary hypertension with corticosteroids. Chest 1990;97:500–502.

104 Baughman RP, Judson MA, Lower EE, et al: Inhaled iloprost for sarcoidosis associated pulmonary hypertension. Sarcoidosis Vasc Diffuse Lung Dis 2009;26:110–120.

105 Milman N, Burton CM, Iversen M, Videbaek R, Jensen CV, Carlsen J: Pulmonary hypertension in end-stage pulmonary sarcoidosis: therapeutic effect of sildenafil? J Heart Lung Transplant 2008;27:329–334.

106 Corte TJ, Gatzoulis MA, Parfitt L, Harries C, Wells AU, Wort SJ: The use of sildenafil to treat pulmonary hypertension associated with interstitial lung disease. Respirology 15:1226–1232.

107 Tazi A: Adult pulmonary Langerhans' cell histiocytosis. Eur Respir J 2006;27:1272–1285.

108 Dauriat G, Mal H, Thabut G, et al: Lung transplantation for pulmonary Langerhans' cell histiocytosis: a multicenter analysis. Transplantation 2006;81:746–750.

109 Chaowalit N, Pellikka PA, Decker PA, et al: Echocardiographic and clinical characteristics of pulmonary hypertension complicating pulmonary Langerhans cell histiocytosis. Mayo Clin Proc 2004;79:1269–1275.

110 Harari S, Simonneau G, De Juli E, et al: Prognostic value of pulmonary hypertension in patients with chronic interstitial lung disease referred for lung or heart-lung transplantation. J Heart Lung Transplant 1997;16:460–463.

111 Harari S, Brenot F, Barberis M, Simmoneau G: Advanced pulmonary histiocytosis X is associated with severe pulmonary hypertension. Chest 1997;111:1142–1144.

112 Crausman RS, Jennings CA, Tuder RM, Ackerson LM, Irvin CG, King TE Jr: Pulmonary histiocytosis X: pulmonary function and exercise pathophysiology. Am J Respir Crit Care Med 1996;153:426–435.

113 Basset F, Corrin B, Spencer H, et al: Pulmonary histiocytosis X. Am Rev Respir Dis 1978;118:811–820.

114 Friedman PJ, Liebow AA, Sokoloff J: Eosinophilic granuloma of lung. Clinical aspects of primary histiocytosis in the adult. Medicine (Baltimore) 1981;60:385–396.

115 Travis WD, Borok Z, Roum JH, et al: Pulmonary Langerhans cell granulomatosis (histiocytosis X). A clinicopathologic study of 48 cases. Am J Surg Pathol 1993;17:971–986.

116 Hamada K, Teramoto S, Narita N, Yamada E, Teramoto K, Kobzik L: Pulmonary veno-occlusive disease in pulmonary Langerhans' cell granulomatosis. Eur Respir J 2000;15:421–423.

117 Tazi A, Moreau J, Bergeron A, Dominique S, Hance AJ, Soler P: Evidence that Langerhans cells in adult pulmonary Langerhans cell histiocytosis are mature dendritic cells: importance of the cytokine microenvironment. J Immunol 1999;163:3511–3515.

118 Asakura S, Colby TV, Limper AH: Tissue localization of transforming growth factor-beta1 in pulmonary eosinophilic granuloma. Am J Respir Crit Care Med 1996;154:1525–1530.

119 Benyounes B, Crestani B, Couvelard A, Vissuzaine C, Aubier M: Steroid-responsive pulmonary hypertension in a patient with Langerhans' cell granulomatosis (histiocytosis X). Chest 1996;110:284–286.

120 Kiakouama L, Cottin V, Etienne-Mastroianni B, Khouatra C, Humbert M, Cordier JF: Severe pulmonary hypertension in histiocytosis X: long-term improvement with bosentan. Eur Respir J 2010;36:202–204.

121 Taveira-DaSilva AM, Hathaway OM, Sachdev V, Shizukuda Y, Birdsall CW, Moss J: Pulmonary artery pressure in lymphangioleiomyomatosis: an echocardiographic study. Chest 2007;132:1573–1578.

Hilario Nunes
Service de Pneumologie, Hôpital Avicenne
125 rue de Stalingrad
FR–93009 Bobigny (France)
Tel. +33 1 48 95 51 21, E-Mail hilario.nunes@avc.aphp.fr

Chapter 20

Humbert M, Souza R, Simonneau G (eds): Pulmonary Vascular Disorders.
Prog Respir Res. Basel, Karger, 2012, vol 41, pp 199–206

High-Altitude Pulmonary Hypertension

Ruo-Min Di · Zhi-Cheng Jing

Department of Cardio-Pulmonary Circulation, Shanghai Pulmonary Hospital, Tongji University School of Medicine, Shanghai, PR China

Abstract

High-altitude pulmonary hypertension (HAPH) is a specific disease affecting populations that live at high elevations. The prevalence of HAPH among those residing at high altitudes needs to be further defined. Whereas reduction in nitric oxide production may be one mechanism in the development of HAPH, the roles of endothelin-1 and prostaglandin I_2 pathways in the pathogenesis of HAPH deserve further study. Although some studies have suggested that genetic factors contribute to the pathogenesis of HAPH, data published to date are insufficient for the identification of a significant number of gene polymorphisms in HAPH. The clinical presentation of HAPH is nonspecific. Exertional dyspnea is the most common symptom and signs related to right heart failure are common in late stages of HAPH. Echocardiography is the most useful screening tool and right heart catheterization is the gold standard for the diagnosis of HAPH. The ideal management for HAPH is migration to lower altitudes. Phosphodiesterase-5 is an attractive drug target for the treatment of HAPH. In addition, acetazolamide is a promising therapeutic agent for HAPH. To date, no evidence has confirmed whether endothelin receptor antagonists have efficacy in the treatment of HAPH.

High-altitude exposure is a worldwide problem. In South America, the capitals of three of the four main Andean countries (Bolivia, Colombia, Ecuador, and Peru) are at high altitudes. In South America, some 35 million people live above 2,500 m. In Asia, the countries of Afghanistan, Bhutan, China, India, Kyrgyzstan, and Nepal have 2–45% of their populations living above 2,500 m. In China alone, there are four high plateaus (Qinghai-Tibet, Inner Mongolia, Yun-Gui, and the Yellow Land) with a total population of nearly 80 million people. In North America, Mexico and the western United States have relatively smaller, but increasing, high-altitude populations. It is estimated that more than 140 million people live 2,500 m above sea level, and the number of temporary visitors to mountains is close to 40 million [1]. There are several specific locations where high-altitude studies have recently been performed: (1) the Himalayas of Asia, (2) the Andes of South America, (3) the Rocky Mountains of North America, (4) the Tian Shan and Pamir mountain ranges of central Asia, and (5) the Ethiopian Highlands in East Africa. It is estimated that up to 5–10% of high-altitude inhabitants may develop chronic mountain syndrome (CMS) or high-altitude pulmonary hypertension (HAPH) [2]. As a consequence, high altitude-related diseases are public health concerns in mountainous regions of the world. The present review will focus on the epidemiology, pathophysiology, pathogenesis, clinical characteristics, and treatment of HAPH.

Definition

A uniform description of altitude-related illnesses has been lacking, with the result that nomenclatures and diagnostic criteria have varied over time and in different high-altitude regions of the world. A consensus that develops a consistent nomenclature and diagnostic criteria could quickly improve public health in high-altitude areas and facilitate high altitude-related disease research.

High-altitude stress is primarily due to the hypoxia of low atmospheric pressure; however, dry air, intense solar radiation, extreme cold, and exercise contribute to acute and chronic disorders. Acute mountain sickness is a clinical syndrome occurring in otherwise healthy normal individuals who ascend rapidly to high altitudes. Symptoms develop over a period of a few hours to days. The usual symptoms include headache, anorexia, nausea, vomiting, lethargy, unsteadiness of gait, undue dyspnea on moderate exertion, and interrupted sleep. Acute pulmonary edema and cerebral edema of high altitude are malignant forms of acute mountain sickness. Of these, high-altitude pulmonary edema (HAPE) is highly correlated with acute pulmonary hypertension [3]. However, the study by Maggiorini et al. [4] indicated HAPE is initially a hydrostatic-type pulmonary edema caused by an increase in pulmonary capillary pressure.

Monge [5] originally used the name 'subacute mountain sickness' (SMS) to describe the persistence of headache, anorexia, nausea, dizziness, and difficulty to sleep – the usual symptoms of acute mountain sickness – during the weeks and months after arrival to high-altitude locations. Typically, in all these patients, mainly miners of the Peruvian Andes, physical findings suggesting congestive failure of the right heart were absent. The name 'SMS' has also recently been used to describe the rapid (within a few weeks or months after ascent to high altitude) development of congestive right heart failure in Han Chinese infants and Indian soldiers [6, 7]. In this setting, SMS is an exaggerated pulmonary hypertensive response to high-altitude hypoxia.

Two separate entities of subacute nature have been described in infants and adults. Subacute infantile mountain sickness is a condition seen predominantly in Han Chinese infants living in Tibet, although it has been described in other high-altitude communities as well. It came into prominence only after the large-scale migration of Chinese population from low altitudes in mainland China to the high altitudes of the Qinghai-Tibetan plateau. The condition is characterized by features of severe hypoxic pulmonary hypertension and heart failure. Pulmonary histology is consistent with muscularization of the pulmonary arterioles, but no intimal proliferation or plexiform lesions are seen. The second syndrome, adult SMS, has been described almost exclusively in Indian soldiers living at extreme altitudes for prolonged periods of time. In this condition as well, hypoxic pulmonary hypertension appears to be the dominant factor responsible for severe congestive heart failure.

Both of these conditions have several similarities with brisket disease in cattle; hypoxic pulmonary vasoconstriction plays an important role in the pathogenesis, and removal from high altitude results in complete resolution. Thus, it appears that both these syndromes are human counterparts of brisket disease in cattle [8]. According to the authors' concept, the name 'SMS' should be reserved for the description of the original syndrome published in 1937, and the name 'cardiac SMS' should be used to describe the syndrome described by Anand et al. [8]. According to the 6th World Congress on Mountain Medicine and High Altitude Physiology held in 2004, cardiac SMS was included in HAPH (as defined in the HAPH section) [2].

Monge and Whittembury [6] originally described chronic mountain sickness as a syndrome characterized by a triad of excessive erythrocytosis, severe hypoxemia, and impaired mental function. Right heart failure was not included in the triad because in the Andes it is a rare complication in the end-stage of the disease. Therefore, in analogy to the condition of SMS, the authors proposed to name the condition of congestive right heart failure without excessive erythrocytosis as 'cardiac chronic mountain sickness' because it is mainly observed in immigrants born at low altitude after years of residence at high altitude. Consequently, the names 'chronic mountain sickness' and 'Monge's disease' should be reserved to describe chronic high-altitude disease associated with excessive erythrocytosis, severe hypoxemia, and hypercapnia at the given altitude, with or without the development of congestive failure of the right heart in its end-stage. An international consensus statement on chronic and subacute high-altitude diseases has been published, and the definition of CMS has been established as follows:

> A clinical syndrome that occurs to native or long-life residents above 2,500 m. It is characterized by excessive erythrocytosis (females, Hb ≥19 g/dl; males, Hb ≥21 g/dl), severe hypoxemia, and in some cases moderate or severe PH, which may evolve to cor pulmonale, leading to congestive HF. The clinical picture of CMS gradually disappears after descending to low altitude and reappears after returning to HA [2].

The clinical symptoms of CMS include headache, dizziness, breathlessness and/or palpitations, sleep disturbance, fatigue, localized cyanosis, burning in the palms of the hands and soles of the feet and dilatation of the veins, muscle and joint pain, loss of appetite, lack of mental concentration, and alterations of memory. Clinical signs include excessive erythrocytosis, severe hypoxemia, pulmonary hypertension (not mandatory), and heart failure (not mandatory). The prevalence of chronic mountain sickness in high-altitude dwellers ranges from 1.2% in native Tibetans to 5.6% in Chinese Han, 6–8% in male residents of La Paz, Bolivia, and 15.6% in the Andes [7].

The definition and diagnostic criteria of HAPH remain somewhat vague. According to the 6th World Congress on Mountain Medicine and High Altitude Physiology held in 2004 and the 4th World Symposium on Pulmonary

Hypertension held in 2008, HAPH is a clinical syndrome that occurs in children and adults residing above 2,500 m and is classified in the third group of PH [9]. It is a hemodynamic and pathophysiological condition defined as an increase in mean pulmonary arterial pressure (PAP) ≥25 mm Hg at rest as assessed by right heart catheterization measured at the altitude of residence, and characterized by right ventricular hypertrophy, heart failure, moderate hypoxemia, and the absence of excessive erythrocytosis (females, Hb <19 g/dl; males, Hb <21 g/dl). Historical terms of HAPH include: chronic mountain sickness of the vascular type, high-altitude heart disease (HAHD), hypoxic cor pulmonale, infant SMS, pediatric high-altitude heart disease, and adult SMS. The following disorders should be ruled out: (1) other causes of pulmonary hypertension, including persistent pulmonary hypertension of the new born; (2) chronic obstructive pulmonary diseases such as chronic bronchitis, chronic obstructive emphysema, and chronic cor pulmonale; (3) interstitial lung disease, including pneumoconiosis; (4) other cardiovascular diseases complicated with pulmonary hypertension, such as coronary heart disease, valvular heart disease, dilative and hypertensive cardiomyopathy, and congenital heart diseases. Thus, pulmonary hypertension is a hallmark of HAPE and congestive right heart failure in SMS and CMS in the Himalayas and in the end-stage of CMS (Monge's disease) in the Andes. The terminology of HAPH may include HAPE, cardiac SMS, and cardiac CMS. For screening, pulmonary artery pressure is assessed using echocardiography. For confirmation of the diagnosis, as well as to exclude pulmonary hypertension due to heart diseases, right heart catheterization is required.

Epidemiology

Although HAPH is not a rare disorder in high-altitude residents and systolic pulmonary pressure can be evaluated easily, pulmonary hypertension is infrequently noted in most CMS studies. As a result, the prevalence of HAPH among general highland residents is still unknown.

Aldashev et al. [10] estimated the prevalence of HAPH among the high-altitude inhabitants of the Tien-Shan and Pamir mountains of Kyrgyzstan by the frequency of electrocardiographic (ECG) signs of cor pulmonale and pulmonary hemodynamics measured during right heart catheterization. An ECG survey of 741 highlanders demonstrated ECG signs of cor pulmonale in 14% of subjects. Indeed, the frequency of ECG signs is likely to underestimate the true prevalence of pulmonary hypertension and right ventricular hypertrophy because the sensitivity of ECG in the diagnosis of right ventricular hypertrophy is as low as 20%, depending on the criterion used. The pulmonary artery hemodynamics measured in an independent group of 136 male highlanders with symptoms of dyspnea at altitude revealed established pulmonary hypertension (mean PAP ≥25 mm Hg) in 20%. However, their measurements of pulmonary hemodynamics in highlanders are likely to overestimate the true prevalence of HAPH in highlanders because they selected subjects with exertional dyspnea. Kyrgyz studies reported the HAPH prevalence is 4.6% in the male population who live at the high altitudes of the Tien-Shan and Pamir mountains (3,000–4,200 m) [10]. Wu [11, 12] reported that in the Qinghai Province of China, HAPH is more common in children than adults and the enhanced incidence of HAPH with increasing altitude is more pronounced in children than adults. However, fewer HAPH patients were found among both children and adults in a population of Tibetan natives.

Pathology

HAPH is characterized by increased pulmonary vascular resistance secondary to hypoxia-induced pulmonary vasoconstriction and vascular remodeling of pulmonary arterioles [13]. The vascular alterations involve all elements of the vessel wall and include endothelial dysfunction, extension of smooth muscle into previously nonmuscular vessels, and adventitial thickening. Sites of hypoxic pulmonary vasoconstriction are small pulmonary arterioles and veins with a diameter of <900 μm. Venous changes account for 20% of the total increase in pulmonary vascular resistance caused by hypoxia [14]. The result of these changes is an increased pressure load on the right ventricle leading to reduced exercise capacity and premature death from right ventricular failure. The structural changes in the pulmonary vasculature are due, at least in part, to hypoxia-associated smooth muscle cell proliferation and, together with increased pulmonary vascular tone, represent targets for therapeutic intervention [10].

Histological examination of the pulmonary vessels in high-altitude residents who died from causes other than CMS showed persistence of the typical fetal patterns (thickened media) [15]. The fact that high altitude-induced changes of the pulmonary vasculature and right heart are reversible upon relocation to a lower altitude suggests a rapid remodeling process of the pulmonary vessels in response to changes in atmospheric oxygen content. Moreover, the fact that at high altitude supplemental oxygen significantly decreases PAP, both in acclimatized healthy subjects and long-term high-altitude residents, also supports this remodeling concept. The study by Li and Sui [16] reported autopsy results of 20 adults and 100 infants from Tibet who had died of HAPH. The major findings included dilatation of the pulmonary artery trunk, atheromas and thrombosis of the pulmonary artery, and hypertrophy and dilatation of the right ventricle and right atrium. Hypertrophy of both ventricles was also found in some cases. Compared with the normal age-matched controls, the ratio of right-to-left ventricular weight of these patients was significantly greater and the weight of the right ventricle even exceeded the left ventricle in some cases. Severe medial hypertrophy of the small pulmonary arteries with crenation of the elastic laminae was the most significant histological finding in the pulmonary vasculature. Singh et al. [17] reported the presence of numerous occluding fibrin thrombi in the smaller branches of the pulmonary vasculature based on necropsy findings in HAPH.

Pathophysiology

The partial pressure of oxygen in inspired air falls with increasing terrestrial elevation above sea level. As a consequence of the hypobaric hypoxic environments, human residents at high altitudes develop numerous physiologic responses, including (in particular), increases in hemoglobin concentration and PAP. In severely hypoxic residents, large increases in hemoglobin and/or PAP may be associated with potentially fatal illnesses. Sustained alveolar hypoxia, such as that experienced by high-altitude residents, has a marked physiological impact on the pulmonary vasculature. The hemodynamic outcome (i.e. increased PAP) is due to enhanced pulmonary vasoconstriction and pulmonary vascular remodeling, both of which cause reduction of the vascular lumen diameter and an increase in pulmonary vascular resistance [14]. In rats exposed to hypoxia, precapillary vessels of a diameter of approximately 25 mm, which normally do not have smooth muscle cells, begin to generate from adventitial fibroblasts within 24 h [18]. Light microscopic examination of nonmuscular arterioles after exposure to hypoxia shows that smooth muscle begins to appear by day 2 at simulated altitude, with the proportion of muscularized arterioles corresponding to the increasing PAP. Interestingly, these previous studies show that after returning to normoxia, smooth muscle cells persisted in normally nonmuscularized arterioles, suggesting that the histological changes may persist for a very long time after chronic exposure to hypoxia.

Taken together, these findings suggest that hypoxia-associated smooth muscle proliferation in originally weakly muscularized arterioles and normally nonmuscular pulmonary vessels is likely to be a major pathophysiological mechanism for the development of HAPH. Vasoconstriction is a secondary factor because the administration of oxygen decreases the PAP only by 15–20%. A previous study showed blood coagulation changes at high altitude predisposing to pulmonary hypertension [19]. Subjects who had developed pulmonary hypertension at high altitude showed a significant increase of plasma fibrinogen, fibrinolytic activity, platelet adhesiveness, platelet factor 3, factor V, and factor VIII. In subjects who did not develop pulmonary hypertension, however, there was a significant increase of plasma fibrinogen and fibrinolytic activity only. Hypervolemia, polycythemia, and increased blood viscosity are all considered secondary causal factors.

Pathogenesis

The intracellular mechanisms underlying the pathogenesis of HAPH are poorly understood, but a reduction in nitric oxide (NO) production is thought to play a role [20]. Animal studies showed that the absence of endothelial NO synthase increased susceptibility to HAPH. Anand et al. [21] demonstrated that inhaled NO can cause an acute decrease in PAP, intrapulmonary shunting, and improvement in oxygenation in HAPE. The roles of endothelin-1 and prostaglandin I_2 pathways in the pathogenesis of HAPH are still not well characterized.

In the pulmonary vasculature, it appears that transmembrane ion flux plays an important role in controlling the cellular processes that underlie both vasoconstriction and medial hypertrophy and hyperplasia during hypoxic exposure [22]. Alteration in the transport of K^+ and Ca^{2+} through their respective ion channels modulates these processes by affecting cell volume, membrane potential, cytosolic Ca^{2+} concentration, gene transcription, apoptosis, and cell-cycle progression. Precisely how K^+ and Ca^{2+} channels 'sense' changes in oxygen tension or how their activity and expression somehow 'adapt' at higher altitudes is unclear. Although pulmonary physiologists are attempting to define this mechanism, it is becoming increasingly apparent that ion channels themselves are probably not the actual oxygen sensors.

Genetics

It is possible that individuals who develop high-altitude PH share common and, as yet, unidentified genes that influence the pulmonary arteriolar and/or venous response to hypoxia and the generation of smooth muscle cells from adventitial fibroblasts in weakly and nonmuscularized pulmonary vessels. Previous studies have shown that Tibetan-native Chinese, compared to Han Chinese or South American high-altitude natives, have a remarkable lack of muscularization of pulmonary arteries, and lower hypoxic pulmonary vasoconstrictive response and hemoglobin concentration [23]. This suggests that Tibetans' protection from high altitude-related illnesses might be due to genetic factors. The association of high-altitude disorders with polymorphisms in genes has been investigated in recent years. These genes includes endothelial NO synthase, β_2-adrenergic receptor, angiotensin-converting enzyme I, bone morphogenetic protein receptor type 2, activin receptor-like kinase 1, 5-hydroxytryptamine transporter, and hypoxia-inducible factor 1. León-Velarde and Mejia [24] summarized the available data on genes known to be regulated by hypoxia-inducible factor-1 and/or by hypoxia that have been studied in populations from high-altitude regions suffering from HAPH. Even though some alleles are more prevalent (G allele of endothelial NO synthase polymorphism Glu298Asp in Sherpas and angiotensin-converting enzyme I allele in HAPH Kyrgyz) or less prevalent (angiotensin-converting enzyme D allele in high-altitude Andeans) in the different high-altitude populations, data published to date are inconclusive regarding these gene polymorphisms in HAPH [25, 26]. Genetic understanding of these disorders is still in its infancy.

Clinical Presentations

Symptoms
Polycythemia, hypoxemia, and pulmonary arterial hypertension are principal characteristics of CMS. At an early stage, PH may be asymptomatic, but as the condition progresses exertional dyspnea becomes the most frequent presenting symptom. Moreover, fatigue, weakness, anginal chest pain, syncope, and exercise intolerance are also common complaints. In addition to these symptoms of PH, HAPH patients may also manifest common symptoms of CMS, such as headache, dizziness, insomnia, cognitive dysfunction, somnolence, slowed mental function, confusion, and impaired memory.

Physical Examination
Episodes suggestive of right heart failure with dyspnea, cough, turgid jugular veins, and peripheral edema follow the initial symptoms within a few years in Han Chinese subjects [27], but are rare in high-altitude residents in the Andes. In both populations, marked cyanosis of the face and fingers, clubbing of the digits, hepatomegaly, and ascites may be present in the late stage of the disease.

Electrocardiogram
Indices of right ventricular hypertrophy can be seen on electrocardiography, including right axis deviation, defined as a frontal plane QRS axis of ≥90 (pattern A); R wave in lead V1 of ≥5 mm, an R/S ratio of >1, and S > R in V5 or V6 (pattern B); and a leftward shift in the transition zone (pattern C).

The study by Kojonazarov et al. [28] evaluated electrocardiography for the detection of pulmonary hypertension in high-altitude inhabitants. In 44 subjects with one or more ECG-RVH patterns, the right ventricular anterior wall thickness was >0.5 cm on echocardiographic study in 22 subjects, giving an ECG sensitivity of 50% for diagnosing RVH. In 16 subjects with a normal electrocardiogram, the right ventricular wall thickness was normal (0.4 ± 0.05 cm), giving a specificity of 100%. Negative predictive value by electrocardiography was 42% and positive predictive value was 100%. In 44 subjects with electrocardiography-defined RVH, pulmonary hypertension was confirmed by direct invasive measurement in 26 subjects. Thus, the sensitivity of electrocardiography for detecting HAPH was 59%. In 16 subjects with a normal electrocardiogram, pulmonary hypertension was diagnosed at right heart catheterization in 3 subjects, giving a specificity for ECG of 81%. Negative predictive value of electrocardiography was 42% and positive predictive value was 90%.

Pulmonary Function Test
Patients with HAPH are usually more hypoxemic than normal high-altitude residents, in part because of hypoventilation during both awake and sleep states. Compared with residents living at sea level, it has been found that both healthy residents at high altitude and patients with HAPH present a decreased ventilatory response to hypoxia, with the difference between those with and without HAPH not being statistically significant [29]. However, compared with healthy high-altitude residents, patients with HAPH present higher end-tidal carbon dioxide tension and lower end-tidal oxygen tension, suggesting a lower level of alveolar ventilation rather than a hypoxic ventilatory response in these subjects [29]. Thus, from the results of these studies, it may

be concluded that a lower level of alveolar ventilation rather than a reduced peripheral chemosensitivity to hypoxia is the primary mechanism leading to hypoxemia.

Chest Radiography

Enlargement of the heart, dilatation of the pulmonary trunk, and general dilatation of the small lung vessels were found on chest radiography and reported in Han Chinese and South Americans. Kerley's B lines are characteristically absent in HAPH patients [30]. These symptoms suggest that congestive right heart failure is associated with excessively elevated PAP in both populations.

Echocardiography

Echocardiography can provide both estimates of PAP and an assessment of cardiac structure and function. These features justify its application as the most commonly used screening tool in assessing patients with suspected HAPH. Systolic PAP is calculated by adding the estimated right atrial pressure to the pressure gradient between the right ventricle and the right atrium (ΔP-RV/RA) using the modified Bernoulli equation ($\Delta P\text{-}RV/RA = 4V^2$) where V is the peak velocity of the regurgitant jet across the tricuspid valve and Δ indicates change.

The study by Kojonazarov et al. [28] evaluated Doppler echocardiography for the detection of pulmonary hypertension in high-altitude inhabitants. All subjects underwent Doppler echocardiography followed by a cardiac catheterization within 7 days of arrival in Bishkek (Kyrgyzstan; altitude 760 m). Pulmonary flow acceleration time and the maximum velocity of tricuspid regurgitation were measured. Sufficient quality tricuspid regurgitant jets were recovered in only 28% of the patients. Therefore, PAP was estimated from the pulmonary flow acceleration time, which was recovered in 100% of the patients. Thirty-seven patients had pulmonary hypertension on echocardiography. Pulmonary hypertension was confirmed in 29 patients on catheterization. Pulmonary hypertension was detected with 70% sensitivity and 88% specificity by echocardiography. The correlation coefficient between echocardiography and catheterization studies was $r^2 = 0.78$.

Right Heart Catheterization

For the purposes of confirming the diagnosis, as well as excluding PH due to other causes, right heart catheterization measure of PAP is recommended [31]. The level of altitude has an inverse relation to arterial oxygen saturation (SaO_2) and a direct relationship to the PAP. Mild or moderate increases of altitude above 3,000 m are associated with important changes in SaO_2 and PAP. PPA values of ≈22 mm Hg and SaO_2 values of 85–90% have been found in cities between 3,500 and 3,700 m. Higher PPA values between 23 and 28 mm Hg and SaO_2 values between 78 and 81% have been described in Chengdou in Qinghai, China, located at ≈4,000 m, and in the Andean towns of Morococha and Cerro de Pasco, located at >4,000 m [32]. Pulmonary hemodynamic measurements performed in children and young adults show persistence of elevated PAP at high altitude for weeks, months, or years [33]. Performance of right heart catheterization was reported in Han Chinese subjects who developed HAPH after residing in Lhasa at an elevation 3,658 m for 11–36 years, as well as in Andes natives residing at an elevation of approximately 4,300 m. The hemodynamic data show the mPAP averaged 45 mm Hg in Andes natives and 40 mm Hg in Han Chinese subjects. In all subjects, right atrial pressure, pulmonary artery occlusion pressure, and cardiac output were normal. Currently, there is no available information that indicates significant differences of pulmonary hemodynamics among CMS, high-altitude heart disease, and high-altitude cor pulmonale. Most publications describe moderate degrees of pulmonary hypertension in these entities. Severe degrees of PH (PPA >40 mm Hg) have only been reported in CMS.

Treatments

The ideal management for HAPH is migration to low altitude. However, for patients who choose to remain at high altitude, other means of reducing PH may be attempted, although their efficacy has not been fully established.

A number of treatments including oxygen supplementation, calcium channel blockers (such as nifedipine), NO inhalation, prostacyclins, and endothelin receptor antagonists, as well as phosphodiesterase (PDE) inhibitors, have been demonstrated to decrease hypoxemia, PH, and the alveolar-arterial gradient in pulmonary arterial hypertension. However, the efficacy of these treatments for HAPH needs to be further evaluated.

NO has vasorelaxant and antiproliferative effects that are mediated by cyclic guanosine monophosphate, which is hydrolyzed by PDEs. PDE5 is the major PDE subtype present in the pulmonary vasculature and is more abundant in the lungs than in other tissues [34]. This abundance of PDE5 in the lungs provides a mechanism for relatively selective pulmonary vasodilatation with little systemic hypotension. Aldashev et al. [35] studied the effects of sildenafil in 14 HAPH patients and reported a reduction in mPAP, with an improvement in 6-min walk distance and an increase in cardiac index after 3 months. The meta-analysis by Jin et al. [36] indicates that treatment with PDE5 inhibitors can markedly attenuate altitude-induced pulmonary hypertension without significantly affecting systolic blood pressure, heart rate, and SaO_2 under rest and exercise conditions. Therefore, PDE5 is an attractive drug target for the treatment of HAPH. Long-term treatment with a PDE5 inhibitor, such as sildenafil, may be a promising therapy for HAPH.

Although endothelin receptor antagonists have been proven to reduce PAP and increase exercise capacity in patients with pulmonary arterial hypertension, their effects on exercise capacity at altitude are unknown. Recently, Seheult et al. [37] demonstrated that bosentan therapy initiated 5 days prior to ascent to high altitude did not improve exercise capacity or reduce systolic pulmonary arterial hypertension, and worsened arterial oxygen saturation measured by pulse oximetry during high-intensity exercise at altitude. Modesti et al. [38] demonstrated that the use of a mixed ET_A/ET_B antagonist (bosentan) at high altitudes effectively controls the hypoxia-induced increase in pulmonary blood pressure [32].

A number of studies have emphasized the mechanisms by which acetazolamide and angiotensin-converting enzyme inhibitors may be effective agents for the treatment of HAPH. Richalet et al. [39] demonstrated that acetazolamide reduces hypoventilation, improves pulmonary circulation, and decreases erythropoiesis. Its use as a chronic treatment for HAPH has been shown to be efficacious and safe. The low cost of acetazolamide may allow for wide adoption with a considerable positive impact on public health in high-altitude regions. Niazova [40] investigated the effect of captopril on both systemic and pulmonary arterial pressures in patients with HAPH and the result showed captopril significantly decreases systemic and pulmonary arterial pressures. The efficacy of acetazolamide and angiotensin-converting enzyme inhibitors in HAPH need to be further studied.

Future Directions

The prevalence of HAPH among general highland residents is still unknown. Deciphering the molecular mechanisms of pulmonary vascular remodeling in HAPH appears to be a fascinating journey ahead. Further work to discover genomic susceptibility is needed because signaling consequences of common polymorphisms can be overcome by appropriate pharmacological approaches in many cases. There is an urgent need for larger scale, prospectively designed, randomized, double-blind trials using calcium channel blockers, endothelin receptor antagonists, prostaglandins, or PDE5 inhibitors in HAPH.

References

1 Moore LG, Niermeyer S, Zamudio S: Human adaptation to high altitude: regional and life-cycle perspectives. Am J Phys Anthropol Suppl 1998; 27:25–64.

2 León-Velarde F, et al: Consensus statement on chronic and subacute high altitude diseases. High Alt Med Biol 2005;6:147–157.

3 Johnson TS, Rock PB: Acute mountain sickness. N Engl J Med 1998;319:841–845.

4 Maggiorini M, Mélot C, Pierre S, Pfeiffer F, Greve I, Sartori C, Lepori M, Hauser M, Scherrer U, Naeije R: High-altitude pulmonary edema is initially caused by an increase in capillary pressure. Circulation 2001;103:2078–2083.

5 Monge C: High altitude disease. Arch Intern Med 1937;59:32.

6 Monge C, Whittembury J: Chronic mountain sickness. Johns Hopkins Med J 1976;139:87.

7 Pasha MA, Newman JH: High-altitude disorders: pulmonary hypertension: pulmonary vascular disease: the global perspective. Chest 2010; 137:13S–19S.

8 Anand IS, Wu T: Syndromes of subacute mountain sickness. High Alt Med Biol 2004;5:156–170.

9 McLaughlin VV, Archer SL, Badesch DB, Barst RJ, Farber HW, Lindner JR, Mathier MA, McGoon MD, Park MH, Rosenson RS, Rubin LJ, Tapson VF, Varga J: ACCF/AHA 2009 expert consensus document on pulmonary hypertension: a report of the American College of Cardiology Foundation Task Force on Expert Consensus Documents and the American Heart Association developed in collaboration with the American College of Chest Physicians; American Thoracic Society, Inc.; and the Pulmonary Hypertension Association. J Am Coll Cardiol 2009;53:1573–1619.

10 Aldashev AA, Sarybaev AS, Sydykov AS, Kalmyrzaev BB, Kim EV, Mamanova LB, Maripov R, Kojonazarov BK, Mirrakhimov MM, Wilkins MR, Morrell NW: Characterization of high-altitude pulmonary hypertension in the Kyrgyz: association with angiotensin-converting enzyme genotype. Am J Respir Crit Care Med 2002; 166:1396–1402.

11 Wu TY: An investigation on high altitude heart disease (in Chinese). Zhonghua Yi Xue Za Zhi 1983;63:90–92.

12 Wu T: An epidemiological study on high altitude disease at Qinghai-Xizang (Tibet) plateau (in Chinese). Zhonghua Liu Xing Bing Xue Za Zhi 1987;8:65–69.

13 Maggiorini M, Leon-Velarde F: High-altitude pulmonary hypertension: a pathophysiological entity to different diseases. Eur Respir J 2003;22:1019–1025.

14 Hakim TS, Michel RP, Minami H, Chang HK: Site of pulmonary hypoxic vasoconstriction studied with arterial and venous occlusion. J Appl Physiol 1983;54:1298–1302.

15 Gamboa R, Marticorena E: The ductus arteriosus in the newborn infant at high altitude. Vasa 1972;1:192–195.

16 Li JB, Sui GJ: Pathological findings in high-altitude heart disease. Applied High-altitude Medicine. Lhasa, Tibet, Tibet Press, 1984; pp. 288–305.

17 Singh I, Khanna P, Hoon R, Lal M, Rao B: High-altitude pulmonary hypertension. Lancet 1965;286:146–150.

18 Sobin SS, Tremer HM, Hardy JD, Chiodi HP: Changes in arteriole in acute and chronic hypoxic pulmonary hypertension and recovery in rat. J Appl Physiol 1983;55:1445–1455.

19 Singh I, Chohan I: Blood coagulation changes at high altitude predisposing to pulmonary hypertension. Br Heart J 1972;34:611.
20 Beall CM, Laskowski D, Strohl KP, Soria R, Villena M, Vargas E, Alarcon AM, Gonzales C, Erzurum SC: Pulmonary nitric oxide in mountain dwellers. Nature 2001;414:411–412.
21 Anand IS, Prasad BA, Chugh SS, Rao KR, Cornfield DN, Milla CE, Singh N, Singh S, Selvamurthy W: Effects of inhaled nitric oxide and oxygen in high-altitude pulmonary edema. Circulation 1998;98:2441–2445.
22 Remillard CV, Yuan JX: High altitude pulmonary hypertension: role of K^+ and Ca^{2+} channels. High Alt Med Biol 2005;6:133–146.
23 Groves BM, Droma T, Sutton JR, McCullough RG, McCullough RE, Zhuang J, Rapmund G, Sun S, Janes C, Moore LG: Minimal hypoxic pulmonary hypertension in normal Tibetans at 3,658 m. J Appl Physiol 1993;74:312–318.
24 León-Velarde F, Mejia O: Gene expression in chronic high altitude diseases. High Alt Med Biol 2008;9:130–139.
25 Droma Y, Hanaoka M, Ota M, Katsuyama Y, Koizumi T, Fujimoto K, Kobayashi T, Kubo K: Positive association of the endothelial nitric oxide synthase gene polymorphisms with high-altitude pulmonary edema. Circulation 2002;106:826–830.
26 Morrell NW, Sarybaev AS, Alikhan A, Mirrakhimov MM, Aldashev AA: ACE genotype and risk of high altitude pulmonary hypertension in Kyrghyz highlanders. Lancet 1999;353:814.
27 Ge RL, Helun G: Current concept of chronic mountain sickness: pulmonary hypertension-related high-altitude heart disease. Wilderness Environ Med 2001;12:190–194.
28 Kojonazarov B, Imanov BZ, Amatov TA, Mirrakhimov MM, Naeije R, Wilkins MR, Aldashev AA: Noninvasive and invasive evaluation of pulmonary arterial pressure in highlanders. Eur Respir J 2007;29:352–356.
29 León-Velarde F, Gamboa A, Rivera-Ch M, Palacios JA, Robbins PA: Selected contribution: peripheral chemoreflex function in high-altitude natives and patients with chronic mountain sickness. J Appl Physiol 2003;94:1269–1278, discussion 1253–1264.
30 Pei SX, Chen XJ, Si Ren BZ, Liu YH, Cheng XS, Harris EM, Anand IS, Harris PC: Chronic mountain sickness in Tibet. Q J Med 1989;71:555–574.
31 McGoon M, Gutterman D, Steen V, Barst R, McCrory DC, Fortin TA, Loyd JE, American College of Chest Physicians: Screening, early detection, and diagnosis of pulmonary arterial hypertension: ACCP evidence-based clinical practice guidelines. Chest 2004;126:14S–34S.
32 Penaloza D, Arias-Stella J: The heart and pulmonary circulation at high altitudes: healthy highlanders and chronic mountain sickness. Circulation 2007;115:1132–1146.
33 Sime F, Banchero N, Penaloza D, Gamboa R, Cruz J, Marticorena E: Pulmonary hypertension in children born and living at high altitudes. Am J Cardiol 1963;11:143–149.
34 Clarke WR, Uezono S, Chambers A, Doepfner P: The type III phosphodiesterase inhibitor milrinone and type V PDE inhibitor dipyridamole individually and synergistically reduce elevated pulmonary vascular resistance. Pulm Pharmacol 1994;7:81–89.
35 Aldashev AA, Kojonazarov BK, Amatov TA, Sooronbaev TM, Mirrakhimov MM, Morrell NW, Wharton J, Wilkins MR: Phosphodiesterase type 5 and high altitude pulmonary hypertension. Thorax 2005;60:683–687.
36 Jin B, Luo XP, Ni HC, Shi HM: Phosphodiesterase type 5 inhibitors for high-altitude pulmonary hypertension: a meta-analysis. Clin Drug Investig 2010;30:259–265.
37 Seheult RD, Ruh K, Foster GP, Anholm JD: Prophylactic bosentan does not improve exercise capacity or lower pulmonary artery systolic pressure at high altitude. Respir Physiol Neurobiol 2009;165:123–130.
38 Modesti PA, Vanni S, Morabito M, Modesti A, Marchetta M, Gamberi T, Sofi F, Savia G, Mancia G, Gensini GF, Parati G: Role of endothelin-1 in exposure to high altitude: Acute Mountain Sickness and Endothelin-1 (ACME-1) study. Circulation 2006;114:1410–1416.
39 Richalet JP, Rivera-Ch M, Maignan M, Privat C, Pham I, Macarlupu JL, Petitjean O, León-Velarde F: Acetazolamide for Monge's disease: efficiency and tolerance of 6-month treatment. Am J Respir Crit Care Med 2008;177:1370–1376.
40 Niazova ZA, Batyraliev TA, Aikimbaev KS, Kudaiberdieva GZ, Akgul F, Soodanbekova YK, Birand A: High-altitude pulmonary hypertension: effects of captopril on pulmonary and systemic arterial pressures. J Hum Hypertens 1996;10(Suppl 3):S141–S142.

Prof. Zhi-Cheng Jing, MD
Department of Cardio-Pulmonary Circulation, Shanghai Pulmonary Hospital, Tongji University School of Medicine
507 Zhengmin Road
Shanghai 200433 (PR China)
Tel. +86 21 65115006 2110, E-Mail jingzhicheng@gmail.com

Chapter 21

Humbert M, Souza R, Simonneau G (eds): Pulmonary Vascular Disorders.
Prog Respir Res. Basel, Karger, 2012, vol 41, pp 207–217

Acute Pulmonary Venous Thromboembolic Disease

Olivier Sanchez[a,b] · Guy Meyer[a,b]

[a]Université Paris Descartes, Sorbonne Paris Cité, [b]Service de Pneumologie et Soins Intensifs, Hôpital Européen Georges Pompidou, Assistance Publique Hôpitaux de Paris, Paris, France

Abstract

Venous thromboembolism (VTE) is a common disease considered to be the result of the interaction between patient-related and setting-related risk factors. Several diagnostic algorithms combining clinical probability assessment, D-dimer testing, and imaging have been validated. The adherence to these algorithms appears important, as inappropriate use can increase the recurrence of VTE and death. Clinical assessment of hemodynamic tolerance remains the cornerstone of risk stratification for patients with pulmonary embolism (PE). The presence of shock defines patients with high-risk PE. Thrombolytic treatment associated with anticoagulants is the first-line treatment in these patients. Patients with normotensive PE and normal right ventricular function are at low-risk and have good outcome with anticoagulant therapy alone. Outpatient management appears safe and feasible for selected low-risk patients. The presence of right ventricular dysfunction seems to identify intermediate-risk patients among those with normal blood pressure. The use of thrombolytic treatment is highly controversial in these patients. A large randomized placebo-controlled trial is currently under way to clarify this question. The risk of recurrent VTE after anticoagulant treatment varies largely between studies. A significant proportion of patients have residual perfusion defects several months after the diagnosis of PE. The long-term clinical significance of this finding remains to be evaluated.

The annual incidence of venous thromboembolism (VTE) is around 1–2 cases per 1,000 persons and is strongly age-dependent since it rises to nearly 1% per year after 75 years. VTE is a major public health burden with an estimated 370,000 related deaths in 2004 in 6 European countries. Recent published data on risk factors, diagnosis, prognosis, and long-term prognosis of acute pulmonary embolism (PE) is the main focus of this review.

Risk Factors

VTE is currently considered a result of the interaction between patient-related and setting-related risk factors. However, VTE can occur in patients without any identifiable predisposing factor.

Pregnancy and Postpartum Period

VTE is one of the leading causes of maternal morbidity and mortality. About two thirds of VTE occur during pregnancy and one third postpartum. As compared with nonpregnant women, the risk of VTE is increased 5-fold during pregnancy and 60-fold during the first 3 months after delivery. The risk is highest in the third trimester of pregnancy and during the first 6 weeks after delivery. The risk of thrombosis during pregnancy is affected by the presence of prothrombotic abnormalities. Women with factor V Leiden or prothrombin 20210A have a 30- to 50-fold increased risk of VTE during pregnancy and postpartum compared to nonpregnant noncarriers.

Cancer

In patients with cancer, VTE is a common complication. Compared with persons without malignancy, the risk of developing symptomatic VTE is 7-fold higher in patients with cancer. Hematologic malignancies; tumors of the pancreas, brain, and lung; and gastrointestinal cancers have the highest risk of VTE. Adjusting for age, race, and stage, diagnosis of VTE is a significant predictor of death during the first year for all cancer types.

In patients with symptomatic VTE, the prevalence of previously unsuspected concomitant cancer, discovered by routine investigation at the time of VTE diagnosis, varies between 4 and 12%. The risk of occult cancer is increased 3- to 4-fold in idiopathic VTE compared with secondary VTE. Considering the high incidence of cancer in the first months after VTE, screening for an underlying malignancy may be clinically relevant. The usefulness of extensive screening for occult malignancy after VTE is still unconfirmed. Current data also suggest that more malignancies are detected in studies using an extensive screening strategy (CT of the abdomen and pelvis, etc.) as compared to studies using a limited screening strategy [1]. In one study, 201 patients with idiopathic deep venous thrombosis (DVT) were randomized either to extensive or limited screening for underlying cancer. Cancer was discovered during hospitalization in 13% of the patients who underwent extensive screening, but in none of the control group with limited screening. During follow-up, only one cancer developed in the group with extensive screening and 10 occurred in the control group. Overall mortality and cancer-related mortality (the primary endpoint of the study) did not differ between groups. More recently, a Dutch group enrolled 630 patients with unprovoked VTE in a cohort study with concurrent control where patients had a limited or extensive cancer screening depending on their hospital [2]. Cancer was found using clinically oriented screening in 12 of 342 patients in the extensive screening group and in 7 of the 288 patients included in the control group. Six additional cancers were detected by systematic abdominal and chest CT in the extensive screening group. During follow-up, 12 and 14 cancers were diagnosed in the extensive and limited screening groups, respectively. No difference was observed in total or cancer-related mortality [2]. These results do not support the use of a systematic extensive screening for underlying cancer in patients with unprovoked VTE.

Hormone Replacement Therapy and Oral Contraceptive Therapy

Most oral contraceptives consist of a combination of an estrogen and a progestogen. The reduction in the dose of estrogen over time has reduced the risk of VTE in users, although there is still a 2- to 5-fold increased risk. Since the absolute risk of VTE is low in young women, the annual risk in users of oral contraceptives remains low, at 2–3 per 10,000. The risk is highest during the first year of use. The type of progestogen affects the risk of venous thrombosis, with a 2-fold higher risk for contraceptives containing a third generation (i.e. desogestrel, gestodene) than a second generation (levonorgestrel) progestogens.

Hormone replacement therapy is prescribed for the treatment of symptoms of menopause. It increases the risk of VTE 2- to 4-fold [3]. However, in contrast to the oral course, transdermal estrogen does not have a first-pass effect through the liver, and it has been suggested that this might lead to less risk of thrombosis. Recently, a large multicenter case-control study and a meta-analysis showed that oral estrogen, but not transdermal estrogen, increased the risk of VTE [3]. Compared with nonusers of estrogen, the OR of first VTE in current users of oral estrogen was 2.5 (95% CI: 1.9–3.4) as compared to 1.2 (95% CI: 0.9–1.7) in current users of transdermal estrogen [3]. The risk of VTE in women using oral estrogen was higher in the first year of treatment (4.0, 95% CI: 2.9–5.7) compared with treatment for more than 1 year (2.1, 95% CI: 1.3–3.8; $p < 0.05$) [3].

Inherited Causes

Deficiencies of natural coagulation inhibitors such as antithrombin, protein C, and protein S are strong risk factors for VTE, but these deficiencies are rare and explain only 1% of all VTE. Factor V Leiden and prothrombin (factor II) G20210A are two more common genetic variants which have been consistently found to be associated with VTE, but still only explain a fraction of VTE. Since genetic risk factors are either rare or have a weak overall effect, their usefulness for clinical practice is still minimal and rarely affect treatment. The search of thrombophilia is not indicated when an acquired risk factor is identified (i.e. surgery, cancer, etc.) and should be restricted in idiopathic VTE in young patients (<60 years) or patients with recurrent VTE.

Diagnosis

Over the last two decades, many new diagnostic tests and strategies have been introduced for the diagnostic work-up of patients with suspected PE. To enforce an accurate diagnosis, diagnostic tests have now been integrated in algorithms consisting of clinical pretest probability and D-dimer testing followed by imaging.

Clinical Probability

Clinical probability assessment has become a mandatory step in the investigation of patients with clinically suspected PE. Clinical pretest probability of PE can be assessed empirically by taking into account the patient's medical history and risk factors for VTE, clinical signs, and routine laboratory tests. Several clinical prediction rules are available for PE diagnosis [4]. Two clinical prediction rules have been widely used and validated in diagnostic studies: the Wells' score and the Geneva score (table 1). The revised Geneva

Table 1. Clinical prediction rules for PE: the Wells' score and the revised Geneva score

Wells' score		Revised Geneva score	
Variable	Points	Variable	Points
Active cancer	+1	Age > 65 years	+1
Hemoptysis	+1	Active cancer	+2
Previous DVT or PE	+1.5	Hemoptysis	+2
Heart rate >100/min	+1.5	Previous DVT or PE	+3
Surgery or bed rest ≥3 days within 1 month	+1.5	Surgery or lower limb fracture within 1 month	+2
Clinical signs of DVT	+3	Unilateral edema and pain at palpation	+4
No alternative diagnosis as more likely than PE	+3	Spontaneously reported calf pain	+3
		Heart rate 75–94/min	+3
		Heart rate ≥95/min	+5

Clinical probability	Points	PE% (95% CI)	Clinical probability	Points	PE% (95% CI)
Low	< 2	6% (4–8)	Low	≤ 3	9% (8–11)
Intermediate	2–6	23% (18–28)	Intermediate	4–10	26% (24–28)
High	≥7	49% (43–56)	High	≥ 11	76% (69–82)
Clinical probability (dichotomized)					
PE unlikely	≤ 4	8% (6–11)			
PE likely	>4	34% (29–40)			

score provides a model that is independent of clinical judgement and the results of chest X-ray and arterial blood gases (table 1). Recently, it has been proposed to further simplify the computation of these scores, attributing one point to all criteria whatever the weight they carried in the original model [4]. The diagnostic accuracy of these rules has been shown to be comparable [4]. Whichever rule is used, the prevalence of confirmed PE is around 10% in the low probability category, 30% in the moderate category, and 70% in the high clinical category (table 1).

D-Dimer Testing

With its high negative predictive value, D-dimer testing represents an excellent noninvasive triage test in patients with suspected PE. A large variety of D-dimer assays has been evaluated with substantial variation in the diagnostic performance from one assay to another. In a meta-analysis, after adjustment for study characteristics, the sensitivities of the D-dimer enzyme-linked immunofluorescence assay (Vidas; 97%), microplate enzyme-linked immunosorbent assay (Asserachrome; 95%), and latex quantitative assay (Tinaquant, STA-Liatest; 95%) were superior to those of the whole-blood D-dimer assay (SimpliRed; 87%), latex semiquantitative assay (88%), and latex qualitative assay (75%) [5]. A systematic review of management outcome studies showed that the 3-month thromboembolic risk in patients left untreated on the basis of a non-high clinical probability, using the Wells' or Geneva scores, or unlikely clinical probability, using the dichotomized Wells' score, and a negative Vidas D-dimer test was 3 in 2,166 (0.14%, 95% CI: 0.05–0.41) [6]. Therefore, the combination of a negative Vidas D-dimer test and a non-high clinical probability effectively and safely excludes PE [6]. The whole-blood D-dimer assay SimpliRed allows ruling out PE only in patients with low clinical probability with a 3-month thromboembolic risk of 0.2%. In patients with high clinical probability of PE, a D-dimer test should not be performed due to the limited negative predictive value of the test in patients with a high pretest probability in this category. D-dimer tests have low specificity, leading to false-positive result rates of 50% or more and low positive predictive value [5].

Indeed, D-dimers are elevated in a wide variety of conditions including cancer, inflammation, infection, and others. Because positive D-dimer results are usually followed by costly additional tests, the pulmonary embolism rule-out criteria (PERC) rule was developed to identify patients at such a low pretest risk for PE in whom PE can safely be excluded without the need for D-dimer testing, thus avoiding false-positive D-dimer results and the risks of unnecessary imaging testing. The rule is based on eight clinical criteria. In the original study, patients who meet these eight criteria are identified as PERC-negative and appear to have a very low pretest probability of PE, with a residual risk of PE, varying between 0 and 1.4%, similar to the risk after a normal pulmonary angiogram. Recently, Hugli et al. [7] sought to externally validate the diagnostic performance of the PERC rule alone and combined with clinical probability assessment based on the revised Geneva score. Overall, the prevalence of PE was 21.3%. The prevalence of PE was 5.4% (95% CI: 3.1–9.3) among PERC-negative patients and 6.4% (95% CI: 3.7–10.8) among the PERC-negative patients with a low clinical pretest probability of PE [7]. Thus, the PERC rule alone or combined with another clinical decision rule cannot safely identify very-low-risk patients in whom PE can be ruled out without additional testing, at least in populations with a relatively high prevalence of PE [7].

What other options do clinicians have to avoid false-positive D-dimer results? Preliminary evidence suggests that the threshold for defining an abnormal D-dimer result can be increased in elderly patients, without compromising patient safety. In a retrospective analysis, a D-dimer cutoff of 10 × age in patients over 50 years safely reduced the number of false-positive D-dimer results by up to 18%, resulting in a decrease in the number needed to test to exclude one PE [8]. However, the safety of age-adjusted D-dimer cutoffs needs to be prospectively validated before its use can be recommended in clinical practice.

Compression Ultrasonography

Compression ultrasonography (CUS) of the lower limb veins is used as an indirect method to diagnose PE, and finding a proximal DVT in patients with suspected PE is sufficient to warrant anticoagulant treatment without further testing [9]. The only validated diagnostic criterion for DVT is incomplete compressibility of the vein, which indicates the presence of clots [9]. The specificity of CUS in proximal lower limb veins is high (about 95%). Therefore, a positive proximal CUS confirms the diagnosis of proximal DVT. The sensitivity of CUS for diagnosing PE is only approximately 40–50% and a negative proximal CUS cannot rule out PE [9]. The diagnostic yield of CUS in patients suspected of PE might be raised by performing complete ultrasonography, including the distal veins. A recent study aimed to assess whether performing such complete CUS would increase the diagnostic yield of the test in 855 outpatients suspected of PE [10]. Proximal CUS was completed by an examination of the distal veins, the result of which was not disclosed to the physician in charge of the patient. CUS was positive in 21% of patients, of whom 10% had proximal DVT and 11% isolated distal DVT. Of the 59 patients with distal DVT, 21 (36%) had no PE on multidetector helical CT (MDCT) [10]. Twenty of those 21 patients were not given anticoagulant therapy and had an uneventful follow-up. Distal CUS has limited diagnostic performance for the diagnosis of PE [sensitivity 22% (95% CI: 17–29) and specificity 94% (95% CI: 91–96)] [10]. Moreover, it carries a high false-positive rate which might result in overdiagnosis of PE and unnecessary anticoagulant treatment, impeding the use of distal CUS as a confirmatory test for PE [10]. Therefore, it appears that proximal CUS can be performed to avoid CT when positive in patients with contraindications to contrast dye and/or irradiation [9].

Computed Tomography

Over the last two decades, helical CT of the chest has become the procedure of choice for PE diagnosis. MDCT has improved the visualization of the segmental and subsegmental pulmonary arteries. The PIOPED II study reported a sensitivity of MDCT of 83% (95% CI: 76–92) and a specificity of 96% (95% CI: 93–97) [11]. This study also demonstrated that predictive values varied substantially when clinical probability of PE was taken into account. In patients with high or intermediate clinical probability, the positive predictive value of MDCT was high (96 and 92%, respectively), but decreased to 58% in cases of low clinical probability [11]. Negative predictive value of MDCT was high in patients with a low or intermediate clinical probability (96 and 89%, respectively), but was lower in patients with a high clinical probability (60%) [11]. Several outcome studies have assessed the clinical effectiveness of MDCT [12–14]. In one study which included 756 consecutive patients with clinically suspected PE, all patients with high clinical probability or non-high clinical probability and positive D-dimer testing underwent both proximal CUS and MDCT [12]. The overall failure rate of the diagnostic strategy (D-dimer plus MDCT) during 3-month follow-up was 1.5% (8/523; 95% CI: 0.9–2.7) [12]. The Christopher study included 3,306 patients with clinically suspected PE [14]. All patients categorized as 'PE likely' based on the dichotomized Wells' clinical rule and those with positive D-dimer and 'PE unlikely' underwent a MDCT. The 3-month risk of VTE in

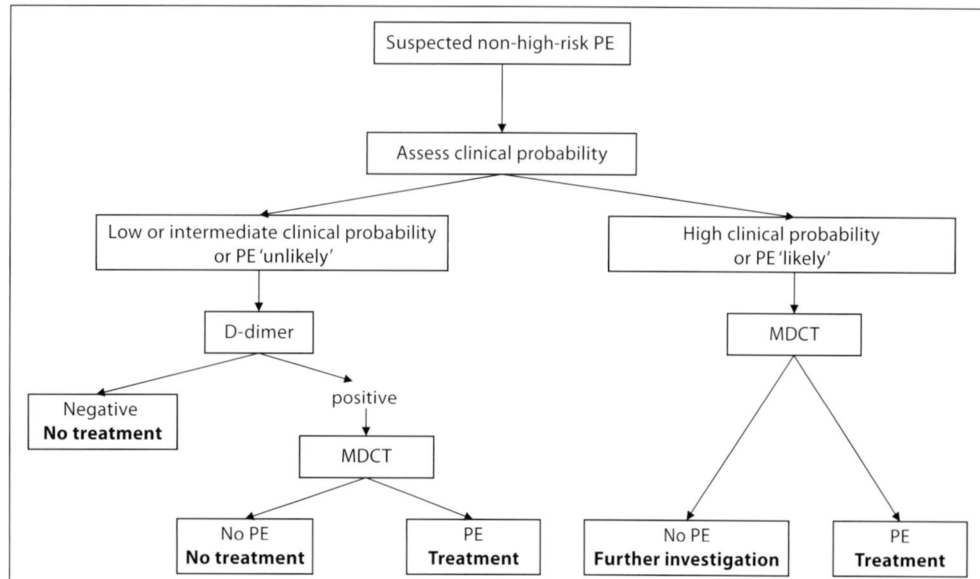

Fig. 1. Diagnostic algorithm for patients with suspected non-high-risk PE (adapted from Torbicki et al. [9]).

patients left untreated by anticoagulant on the basis of negative MDCT was 1.3% (95% CI: 0.7–2.0) [14].

Taken together, these two studies suggest that MDCT alone could be used without addition of CUS to exclude PE. This was definitively confirmed in a multicenter randomized noninferiority trial that included 1,819 patients and compared two strategies: D-dimer-MDCT with and without CUS [13]. The 3-month VTE risk was 0.3% (95% CI: 0.1–1.1) in the D-dimer-CUS-MDCT group and 0.3% (95% CI: 0.1–1.2) in the D-dimer-MDCT group [difference 0.0% (95% CI: –0.9 to 0.8)] [13]. Therefore, it appears that a negative MDCT can exclude PE in patients with non-high clinical probability [9]. In patients with high clinical probability, it is suggested to further investigate with CUS, ventilation perfusion scintigraphy, or pulmonary angiography [9].

The role of CT venography remains controversial. In the PIOPED II study, the sensitivity increases from 83% for MDCT alone to 90% for MDCT combined with CT venography with a similar specificity [11]. However, the clinical usefulness of additional CT venography is questionable since less than 1% of patients clinically suspected of PE and negative thoracic MDCT have DVT on CUS [12]. Moreover, CT venography substantially increases the overall examination radiation.

Diagnostic Algorithms

Various combinations of clinical probability, D-dimer, CUS, ventilation perfusion lung scintigraphy, and helical CT have been evaluated. Roy et al. [15] aimed to assess whether physicians in routine clinical practice used evidence-based diagnostic criteria for managing patients with suspected PE. They showed that diagnostic management was inappropriate in 43% [15]. When PE was excluded on an inappropriate basis, the risk for VTE during follow-up was 6-fold higher than after an appropriate diagnostic management [15]. Age >75 years, known heart failure, chronic lung disease, pregnancy, current anticoagulant treatment, and lack of a written diagnostic protocol for diagnosing PE in the emergency department were identified as independent risk factors for inappropriate management [15]. The European Society of Cardiology has proposed diagnostic algorithms for patients with suspected high-risk and non-high risk PE (fig. 1) [9].

Recently, Roy et al. [16] assessed the effectiveness of a handheld clinical decision support system to improve the diagnostic work-up of outpatients with suspicion of PE. The main outcome was the appropriateness of diagnostic work-up defined as any sequence of tests that yielded a posttest probability less than 5% or greater than 85%. The authors demonstrated that the proportion of patients who received appropriate diagnostic work-ups increased significantly more from the preinterventional period to the interventional period in the computer-based guidelines group ($p = 0.023$) [16]. Moreover, among patients who received appropriate work-ups, those in the computer-based guidelines group received slightly fewer tests than did patients in the paper guidelines group [16].

Magnetic Resonance Imaging

MRI is another possible approach for diagnosis of suspected PE. The PIOPED III study is the first large multicenter study evaluating MRI (n = 371 patients) [17]. Prior to its publication, MRI studies on PE included small numbers of patients or were not prospectively conducted. In these case series, the sensitivity of gadolinium-enhanced MR angiography (MRA) ranged from 77 to 100%, and the specificity ranged from 95 to 98%. In the PIOPED III study, the authors investigated the diagnostic performances of MRA with or without MR venography by comparing independently read MRI with the reference standard for diagnosing PE (D-dimer, MDCT, etc.) [17]. According to the reference test, PE was diagnosed in 104 of the 371 included patients (28%) and was mainly proximal (main or lobar pulmonary artery in 90% of cases) [17]. MRA was technically inadequate in 25% of patients. After exclusion of these inconclusive MRA examinations, technically adequate MRA had a sensitivity of 78% (95% CI: 67–86) and a specificity of 99% (95% CI: 96–100) [17]. When technically inadequate MRA was included as a negative result, MRA had a sensitivity of 57% (95% CI: 47–66) and a specificity of 75% (95% CI: 70–80) [17]. Thus, these results show that MRI has a high specificity for diagnosing PE. However, the rate of technically inadequate images is high and its sensitivity remains limited even when MRA is combined with MR venography. Therefore, MRI still cannot be used as a stand-alone test to exclude PE.

Table 2. PESI and simplified PESI score (18)

Variable	Original PESI	Simplified PESI
Age >80 years	1/year	1
Male sex	10	
Cancer	30	1
Heart failure	10	1
Chronic lung disease	10	
Heart rate >110/min	20	1
Systolic blood pressure <100 mm Hg	30	1
Respiratory rate ≥30 / min	20	
Body temperature <36°C	20	
Disorientation, lethargy, stupor, coma	60	
SaO_2 < 90%	20	1
Risk categories	30-day all-cause mortality, %	
Original PESI		
Class I (< 65 points)	0	
Class II (66–85 points)	1	
Class III (86–105 points)	3.1	
Class IV (106–125 points)	10.4	
Class V (>125 points)	24.4	
Low risk = classes I and II	0–1	
Simplified PESI		
Low risk (0 point)	1.1	
High risk (≥1 point)	8.9	

Risk Stratification

PE can be stratified into several levels of early death rates based on the presence or the absence of risk markers [9]. Several prognostic markers have been proposed.

Clinical Markers

It has been repeatedly shown that the short-term prognosis of PE depends on hemodynamic status. Hemodynamic instability is defined either as systolic blood pressure (SBP) <90 mm Hg or a reduction of at least 40 mm Hg for at least 15 min, or as SBP <100 mm Hg or as a shock index (cardiac frequency divided by SBP) ≥1 [9].

Short-term prognosis of PE also depends on underlying diseases. Using data from patients with PE hospitalized in the USA, Aujesky and colleagues [18] derived and validated the Pulmonary Embolism Severity Index (PESI) score (table 2). Several retrospective and prospective studies have validated PESI as a tool that can accurately identify patients at low risk of death. Lastly, a simplified version of PESI was recently derived and validated (table 2) [18].

Markers of Right Ventricular Dysfunction

Right ventricular dysfunction as evaluated by echocardiography is associated with a high risk of mortality in patients with acute PE. A right-to-left ventricular end-diastolic diameter ratio (RV/LV) ≥0.9 was shown to be an independent predictor of in-hospital death in a monocentric registry, which included 950 patients with acute PE who underwent echocardiography on admission. This association was confirmed in patients with PE and normal blood pressure in a meta-analysis [19]. However, echocardiographic criteria for right ventricular dysfunction differed widely from one study to another.

Recent improvements in CT technology (i.e. MDCT, ECG-gated helical MDCT) provide information on right ventricular dilatation. Two recent studies emphasized the prognostic role of right ventricular dysfunction measured on MDCT [20]. Becattini et al. [20] included 460 patients with acute PE confirmed by MDCT who had transthoracic echocardiography and serum troponin at admission. The diagnostic accuracy of MDCT for detecting right ventricular dysfunction, using echocardiography as the reference standard, shown by the area under the receiver operator characteristic curve (AUC) was 0.86 (95% CI: 0.82–0.91) [20]. A right-to-left ventricular ratio ≥0.9 was identified as a high-sensitivity cutoff for right ventricular dysfunction at MDCT [20]. In multivariable analysis, right ventricular dysfunction as assessed by MDCT was associated with an increased risk for death or clinical deterioration after adjusting for age and gender [20]. Similar results were reported in patients with hemodynamically stable PE [20].

Brain Natriuretic Peptides
Brain natriuretic peptide (BNP) and N-terminal proBNP (NT-proBNP) are two specific markers of wall ventricular stress. A strong correlation between levels of BNP or NT-proBNP and right ventricular dysfunction as assessed by echocardiography has been demonstrated. Three meta-analyses demonstrated a significant relation between high levels of BNP or NT-proBNP and short-term death or a short-term adverse event in patients with PE. Patients with PE and high levels of BNP or NT-proBNP were at higher risk of in-hospital adverse events and 30-day all-cause mortality. This association was also demonstrated in patients with normotensive PE [19].

Cardiac Troponins
Both cardiac troponins T and I have been reported to be elevated in acute PE. The prognostic value of troponins was evaluated in several studies that have been pooled in meta-analyses [19, 21]. They show that elevated levels of troponin were associated with an increased risk of short-term death and adverse outcome events [19, 21]. Conventional troponin assays are characterized by inadequate precision at the lower detection limit. A new generation of highly sensitive troponin assays have been developed which are capable of defining the 99th percentile of a normal (healthy) reference population with a low coefficient of variation. Lankeit et al. [22] assessed the prognostic value of baseline cardiac troponin T levels measured by a highly sensitive assay in 156 normotensive patients with acute PE. Highly sensitive troponin T values ranged from 0.001 to 357.2 pg/ml [median: 27.2 pg/ml (25th to 75th percentile: 9.4–69.4)] [22]. Baseline highly sensitive troponin T was higher in patients with a 30-day adverse outcome compared with patients with an uncomplicated course [71.7 pg/ml (35.5–117.9) vs. 26.4 (9.2–68.2); $p = 0.027$] [22].

Combination of Prognostic Tools
Until recently, little was known about the combination of clinical data, echocardiography, and biomarkers. A multicenter prospective observational study including 570 patients with objectively confirmed PE has recently been conducted in order to address this issue [23]. Echocardiography, BNP, NT-proBNP, and cardiac troponin I measurements were performed on admission. At 30 days, 42 patients (7.4%) had adverse events defined as death, secondary cardiogenic shock, or recurrent VTE [23]. Seventeen of the 41 patients (41.5%) with cardiogenic shock on admission experienced an adverse event, whereas such events were observed in only 25 of the 529 (4.7%) clinically stable patients ($p < 0.0001$). The 30-day mortality rate was also higher in patients with shock (26.8%) than in clinically stable patients (2.8%; $p < 0.0001$) [23]. On multivariate analysis, altered mental state, shock on admission, cancer, BNP, and RV/LV were associated with an adverse outcome at 30 days [23]. A practical prognostic score for use as a bedside tool was derived [23]. In another study, Jimenez et al. [24] assessed the prognostic value of three tests (cardiac troponin I, echocardiography, and lower limbs compression ultrasound) alone or in combination in 591 patients with normotensive PE. The primary outcome (PE-related mortality, hemodynamic collapse, or recurrence of PE within 30 days of follow-up) occurred in 59 patients (10%; PE-related death n = 37, 6.3%). On multivariate analysis, cardiac troponin I >0.1 ng/ml, right ventricular dysfunction on echocardiography, and presence of DVT on CUS were associated with 30-day PE-related mortality [24]. The use of any combination of a two-test strategy improved prognostication of patients with normotensive PE compared with the use of any test alone [24].

New Markers of Myocardial Injury
Heart-type fatty acid binding protein (H-FABP) is abundantly expressed in tissues with active fatty acid metabolism, such as heart and liver. Because of its small weight, it appears in the circulation shortly after cell damage and demonstrates both high sensitivity and specificity in the detection of myocardial injury. Several studies have investigated the prognostic value of H-FABP in patients with acute PE [25]. These studies reported that H-FABP was superior to troponin, NT-proBNP, or myoglobin for risk stratification of PE [25]. A high level of H-FABP (>6 ng/ml) had a high negative predictive value for PE-related death or complication. These preliminary promising data need to be confirmed in larger studies.

Growth differentiation factor (GDF)-15 is a distant member of the transforming growth factor-β family. Under normal conditions, the myocardium does not produce GDF-15, but its cardiac expression sharply increases after pressure overload and ischemia. The prognostic value of GDF-15 was investigated in a study including 123 patients with acute PE [26]. On multivariate analysis, cardiogenic shock on admission, cardiac troponin I, and GDF-15 were independently associated with 30-day complicated outcome [26]. Further studies are needed to confirm these preliminary results.

Treatment

Anticoagulation is the main therapy for acute PE. Anticoagulation should be started as soon as PE is suspected, before objective confirmation (at least in patients with a high clinical probability).

Thrombolytic Treatment
There is good evidence that thrombolytic therapy accelerates resolution of PE and results in a more rapid hemodynamic improvement than heparin alone. The evidence that thrombolytic therapy improves clinical outcome remains controversial. During the past 30 years, several randomized trials including less than 800 patients have compared the efficacy and the safety of thrombolytic therapy plus anticoagulation versus anticoagulation alone. The results of these studies have been summarized in a recent meta-analysis which included 11 studies totaling 748 patients with PE of varying severity [27]. Pooled data from five studies (254 patients) that included at least some hemodynamically unstable patients suggest a trend toward reduction of recurrent PE (3.9 vs. 7.1%; OR: 0.61, 95% CI: 0.23–1.62) and death (6.2 vs. 12.7%; OR: 0.47, 95% CI: 0.2–1.1) and an increase of major bleeding (21.9 vs. 11.9%; OR: 1.98, 95% CI: 1.00–3.92) with fibrinolysis [27]. The reduction was statistically significant when combining recurrent PE or death (9.4 vs. 19.0%; OR: 0.45; 95% CI: 0.22–0.92) [27]. Therefore, thrombolysis should be given in patients with high-risk PE unless there are absolute contraindications to its use [9].

Patients with low-risk PE have a good short-term prognosis under anticoagulant treatment. The results from pooled studies that included exclusively patients with normal blood pressure revealed no clinical benefit in this group [27]. To date, the largest and most recent randomized trial of thrombolytic therapy versus heparin alone included 256 patients with normotensive PE and evidence of right ventricular dysfunction on echocardiography or ECG [28]. The primary endpoint was in-hospital death or clinical deterioration requiring an escalation of treatment. The incidence of the primary endpoint was significantly higher in the heparin plus placebo group than in the heparin plus alteplase group ($p = 0.006$) [28]. However, open-label thrombolysis as rescue therapy was by far the most frequent form of escalation of therapy, and as the decision to use open-label rescue thrombolysis was subjective and could be made after unblinding, this component of the primary outcome has been severely criticized. Therefore, further studies are required to determine the risks and benefits of thrombolytic treatment in patients with normotensive PE and right ventricular dysfunction. A large international multicenter double-blind placebo-controlled trial (PEITHO study: ClinicalTrials.gov Identifier: NCT00639743) has been initiated and is currently under way. This study will randomize 1,000 patients with normotensive PE, right ventricular enlargement on echocardiography (RV/LV >0.9), and elevated level of cardiac troponin to receive either a bolus regimen of tenecteplase plus heparin or heparin and placebo. Therefore, until the results of this trial are published, the use of thrombolytic treatment in patients with intermediate-risk PE should not be generalized, but discussed on a case-by-case basis [9].

Is It Possible to Treat Some Patients with Pulmonary Embolism at Home?
Randomized controlled trials have shown that the treatment of DVT with low-molecular-weight heparin administered primarily at home is as safe as treatment with unfractionated heparin in hospital. Two recent retrospective monocentric studies assessed the safety and efficacy of ambulatory management of patients with PE [29, 30]. Patients were eligible for outpatient management of PE if they were hemodynamically stable, did not require oxygen therapy, did not require parenteral narcotics for pain management, and were not felt to be at high risk for a major hemorrhage. Patients were assessed at 3 months for thrombosis recurrence and major bleeding episodes. In the first study, 639 patients were included, of which 314 were managed as outpatients. Among these, there were three (0.95%; 95% CI: 0.25, 3) thrombotic recurrences, three hemorrhagic events, and nine deaths (2.9%; 95% CI: 1.4, 5.6), all due to underlying cancer and all occurring after the first 7 days of treatment [29]. In the second study, 473 patients with acute PE were included, of which 260 (55.0%) were treated as outpatients [29]. No outpatient died of fatal PE during the 3-month follow-up period. The rates of recurrent VTE in outpatients were 0.4% (95% CI: 0.0–2.1) and 3.8% (95% CI 1.9–7.0) within 14 days and 3 months, respectively. The rates of major bleeding episodes were 0% (95% CI: 0–1.4) and 1.5% (95% CI: 0.4–3.9) within 14 days and 3 months, respectively [29].

Recently, Aujesky et al. [31] undertook an open randomized multicenter noninferiority trial. They randomly assigned 344 patients with acute symptomatic PE and a low risk of death (PESI classes I or II) to initial outpatient (i.e. discharged from hospital ≤24 h after randomization) or inpatient treatment. The primary outcome was symptomatic recurrent VTE within 90 days; safety outcomes included major bleeding within 14 or 90 days and mortality within 90 days. One (0.6%) of the 171 outpatients developed recurrent VTE within 90 days compared with none of the 168 inpatients [95% upper confidence limit (UCL): 2.7%; p = 0.011], reaching the prespecified criterion for noninferiority [31]. Only one patient (0.6%) in each treatment group died within 90 days (95% UCL: 2.1%; p = 0.005 for noninferiority) [31]. Two (1.2%) of the 171 outpatients, but no inpatients, had major bleeding within 14 days (95% UCL: 3.6%; p = 0.031 for noninferiority). However, because one additional outpatient developed major bleeding within 90 days, the noninferiority threshold (4%) was slightly exceeded [3 outpatients (1.8%) vs. no inpatients (95% UCL: 4.5%; p = 0.086)] [31]. These results suggest that, in selected low-risk patients identified by use of the PESI, outpatient treatment is not inferior to inpatient treatment in terms of efficacy and safety, and reduces time spent in hospital [31].

Inferior Vena Cava Filter
Only one published randomized controlled trial included 400 patients with proximal DVT at high risk for PE in a 2-by-2 factorial design to receive unfractionated heparin versus low-molecular-weight heparin, with or without an inferior vena cava (IVC) filter [32]. IVC filters significantly reduced the incidence of recurrent PE at 12 days (1.1 vs. 4.8%; p = 0.03) and at 8 years (6.2 vs. 15.1%; p = 0.008), but not at 2 years (3.4 vs. 6.3%; p = 0.16), and were associated with an increased incidence of recurrent DVT at 8 years (35.7 vs. 27.5%; p = 0.042) resulting in no difference for recurrent VTE between the groups: 58 (36.4%) and 55 (35.4%) in the filter and nonfilter groups, respectively [HR: 1.12 (0.78–1.62); p = 0.54] [32]. More recently, optional vena cava filters are available for clinical use. These filters are designed to be either left in place permanently or retrieved for patients who no longer require vena cava interruption. However, the exact risk/benefit ratio of optional IVC filters is difficult to determine because only retrospective studies or small prospective cohorts have been conducted to date. A large multicenter randomized controlled trial evaluating the risk/benefit ratio of optional IVC filter in patients with DVT and PE and high risk of fatal PE during anticoagulant treatment is currently under way in France (PREPIC 2 study, ClinicalTrials.gov Identifier: NCT00457158). Therefore, until the results of this trial are published, IVC filters are not recommended in the general population of patients with VTE. An IVC filter may be used in case of absolute or temporary contraindication to anticoagulation in patients with a high risk of VTE recurrence, and in case of objectively proven recurrence of VTE despite therapeutic anticoagulation [9].

Long-Term Outcome

Long-Term Mortality
Several studies have investigated the long-term mortality in patients with PE [33]. Agnelli et al. [35] randomized 326 patients with a first episode of PE who had sustained an uneventful 3-month anticoagulant treatment. Anticoagulation therapy was stopped after 3 months in one group, and continued for a further 3–9 months in the other. Nineteen patients (5.8%) died after a mean follow-up of 33.8 months. Pengo et al. [36] reported data for 223 patients followed for a mean period of 94.3 months. The cumulative mortality rate was 10.3% (95% CI: 6.3–14.4) at 3 months, 13.4% at 1 year, and 25.1% (95% CI: 14.2–36.0) at 10 years. Douketis et al. [37] reported the outcome of 602 patients with symptomatic PE who were followed for a total of 2,437 person-years. Patients were followed after the resumption of oral anticoagulant treatment and the rate of subsequent fatal recurrences of PE was assessed. The frequency of definite or probable fatal PE was 0.20 per 100 person-years of follow-up and the case fatality rate of recurrent venous thromboembolism was 3.9%.

Recurrent Venous Thromboembolic Disease during Long-Term Follow-Up
Agnelli et al. [35] reported a recurrence rate for VTE of 3.1 and 3.8% per patient-year after the cessation of anticoagulant treatment [33]. In the van Gogh extension study, 1,215 patients with VTE who had completed 6 months of anticoagulant treatment were allocated to receive either idraparinux or placebo for a further period of 6 months. Among the 587 patients with an initial PE, 283 received idraparinux and 3 of these patients had a recurrent event (1.1%). By contrast, 13 of the 304 patients given placebo had recurrent VTE during the 6-month treatment period (8.6% per patient-year recurrence rate) [33]. In the report by Pengo et al. [36], the cumulative incidence of recurrent VTE was 29.1% (95% CI: 16.9–41.3) after 10 years of follow-up. In the study by Schulman et al. [38], the cumulative 10-year recurrence rate after 6 weeks or 6 months of anticoagulant therapy for a first

episode of VTE was 34.5% for the 107 patients who had PE at inclusion.

Persistent Perfusion Defects

Residual abnormalities have been described on repeated venous ultrasound examinations of patients with DVT and may be associated with a higher risk of recurrent DVT after anticoagulant treatment has been stopped. Data on the long-term outcome of PE are rarer, but recent results suggest that more than 50% of patients with PE still have perfusion defects after 6 months of anticoagulant treatment. In a recent cohort study including 226 patients with symptomatic PE who underwent perfusion lung scans 6–12 months after diagnosis, residual perfusion defects were observed in 29% of the patients [34]. Patients with persistent perfusion defects were more likely to have dyspnea, had higher systolic pulmonary arterial pressure, and walked a shorter distance during the 6-min walk test [34]. Age, the time interval between symptom onset and diagnosis, pulmonary vascular obstruction at the onset of PE, and previous VTE were independent predictors of perfusion defect after treatment of acute PE [34]. The long-term clinical significance of these findings, in terms of recurrent PE and occurrence of chronic thromboembolic pulmonary hypertension, remains unknown.

References

1 Carrier M, Le Gal G, Wells PS, Fergusson D, Ramsay T, Rodger MA: Systematic review: the Trousseau syndrome revisited: should we screen extensively for cancer in patients with venous thromboembolism? Ann Intern Med 2008;149:323–333.

2 Van Doormaal FF, Terpstra W, Van Der Griend R, Prins MH, Nijziel MR, Van De Ree MA, Buller HR, Dutilh JC, ten Cate-Hoek A, Van Den Heiligenberg SM, Van Der Meer J, Otten JM: Is extensive screening for cancer in idiopathic venous thromboembolism warranted? J Thromb Haemost 2011;9:79–84.

3 Canonico M, Plu-Bureau G, Lowe GD, Scarabin PY: Hormone replacement therapy and risk of venous thromboembolism in postmenopausal women: systematic review and meta-analysis. BMJ 2008;336:1227–1231.

4 Ceriani E, Combescure C, Le Gal G, Nendaz M, Perneger T, Bounameaux H, Perrier A, Righini M: Clinical prediction rules for pulmonary embolism: a systematic review and meta-analysis. J Thromb Haemost 2010;8:957–970.

5 Di Nisio M, Squizzato A, Rutjes AW, Buller HR, Zwinderman AH, Bossuyt PM: Diagnostic accuracy of D-dimer test for exclusion of venous thromboembolism: a systematic review. J Thromb Haemost 2007;5:296–304.

6 Carrier M, Righini M, Djurabi RK, Huisman MV, Perrier A, Wells PS, Rodger M, Wuillemin WA, Le Gal G: VIDAS D-dimer in combination with clinical pre-test probability to rule out pulmonary embolism. A systematic review of management outcome studies. Thromb Haemost 2009;101:886–892.

7 Hugli O, Righini M, Le Gal G, Roy PM, Sanchez O, Verschuren F, Meyer G, Bounameaux H, Aujesky D: The pulmonary embolism rule-out criteria (PERC) rule does not safely exclude pulmonary embolism. J Thromb Haemost 2011;9:300–304.

8 Douma RA, le Gal G, Sohne M, Righini M, Kamphuisen PW, Perrier A, Kruip MJ, Bounameaux H, Buller HR, Roy PM: Potential of an age adjusted D-dimer cut-off value to improve the exclusion of pulmonary embolism in older patients: a retrospective analysis of three large cohorts. BMJ 2010;340:c1475.

9 Torbicki A, Perrier A, Konstantinides S, Agnelli G, Galie N, Pruszczyk P, Bengel F, Brady AJ, Ferreira D, Janssens U, Klepetko W, Mayer E, Remy-Jardin M, Bassand JP, Vahanian A, Camm J, De Caterina R, Dean V, Dickstein K, Filippatos G, Funck-Brentano C, Hellemans I, Kristensen SD, McGregor K, Sechtem U, Silber S, Tendera M, Widimsky P, Zamorano JL, Zamorano JL, Andreotti F, Ascherman M, Athanassopoulos G, De Sutter J, Fitzmaurice D, Forster T, Heras M, Jondeau G, Kjeldsen K, Knuuti J, Lang I, Lenzen M, Lopez-Sendon J, Nihoyannopoulos P, Perez Isla L, Schwehr U, Torraca L, Vachiery JL: Guidelines on the diagnosis and management of acute pulmonary embolism: the Task Force for the Diagnosis and Management of Acute Pulmonary Embolism of the European Society of Cardiology (ESC). Eur Heart J 2008;29:2276–2315.

10 Righini M, Le Gal G, Aujesky D, Roy PM, Sanchez O, Verschuren F, Kossovsky M, Bressollette L, Meyer G, Perrier A, Bounameaux H: Complete venous ultrasound in outpatients with suspected pulmonary embolism. J Thromb Haemost 2009;7:406–412.

11 Stein PD, Fowler SE, Goodman LR, Gottschalk A, Hales CA, Hull RD, Leeper KV Jr, Popovich J Jr, Quinn DA, Sos TA, Sostman HD, Tapson VF, Wakefield TW, Weg JG, Woodard PK: Multidetector computed tomography for acute pulmonary embolism. N Engl J Med 2006;354:2317–2327.

12 Perrier A, Roy PM, Sanchez O, Le Gal G, Meyer G, Gourdier AL, Furber A, Revel MP, Howarth N, Davido A, Bounameaux H: Multidetector-row computed tomography in suspected pulmonary embolism. N Engl J Med 2005;352:1760–1768.

13 Righini M, Le Gal G, Aujesky D, Roy PM, Sanchez O, Verschuren F, Rutschmann O, Nonent M, Cornuz J, Thys F, Le Manach CP, Revel MP, Poletti PA, Meyer G, Mottier D, Perneger T, Bounameaux H, Perrier A: Diagnosis of pulmonary embolism by multidetector CT alone or combined with venous ultrasonography of the leg: a randomised non-inferiority trial. Lancet 2008;371:1343–1352.

14 van Belle A, Buller HR, Huisman MV, Huisman PM, Kaasjager K, Kamphuisen PW, Kramer MH, Kruip MJ, Kwakkel-van Erp JM, Leebeek FW, Nijkeuter M, Prins MH, Sohne M, Tick LW: Effectiveness of managing suspected pulmonary embolism using an algorithm combining clinical probability, D-dimer testing, and computed tomography. JAMA 2006;295:172–179.

15 Roy PM, Meyer G, Vielle B, Le Gall C, Verschuren F, Carpentier F, Leveau P, Furber A: Appropriateness of diagnostic management and outcomes of suspected pulmonary embolism. Ann Intern Med 2006;144:157–164.

16 Roy PM, Durieux P, Gillaizeau F, Legall C, Armand-Perroux A, Martino L, Hachelaf M, Dubart AE, Schmidt J, Cristiano M, Chretien JM, Perrier A, Meyer G: A computerized handheld decision-support system to improve pulmonary embolism diagnosis: a randomized trial. Ann Intern Med 2009;151:677–686.

17 Stein PD, Chenevert TL, Fowler SE, Goodman LR, Gottschalk A, Hales CA, Hull RD, Jablonski KA, Leeper KV Jr, Naidich DP, Sak DJ, Sostman HD, Tapson VF, Weg JG, Woodard PK: Gadolinium-enhanced magnetic resonance angiography for pulmonary embolism: a multicenter prospective study (PIOPED III). Ann Intern Med 2010;152:434–443.

18 Jimenez D, Aujesky D, Moores L, Gomez V, Lobo JL, Uresandi F, Otero R, Monreal M, Muriel A, Yusen RD: Simplification of the Pulmonary Embolism Severity Index for prognostication in patients with acute symptomatic pulmonary embolism. Arch Intern Med 2010;170:1383–1389.

19 Sanchez O, Trinquart L, Colombet I, Durieux P, Huisman MV, Chatellier G, Meyer G: Prognostic value of right ventricular dysfunction in patients with haemodynamically stable pulmonary embolism: a systematic review. Eur Heart J 2008;29:1569–1577.

20 Becattini C, Agnelli G, Vedovati MC, Pruszczyk P, Casazza F, Grifoni S, Salvi A, Bianchi M, Douma R, Konstantinides S, Lankeit M, Duranti M: Multidetector computed tomography for acute pulmonary embolism: diagnosis and risk stratification in a single test. Eur Heart J 2011;32:1657–1663.

21 Becattini C, Vedovati MC, Agnelli G: Prognostic value of troponins in acute pulmonary embolism: a meta-analysis. Circulation 2007;116:427–433.

22 Lankeit M, Friesen D, Aschoff J, Dellas C, Hasenfuss G, Katus H, Konstantinides S, Giannitsis E: Highly sensitive troponin T assay in normotensive patients with acute pulmonary embolism. Eur Heart J 2010;31:1836–1844.

23 Sanchez O, Trinquart L, Caille V, Couturaud F, Pacouret G, Meneveau N, Verschuren F, Roy PM, Parent F, Righini M, Perrier A, Lorut C, Tardy B, Benoit MO, Chatellier G, Meyer G: Prognostic factors for pulmonary embolism: the prep study, a prospective multicenter cohort study. Am J Respir Crit Care Med 2010;181:168–173.

24 Jimenez D, Aujesky D, Moores L, Gomez V, Marti D, Briongos S, Monreal M, Barrios V, Konstantinides S, Yusen RD: Combinations of prognostic tools for identification of high-risk normotensive patients with acute symptomatic pulmonary embolism. Thorax 2011;66:75–81.

25 Dellas C, Puls M, Lankeit M, Schafer K, Cuny M, Berner M, Hasenfuss G, Konstantinides S: Elevated heart-type fatty acid-binding protein levels on admission predict an adverse outcome in normotensive patients with acute pulmonary embolism. J Am Coll Cardiol 2010;55: 2150–2157.

26 Lankeit M, Kempf T, Dellas C, Cuny M, Tapken H, Peter T, Olschewski M, Konstantinides S, Wollert KC: Growth differentiation factor-15 for prognostic assessment of patients with acute pulmonary embolism. Am J Respir Crit Care Med 2008;177:1018–1025.

27 Wan S, Quinlan DJ, Agnelli G, Eikelboom JW: Thrombolysis compared with heparin for the initial treatment of pulmonary embolism: a meta-analysis of the randomized controlled trials. Circulation 2004;110:744–749.

28 Konstantinides S, Geibel A, Heusel G, Heinrich F, Kasper W: Heparin plus alteplase compared with heparin alone in patients with submassive pulmonary embolism. N Engl J Med 2002;347:1143–1150.

29 Erkens PM, Gandara E, Wells P, Shen AY, Bose G, Le Gal G, Rodger M, Prins MH, Carrier M: Safety of outpatient treatment in acute pulmonary embolism. J Thromb Haemost 2010;8:2412–2417.

30 Kovacs MJ, Hawel JD, Rekman JF, Lazo-Langner A: Ambulatory management of pulmonary embolism: a pragmatic evaluation. J Thromb Haemost 2010;8:2406–2411.

31 Aujesky D, Roy PM, Verschuren F, Righini M, Osterwalder J, Egloff M, Renaud B, Verhamme P, Stone RA, Legall C, Sanchez O, Pugh NA, N'gako A, Cornuz J, Hugli O, Beer H-J, Perrier A, Fine MJ, Yealy DM: Outpatient versus inpatient treatment for patients with acute pulmonary embolism: an international, open-label, randomised, non-inferiority trial. Lancet 2011;378:41–48.

32 The PREPIC Study Group: Eight-year follow-up of patients with permanent vena cava filters in the prevention of pulmonary embolism: the PREPIC (Prevention du Risque d'Embolie Pulmonaire par Interruption Cave) randomized study. Circulation 2005;112:416–422.

33 Meyer G, Planquette B, Sanchez O: Long-term outcome of pulmonary embolism. Curr Opin Hematol 2008;15:499–503.

34 Sanchez O, Helley D, Couchon S, Roux A, Delaval A, Trinquart L, Collignon MA, Fischer AM, Meyer G: Perfusion defects after pulmonary embolism: risk factors and clinical significance. J Thromb Haemost 2010;8:1248–1255.

35 Agnelli G, Prandoni P, Becattini C, Silingardi M, Taliani MR, Miccio M, Imberti D, Poggio R, Ageno W, Pogliani E, Porro F, Zonzin P: Extended oral anticoagulant therapy after a first episode of pulmonary embolism. Ann Intern Med 2003; 139:19–25.

36 Pengo V, Lensing AW, Prins MH, Marchiori A, Davidson BL, Tiozzo F, Albanese P, Biasiolo A, Pegoraro C, Iliceto S, Prandoni P: Incidence of chronic thromboembolic pulmonary hypertension after pulmonary embolism. N Engl J Med 2004;350:2257–2264.

37 Douketis JD, Gu CS, Schulman S, Ghirarduzzi A, Pengo V, Prandoni P: The risk for fatal pulmonary embolism after discontinuing anticoagulant therapy for venous thromboembolism. Ann Intern Med 2007;147:766–774.

38 Schulman S, Lindmarker P, Holmstrom M, Larfars G, Carlsson A, Nicol P, Svensson E, Ljungberg B, Viering S, Nordlander S, Leijd B, Jahed K, Hjorth M, Linder O, Beckman M: Post-thrombotic syndrome, recurrence, and death 10 years after the first episode of venous thromboembolism treated with warfarin for 6 weeks or 6 months. J Thromb Haemost 2006;4:734–742.

Olivier Sanchez
Service de Pneumologie et Soins Intensifs
Hôpital Européen Georges Pompidou
20 rue Leblanc, FR–75015 Paris (France)
Tel. +33 1 56 09 34 61, E-Mail olivier.sanchez@egp.aphp.fr

Chapter 22
Humbert M, Souza R, Simonneau G (eds): Pulmonary Vascular Disorders.
Prog Respir Res. Basel, Karger, 2012, vol 41, pp 218–225

Anticoagulation for Venous Thromboembolism in the Modern Management Era

Grégoire Le Gal[a,b] · Christophe Leroyer[a,b] · Dominique Mottier[a,b]

[a]EA3878 (GETBO) IFR 148, Université de Brest, [b]Département de médecine interne et de pneumologie, CHU de la Cavale Blanche, Brest, France

Abstract

Over the last decades, several major improvements in anticoagulant therapy strongly modified the management of venous thromboembolism (VTE) patients. Current research focuses on the development of new anticoagulant drugs, personalized therapeutic strategies based on individual risks of recurrent VTE, bleeding, and the values and preferences of the patients. Studies show that novel oral anticoagulants have less food and drug interactions than vitamin K antagonists. New oral drugs have been tested in noninferiority trials, either as a single-drug approach treatment (e.g. rivaroxaban or apixaban), or challenge vitamin K antagonists (e.g. dabigatran or edoxaban) after an initial course of low-molecular-weight heparin. Little is known about their potential in specific populations, such as cancer or elderly patients. The long-term decision concerning anticoagulation focuses on estimating individual risks of recurrent VTE and bleeding; several clinical and/or biological criteria are currently being tested as potential predictors of recurrence. The lack of monitoring of new oral anticoagulants suppresses the feedback of the international normalized ratio. Evaluation of both adherence and quality of life in patients receiving new drugs will be important. It is likely that educational efforts will need to be maintained or even reinforced in the future anticoagulant era.

This chapter deals with the anticoagulant treatment of non-severe venous thromboembolism (VTE); the use of thrombolysis in massive pulmonary embolism (PE) will not be discussed herein. Anticoagulant therapy is the cornerstone of the management of patients with VTE, and aims to (1) avoid the extension of the thrombotic process, (2) prevent migration of a lower limb vein thrombus to the lung, (3) prevent VTE recurrence, and (4) prevent long-term complications of VTE, i.e. postthrombotic syndrome and chronic thromboembolic pulmonary hypertension.

Over the last decades, several major improvements in anticoagulant therapy strongly modified the management of VTE patients. Current research focuses on the development of new anticoagulant drugs and personalized therapeutic strategies based on individual risks of recurrent VTE, bleeding, and the values and preferences of the patients.

Current Management of Venous Thromboembolism

Available Anticoagulant Drugs

Parenteral unfractionated heparin (UFH), low-molecular-weight heparin (LMWH), and fondaparinux are fast-acting anticoagulant drugs used to prevent thrombus extension in the initial treatment phase. Oral vitamin K antagonists (VKAs) require several days of treatment to become active, and hence are used for VTE secondary prevention. Parenteral danaparoid, lepirudin, and argatroban are mainly used for the treatment of heparin-induced thrombocytopenia, a rare but potentially severe complication of heparin use.

Unfractionated Heparin

Heparin is a highly sulfated mucopolysaccharide, extracted from porcine intestine. It is a mixture of molecules with heterogeneous size, anticoagulant activity, and pharmacokinetic properties. Not all heparin molecules possess the pentasaccharide sequence that provides the anticoagulant activity through a liaison to antithrombin. Heparin increases the natural anticoagulant activity of antithrombin against activated coagulation factors II (thrombin) and X. It may be administered intravenously or subcutaneously. Apart from bleeding, the adverse effects of heparin are the ability to induce osteoporosis and heparin-induced thrombocytopenia, requiring regular platelet count monitoring while on treatment; the longer the chain of heparin, the higher the risk of such complications. The length of heparin's chains is also associated with variable ways of elimination: longer chains have tissue clearance, while shorter chains have renal clearance. These variations in pharmacokinetics necessitate the monitoring of the anticoagulant activity of UFH by biological tests and subsequent frequent dose adjustments. In case of bleeding, emergency reversal of UFH may be obtained by the perfusion of protamine sulfate.

UFH is the only anticoagulant treatment that has been evaluated against placebo in the landmark randomized controlled trial published by Barrit and Jordan in 1960 [1]. In this trial, 35 patients were randomized between a control group and an intravenous UFH group. Half of the patients in the control group died, as compared with none of the patients on UFH. UFH became the reference initial treatment for VTE.

Low-Molecular-Weight Heparins

LMWHs are obtained through depolymerization of heparin chains. This lower and more homogeneous molecular weight explains a predominant anti-Xa over the anti-IIa activity, more predictable pharmacokinetics allowing the use of a subcutaneous fixed dose according to patient weight with no need to monitor the anticoagulant activity. Finally, the risk of osteoporosis and heparin-induced thrombocytopenia is lower with LMWH as compared with UFH, which allows avoiding platelet monitoring. On the other hand, LMWHs are mainly eliminated through the kidney, limiting their use in patients with renal failure. Moreover, protamine sulfate is less effective in antagonizing LWMH than UFH.

The advantages of LMWH over UFH led investigators to evaluate its use in the management of VTE. Many clinical trials confirmed the similar efficacy and safety of LMWH as compared with UFH for the treatment of deep vein thrombosis (DVT) and/or PE [2]. Several LMWHs exist: certoparin, dalteparin, enoxaparin, nadroparin, reviparin, and tinzaparin. They have replaced UFH in the initial management of patients with VTE, except in patients with severe renal failure or severe VTE.

Fondaparinux

Fondaparinux is an antithrombin-dependent synthetic pentasaccharide with exclusive anti-Xa activity. It has several advantages over LMWH: a fixed subcutaneous therapeutic dose of 7.5 mg for patients with body weight between 50 and 100 kg, 5 mg in patients with a body weight below 50, and 10 mg in patients with a body weight above 100 kg. There is no need for biological monitoring with fondaparinux, neither for efficacy (anticoagulant activity) nor for safety (platelet count) concerns. Its synthetic nature excludes the theoretical risk of infectious contamination of animal originated drugs (UFH, LMWH). On the other hand, similar to LMWHs, the renal clearance of fondaparinux contraindicates its use in patients with renal failure. Moreover, unlike heparins, fondaparinux has no specific antidote. Nonspecific drugs may be used if an urgent reversal is needed, such as recombinant activated factor VII.

The efficacy and safety of fondaparinux at the initial treatment phase of VTE was demonstrated in the MATISSE-DVT [3] and MATISSE-PE [4] trials.

Vitamin K Antagonists

VKAs can be administered orally. VKAs inhibit the synthesis of coagulation factors by the liver. It inhibits synthesis of factors II, VII, IX, and X, but also the synthesis of natural anticoagulant proteins C and S. Unlike heparins, they have no activity on activated coagulation factors. This, along with the long half-life of factor II (i.e. prothrombin) responsible for a delayed onset of action, explains why VKAs cannot be used alone in the acute phase of VTE. Their use is complicated by a narrow therapeutic window and great interindividual and intraindividual variabilities over time. Interindividual variability is explained by important variations in genes involved in the metabolism of vitamin K and of VKAs, while intraindividual variability over time is explained by numerous drug and food interactions, as well as comorbidities.

Whenever possible, VKAs should be started together with a fast-acting anticoagulant on the first treatment day. Their efficacy is monitored by the international normalized ratio (INR). The therapeutic target range for VTE is between 2.0 and 3.0. Under- and overdosing exposes patients to the risks of recurrent VTE and of bleeding, respectively. VKAs have a long duration of action. However, when urgent reversal is needed, for example in patients with bleeding or need for urgent surgery, the use of vitamin K and prothrombin complex concentrates allows a prompt restoration of hemostasis. Vitamin K can also be used to correct high INR values [5].

Practical Management

Initiation of Treatment

An injection of a fast-acting anticoagulant drug (UFH, LMWH, or fondaparinux) should be performed in patients with suspected VTE at the time of clinical suspicion while awaiting the results of diagnostic tests if the clinical suspicion is high [6]. Once the diagnosis is confirmed, short-term treatment should be performed with subcutaneous LMWH, intravenous UFH, subcutaneous UFH, or subcutaneous fondaparinux. In case of renal failure, only UFH should be used. Short-term treatment should be continued for at least 5 days and until the INR is >2.0 for 24 h. VKA should be initiated together with LMWH, UFH, or fondaparinux on the first treatment day. A first INR should be performed on day 2 or 3. Dose adjustment can be performed using a validated initiation nomogram. Once a stable dose of VKA has been reached, INR monitoring may be performed each month, and in the interval in case of change in medication of medical condition [6].

Duration of Anticoagulant Therapy

After a first episode of VTE, determination of the optimal duration for oral anticoagulant therapy (OAT) is based on the risk of recurrent VTE after OAT discontinuation and on the risk of bleeding while on OAT.

Risk of Recurrent Venous Thromboembolism. The main determinant of the risk of recurrent VTE is the circumstance in which VTE occurred. In fact, VTE is classified on the basis of the presence or absence of precipitating (or provoking) factors, such as whether it is provoked (due to a transient reversible risk factor, e.g. cast, surgery, immobilization, recent trauma), malignancy-associated, or unprovoked. Patients with provoked VTE have a very low risk of recurrent VTE after 3 months of OAT and can safely discontinue OAT. Conversely, patients with unprovoked VTE have a 5–27% risk of recurrent VTE during the first year after OAT discontinuation [7]. Finally, patients with malignancy-associated VTE have a very high risk of recurrent VTE at OAT discontinuation, and should be treated as long as the cancer is active (see below). The presence of major inherited or acquired thrombophilia such as antithrombin deficiency or antiphospholipid antibodies syndrome is associated with a very high risk of recurrent VTE and justifies long-term treatment.

Risk of Bleeding. Bleeding is the main complication of OAT. The annual incidence of major bleeding is estimated between 2.4 and 5% per year, and the incidence of fatal bleeding between 0.4 and 0.8% per year [8]. Some risk factors are associated with an increased risk of bleeding: age, a history of previous stroke or gastrointestinal bleeding, uncontrolled hypertension, and the presence of concomitant comorbidities. The risk of bleeding is increased when the INR is above 3. This increased risk is more pronounced in patients with an INR above 4.5. Some medications increase the risk of bleeding, either through a pharmacokinetic interaction with VKA or through pharmacodynamic interaction (antiplatelet or nonsteroid anti-inflammatory agents).

Recommendations. Current recommendations are mainly based on the 8th American College of Chest Physicians (ACCP) guidelines on antithrombotic and thrombolytic therapy published in 2008 [6]. For patients with provoked VTE, current recommendations are to treat with VKA for 3 months. For patients with unprovoked VTE, the ACCP recommendation is to treat with a VKA for at least 3 months. After 3 months of anticoagulant therapy, all patients with unprovoked VTE should be evaluated for the risk-benefit ratio of long-term therapy. The ACCP recommend long-term treatment for patients with a first unprovoked VTE, in whom risk factors for bleeding are absent and for whom good anticoagulant monitoring is achievable. This stresses the need for validated tools to assess the individual risk-benefit ratio. For patients with a first episode that was associated with a major inherited or acquired thrombophilia (i.e. antiphospholipid antibody syndrome or antithrombin deficiency), long-term treatment is recommended. Finally, for patients with a second episode of unprovoked VTE, long-term treatment is recommended.

Specific Clinical Settings

Patients with Active Malignancy. Cancer is one of the main risk factors for VTE. VTE may be the manifestation of an occult cancer, and 10% of patients with unprovoked VTE will have a cancer diagnosed in the year following the thrombotic episode [9]. VTE is a major prognostic factor in cancer patients, and significantly increases the risk of death, mainly in patients with localized malignancy. The use of VKA has several limitations in cancer patients: numerous interactions, digestive disorders, frequent need for VKA interruption due to thrombocytopenia or invasive procedures, etc. In patients with malignancy who develop VTE, the risk of bleeding and of recurrent VTE on OAT is higher than in noncancer patients. Several randomized controlled trials have demonstrated that the use of long-term LMWH therapy halves the risk of recurrent VTE, with no increase in the risk of bleeding. Current recommendations are to treat VTE in cancer patients with daily injections of LMWH for at least 3 months [6]. These patients should receive subsequent anticoagulant therapy with LMWH or VKA indefinitely or as long as the cancer is active.

Pregnancy. Pregnancy is another risk factor for VTE. Venous stasis is increased due to vein compression by the gravid uterus. Coagulation is globally enhanced due to estrogen impregnation: increase in coagulation factors, and decrease in the performance of natural anticoagulant system. VKAs are contraindicated during the first and third trimester of pregnancy. Current recommendations are to treat pregnant women who develop VTE while pregnant with UFH or LMWH throughout pregnancy and to continue the anticoagulant therapy for 6 weeks postpartum for a minimum duration of 6 months [10]. During the postpartum period women may be switched to VKA, using warfarin in the case of breastfeeding.

Recent Improvements and Unresolved Issues

New Anticoagulant Drugs

New drugs under development have the potential to act on two distinct targets: activated thrombin for orally available dabigatran etexilate, and activated factor Xa either through antithrombin for subcutaneously administered idraparinux or directly for oral rivaroxaban, apixaban, or edoxaban. These new drugs may be less affected by diet and genetics and have less drug interactions compared to VKAs [11]. The first stages of clinical development focused on primary prevention of VTE in surgical patients. The new drugs have been tested either as a single-drug approach treatment for VTE (e.g. rivaroxaban) or challenge VKAs (e.g. dabigatran or edoxaban) after an initial course of LMWH. The single-drug approach has the potential to eliminate the risk of heparin-induced thrombocytopenia. Of note, all new drugs were compared to reference treatment, but no face-to-face comparison between two new anticoagulant drugs is ongoing. Data from studies in prevention of stroke in atrial fibrillation patients or in acute coronary syndrome patients are not discussed in this chapter, but add to the assessment of safety profile.

From Clinical Trials to Practice

To better understand ongoing developments, some issues need to be addressed regarding study methods and interpretation.

Study Design. The development of new anticoagulant drugs is mainly based on noninferiority trials [12]. In fact, the objective of these new drugs is usually not to gain in efficacy, but to demonstrate a similar efficacy while bringing about better safety and ease of management. The goal of such a trial is to demonstrate that the new drug is not inferior to the reference treatment. A noninferiority margin is determined, which corresponds to the maximum loss of efficacy that is accepted to conclude to noninferiority. The definition of this margin is a matter of controversy. There is consensus that it should ensure the preservation of at least three quarters of the efficacy of the reference treatment as compared with placebo. Another difference with superiority trials is the importance of a per protocol analysis because the intention to treat analysis favors noninferiority. Admittedly, the intention to treat analysis remains the main analysis because it preserves the benefit of patient randomization. Also, there is a debate about whether a double-blind or an open-label design should be used in noninferiority trials. Although open-label trials are 'closer to reality', the double-blind design is crucial to ensure that the placebo effect is similar in the two arms, as such a placebo can strongly favor noninferiority.

Patient Selection. Patients included in clinical trials should have similar characteristics as patients for whom the treatment will be used in clinical practice. This has been an issue in recent trials on new anticoagulant drugs. Most of them had many exclusion criteria which selected patients with a lower risk of bleeding and of recurrent VTE. As a result, the mean age of patients included in these trials was at least 10 years younger than that of real-life patients. The need for signed informed consent impedes the inclusion of patients with impaired cognitive function, though VTE mainly affects elderly patients with a different risk profile. Finally, few cancer patients were included, and no patients with renal or hepatic failure. This raises issues on the generalizability of the results to the general population.

Study Outcome. Endpoints in clinical trials on new anticoagulant treatment aim at comparing the safety and efficacy of the two compared drugs. Most studies use an efficacy primary study outcome that combines death due to fatal PE and objectively confirmed recurrent VTE. Bleeding is used as the main safety outcome. An issue is that it is not easy to balance the absolute risks of recurrent VTE and bleeding. Not all recurrent VTE and bleeding events share the same prognosis. The definition of major bleeding by the International Society of Thrombosis and Haemostasis [13] comprises very different clinical scenarios with different clinical consequences and prognosis. The case fatality rate of each of these thrombotic and bleeding complications needs to be considered. Moreover, most trials have a short follow-up duration and hence never take into account the delayed complications of VTE such as postthrombotic syndrome and chronic thromboembolic pulmonary hypertension.

New Drugs in Development

Dabigatran. Orally administrated dabigatran etexilate is rapidly converted by esterases to the active drug dabigatran, which acts as a direct inhibitor of thrombin. Plasma levels of dabigatran peak at 2 h after administration and the drug is excreted by the kidney with approximately 80% of the drug

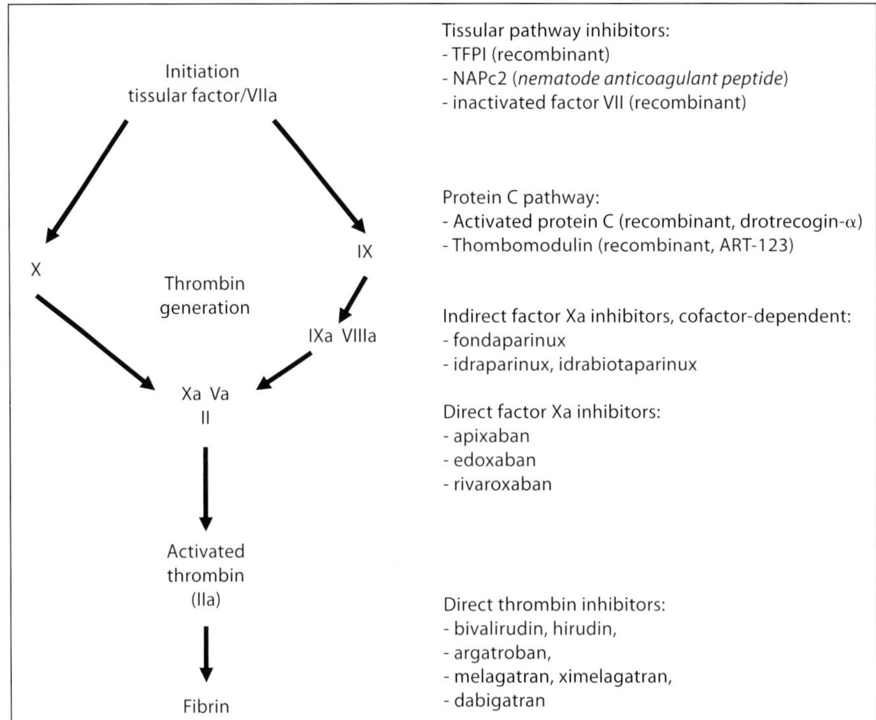

Fig. 1. Steps in blood coagulation and new anticoagulants.

unchanged in the urine. The predictable pharmacokinetics and the half-life of 12–17 h allow for a once or twice daily administration at fixed doses. Administration of dabigatran with P-glycoprotein inhibitors, such as quinidine, verapamil, or amiodarone is contraindicated.

The phase III RE-COVER trial has evaluated dabigatran etexilate for the treatment of acute symptomatic VTE (proximal DVT or PE), in a randomized double-blind noninferiority trial with warfarin as the comparator after an initial course of parenteral anticoagulation therapy. Oral dabigatran was given at a fixed dose of 150 mg twice daily. The primary outcome was the 6-month incidence of recurrent VTE and related deaths, confirmed following central adjudication. The primary outcome was confirmed in 2.4% of 1,274 patients randomly assessed to dabigatran and 2.1% of 1,265 patients randomly assessed to warfarin (HR with dabigatran of 1.1, 95% CI: 0.65–1.84). Bleeding occurred in 5.6% of patients in the dabigatran group and 8.8% in the warfarin group (HR: 0.63, 95% CI: 0.47–0.84). Dyspepsia was more frequent in the dabigatran group (2.9 vs. 0.6%, $p < 0.001$) [12]. In contrast to what was observed with exposure to ximelagatran, there was no evidence of hepatic toxic effects associated with dabigatran. A second trial with the same study design is ongoing (www.clinicaltrials.gov: NCT00680186).

The next steps of dabigatran development in VTE include the long-term secondary prevention of recurrent VTE over 18 months in patients who have completed a course of conventional anticoagulant treatment with a VKA for 6–18 months (RE-MEDY; www.clinicaltrials.gov: NCT00558259) or 3–6 months (RE-SOLVE; www.clinicaltrials.gov: NCT00329238).

Idraparinux and Idrabiotaparinux. Idraparinux is a long-acting inhibitor of factor-Xa administrated subcutaneously once a week. Initial trials showed noninferiority to standard therapy for DVT, but inferiority for PE [14]. Moreover, in the atrial fibrillation study, long-term treatment was associated with an increased risk of major bleeding [15]. Consequently, the development of idraparinux was stopped. The drug was modified by attaching biotin moiety at the nonreducing end unit ('idrabiotaparinux'), which allows, in case of bleeding, the neutralization of the drug with avidin, an egg-derived protein with low antigenicity. Idrabiotaparinux was compared to idraparinux in a bioequivalence randomized double-blind trial in DVT patients. In that trial, idrabiotaparinux had a similar time course of factor-Xa inhibition, efficacy, and safety as idraparinux [16].

Oral Direct Anti-Xa Inhibitors: Rivaroxaban, Apixaban, and Edoxaban. The family of oral direct factor Xa

Table 1. New oral anticoagulant regimens as evaluated in clinical trials

Drug	Target	LMWH pre-treatment?	Regimen	Time to peak, h	Half-life, h	Renal excretion, %	Drug interaction
Dabigatran	factor IIa	yes	150 mg b.i.d.	1.5	14–17	>80	P-glycoprotein inhibitor quinidine contraindicated
Rivaroxaban	factor Xa	no	15 mg b.i.d. × 3 weeks, then 20 mg o.d.	2–3	7–11	33	inhibitors of both CYP3A4 and P-glycoprotein (ketoconazole and ritonavir contraindicated)
Apixaban	factor Xa	no	10 mg b.i.d. × 7 days, then 5 mg b.i.d.	1–2	8–14	25	_
Edoxaban	factor Xa	yes	60 mg o.d.; dose reduction: 30 mg o.d. in patients with body weight <60 kg, GFR 30–60 ml/min, P-glycoprotein inhibitor use	1–2	8–11	35	P-glycoprotein inhibitors (verapamil, quinidine)

inhibitors comprises several drugs: rivaroxaban, apixaban, and edoxaban. These three drugs have a direct effect on factor Xa independent from antithrombin. Results of phase 3 clinical trials of rivaroxaban in VTE patients have already been reported. Plasma levels peak at 3 h after administration, and one third is excreted unchanged by the kidneys, one third by the liver (CYP3A4-dependent and independent pathways) and excreted via the fecal route, and the remaining, being inactive metabolites, is eliminated by the kidneys. Rivaroxaban has a bioavailability of about 80%, a half-life of 5–9 h in young people and 11–13 h in the elderly, allowing a once daily administration. Administration of rivaroxaban with inhibitors of both CYP3A4 and P-glycoprotein, such as ketoconazole and ritonavir, is contraindicated.

The phase III EINSTEIN-DVT trial compared rivaroxaban 15 mg b.i.d. for 3 weeks followed by 20 mg o.d. with LMWH and VKA for treatment of symptomatic DVT in a noninferiority open-label randomized trial. The primary outcome was the incidence of symptomatic recurrent VTE, recurrent DVT, and nonfatal and fatal PE, and confirmed following central adjudication. The primary outcome was confirmed in 2.1% of 1,731 patients randomly assessed to rivaroxaban and 3.0% of 1,717 patients randomly assessed to warfarin (HR with rivaroxaban of 0.68, 95% CI: 0.44–1.04). Bleeding occurred in 8.1% of patients in the dabigatran group and 8.1% in the warfarin group (HR: 0.97, 95% CI: 0.76–1.22). No difference in any adverse events was found between the two groups [17].

Challenges

Several challenges arise from the development of the new anticoagulant drugs. Even if new anticoagulant drugs will simplify the management of patients with VTE, regimens evaluated in clinical trials differ widely between drugs. Some include pretreatment with LMWH, while others do not, and some drugs are prescribed at a higher dose for a variable period of time (e.g. 3 weeks for rivaroxaban, 1 for apixaban). Finally, a lower dose of edoxaban has been evaluated in a subgroup of patients (table 1).

One of the main concerns is the lack of a specific antidote. Although the short half-life of the new anticoagulant drugs limit the need for antidote use, rapid reversal is necessary in patients with life-threatening bleedings or who require rapid surgical intervention. Some antidotes are under development, in particular a modified factor Xa with no catalytic activity [18].

No monitoring tests are currently available for the new anticoagulant drugs. The efficacy and safety of these drugs were demonstrated in clinical trials in which no monitoring or dose adjustments were performed. However, it may be useful to appraise the anticoagulant activity in treated patients in case of recurrent VTE or bleeding events, and before surgical intervention. Adherence to treatment is discussed below.

Personalized Care

Achieving Better Control of Oral Anticoagulant Therapy

VKA monitoring is of utmost importance. In routine practice, half of recurrent VTE on treatment occurs in patients with infratherapeutic INR values, and half of the bleeding episodes on VKA occurs in patients with supratherapeutic INR values. Even in clinical trials with selected and frequently monitored patients, the proportion of time spent within the therapeutic range is barely above 60%. Several approaches have been tested to improve this issue. Online open access 'summary for patients' or booklets regularly updated by scientific societies are available worldwide with patient information. In a recent hospital-based survey on thromboprophylaxis, however, participants reported hearing about VTE more frequently from friends, relatives, or the media than from healthcare providers [19]. Eliciting patient preferences is a prerequisite, especially when faced with the recommendation of long-term treatment. Data suggest that side effects, such as major bleeding events, are not systematically associated with a preference for treatment cessation [20]. Lower mental status functioning and poor cognitive functioning have been identified as risk factors of poor adherence to long-term OAT. Higher education status, possibly linked to independent decision making or distrust in healthcare providers, may be associated with poor adherence to long-term OAT [21]. Altogether, these findings suggest both a dramatic interindividual variability around perceptions and preferences for OAT [22] and an inability to improve adherence through increasing patient knowledge only.

Most structured educational interventions have been developed for patients on VKAs, irrespective of indication. Anticoagulant clinics are facilities in charge of monitoring patients and performing dose adjustments with the help of dedicated personnel and software [23]. New devices are available that offer patients the possibility of monitoring their VKA treatment themselves [24]. Almost all published interventions show that self-management of VKAs, compared to usual care, leads to a better control of INR values within the therapeutic range [25]. Studies also suggest that educational interventions have the potential to reduce rates of bleeding events [26–27].

Newer oral anticoagulants may become promising alternatives to VKAs, with the advantage of fixed doses and no blood sampling. Whether discontinuation of therapy is lowered by the use new oral anticoagulants is unclear from available published randomized trials. Conversely, using an oral drug with no initial injection and no mention of a narrow therapeutic window could lead to 'trivialization' of anticoagulation. Moreover, the lack of monitoring suppresses a potential adherence tool, INR monitoring allowing giving feedback to patients on the way they manage their therapy. Finally, unlike VKAs, the action of which lasts several days, the short half-life of new oral anticoagulant drugs might render crucial the day-to-day compliance to the treatment. Evaluation of both adherence and quality of life in patients receiving new OAT will be important. It is likely that educational efforts will need to be maintained or even reinforced in the future anticoagulant era.

Predicting Individual Risks of Recurrent VTE and Bleeding

The risk-benefit balance of anticoagulant treatment after 3–6 months of treatment of a first unprovoked VTE is unclear. This long-term decision should be based on balancing the long-term mortality risk from recurrent VTE, largely preventable with OAT, against the long-term mortality risk of major bleeding, the principal complication of OAT. There are important knowledge gaps in estimating the long-term mortality risk of recurrent VTE in patients with unprovoked VTE who discontinue therapy and the long-term mortality risk from major bleeding in those who continue OAT [28]. Current approaches focus on estimating individual risks of recurrent VTE and bleeding. Male gender, older age, postthrombotic syndrome, elevated D-dimer levels, elevated factor VIII levels after discontinuation of OAT, thrombophilia, and persistent abnormalities on diagnostic imaging have been reported as being predictors of recurrence. Clinical prediction rules integrating most discriminant predictors both for bleeding and recurrent VTE may help in resolving these issues [29].

Conclusion

Numerous new anticoagulant drugs are currently under study on phase 3 clinical trials. The first published studies suggest that most of them may be noninferior to conventional therapeutic strategies both in terms of efficacy and safety. Therefore, they might replace LMWH and VKAs in the management of VTE. Of note, new drugs have not yet been fully evaluated in several subgroups of patients frequently encountered in daily practice (e.g. elderly and cancer patients). Furthermore, the risk-benefit ratio may not be different enough to lead to deep modifications in treatment duration or indication. Cost-effective analyses should pay attention to the need for reinforced patient education strategies in the future anticoagulation era.

Acknowledgement

The authors would like to thank Mrs. Alavi for her help in preparing this manuscript.

References

1 Barritt DW, Jordan SC: Anticoagulant drugs in the treatment of pulmonary embolism. A controlled trial. Lancet 1960;1:1309–1312.

2 Quinlan D, McQuillan A, Eikelboom J: Low-molecular-weight heparin compared with intravenous unfractionated heparin for treatment of pulmonary embolism: a meta-analysis of randomized, controlled trials. Ann Intern Med 2004;140:175–183.

3 Buller HR, Davidson BL, Decousus H, Gallus A, Gent M, Piovella F, Prins MH, Raskob G, Segers AE, Cariou R, Leeuwenkamp O, Lensing AW: Fondaparinux or enoxaparin for the initial treatment of symptomatic deep venous thrombosis: a randomized trial. Ann Intern Med 2004;140: 867–873.

4 The MATISSE Investigators: Subcutaneous fondaparinux versus intravenous unfractionated heparin in the initial treatment of pulmonary embolism. N Engl J Med 2003;349:1695–1702.

5 Ansell J, Hirsh J, Hylek E, Jacobson A, Crowther M, Palareti G: Pharmacology and management of the vitamin K antagonists: American College of Chest Physicians Evidence-Based Clinical Practice Guidelines (8th Edition). Chest 2008; 133:160S–198S.

6 Kearon C, Kahn SR, Agnelli G, Goldhaber SZ, Raskob GE, Comerota AJ: Antithrombotic therapy for venous thromboembolic disease: American College of Chest Physicians Evidence-Based Clinical Practice Guidelines (8th edition). Chest 2008;133:454S–545S.

7 Rodger M, Carrier M, Gandara E, Le Gal G: Unprovoked venous thromboembolism: Short term or indefinite anticoagulation? Balancing long-term risk and benefit. Blood Rev 2010;24:171–178.

8 Landefeld C, Beyth R: Anticoagulant-related bleeding: clinical epidemiology, prediction, and prevention. Am J Med 1993;95:315–328.

9 Carrier M, Le Gal G, Wells PS, Fergusson D, Ramsay T, Rodger MA: Systematic review: the Trousseau syndrome revisited: should we screen extensively for cancer in patients with venous thromboembolism? Ann Intern Med 2008;149: 323–333.

10 Bates SM, Greer IA, Pabinger I, Sofaer S, Hirsh J: Venous thromboembolism, thrombophilia, antithrombotic therapy, and pregnancy: American College of Chest Physicians Evidence-Based Clinical Practice Guidelines (8th edition). Chest 2008;133:844S–886S.

11 Linkins LA, Weitz JI: New and emerging anticoagulant therapies for venous thromboembolism. Curr Treat Options Cardiovasc Med 2010;12:142–155.

12 Schulman S, Kearon C, Kakkar AK, Mismetti P, Schellong S, Eriksson H, Baanstra D, Schnee J, Goldhaber SZ: Dabigatran versus warfarin in the treatment of acute venous thromboembolism. N Engl J Med 2009;361:2342–2352.

13 Schulman S, Angeras U, Bergqvist D, Eriksson B, Lassen MR, Fisher W: Definition of major bleeding in clinical investigations of antihemostatic medicinal products in surgical patients. J Thromb Haemost 2010;8:202–204.

14 Buller HR, Cohen AT, Davidson B, Decousus H, Gallus AS, Gent M, Pillion G, Piovella F, Prins MH, Raskob GE: Idraparinux versus standard therapy for venous thromboembolic disease. N Engl J Med 2007;357:1094–1104.

15 Bousser MG, Bouthier J, Buller HR, Cohen AT, Crijns H, Davidson BL, Halperin J, Hankey G, Levy S, Pengo V, Prandoni P, Prins MH, Tomkowski W, Torp-Pedersen C, Wyse DG: Comparison of idraparinux with vitamin K antagonists for prevention of thromboembolism in patients with atrial fibrillation: a randomised, open-label, non-inferiority trial. Lancet 2008;371:315–321.

16 Efficacy and safety of once weekly subcutaneous idrabiotaparinux in the treatment of patients with symptomatic deep venous thrombosis. J Thromb Haemost 2011;9:92–99.

17 Bauersachs R, Berkowitz SD, Brenner B, Buller HR, Decousus H, Gallus AS, Lensing AW, Misselwitz F, Prins MH, Raskob GE, Segers A, Verhamme P, Wells P, Agnelli G, Bounameaux H, Cohen A, Davidson BL, Piovella F, Schellong S: Oral rivaroxaban for symptomatic venous thromboembolism. N Engl J Med 2010;363:2499–2510.

18 Lu G, DeGuzman FR, Lakhotia S, Hollenbach SJ, Phillips DR, Sinha U: Recombinant antidote for reversal of anticoagulation by factor Xa inhibitors. ASH Annual Meeting Abstracts 2008;112: 983.

19 Le Sage S, McGee M, Emed JD: Knowledge of venous thromboembolism (VTE) prevention among hospitalized patients. J Vasc Nurs 2008; 26:109–117.

20 Locadia M, Bossuyt PM, Stalmeier PF, Sprangers MA, van Dongen CJ, Middeldorp S, Bank I, van der Meer J, Hamulyak K, Prins MH: Treatment of venous thromboembolism with vitamin K antagonists: patients' health state valuations and treatment preferences. Thromb Haemost 2004;92: 1336–1341.

21 Arnsten JH, Gelfand JM, Singer DE: Determinants of compliance with anticoagulation: a case-control study. Am J Med 1997;103:11–17.

22 Kneeland PP, Fang MC: Current issues in patient adherence and persistence: focus on anticoagulants for the treatment and prevention of thromboembolism. Patient Prefer Adherence 2010;4: 51–60.

23 Poller L, Shiach C, MacCallum P, Johansen A, Munster A, Magalhaes A, Jespersen J: Multicentre randomised study of computerised anticoagulant dosage. European Concerted Action on Anticoagulation. Lancet 1998;352:1505–1509.

24 Sawicki P: A structured teaching and self-management program for patients receiving oral anticoagulation: a randomized controlled trial. Working Group for the Study of Patient Self-Management of Oral Anticoagulation. JAMA 1999;281:145–150.

25 Siebenhofer A, Berghold A, Sawicki PT: Systematic review of studies of self-management of oral anticoagulation. Thromb Haemost 2004;91:225–232.

26 Beyth RJ, Quinn L, Landefeld CS: A multicomponent intervention to prevent major bleeding complications in older patients receiving warfarin. A randomized, controlled trial. Ann Intern Med 2000;133:687–695.

27 Pernod G, Labarere J, Yver J, Satger B, Allenet B, Berremili T, Fontaine M, Franco G, Bosson JL: EDUC'AVK: reduction of oral anticoagulant-related adverse events after patient education: a prospective multicenter open randomized study. J Gen Intern Med 2008;23:1441–1446.

28 Carrier M, Le Gal G, Wells PS, Rodger MA: Systematic review: case-fatality rates of recurrent venous thromboembolism and major bleeding events among patients treated for venous thromboembolism. Ann Intern Med 2010;152:578–589.

29 Rodger MA, Kahn SR, Wells PS, Anderson DA, Chagnon I, Le Gal G, Solymoss S, Crowther M, Perrier A, White R, Vickars L, Ramsay T, Betancourt MT, Kovacs MJ: Identifying unprovoked thromboembolism patients at low risk for recurrence who can discontinue anticoagulant therapy. CMAJ 2008;179:417–426.

Prof. Grégoire Le Gal, MD, PhD
Department of Internal Medicine and Chest Diseases
Brest University Hospital, Boulevard Tanguy Prigent
FR–29609 Brest Cedex (France)
Tel. +33 2 98 34 73 36, E-Mail gregoire.legal@chu-brest.fr

Chapter 23

Humbert M, Souza R, Simonneau G (eds): Pulmonary Vascular Disorders.
Prog Respir Res. Basel, Karger, 2012, vol 41, pp 226–236

Chronic Thromboembolic Pulmonary Hypertension

Irene M. Lang[a] · Xavier Jais[b]

[a]Medical University of Vienna, Vienna, Austria; [b]University Paris Sud (Paris XI), INSERM U 999, Hôpital Antoine Béclère, Clamart, France

Abstract

Chronic thromboembolic pulmonary hypertension (CTEPH) is a dual pulmonary vascular disease comprising major vessel thrombotic obstruction, and classical small-vessel arteriopathy. In general, only a few patients who have survived an acute thromboembolic event continue to develop CTEPH. However, approximately 25% of patients with CTEPH have never experienced symptomatic venous thromboembolism, suggesting that the true incidence of the disorder may still be underestimated. Splenectomy, infected ventriculoatrial shunt, inflammatory bowel disease, thyroid hormone replacement therapy, having survived cancer, and non-0 blood groups have been identified as CTEPH-associated conditions, while chronic obstructive pulmonary disease is the most common other reported cause for pulmonary hypertension in CTEPH. Misguided thrombus resolution as a variant of pulmonary arterial vascular remodeling, lysis-resistant fibrin/fibrinogen, an abnormal acute-phase response driven by Th1 lymphokines, and a platelet-derived growth factor-dependent vascular proliferative process are thought to be basic mechanisms of disease [Pepke-Zaba et al: Circulation 2011;124:1973–1981]. The primary treatment of CTEPH remains surgical pulmonary endarterectomy. Recent data from the European CTEPH registry indicate that on average 36.6% of patients are nonoperable. Based on the concept of a disorder that involves small pulmonary arterioles, vasodilator therapy has been proposed for those patients. The BENEFIT study, the first multicenter randomized controlled trial of the dual endothelin receptor antagonist bosentan in nonoperable CTEPH patients failed to achieve the second component of the coprimary endpoint. Further trials and the availability of novel treatment concepts raise hope for medical treatments of nonoperable CTEPH patients.

Chronic thromboembolic pulmonary hypertension (CTEPH) results from obstruction of the pulmonary vascular bed by nonresolving thromboemboli. Increased pulmonary vascular resistance (PVR) subsequently leads to progressive pulmonary hypertension (PH) and right heart failure. In the nonoccluded areas, pulmonary arteriopathy indistinguishable from that of pulmonary arterial hypertension (PAH) can develop and contribute to disease progression [1–3]. In general, only few patients who have survived an acute thromboembolic event continue to develop CTEPH. However, about one third of patients with CTEPH have never experienced symptomatic venous thromboembolism, suggesting that the true incidence of the disorder may still be underestimated. In the 2008 World Symposium on Pulmonary Hypertension, CTEPH was labeled as Group IV, without further subclassification. Recently, the Association for Research in CTEPH has collected 679 patients within the European CTEPH Registry to obtain observational data on incidence, prevalence, clinical symptoms, etiologies, associated conditions, treatments, and outcomes. From these recent data and from previous experience, it has become evident that operability, which is the center-specific evaluation of suitability for pulmonary endarterectomy (PEA), is a key determinant of prognosis. Therefore, the distinction of operable versus nonoperable disease has been chosen as a prespecified criterion for statistical analysis of the European database [4].

Definition

CTEPH is defined by the following observations that are made after at least 3 months of effective anticoagulation [5]: (1) a mean pulmonary arterial pressure >25 mm Hg with a pulmonary capillary wedge pressure ≤15 mm Hg, and (2) one or more mismatched segmental or larger perfusion defects detected by ventilation-perfusion lung scanning/

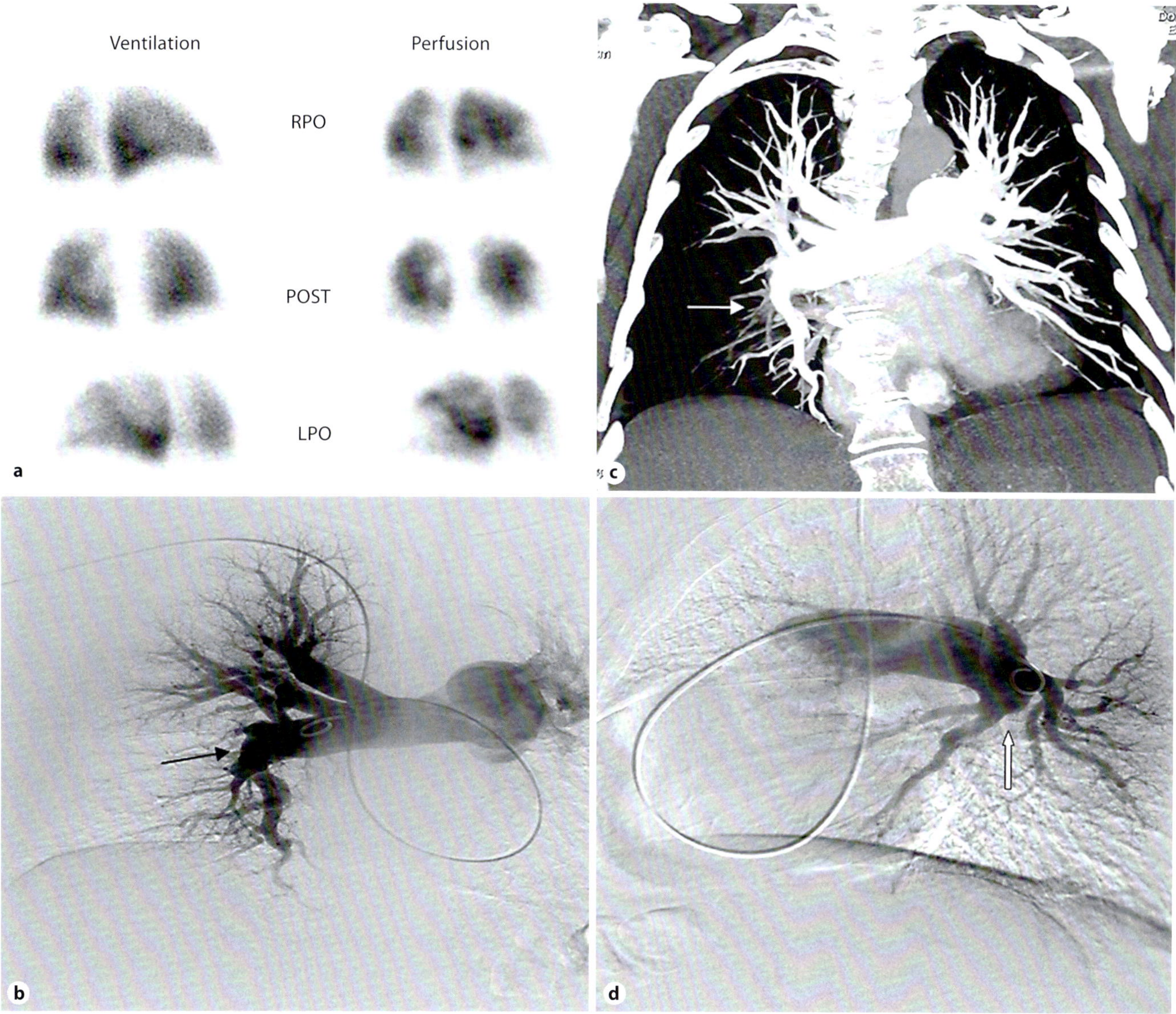

Fig. 1. CTEPH in a 60-year-old woman. **a** Ventilation-perfusion lung scan reveals several segmental mismatched perfusion defects. RPO = Right posterior oblique view; POST = posterior view; LPO = left posterior oblique view. **b** Right anteroposterior pulmonary angiogram shows multiple intimal irregularities (arrow) and obstruction of multiple segmental arteries. **c** Coronal reformatted multidetector CT angiography shows organized thrombus (arrow) as cause of intimal irregularities. **d** Left lateral pulmonary angiogram demonstrates absent flow to posterior basal segment arteries (arrow).

multidetector computed tomographic angiography/pulmonary angiography (fig. 1).

Epidemiology and Natural History

The incidence and prevalence of CTEPH are unknown. Classical estimates of disease frequency refer to the number of CTEPH cases per survived pulmonary thromboembolic events. However, 25–30% of affected patients deny previous symptoms or a diagnosis of previous acute venous thromboembolism [6], suggesting a higher prevalence than estimated from pulmonary embolism (PE) registries [3].

According to most recent data, the incidence of CTEPH in patients who suffered from acute PE has been reported to be in the range of 0.1–9.1%, depending on the selection criteria applied in the individual studies [7–12]. The difficulty to acutely recognize CTEPH in clinical disguise of acute PE has accounted for the highly variable incidences of CTEPH following acute PE.

The natural history of CTEPH usually includes a 'honeymoon' period following acute PE during which symptoms are absent despite significant PH. The diagnosis of CTEPH is commonly made when PH is advanced and causes dyspnea, hypoxemia, and right ventricular failure. The clinical presentation of CTEPH is characterized by nonspecific symptoms and include exercise intolerance and dyspnea, fatigue, chest pain, and exertional syncope. These symptoms are also consistent with other more common cardiopulmonary conditions such as asthma, chronic obstructive pulmonary disease, interstitial lung disease, coronary artery disease, cardiac arrhythmia, and heart failure, which make clinical diagnosis difficult.

Risk Factors

In recent years, a number of apparently unrelated conditions have been identified as risk factors for CTEPH. Populations at risk are those with a history of splenectomy [11–13]; carriers of ventriculoatrial (VA) shunts for the treatment of hydrocephalus or carriers of pacemakers with a history of device infection [6, 14]; patients with inflammatory bowel disease [14], thyroid hormone replacement [6], and circulating antiphospholipid antibodies [6, 15, 16]; those who have survived cancer [6]; individuals with non-0 blood groups [6, 17] and elevated plasma coagulation factor VIII [17]; and carriers of the fibrinogen Aα Thr312Ala polymorphism [18]. Evidence on reported risk factors mainly originates from observational case-control analyses of CTEPH patients that employed survivors of major PE or PAH patients as controls [6, 14]. A substudy of the multicenter prospective CTEPH registry is under way and will elucidate risk factor profiles in comparison with idiopathic PAH (IPAH).

Etiology and Pathophysiology

CTEPH results from recurrent pulmonary emboli arising from sites of venous thrombosis. The current concept is that failing thrombus resolution, fibrous obstruction, and secondary remodeling processes of the pulmonary vascular bed lead to an increase in PVR, progressive right heart failure, and death.

Although CTEPH is understood as a thromboembolic disorder, neither classical plasmatic risk factors for venous thromboembolism nor defects in fibrinolysis are associated with CTEPH. Compared with the general population, no increased prevalence of the factor V Leiden mutation was found [16, 19]. Other hereditary thrombotic risk factors, such as deficiencies in antithrombin, protein C, protein S, or the prothrombin gene mutation [20, 21] lack a systematic association with CTEPH. Efforts to identify functional defects [22, 23] or gene polymorphisms [18] in the pulmonary vascular fibrinolytic system of affected individuals have failed. Neither alterations in plasma levels of type 1 plasminogen activator inhibitor nor tissue-type plasminogen activator could be linked with CTEPH [24].

The identification of clinical risk factors for CTEPH has shed new light on molecular mechanisms underlying thrombus persistence and its fibrous transformation. The observation that carriers of VA shunts represent a CTEPH risk population [6, 14] has stimulated experimental research. Shunt infection is common in patients with VA shunts, and *Staphylococcus aureus* or *epidermidis* is responsible for up to one half of these infections [25], leading to thrombosis and device failure [26]. The majority of CTEPH patients carrying either a VA shunt or pacemaker had a history of device infection. Indeed, staphylococcal DNA was present in 6 of 7 PEA specimens from VA shunt/pacemaker carriers. In a murine model of stagnant-flow venous thrombosis, staphylococcal infection delayed thrombus resolution in parallel with an upregulation of profibrotic molecules, such as transforming growth factor-β and connective tissue growth factor [27]. Based on the available data, it cannot be said whether the risk to develop CTEPH is to be attributed to hypothyroidism or thyroid hormone replacement therapy, or both. In tumor survivors, the interaction of tissue factor, thrombin, and other coagulation factors with protease activated receptor proteins expressed by tumor cells and host vascular cells may have led to the induction of genes related to angiogenesis, cell survival, cell adhesion, and migration. Of note, time delays between the occurrence of a CTEPH-associated medical condition and manifestation of CTEPH is in the order of 2–40 years [14].

Pulmonary vascular remodeling is believed to occur in areas free of thrombosis and is histologically indistinguishable from other forms of PH [28–31]. There is a broad individual variation with respect to the degree of pulmonary arteriopathy, which was originally labeled as 'secondary vascular changes' by Moser et al. [5]. Although concomitant pulmonary vascular disease predicts adverse outcome [32, 33], biological mechanisms that predict the degree of vascular involvement have not been identified. Mutations in the type-2 bone morphogenetic protein receptor gene that have been linked to the development of pulmonary vascular disease in familial PAH and IPAH [34, 35] were not related to CTEPH [36]. Interestingly, CTEPH patients with a history of splenectomy, infected VA shunt, inflammatory bowel disease, or osteomyelitis face an adverse outcome as compared to affected patients without a clinical risk factor [37]. This finding has been attributed to more severe small vessel pathology, although the exact mechanisms remain unclear.

Clinical Presentation

Symptoms and Physical Signs
Similar to patients with other subsets of PH, CTEPH patients suffer from symptoms of progressive right heart failure. In earlier stages of disease, typical patient complaints are dyspnea on exertion, fatigue, and rapid exhaustion. Symptoms of overt right heart failure in advanced stages of disease are resting dyspnea and fluid retention. Physical findings are often subtle and may include a prominent pulmonary component of S2, left parasternal heave, and a systolic murmur if tricuspid regurgitation is present. Typical clinical signs of right heart failure are extended neck veins, leg edema, ascites, hepatomegaly, and acrocyanosis. A rare but typical clinical finding is bruits over peripheral lung fields [38]. This acoustic phenomenon is thought to occur in approximately 10% of CTEPH patients and has been attributed to turbulent blood flow in partially occluded pulmonary vessels [8].

Clinical Course

Despite similarities in symptoms and physical signs, the course of CTEPH is clearly different from nonthromboembolic PH. A major difference is encountered in the age of disease onset. On average, CTEPH patients are 7 years older at the time of diagnosis, with the majority of patients presenting between the sixth and seventh life decade [1, 6, 39]. In contrast to a progressive course of PAH, CTEPH progresses episodically with ‘honeymoon periods’ lasting anywhere from a few months to several years between episodes of severe desaturation and deterioration. A study from Japan reported a mean survival of 6.8 years after diagnosis in CTEPH patients if left untreated [40]. For comparison, patients with IPAH face an untreated median survival of less than 3 years after diagnosis [41].

Diagnosis

CTEPH that is successfully subjected to bilateral surgical PEA regains near-normal functional capacity [42, 43]. Thus, a major goal in the diagnostic work-up of patients presenting with PH is to exclude CTEPH and explore operability. Imaging has become central to the diagnosis of CTEPH and assessment of operability. Although visualization of the thrombus site and extent may serve as surgical ‘road map’, the operability statement is complex and hardly standardized. It is determined by thrombus location, underlying disease modifying factors, general comorbidities, the status of the lung parenchyma, hemodynamics in absolute numbers (i.e. PVR above 1,000 dyn•s•cm^{-5} confers increased risk), the relation of hemodynamic compromise and thrombus extension, previous cardiothoracic surgeries, hemodynamics after a previous PEA, experience of the surgeon, unilateral versus bilateral disease, the response to nitric oxide during acute testing [33], upstream resistance [44], and plasma levels of biomarkers, i.e. ADMA [45] and FABP [46]. Because the degree of concomitant small vessel arteriopathy has a major impact on PEA outcome, a series of techniques have been developed that may help to assess the functional status of the distal pulmonary vascular bed [32, 33].

Imaging

In experienced PEA centers in Europe and the United States, available imaging techniques are used complementarily. Traditionally, ventilation-perfusion scanning and pulmonary angiography have been key diagnostic tools for CTEPH. In light of the technical evolution, multidetector computed tomographic angiography and magnetic resonance angiography may eventually supersede traditional imaging techniques [47].

Ventilation-Perfusion Scanning
Ventilation-perfusion lung scanning represents a mainstay in the diagnostic work-up of PH patients. A normal ventilation-perfusion scintigram virtually rules out CTEPH [7, 48–51]; however, in the presence of PH, one or more mismatched segmental or larger defects generally indicate CTEPH [50]. In clinical routine, an abnormal perfusion scan alone is diagnostic in the absence of severe pulmonary parenchymal disease.

Pulmonary Angiography
Visualization of thromboembolic occlusions proximal and in the distality of the pulmonary vascular tree makes pulmonary angiography the established gold standard in CTEPH diagnosis, and the most important resource for the assessment of operability [52–54]. Major drawbacks of this technique are

its invasiveness and limited access, which results in limited expertise, especially in low-volume centers.

Hemodynamic Evaluation
Concomitant pulmonary vascular disease is a predictor of adverse surgical outcome in patients with CTEPH [32, 33]. Kim et al. [32] invasively analyzed pulmonary arterial occlusion pressure waveforms, a technique that has been used for partitioning PVR. Preoperative assessment of upstream resistance in 26 CTEPH patients correlated with both postoperative total pulmonary resistance index and postoperative mean pulmonary arterial pressure. More recently, Skoro-Sajer et al. [33] demonstrated that acute vasoreactivity testing with nitric oxide predicts surgical outcome. Sixty-two patients were followed for a median of 70.9 months after PEA. Those who experienced a reduction in mean pulmonary arterial pressure >10.4% with nitric oxide inhalation had lower postoperative pulmonary pressures and a clear long-term survival benefit as opposed to patients with acute vasoreactivity below this threshold.

Treatment

The most effective therapy for CTEPH is PEA. Successful PEA results in marked improvements in mean pulmonary arterial pressure, PVR, and cardiac output [55–57]. Improved hemodynamics after successful PEA results in substantial reverse right ventricular remodeling with reductions in tricuspid regurgitation and a return of parameters of right ventricular systolic and diastolic function towards normal [58–60]. Symptoms [61–63] and measures of functional capacity, such as 6-min walking distance and New York Heart Association (NYHA) functional class markedly improve after PEA, and the beneficial effect persists over time [57, 64].

However, surgical success largely depends on patient suitability. Beyond established standards and parameters that predict surgical success [62], operability is dependent on the expertise of the surgical team and available resources. Thus, the proportion of CTEPH patients not suitable for PEA varies from center to center, and may be as high as 50%.

Current criteria for PEA include confirmed diagnosis of CTEPH in NYHA functional classes II, III, or IV; a preoperative PVR >300 dyn•s•cm^{-5}; surgical accessibility of thrombi in the main, lobar, or segmental pulmonary arteries; absence of severe comorbidities; and patient consent [65].

A crucial issue in the preoperative assessment of CTEPH patients is the definition of the degree of secondary arteriopathy and its contribution to overall PVR. Interestingly, patients with a history of deep vein thrombosis and a plasmatic thrombophilia are more likely to be surgical candidates (CTEPH Registry, unpubl.). Patients with thromboembolic defects in the main, lobar, or proximal segmental level are characterized as having proximal disease and represent the main target population for PEA. In contrast, patients with significant PH, but little or no visible evidence of thromboembolic pathology, are considered poor candidates for surgery [44]. This latter group is usually characterized by severe pulmonary arteriopathy. Operability remains a center-specific assessment and may vary largely.

In fact, patients who do not undergo surgery or suffer from persistent or residual PH after PEA face a poor prognosis. Particularly in patients with a mean pulmonary artery pressure >50 mm Hg, 5-year survival rates are as low as 10% [39, 66–68]. Medical therapies currently used in the management of CTEPH come from a number of drug classes, such as anticoagulants, diuretics, or digitalis. Supportive treatment with anticoagulants reduces the risk of recurrent pulmonary thromboembolic events, and maintenance of lifelong anticoagulation is recommended [8]. Diuretics may be used in conditions of fluid overload, and chronic oxygen supplementation is used for the treatment of hypoxemia.

The evidence for pathogenic mechanisms held in common between nonthromboembolic PH and CTEPH provides a strong rationale for the usefulness of vasodilator drugs in CTEPH patients. Pharmacotherapy is currently not approved, but justified for 'compassionate use' in nonoperable patients. It can also be used as a 'therapeutic bridge' to PEA in patients considered at high risk due to poor hemodynamics, in patients with persistent or residual PH after PEA, or when surgery is contraindicated due to a significant comorbidity.

Current knowledge on the effects of vasodilator treatment in patients with CTEPH primarily originates from uncontrolled single-center experiences, retrospective evaluations, and trials primarily assessing nonthromboembolic PH that included, but did not exclusively evaluate, patients with CTEPH. Prostacyclin and -analogues, endothelin receptor antagonists, and phosphodiesterase-5 inhibitors were employed.

Surgical Technique

PEA is performed under cardiopulmonary bypass with intermittent circulatory arrest to permit medial dissection from the main pulmonary arteries to the subsegmental branches.

Inferior vena cava filters are routinely implanted perioperatively in the USA, but no particular benefit has been demonstrated; filter implantation has been abandoned in many European PEA centers and remains a matter of debate [69]. Out of 384 evaluable operated patients in the European CTEPH registry, 189 (49.2%) had a perioperative complication including infection (18.8%, of which 65.7% had ventilator-acquired pneumonia, 6.0% mediastinitis, 4.5% catheter-related sepsis, and 31.3% other), persistent PH (16.7%), neurological (11.2%) or bleeding (10.2%) complications, pulmonary reperfusion edema (9.6%), pericardial effusion (8.3%), or need for extracorporeal membrane oxygenation (3.1%). The occurrence of neurological complications increased with increasing circulatory arrest time. The duration of circulatory arrest was a risk factor for developing neurological complications: the odds ratio for comparison of circulatory arrest time less than 20 min with more than 60 min was 0.09 (95% CL: 0.01, 0.74). Three patients had irreversible complications [cerebrovascular accident (n = 2), worsening of pre-existing schizophrenia (n = 1)] despite circulatory arrest durations comparable with the median observed for the whole population [4].

In the European database, in-hospital mortality due to perioperative complications was 4.7%, and documented 1-year mortality was 7%, appearing low compared with 30-day mortality ranges between 5 and 10% as reported in previous years [56, 57, 64]. Residual PH which may result from incomplete endarterectomy or small-vessel arteriopathy is an important predictor of late postoperative adverse events [57, 67]. Postoperative NYHA class III-IV symptoms, unsuccessful pulmonary thromboendarterectomy, high PVR, and persistent abnormalities of gas exchange are associated with an increased risk of late adverse events [57]. In the European CTEPH registry, exercise capacity predicted 1-year mortality and postoperative PVR was a predictor of in-hospital and 1-year mortality [4].

Balloon Pulmonary Angioplasty

For patients who have nonoperable disease due to distal surgically inaccessible disease or who have persistent or recurrent PH after PEA, balloon pulmonary angioplasty offers an alternative therapy. Balloon pulmonary angioplasty can significantly reduce pulmonary artery pressure in patients with CTEPH. Improvement in NYHA functional class and 6-min walk capacity has been observed after successful balloon pulmonary angioplasty [70]. However, experience is very limited and the procedure is not generally recommended.

Medical Therapy

Anticoagulation is used in most patients with CTEPH because of a history of PE in 74.8% [1]. The rationale for the utility of medical therapy with pulmonary vasodilators in CTEPH is based upon recent pathophysiologic observations that suggest similarities to IPAH. Histological examination of patients with CTEPH has demonstrated vessel morphology that resembles that of IPAH, suggesting a degree of shared pathophysiology with PAH. Patients with CTEPH do show acute vasoreactivity to inhaled pulmonary vasodilators, which is related to prognosis [33]. The introduction of pulmonary vasodilator therapy for patients with CTEPH has contributed to improved survival in patients with nonoperable disease [13]. Pulmonary vasodilators currently used in CTEPH include the endothelin receptor antagonist bosentan, the phosphodiesterase inhibitor sildenafil, and prostacyclin analogues such as treprostinil. In the European CTEPH registry, roughly 40% of patients had been put on a PAH-specific treatment at the time of diagnosis, regardless of operability (unpubl. data).

Prostacyclin and Prostacyclin Analogues

Beraprost Sodium

Ono et al. [71] studied the efficacy of oral beraprost sodium in nonoperable patients with CTEPH. Patients were classified into two groups, one receiving oral beraprost sodium (n = 20), the other conventional therapy (n = 23). In contrast to the control group, treated patients experienced improvements in NYHA functional class. In a subgroup of patients undergoing hemodynamic evaluation after 2 ± 1 months, oral beraprost sodium treatment resulted in significant improvements in mean pulmonary arterial pressure and total pulmonary resistance, but not cardiac output. Overall, the study suggested that vasodilator treatment on top of conventional therapy improves 1- and 5-year survival. Vizza et al. [72] compared the effects of 6 months of beraprost treatment in 8 patients with distal CTEPH and matched individuals with IPAH. The authors concluded that in patients with CTEPH, beraprost led to similar mid-term clinical and hemodynamic improvements as in patients with nonthromboembolic PH.

Epoprostenol

Beneficial effects were also observed when patients were treated with epoprostenol. Nagaya et al. [73] administered intravenous epoprostenol to 12 CTEPH patients scheduled for PEA. Because of severe PH with PVR values exceeding 1,200 dyn•s•cm^{-5}, these patients were considered high-risk surgical candidates. During a mean follow-up period of 46 ± 12 days, intravenous prostacyclin resulted in a 28% decrease in PVR before surgery. Moreover, plasma brain natriuretic peptide levels markedly decreased, suggesting improvement in right ventricular function. In another retrospective series [74], 9 patients with moderate-to-severe CTEPH were treated with intravenous epoprostenol for 2–26 months before PEA. Six patients experienced either clinical stability or improvement that was associated with a mean reduction in PVR of 28% (range: 0–46). Three patients experienced clinical deterioration during epoprostenol administration, with a significant increase in PVR in 2 patients. Data from an Italian patient cohort [75] comprising 16 patients with nonthromboembolic PH and 11 with surgically untreatable CTEPH suggested that epoprostenol therapy over a median period of 12.4 months improves clinical status, exercise capacity, and NYHA functional class. In a more recent analysis [76], 27 consecutive patients with nonoperable CTEPH were treated with long-term intravenous epoprostenol. After 20 ± 8 months of treatment, there was sustained improvement of exercise capacity and hemodynamic parameters in those who survived.

Treprostinil

In an open-label study of 25 patients with severe nonoperable CTEPH, subcutaneously administered treprostinil resulted in significant improvements in 6-min walking distance, World Health Organization functional class, levels of brain-type natriuretic peptide, cardiac output, and PVR. Treatment with subcutaneously administered treprostinil was associated with improved long-term survival compared with historical controls [77]. Based on these results, and the urgent need for a management strategy in nonoperable patients, a randomized controlled trial has been initiated to evaluate the benefit of subcutaneous treprostinil ('CTREPH trial').

Iloprost

A subgroup of patients enrolled in the AIR (Aerosolized Iloprost Randomized) study, a prospective randomized placebo-controlled trial, suffered from CTEPH. The study failed to demonstrate significant beneficial effects of inhaled iloprost in this subpopulation [78]. Kramm et al. [79] studied the effect of inhaled iloprost administered immediately before PEA, after intensive care unit admission, and 12 h after surgery (n = 10). Preoperative treatment had no significant effect on hemodynamic parameters, but led to detrimental systemic vasodilation and hypotension. Postoperative treatment, however, showed beneficial effects on PVR and mean pulmonary arterial pressure on top of the relief of hemodynamics by PEA. The same investigators administered aerosolized iloprost in a randomized placebo-controlled fashion in the setting of persistent PH in the postoperative period [80]. Iloprost significantly enhanced cardiac index and reduced mean pulmonary arterial pressure and PVR compared with placebo.

Endothelin Receptor Antagonists

Bosentan

The effects of the dual endothelin receptor antagonist bosentan were assessed in 16 nonoperable patients with CTEPH [81]. After 6 months of treatment, NYHA functional class improved in 11 patients. In addition, a significant improvement was encountered in 6-min walking distance, paralleled by a reduction in serum levels of N-terminal brain natriuretic peptide. In the same issue of *Chest*, Hoeper et al. [82] published results from a prospective, multicenter, open-label trial evaluating bosentan treatment in CTEPH patients. At the 3-month follow-up visit, the 6-min walking distance as well as hemodynamic parameters and serum levels of N-terminal brain natriuretic peptide had significantly improved in the treatment groups as compared to controls. Another retrospective, open-label study assessed bosentan treatment in 20 patients with CTEPH [83]. After at least 3 months of treatment, Hughes et al. [83] found significant improvement in the 6-min walking distance as well as in hemodynamic parameters, such as PVR and cardiac index. Mean pulmonary artery pressure was also reduced, but did not reach statistical significance as compared to the baseline value. Moreover, Hughes et al. [84] reported findings from a retrospective open-label study evaluating long-term efficacy and safety of bosentan in CTEPH patients from three European centers (n = 47). A clear improvement was observed in 6-min walking distance at the 1-year follow-up. Twenty-eight patients had undergone right heart catheterization after 1 year, and demonstrated significant improvement in cardiac index and a decrease in total pulmonary resistance. Seyfarth et al. [85] investigated the effect of long-term bosentan treatment on exercise tolerance and right ventricular function, as measured by the Tei index. Twelve consecutive patients with CTEPH not eligible for PEA or following partial or complete failure of PEA were included in a nonrandomized, open-label prospective study. After 24 months of therapy, a beneficial effect on both outcome measures was achieved. The Swiss BOCTEPH study [86] was a national open-label trial assessing the effect of bosentan on hemodynamics, exercise capacity, quality of life, safety, and tolerability in patients with CTEPH. Fifteen patients not eligible or waiting for surgery were enrolled. Similar to previous results, positive effects on all study endpoints could be achieved after 6 months of treatment.

The mainly positive experience gained from these small observational series supported the concept of vasodilator treatment in nonoperable CTEPH patients and led to the first double-blind, randomized, placebo-controlled trial in nonoperable CTEPH. The BENEFIT study investigated the effects of bosentan in nonoperable forms of CTEPH [87]. A total of 157 patients were enrolled and randomized in a 1:1 fashion to receive bosentan or placebo for 16 weeks. The study population consisted of symptomatic patients in WHO functional classes II, III, or IV with a 6-min walking distance <450 m. A diagnosis of CTEPH had to be demonstrated by ventilation-perfusion lung scanning and pulmonary angiography. Patients could only be included if CTEPH had been judged nonoperable because of peripheral localization of thrombotic material, or persistent/recurrent PH after PEA without evidence of recurrent thromboembolism. To select a homogenous population of truly nonoperable subjects, an operability evaluation committee consisting of two specialized pulmonologists and two PEA surgeons adjudicating the inoperability status was formed. Patients who were unanimously judged operable were excluded from the primary analysis.

PVR that directly reflects disease pathobiology and the 6-min walking test as a measure of exercise capacity were chosen as coprimary endpoints. Although a statistically significant treatment effect of bosentan over placebo on PVR could be demonstrated [–24.1% of baseline (95% CI: –31.5 to –16.0%)], the effect on 6-min walking distance was as low as +2.2 m (95% CI: –22.5 to +28.8 m). The reasons for these discrepant results remain unclear. One explanation was advanced age of the patient population enrolled in the BENEFIT trial compared with the typical IPAH patient studied in pivotal vasodilator trials. In addition, comorbid conditions or skeletal muscle deconditioning could prevent or delay recovery of exercise capacity. Another hypothesis was that the duration of the study was not long enough to demonstrate improvement in the 6-min walking distance.

Phosphodiesterase-5 Inhibitors

Sildenafil

Ghofrani et al. [88] assessed sildenafil treatment in 12 patients with nonoperable CTEPH. In this open-label study, acute vasodilator testing with sildenafil showed considerable vasoreactivity, clear hemodynamic improvement, and an increase in 6-min walking distance after a mean treatment duration of 6.5 ± 1.1 months. Sheth et al. [89] investigated 6 patients with nonoperable CTEPH and left ventricular dysfunction. After 6 weeks of sildenafil therapy, beneficial effects on mean pulmonary artery pressure, pulmonary capillary wedge pressure, and NYHA functional class were shown. In a double-blind placebo-controlled pilot study performed by Suntharalingam et al. [90], 19 subjects with nonoperable CTEPH were randomly assigned to sildenafil or placebo for 12 weeks. The primary endpoint was change in 6-min walking distance. Secondary endpoints included changes in World Health Organization class, cardiopulmonary hemodynamics, quality of life scores, and N-terminal brain natriuretic peptide. All subjects were transferred to open-label sildenafil at the end of the study and offered repeat assessment at 12 months. Although the study was not sufficiently powered to test the primary endpoint, it did suggest beneficial effects in favor of sildenafil in several secondary endpoints at both 3 and 12 months.

In an open-label clinical trial, 104 patients with nonoperable CTEPH received treatment with 50 mg of sildenafil three times daily [91]. On follow-up, long-term treatment with sildenafil was associated with significant improvements in PVR, cardiac index, 6-min walking distance, and World Health Organization functional class. In a subset of patients who underwent initial right heart catheterization, the acute response to sildenafil was not predictive of long-term outcome of therapy [91].

The finding of a significant hemodynamic benefit without improvement in exercise capacity fueled a debate over the usefulness of the 6-min walking test in CTEPH patients. Tailoring trial designs to this unique subset of PH will be one of the challenges in the near future. Currently, the effect of other vasodilator compounds, e.g. riociguat (CHEST) or treprostinil (CTREPH), are being tested in multinational placebo-controlled trials.

Prognosis

In contrast to the acute response to inhaled nitric oxide, response to chronic pulmonary vasodilators, such as bosentan, sildenafil, or prostanoids, does not appear to predict outcomes after PEA [92]. The best outcomes are to be expected if the preoperative PVR is <1,000–1,200 $dyn\bullet s\bullet cm^{-5}$ and concordant with anatomic disease, a lack of certain comorbid conditions [37], and when a postoperative PVR of <500 $dyn\bullet s\bullet cm^{-5}$ is reached [69].

Future Directions of Therapy

Successful PEA represents a curative therapy for patients with CTEPH, and will remain the treatment of choice.

However, the assessment and definition of concomitant pulmonary vascular disease that may preclude an adequate relief from PH after PEA and increase perioperative mortality remains undefined in the preoperative diagnostic work-up of CTEPH patients. Promising techniques for the evaluation of the functional status of the distal pulmonary vascular bed have been introduced. One of the future efforts to be undertaken by the scientific community is to standardize approaches. Preoperative quantification of small vessel disease together with a precise estimate of thrombus load may set the stage for a clear-cut differentiation between those who are candidates for PEA and those who are not. At present, none of the vasodilator compounds established in the treatment of PAH have been approved for the treatment of nonoperable CTEPH.

Key Points

- CTEPH is a dual vascular disorder comprising major vessel vascular remodeling of thrombus resolution and a classical small-vessel arteriopathy.
- In general, only a small minority of patients who have survived an acute thromboembolic event continue to develop CTEPH.
- Because of potential surgical curability of the disorder, a diagnosis of PH should always be followed by the search for underlying thromboembolism.
- Comorbid conditions are common.
- Traditional plasmatic prothrombotic risk factors are not risk factors for CTEPH.
- By contrast, splenectomy, infected VA shunt, inflammatory bowel disease, thyroid hormone replacement therapy, or having survived cancer have been identified as CTEPH-associated conditions.
- A average period of 100 months precedes CTEPH manifestation after occurrence of a major risk factor.
- Non-0 blood groups are associated with CTEPH.
- Different major risk factor profiles between operable and nonoperable patients may suggest that these two represent different pathophysiological entities.
- Pulmonary endarterectomy is the treatment of choice in patients with confirmed CTEPH.
- In specialized centers, the surgical management of incident, newly diagnosed CTEPH patients provides in-hospital death rates of <5%; however, at least 36% of all patients are nonoperable.
- About 40% of all newly diagnosed patients are currently started on PAH vasodilator treatments.
- Vasodilator trials in patients with nonoperable CTEPH will clarify whether medical therapy for CTEPH is effective.

References

1 Pepke-Zaba J, Delcroix M, Lang I, et al: Chronic thromboembolic pulmonary hypertension (CTEPH): results from an international prospective registry. Circulation 2011;124:1973–1981.
2 Auger WR, Kim NH, Kerr KM, Test VJ, Fedullo PF: Chronic thromboembolic pulmonary hypertension. Clin Chest Med 2007;28:255–269, x.
3 Lang IM: Chronic thromboembolic pulmonary hypertension – not so rare after all. N Engl J Med 2004;350:2236–2238.
4 Mayer E, Jenkins D, Lindner J, et al: Surgical management and outcome of patients with chronic thromboembolic pulmonary hypertension: results from an international prospective registry. J Thorac Cardiovasc Surg 2011;141:702–710.
5 Moser KM, Auger WR, Fedullo PF: Chronic major-vessel thromboembolic pulmonary hypertension. Circulation 1990;81:1735–1743.
6 Bonderman D, Wilkens H, Wakounig S, et al: Risk factors for chronic thromboembolic pulmonary hypertension. Eur Respir J 2009;33:325–331.
7 Fedullo PF, Auger WR, Kerr KM, Rubin LJ: Chronic thromboembolic pulmonary hypertension. N Engl J Med 2001;345:1465–1472.
8 Hoeper MM, Mayer E, Simonneau G, Rubin LJ: Chronic thromboembolic pulmonary hypertension. Circulation 2006;113:2011–2020.
9 Pengo V, Lensing AW, Prins MH, et al: Incidence of chronic thromboembolic pulmonary hypertension after pulmonary embolism. N Engl J Med 2004;350:2257–2264.
10 Klok FA, van Kralingen KW, van Dijk AP, Heyning FH, Vliegen HW, Huisman MV: Prospective cardiopulmonary screening program to detect chronic thromboembolic pulmonary hypertension in patients after acute pulmonary embolism. Haematologica 2010;95:970–975.
11 Becattini C, Agnelli G, Pesavento R, et al: Incidence of chronic thromboembolic pulmonary hypertension after a first episode of pulmonary embolism. Chest 2006;130:172–175.
12 Marti D, Gomez V, Escobar C, et al: Incidence of symptomatic and asymptomatic chronic thromboembolic pulmonary hypertension (in Spanish). Arch Broncopneumol 2010;46:628–633.
13 Condliffe R, Kiely DG, Gibbs JS, et al: Prognostic and aetiological factors in chronic thromboembolic pulmonary hypertension. Eur Respir J 2008;33:332–338.
14 Bonderman D, Jakowitsch J, Adlbrecht C, et al: Medical conditions increasing the risk of chronic thromboembolic pulmonary hypertension. Thromb Haemost 2005;93:512–516.
15 Auger WR, Permpikul P, Moser KM: Lupus anticoagulant, heparin use, and thrombocytopenia in patients with chronic thromboembolic pulmonary hypertension: a preliminary report. Am J Med 1995;99:392–396.
16 Wolf M, Boyer-Neumann C, Parent F, et al: Thrombotic risk factors in pulmonary hypertension. Eur Respir J 2000;15:395–399.
17 Bonderman D, Turecek PL, Jakowitsch J, et al: High prevalence of elevated clotting factor VIII in chronic thromboembolic pulmonary hypertension. Thromb Haemost 2003;90:372–376.
18 Suntharalingam J, Goldsmith K, van Marion V, et al: Fibrinogen Aalpha Thr312Ala polymorphism is associated with chronic thromboembolic pulmonary hypertension. Eur Respir J 2008;31:736–741.
19 Lang IM, Klepetko W, Pabinger I: No increased prevalence of the factor V Leiden mutation in chronic major vessel thromboembolic pulmonary hypertension (CTEPH). Thromb Haemost 1996;76:476–477.
20 Colorio CC, Martinuzzo ME, Forastiero RR, Pombo G, Adamczuk Y, Carreras LO: Thrombophilic factors in chronic thromboembolic pulmonary hypertension. Blood Coagul Fibrinolysis 2001;12:427–432.
21 Laczika K, Lang IM, Quehenberger P, et al: Unilateral chronic thromboembolic pulmonary disease associated with combined inherited thrombophilia. Chest 2002;121:286–289.
22 Lang IM, Marsh JJ, Olman MA, Moser KM, Loskutoff DJ, Schleef RR: Expression of type 1 plasminogen activator inhibitor in chronic pulmonary thromboemboli. Circulation 1994;89:2715–2721.

23 Lang IM, Marsh JJ, Olman MA, Moser KM, Schleef RR: Parallel analysis of tissue-type plasminogen activator and type 1 plasminogen activator inhibitor in plasma and endothelial cells derived from patients with chronic pulmonary thromboemboli. Circulation 1994;90:706–712.
24 Olman MA, Marsh JJ, Lang IM, Moser KM, Binder BR, Schleef RR: Endogenous fibrinolytic system in chronic large-vessel thromboembolic pulmonary hypertension. Circulation 1992;86:1241–1248.
25 Schoenbaum SC, Gardner P, Shillito J: Infections of cerebrospinal fluid shunts: epidemiology, clinical manifestations, and therapy. J Infect Dis 1975;131:543–552.
26 Colli BO, Starr EM, Martelli N: Surgical treatment of hydrocephalus in children. II. Complications (in Portuguese). Arq Neuropsiquiatr 1981; 39:408–419.
27 Bonderman D, Jakowitsch J, Redwan B, et al: Role for staphylococci in misguided thrombus resolution of chronic thromboembolic pulmonary hypertension. Arterioscler Thromb Vasc Biol 2008;28:678–684.
28 Moser KM, Braunwald NS: Successful surgical intervention in severe chronic thromboembolic pulmonary hypertension. Chest 1973;64:29–35.
29 Moser KM, Bloor CM: Pulmonary vascular lesions occurring in patients with chronic major vessel thromboembolic pulmonary hypertension. Chest 1993;103:685–692.
30 Arbustini E, Morbini P, D'Armini AM, et al: Plaque composition in plexogenic and thromboembolic pulmonary hypertension: the critical role of thrombotic material in pultaceous core formation. Heart 2002;88:177–182.
31 Blauwet LA, Edwards WD, Tazelaar HD, McGregor CG: Surgical pathology of pulmonary thromboendarterectomy: a study of 54 cases from 1990 to 2001. Hum Pathol 2003;34:1290–1298.
32 Kim NH, Fesler P, Channick RN, et al: Preoperative partitioning of pulmonary vascular resistance correlates with early outcome after thromboendarterectomy for chronic thromboembolic pulmonary hypertension. Circulation 2004;109:18–22.
33 Skoro-Sajer N, Hack N, Sadushi-Kolici R, et al: Pulmonary vascular reactivity and prognosis in patients with chronic thromboembolic pulmonary hypertension: a pilot study. Circulation 2009;119:298–305.
34 Deng Z, Morse JH, Slager SL, et al: Familial primary pulmonary hypertension (gene PPH1) is caused by mutations in the bone morphogenetic protein receptor-II gene. Am J Hum Genet 2000;67:737–744.
35 Thomson JR, Machado RD, Pauciulo MW, et al: Sporadic primary pulmonary hypertension is associated with germline mutations of the gene encoding BMPR-II, a receptor member of the TGF-beta family. J Med Genet 2000;37:741–745.
36 Du L, Sullivan CC, Chu D, et al: Signaling molecules in nonfamilial pulmonary hypertension. N Engl J Med 2003;348:500–509.
37 Bonderman D, Skoro-Sajer N, Jakowitsch J, et al: Predictors of outcome in chronic thromboembolic pulmonary hypertension. Circulation 2007; 115:2153–2158.
38 ZuWallack RL, Liss JP, Lahiri B: Acquired continuous murmur associated with acute pulmonary thromboembolism. Chest 1976;70:557–559.
39 Riedel M, Stanek V, Widimsky J, Prerovsky I: Longterm follow-up of patients with pulmonary thromboembolism. Late prognosis and evolution of hemodynamic and respiratory data. Chest 1982;81:151–158.
40 Kunieda T, Nakanishi N, Satoh T, Kyotani S, Okano Y, Nagaya N: Prognoses of primary pulmonary hypertension and chronic majorvessel thromboembolic pulmonary hypertension determined from cumulative survival curves. Intern Med 1999;38:543–546.
41 D'Alonzo GE, Barst RJ, Ayres SM, et al: Survival in patients with primary pulmonary hypertension. Results from a national prospective registry. Ann Intern Med 1991;115:343–349.
42 Mayer E, Klepetko W: Techniques and outcomes of pulmonary endarterectomy for chronic thromboembolic pulmonary hypertension. Proc Am Thorac Soc 2006;3:589–593.
43 Bonderman D, Martischnig AM, Vonbank K, et al: Right ventricular load at exercise is a cause of persistent exercise limitation in patients with normal resting pulmonary vascular resistance after pulmonary endarterectomy. Chest 2011; 139:122–127.
44 Kim NH: Assessment of operability in chronic thromboembolic pulmonary hypertension. Proc Am Thorac Soc 2006;3:584–588.
45 Skoro-Sajer N, Mittermayer F, Panzenboeck A, et al: Asymmetric dimethylarginine is increased in chronic thromboembolic pulmonary hypertension. Am J Respir Crit Care Med 2007;176:1154–1160.
46 Lankeit M, Dellas C, Panzenbock A, et al: Heart-type fatty acid-binding protein for risk assessment of chronic thromboembolic pulmonary hypertension. Eur Respir J 2008;31:1024–1029.
47 Lang IM, Plank C, Sadushi-Kolici R, Jakowitsch J, Klepetko W, Maurer G: Imaging in pulmonary hypertension. JACC Cardiovasc Imaging jjj;3:1287–1295.
48 Fishman AJ, Moser KM, Fedullo PF: Perfusion lung scans vs pulmonary angiography in evaluation of suspected primary pulmonary hypertension. Chest 1983;84:679–683.
49 Moser KM, Page GT, Ashburn WL, Fedullo PF: Perfusion lung scans provide a guide to which patients with apparent primary pulmonary hypertension merit angiography. West J Med 1988;148:167–170.
50 Lisbona R, Kreisman H, Novales-Diaz J, Derbekyan V: Perfusion lung scanning: differentiation of primary from thromboembolic pulmonary hypertension. AJR Am J Roentgenol 1985; 144:27–30.
51 Powe JE, Palevsky HI, McCarthy KE, Alavi A; Pulmonary arterial hypertension: value of perfusion scintigraphy. Radiology 1987;164:727–730.
52 Pitton MB, Duber C, Mayer E, Thelen M: Hemodynamic effects of nonionic contrast bolus injection and oxygen inhalation during pulmonary angiography in patients with chronic major-vessel thromboembolic pulmonary hypertension. Circulation 1996;94:2485–2491.
53 Auger WR, Fedullo PF, Moser KM, Buchbinder M, Peterson KL: Chronic major-vessel thromboembolic pulmonary artery obstruction: appearance at angiography. Radiology 1992;182:393–398.
54 Nicod P, Peterson K, Levine M, et al: Pulmonary angiography in severe chronic pulmonary hypertension. Ann Intern Med 1987;107:565–568.
55 D'Armini AM, Cattadori B, Monterosso C, et al: Pulmonary thromboendarterectomy in patients with chronic thromboembolic pulmonary hypertension: hemodynamic characteristics and changes. Eur J Cardiothorac Surg 2000;18:696–701, discussion 701–702.
56 Piovella F, D'Armini AM, Barone M, Tapson VF: Chronic thromboembolic pulmonary hypertension. Semin Thromb Hemost 2006;32:848–855.
57 Corsico AG, D'Armini AM, Cerveri I, et al: Long-term outcome after pulmonary endarterectomy. Am J Respir Crit Care Med 2008;178:419–424.
58 Reesink HJ, Marcus JT, Tulevski, II, et al: Reverse right ventricular remodeling after pulmonary endarterectomy in patients with chronic thromboembolic pulmonary hypertension: utility of magnetic resonance imaging to demonstrate restoration of the right ventricle. J Thorac Cardiovasc Surg 2007;133:58–64.
59 Iino M, Dymarkowski S, Chaothawee L, Delcroix M, Bogaert J: Time course of reversed cardiac remodeling after pulmonary endarterectomy in patients with chronic pulmonary thromboembolism. Eur Radiol 2008;18:792–799.
60 Casaclang-Verzosa G, McCully RB, Oh JK, Miller FA Jr, McGregor CG: Effects of pulmonary thromboendarterectomy on right-sided echocardiographic parameters in patients with chronic thromboembolic pulmonary hypertension. Mayo Clin Proc 2006;81:777–782.
61 Jamieson SW, Kapelanski DP, Sakakibara N, et al: Pulmonary endarterectomy: experience and lessons learned in 1,500 cases. Ann Thorac Surg 2003;76:1457–1462, discussion 62–64.
62 Klepetko W, Mayer E, Sandoval J, et al: Interventional and surgical modalities of treatment for pulmonary arterial hypertension. J Am Coll Cardiol 2004;43:73S–80S.
63 Dartevelle P, Fadel E, Mussot S, et al: Chronic thromboembolic pulmonary hypertension. Eur Respir J 2004;23:637–648.
64 Matsuda H, Ogino H, Minatoya K, et al: Long-term recovery of exercise ability after pulmonary endarterectomy for chronic thromboembolic pulmonary hypertension. Ann Thorac Surg 2006;82:1338–1343, discussion 1343.
65 Doyle RL, McCrory D, Channick RN, Simonneau G, Conte J: Surgical treatments/interventions for pulmonary arterial hypertension: ACCP evidence-based clinical practice guidelines. Chest 2004;126:63S–71S.

66 Hartz RS, Byrne JG, Levitsky S, Park J, Rich S: Predictors of mortality in pulmonary thromboendarterectomy. Ann Thorac Surg 1996;62:1255–9, discussion 1259–1260.
67 Archibald CJ, Auger WR, Fedullo PF, et al: Long-term outcome after pulmonary thromboendarterectomy. Am J Respir Crit Care Med 1999;160:523–528.
68 Lewczuk J, Piszko P, Jagas J, et al: Prognostic factors in medically treated patients with chronic pulmonary embolism. Chest 2001;119:818–823.
69 Keogh AM, Mayer E, Benza RL, et al: Interventional and surgical modalities of treatment in pulmonary hypertension. J Am Coll Cardiol 2009;54:S67–S77.
70 Feinstein JA, Goldhaber SZ, Lock JE, Ferndandes SM, Landzberg MJ: Balloon pulmonary angioplasty for treatment of chronic thromboembolic pulmonary hypertension. Circulation 2001;103:10–13.
71 Ono F, Nagaya N, Okumura H, et al: Effect of orally active prostacyclin analogue on survival in patients with chronic thromboembolic pulmonary hypertension without major vessel obstruction. Chest 2003;123:1583–1588.
72 Vizza CD, Badagliacca R, Sciomer S, et al: Mid-term efficacy of beraprost, an oral prostacyclin analog, in the treatment of distal CTEPH: a case control study. Cardiology 2006;106:168–173.
73 Nagaya N, Sasaki N, Ando M, et al: Prostacyclin therapy before pulmonary thromboendarterectomy in patients with chronic thromboembolic pulmonary hypertension. Chest 2003;123:338–343.
74 Bresser P, Fedullo PF, Auger WR, et al: Continuous intravenous epoprostenol for chronic thromboembolic pulmonary hypertension. Eur Respir J 2004;23:595–600.
75 Scelsi L, Ghio S, Campana C, et al: Epoprostenol in chronic thromboembolic pulmonary hypertension with distal lesions. Ital Heart J 2004;5:618–623.
76 Cabrol S, Souza R, Jais X, et al: Intravenous epoprostenol in inoperable chronic thromboembolic pulmonary hypertension. J Heart Lung Transplant 2007;26:357–362.
77 Skoro-Sajer N, Bonderman D, Wiesbauer F, et al: Treprostinil for severe inoperable chronic thromboembolic pulmonary hypertension. J Thromb Haemost 2007;5:483–489.
78 Olschewski H, Simonneau G, Galie N, et al: Inhaled iloprost for severe pulmonary hypertension. N Engl J Med 2002;347:322–329.
79 Kramm T, Eberle B, Krummenauer F, Guth S, Oelert H, Mayer E: Inhaled iloprost in patients with chronic thromboembolic pulmonary hypertension: effects before and after pulmonary thromboendarterectomy. Ann Thorac Surg 2003;76:711–718.
80 Kramm T, Eberle B, Guth S, Mayer E: Inhaled iloprost to control residual pulmonary hypertension following pulmonary endarterectomy. Eur J Cardiothorac Surg 2005;28:882–888.
81 Bonderman D, Nowotny R, Skoro-Sajer N, et al: Bosentan therapy for inoperable chronic thromboembolic pulmonary hypertension. Chest 2005;128:2599–2603.
82 Hoeper MM, Kramm T, Wilkens H, et al: Bosentan therapy for inoperable chronic thromboembolic pulmonary hypertension. Chest 2005;128:2363–2367.
83 Hughes R, George P, Parameshwar J, et al: Bosentan in inoperable chronic thromboembolic pulmonary hypertension. Thorax 2005;60:707.
84 Hughes RJ, Jais X, Bonderman D, et al: The efficacy of bosentan in inoperable chronic thromboembolic pulmonary hypertension: a 1-year follow-up study. Eur Respir J 2006;28:138–143.
85 Seyfarth HJ, Hammerschmidt S, Pankau H, Winkler J, Wirtz H: Long-term bosentan in chronic thromboembolic pulmonary hypertension. Respiration 2007;74:287–292.
86 Ulrich S, Speich R, Domenighetti G, et al: Bosentan therapy for chronic thromboembolic pulmonary hypertension. A national open label study assessing the effect of bosentan on haemodynamics, exercise capacity, quality of life, safety and tolerability in patients with chronic thromboembolic pulmonary hypertension (BOCTEPH-Study). Swiss Med Wkly 2007;137:573–580.
87 Jais X, D'Armini AM, Jansa P, et al: Bosentan for treatment of inoperable chronic thromboembolic pulmonary hypertension: BENEFIT (Bosentan Effects in Inoperable Forms of Chronic Thromboembolic Pulmonary Hypertension), a randomized, placebo-controlled trial. J Am Coll Cardiol 2008;52:2127–2134.
88 Ghofrani HA, Schermuly RT, Rose F, et al: Sildenafil for long-term treatment of nonoperable chronic thromboembolic pulmonary hypertension. Am J Respir Crit Care Med 2003;167:1139–1141.
89 Sheth A, Park JE, Ong YE, Ho TB, Madden BP: Early haemodynamic benefit of sildenafil in patients with coexisting chronic thromboembolic pulmonary hypertension and left ventricular dysfunction. Vascul Pharmacol 2005;42:41–45.
90 Suntharalingam J, Treacy CM, Doughty NJ, et al: Long-term use of sildenafil in inoperable chronic thromboembolic pulmonary hypertension. Chest 2008;134:229–236.
91 Reichenberger F, Voswinckel R, Enke B, et al: Long-term treatment with sildenafil in chronic thromboembolic pulmonary hypertension. Eur Respir J 2007;30:922–927.
92 Jensen KW, Kerr KM, Fedullo PF, et al: Pulmonary hypertensive medical therapy in chronic thromboembolic pulmonary hypertension before pulmonary thromboendarterectomy. Circulation 2009;120:1248–1254.

Irene M. Lang, MD, Professor of Vascular Biology
Department of Internal Medicine II, Division of Cardiology, Medical University of Vienna
Währinger Gürtel 18–20
AT–1090 Vienna (Austria)
Tel. +43 1 40 400 4614, E-Mail irene.lang@meduniwien.ac.at

Chapter 24

Humbert M, Souza R, Simonneau G (eds): Pulmonary Vascular Disorders.
Prog Respir Res. Basel, Karger, 2012, vol 41, pp 237–245

Medical Treatment of Pulmonary Arterial Hypertension

Dermot S. O'Callaghan[a] · Sean P. Gaine[b]

[a]Service de Pneumologie et Réanimation Respiratoire, Centre National de Référence de l'Hypertension Artérielle Pulmonaire Sévère, Hôpital Antoine Béclère, Assistance Publique Hôpitaux de Paris, Université Paris-Sud 11, Clamart, France; [b]National Pulmonary Hypertension Unit, Department of Respiratory Medicine, Mater Misericordiae University Hospital, University College Dublin, Dublin, Ireland

Abstract

Pulmonary arterial hypertension is a rare disease characterized by a sustained increase in pulmonary vascular resistance and pulmonary arterial pressure resulting in progressive right ventricular dysfunctional and premature death. Preclinical and clinical studies on agents acting on the prostacyclin, endothelin-1, and nitric oxide pathways have led to the development of a number of targeted therapies that confer meaningful and durable improvements in important endpoints such as functional class, exercise capacity, and pulmonary hemodynamics and reduce episodes of clinical worsening. As a result, the management of this disorder has become increasingly complex. Although published guidelines provide broad recommendations for optimum approaches according to type and severity of disease, many uncertainties remain. Routine monitoring of response to treatment by clinical, functional, and hemodynamic assessment is critically important in order to guide therapeutic decision-making. When treatment goals are considered to be unmet, escalation of therapy is recommended. However, the optimal timing and type of combination strategies require further study.

Pulmonary arterial hypertension (PAH) is a rare disease characterized by a sustained increase in pulmonary vascular resistance and pulmonary arterial pressure resulting in progressive right ventricular dysfunctional and premature death [1]. In less than 20 years, PAH has been transformed from a disorder characterized by a uniformly poor prognosis due to a lack of treatment alternatives to one for which several pharmacologic agents now exist. Preclinical and clinical studies on agents acting on the prostacyclin, endothelin (ET-1), and nitric oxide (NO) pathways have led to the development of the prostanoid, endothelin receptor antagonist, and phosphodiesterase type-5 (PDE5) inhibitor drug classes, respectively. Accumulated data indicate these various 'specific therapies' confer meaningful and durable improvements in important endpoints such as functional class, exercise capacity, and pulmonary hemodynamics and reduce episodes of clinical worsening [2, 3].

Prostanoids

Endothelium-derived prostaglandin I_2, or prostacyclin, is a potent pulmonary vasodilator that also exerts antithrombotic, antiproliferative, antimitogenic, and immunomodulatory activity. In the pulmonary vasculature and serum of patients with PAH, prostacyclin synthase and prostacyclin metabolites are markedly reduced or absent [4, 5]. The prostanoids are a family of stable prostacyclin analogues available in different formulations that have been developed for treatment of PAH (fig. 1).

Epoprostenol

Epoprostenol, a synthetic sodium salt of naturally occurring prostaglandin I_2, was the first prostanoid to be tested in PAH in the early 1980s. A half-life <5 min mandates an indwelling intravenous central venous catheter and an infusion pump for continuous administration (table 1). Meticulous monitoring is required for epoprostenol-treated patients because of the significant side-effect profile and risk of catheter-related infection. Furthermore, interruption of drug delivery, either due to pump malfunction or catheter obstruction or damage may result in potentially fatal rebound of pulmonary hypertension.

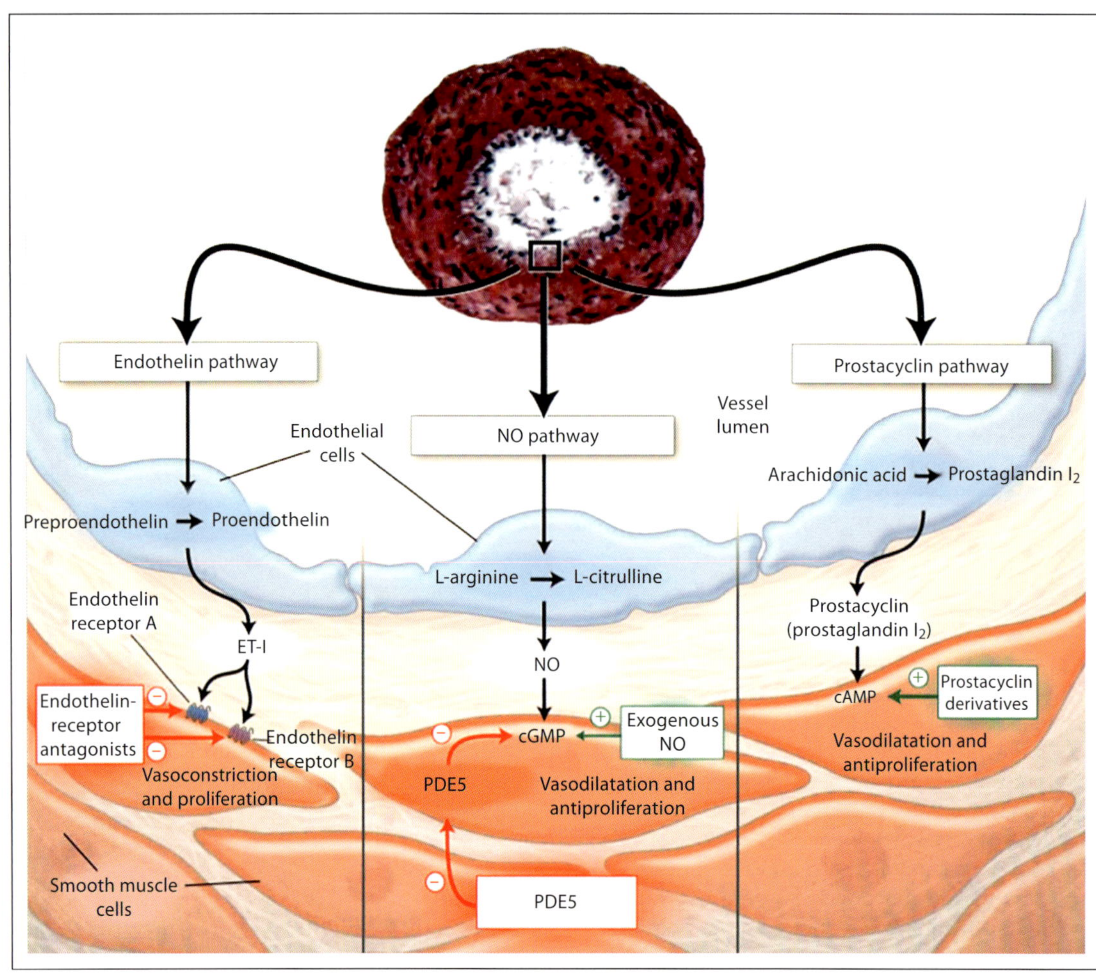

Fig. 1. Therapeutic targets in PAH (reproduced with permission from Humbert et al. [2]). ERA = Endothelin receptor antagonists; s.c. = subcutaneous; i.v. = intravenous; inh. = inhaled.

The clinical efficacy of epoprostenol was examined in three unblinded studies. Rubin et al. [6] reported that pulmonary hemodynamics improved in idiopathic PAH patients after 2 months of therapy, whereas patients receiving conventional treatments showed clinical worsening. Improvements in exercise capacity and pulmonary hemodynamics were sustained for up to a year after initiation of treatment [7]. A subsequent study of epoprostenol among 81 idiopathic PAH patients with modified New York Heart Association (NYHA) functional class III-IV symptoms demonstrated a placebo-adjusted increase of 47 m in 6-min walk distance (6MWD) after 12 weeks [8]. In addition, a survival advantage with therapy was shown, as 8 patients receiving conventional treatment died compared to none among the epoprostenol group.

Subsequent retrospective studies have reported improved survival in epoprostenol-treated patients compared to matched historical controls [9, 10]. Indeed, epoprostenol is the only PAH therapy to have demonstrated a mortality benefit in a randomized trial and on this basis was granted regulatory approval for treatment of patients with NYHA functional class III or IV symptoms (fig. 2). A novel formulation of epoprostenol that is thermostable for up to 24 h without refrigeration has recently been made available.

Treprostinil

Treprostinil is a prostacyclin analogue with greater stability and a longer half-life than epoprostenol that may be delivered by subcutaneous, intravenous, inhaled, or oral routes. The subcutaneous form is stable at room temperature and

Table 1. Currently licensed treatments for PAH

Therapeutic class	Drug	Half-life	Administration	Dosing frequency	NYHA-FC indications[1]	Most common adverse effects
Prostacyclin analogues	epoprostenol	5 min	i.v.	continuous infusion	III–IV	flushing jaw pain headache GI upset hypotension catheter-related BSI (i.v. route) Site pain (s.c. route) Cough (inhaled route)
	treprostinil	4 h	inh.	up to 12 inhalations 4 times per day	III (USA)	
			s.c.	continuous infusion	III (Eur), II–IV (USA), III–IV (Canada)	
			i.v.	continuous infusion	II–IV (USA), III–IV (Canada)	
	iloprost	20–30 min	Inh.	6–9 nebulizations/day	III (Eur), III–IV (USA)	
			i.v.	continuous infusion	III–IV (New Zealand)	
	beraprost	60 min	oral	4 times per day	II–IV (Japan, South Korea)	
Endothelin receptor antagonists	bosentan	5 h	oral	twice daily	II–III (Eur), II–IV (USA, Canada)	transaminase increases teratogenicity headache rhinorrhea/ nasal congestion
	ambrisentan	15 h	oral	once daily		
PDE 5 inhibitors	sildenafil	4 h	oral	3 times per day	II–III (Eur), II–IV (USA, Canada)	headache flushing dyspepsia rhinorrhea/ nasal congestion
	tadalafil	18 h	oral	once daily		

Eur = Europe; i.v. = intravenous; s.c. = subcutaneous; inh. = inhaled.
[1]Indications vary among different European countries

is delivered via a microinfusion pump. In a pivotal 12-week randomized trial of 470 patients with PAH that was idiopathic or associated with connective tissue disease or congenital intracardiac shunt, treprostinil increased 6MWD in a dose-dependent fashion and conferred improvements in symptoms, quality-of-life scores, and hemodynamics [11]. The major limitation of this formulation is infusion site pain, which occurs in most patients.

Treprostinil administered as a continuous intravenous infusion offers the advantage of less frequent need for drug reservoir changing (every 48 h vs. every 12–24 h for epoprostenol) [12]. Transitioning patients from intravenous epoprostenol to intravenous treprostinil is feasible, though may be associated with mild hemodynamic worsening [13]. This formulation of treprostinil is licensed for use in the US only. Concerns have also been expressed regarding

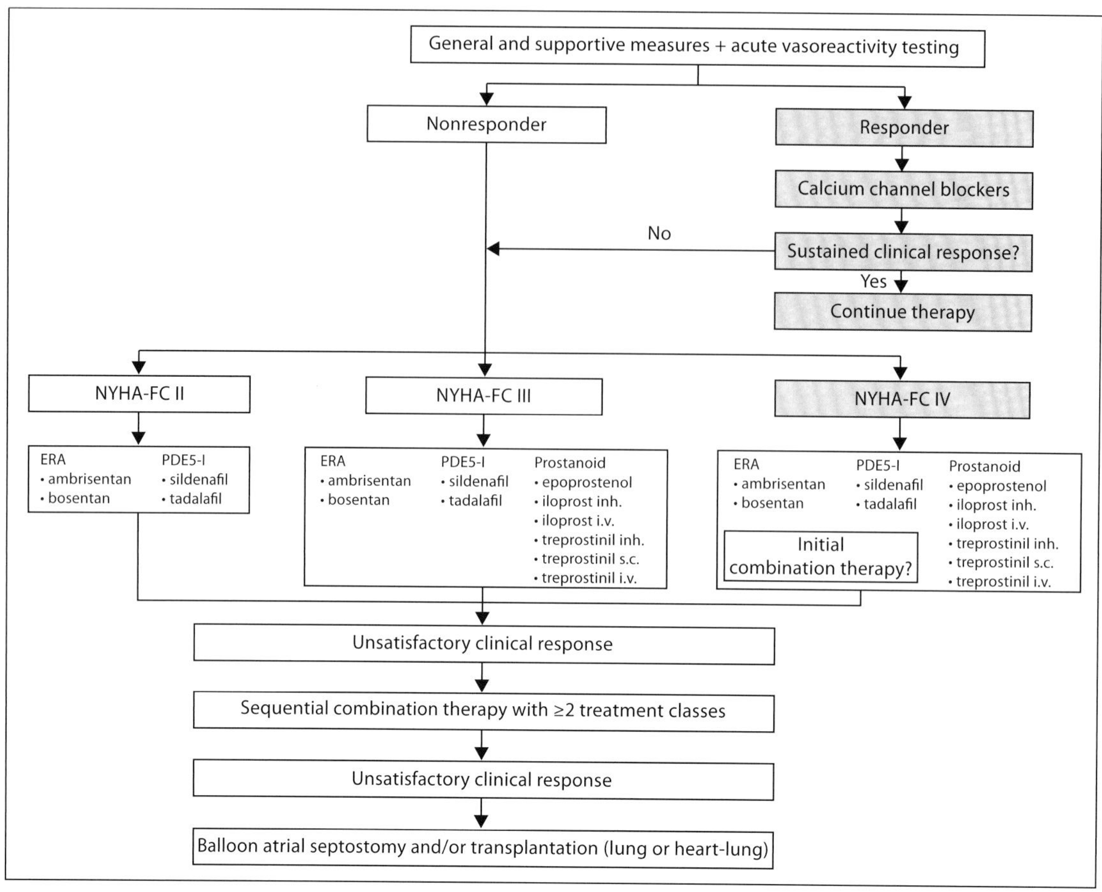

Fig. 2. Treatment algorithm for PAH (reproduced with permission from O'Callaghan [60]).

the relatively higher rate of blood stream infections with intravenous treprostinil compared to epoprostenol [14].

Inhaled treprostinil has been examined as an add-on therapy in PAH. An initial open-label study found that addition of treprostinil conferred improvements in exercise capacity, functional class, and pulmonary hemodynamics in bosentan-treated patients [15]. The subsequent placebo-controlled TRIUMPH-1 study examined the effect of adding inhaled treprostinil to other classes of PAH therapy (endothelin receptor antagonist, PDE5 inhibitor or both) among 235 PAH patients, most of whom had functional class III symptoms [16]. After 12 weeks, treprostinil conferred a median improvement in postdose 6MWD of 20 m. However, there were no improvements in time to clinical worsening, dyspnea scores, or functional class.

The oral form of treprostinil was evaluated in the FREEDOM-C trial, in which 354 patients on stable doses of other classes of oral PAH therapy were randomized to oral treprostinil or placebo, titrated to the maximum tolerated dose [17]. The primary endpoint of change in 6MWD after 16 weeks failed to achieve statistical significance, although patients able to achieve higher treatment doses showed greatest improvement in exercise capacity. Results are awaited from the FREEDOM-M study, which will evaluate the safety and efficacy of oral treprostinil as monotherapy in PAH.

Beraprost

Beraprost is another orally active prostanoid that has demonstrated modest efficacy in PAH. The ALPHABET study randomized 130 patients with PAH to beraprost (median dose: 80 mg four times daily) or placebo [18]. After 12 weeks, the difference between treatment groups in the mean change of 6MWD was +25 m in favor of beraprost ($p = 0.036$), though improvements were only noted in the idiopathic PAH subgroup. Furthermore, NYHA functional class and hemodynamic indices did not significantly change. A subsequent study found that while beraprost improved exercise capacity and reduced risk of disease progression at 6 months, efficacy was not sustained after 1 year of therapy [19].

Iloprost
Iloprost is a stable prostacyclin analogue developed for inhaled and intravenous administration. The pulmonary vasodilatory effects of inhaled iloprost last approximately 1–2 h [20]. Approval for this formulation in PAH was granted on the basis of the AIR study, which compared inhaled iloprost to placebo in 203 patients with idiopathic PAH, anorexigen- or scleroderma-associated PAH, or chronic thromboembolic pulmonary hypertension and associated NYHA functional class III or IV symptoms [21]. Study participants received 6–9 inhalations of 2.5 or 5.0 μg daily of iloprost or placebo. At 12 weeks, 17% of iloprost-treated patients compared with 5% of placebo-treated patients achieved the coprimary endpoint of improvement in functional class and a 10% increase in 6MWD. Postinhalation pulmonary hemodynamic values also improved among those receiving iloprost ($p < 0.001$) and worsened with placebo. Cough, flushing, and jaw pain were the most common adverse events. Interestingly, an open-label German study found that relatively few patients maintain long-term clinical stability when inhaled iloprost is initiated as monotherapy [22].

Nonrandomized study data suggest that intravenous iloprost has efficacy comparable to intravenous epoprostenol [23], greater stability in solution, and a longer plasma half-life. [24] Intravenous iloprost may be considered in patients with advanced disease, though it has not been formally tested in a randomized placebo-controlled trial, and regulatory approval has not yet been granted in the US or Europe.

Endothelin Receptor Antagonists

ET-1 is a potent vasoconstrictor and PASMC mitogen that plays an important pathogenic role in PAH [25]. Its biologic actions are the result of activation of two distinct receptor isoforms, designated endothelin-A (ET_A) and -B (ET_B). In pulmonary arteries, the ET_A subtype is predominantly expressed on PASMCs, whereas the ET_B subtype is mainly found on vascular endothelium, with relatively lesser expression on PASMCs. Binding of ET-1 to ET_A and ET_B receptors on PASMCs promotes vasoconstriction, whereas activation of ET_B receptors on endothelial cells causes vasodilatation via increased prostacyclin and NO levels [26, 27].

Bosentan
Bosentan is a nonselective antagonist of the ET_A and ET_B receptors that was the subject of an initial placebo-controlled study involving 32 patients with idiopathic or scleroderma-related PAH. After 16 weeks, bosentan-treated patients showed a placebo-adjusted increase in 6MWD of 76 m [28]. The efficacy of bosentan was confirmed in the BREATHE-1 study in which 213 patients with functional class III or IV symptoms were randomly assigned twice-daily bosentan or placebo in a 2:1 ratio [29]. Two bosentan dosing schedules were examined to assess the impact of dose ranging. After 16 weeks, placebo-adjusted changes in the primary efficacy endpoint of change in 6MWD of +54 m and +33 m were observed in patients receiving 250 and 125 mg doses of bosentan, respectively, giving an overall change of +44 m in favor of bosentan. No significant difference with respect to change in 6MWD between the two bosentan doses was observed, confirming a lack of a dose-response relationship. Improvements in NYHA functional class were reported in 42% of bosentan-treated patients compared to 30% in the placebo arm. In addition, bosentan-treated patients had overall greater improvements in dyspnea scores and a delayed time to clinical worsening.

A trend toward higher frequency of hepatic injury with bosentan was confirmed in the BREATHE-1 study, with increases in alanine aminotransferase and/or aspartate aminotransferase levels to >3 the upper limit of normal developing in 12 and 14% of the 125 and 250 mg bosentan groups, respectively. Seven patients receiving bosentan experienced transaminase levels of >8 the upper limit of normal, although these episodes were generally self-limiting upon treatment interruption. Monthly monitoring of liver function tests is therefore mandatory and bosentan postmarketing surveillance showed that aspartate aminotransferase/alanine aminotransferase levels >3 the upper limit of normal occur at an annual rate of 10% [30]. Regulatory approval was granted for this agent in the US and Europe in 2001 and 2002, respectively.

The design of the initial bosentan trials precluded a direct analysis of a potential impact on mortality. However, results from subsequently published studies suggest that long-term therapy confers improvements in exercise capacity, functional class, hemodynamics, and possibly survival [31–33]. Data from the EARLY study showed that bosentan use in patients with mildly symptomatic PAH conferred improvements in pulmonary vascular resistance and significantly delayed time to clinical worsening versus placebo [34].

The impact of bosentan in populations with other forms of PAH has also been examined. Significant pulmonary hemodynamic improvements associated with its use were reported in a small randomized, placebo-controlled trial of patients with Eisenmenger's syndrome [35], and beneficial effects were also reported in children with PAH [36] and in patients with HIV infection [37, 38] and portopulmonary hypertension [39, 40]. Data from randomized prospective studies in these populations, however, are lacking.

Ambrisentan

It has been suggested that selective ET_A receptor antagonism may be preferable to nonselective ET_A/ET_B blockade as, in theory, the former approach would block release of pulmonary vasoconstrictors while preserving ET-1-mediated vasodilatory and antimitogenic activity through unimpeded ET_B receptor activation [41]. This hypothesis led to the development and clinical study of the selective ET_A receptor antagonist treatment class [42] in PAH.

Ambrisentan is an orally active, once-daily, highly selective ET_A receptor antagonist that has been evaluated in two randomized, double-blind, placebo-controlled studies. The ARIES-1 and ARIES-2 trials were essentially identical, other than the locations of participating study centers (North America for ARIES-1 and Western Europe for ARIES-2) and ambrisentan doses tested (5 mg and 10 mg in ARIES-1 and 2.5 mg and 5 mg in ARIES-2) [43]. In total, 394 patients with PAH that was idiopathic or associated with anorexigen exposure, connective tissue disease, or HIV infection were evaluated. Combined analysis of the two studies demonstrated that ambrisentan treatment improved 6MWD compared to placebo after 12 weeks (range: +31 to +59 m). The delay in time to clinical worsening was significantly longer among patients randomized to ambrisentan in the ARIES-2, but not ARIES-1 study, whereas improvements in functional class were observed among those receiving the study drug in the ARIES-1 study only. A favorable impact on several secondary endpoints, including dyspnea scores, SF-36 Health Survey, and brain natriuretic peptide levels were also observed among patients receiving ambrisentan. The most common adverse events were peripheral edema, headache, and nasal congestion. No significant increases in liver enzyme levels were observed. The low rate of hepatic injury was confirmed in a recent study that followed 36 patients who initiated ambrisentan after discontinuing bosentan, sitaxsentan (see below), or both due to increased transaminase levels [44]. No episodes of elevated transaminases requiring ambrisentan discontinuation were observed after a median patient drug exposure of 102 weeks. On the basis of the ARIES studies, ambrisentan was granted regulatory approval by the US FDA in 2007 and in Europe in 2008 for PAH associated with functional class II and III symptoms.

Patients from these studies were eligible for inclusion in the ARIES-E (extension) study. At 1 year of treatment, 95% of the patients receiving ambrisentan were still alive with 93% continuing ambrisentan monotherapy [45]. After 2 years of therapy, the mean increase in 6MWD was maintained at +23 and +28 m for the 5 and 10 mg doses, respectively.

The selective ET_A receptor antagonist sitaxsentan was previously approved in Europe, Canada, and Australia. However, following the death of a number of patients from acute liver failure receiving sitaxsentan in a clinical study, the drug was withdrawn from the market worldwide in December 2010.

Phosphodiesterase Type-5 Inhibitors

NO is a potent PASMC relaxant that exerts vasodilatory activity through upregulation of its associated downstream signaling molecule, cyclic guanosine monophosphate, metabolism of which is dependent on the activation of a number of PDEs. Within the pulmonary circulation, PDE5 is the most abundantly expressed isoform. Accordingly, therapeutic strategies that limit cyclic guanosine monophosphate metabolism, thus maintaining the vasodilatory effects of NO, are of interest in treatment of vascular diseases. PAH is associated with abnormally low levels of NO within the pulmonary endothelium, due in part to the reduced expression of NO synthase in the lung microvasculature [46]. In this regard, inhibitors of PDE5 have emerged as an important therapeutic class.

Sildenafil

The first large randomized, placebo-controlled trial evaluating a PDE5 inhibitor was the SUPER study, in which the effects of different doses of sildenafil were tested in 278 patients with PAH that was idiopathic or related to connective tissue disease or surgically corrected left-to-right intracardiac shunts [47]. Most study participants had NYHA functional class II or III symptoms. After 12 weeks of treatment, the mean placebo-adjusted changes in 6MWD for the 20, 40, and 80 mg doses of sildenafil were +45, +46, and +50 m, respectively. Patients in the various sildenafil groups were also more likely to improve by at least one functional class and demonstrate improvement in pulmonary hemodynamics. Adverse events more frequently observed with sildenafil were headache, flushing, and dyspepsia. Long-term follow-up data from 222 patients who completed 1 year of sildenafil monotherapy at the 80-mg dose revealed sustained improvements in exercise capacity, suggesting a durable treatment effect. Furthermore, the calculated survival rate during this extension phase was 97%, a figure substantially greater than the expected survival rate of 71% based on data from historical controls [48].

Tadalafil

Another PDE5 inhibitor, tadalafil, was examined in the PHIRST-1 trial, in which 405 patients who were either treatment-naive or already receiving bosentan were randomized to placebo or one of several doses of tadalafil (2.5, 10, 20, or 40 mg) [49]. After 16 weeks, patients receiving tadalafil showed an overall mean placebo-corrected increase in 6MWD of 33 m, though the improvement was significant only in the 40-mg group. Patients receiving this dose also had both delayed time to clinical worsening and fewer episodes of clinical worsening compared to placebo. Analysis of comparative hemodynamic data from the 93 patients who underwent baseline and follow-up right heart catheterization showed tadalafil conferred significant reductions in mean pulmonary arterial pressure and pulmonary vascular resistance. Favorable effects with tadalafil 40 mg were also demonstrated in patients already receiving background bosentan, though improvements were less marked compared to the treatment-naive cohort [50]. Treatment-related changes in modified NYHA functional class were similar across all groups. Overall, treatment was well tolerated, with most adverse events being of mild-to-moderate severity. Tadalafil, which has the advantage of once-daily dosing, was granted regulatory approval for use in PAH in the US and Europe in 2009.

Combination Treatment

The various specific PAH therapies that act on the prostacyclin, endothelin, and NO pathways have been shown to favorably impact a variety of clinically relevant endpoints. However, disease progression on treatment is frequently observed and use of multidrug regimens in order to simultaneously target different pathways is an appealing concept [51]. Combination approaches using two or more agents from different drug classes are thus recommended for patients in functional class III-IV that fail to improve after initiation of specific therapy, and also for individuals in class II that deteriorate on monotherapy [1]. If there is insufficient clinical improvement despite introduction of a second therapeutic class, triple combinations regimens may be considered. A successful approach employing sequential addition of treatments in order to meet well-defined therapeutic goals has been reported [52] and is advocated in recent guidelines [1]. However, more studies are required to establish whether such a strategy is preferable to upfront double and/or even triple combination approaches [53]. The AMBITION study, which will study outcomes of three patient groups randomized to first-line treatment with ambrisentan, tadalafil, or both, is of particular interest in this regard.

General Measures and Supportive Therapy

A number of important general measures are broadly advocated for patients with pulmonary hypertension in order to provide symptomatic benefit and prevent clinical worsening. Recommendations for these interventions, however, are mostly based on expert consensus or uncontrolled observational studies. Limiting of physical activity to tolerance to avoid potentially dangerous abrupt increases in cardiac demand is advisable.

Administration of medications that may potentially aggravate pulmonary hypertension (such as β-adrenergic receptor blockers [55] or sympathomimetics) should be avoided. Supplemental oxygen may be considered for individuals with resting or exercise-induced hypoxemia in order to maintain oxygen saturation levels at greater than 90%. Oxygen administration during air travel may be warranted, particularly for those with advanced disease. Vaccinations to prevent pneumococcal pneumonia and influenza are also advisable.

Diuretics offer symptomatic benefit in those with volume overload not controlled by dietary measures alone, though there is no evidence for a survival benefit with their use. In the absence of compelling contraindications, oral anticoagulation is recommended in idiopathic or anorexigen-associated PAH as this approach has been shown to be beneficial [56]. An assessment of the risks and benefits of such treatment should be made for other forms of PAH, particularly when an increased risk of bleeding exists.

The additional hemodynamic stresses of pregnancy and labor are poorly tolerated in PAH patients, being associated with an increased rate of potentially fatal clinical worsening

[57]. Female patients of childbearing potential should thus be counseled on appropriate contraception measures. Because effectiveness of hormonal contraception may be reduced with certain PAH-specific treatments, a combination of pharmacologic and mechanical (e.g. intrauterine device) contraception is advised.

In general, 5–10% of patients with PAH that is idiopathic, familial, or associated with anorexigen use will show significant hemodynamic improvements after administration of acute vasodilators at right heart catheterization. Approximately half of these 'responders' benefit from treatment with high-dose calcium channel blockers (usually nifedepine or diltiazem) [58]. Confirmation of a sustained clinical and hemodynamic improvement by repeat catheterization after initiation of these agents is mandatory.

Conclusion

With the ever-increasing number of targeted therapies now available for treatment of PAH, management of this disorder has become increasingly complex. Although published guidelines provide broad recommendations for optimum approaches according to type and severity of disease, many uncertainties remain. Treating clinicians remain charged with selecting the most appropriate agent or agents for individual patients and such choices are additionally influenced by patient preferences and local economic and regulatory considerations. Routine monitoring of response to treatment by clinical, functional, and hemodynamic assessment is critically important in order to guide therapeutic decision-making. When treatment goals are considered to be unmet, escalation of therapy is recommended. However, the optimal timing and type of combination strategies require further study.

References

1 Galiè N, et al: Guidelines for the diagnosis and treatment of pulmonary hypertension. Eur Respir J 2009;34:1219–1263.
2 Humbert M, Sitbon O, Simonneau G: Treatment of pulmonary arterial hypertension. N Engl J Med 2004;351:1425–1436.
3 Galiè N, et al: A meta-analysis of randomized controlled trials in pulmonary arterial hypertension. Eur Heart J 2009;30:394–403.
4 Christman BW, et al: An imbalance between the excretion of thromboxane and prostacyclin metabolites in pulmonary hypertension. N Engl J Med 1992;327:70–75.
5 Tuder RM, et al: Prostacyclin synthase expression is decreased in lungs from patients with severe pulmonary hypertension. Am J Respir Crit Care Med 1999;159:1925–1932.
6 Rubin LJ, et al: Treatment of primary pulmonary hypertension with continuous intravenous prostacyclin (epoprostenol). Results of a randomized trial. Ann Intern Med 1990;112:485–491.
7 Barst RJ, et al: Survival in primary pulmonary hypertension with long-term continuous intravenous prostacyclin. Ann Intern Med 1994;121:409–415.
8 Barst RJ, et al: A comparison of continuous intravenous epoprostenol (prostacyclin) with conventional therapy for primary pulmonary hypertension. The Primary Pulmonary Hypertension Study Group. N Engl J Med 1996;334:296–302.
9 Shapiro SM, et al: Primary pulmonary hypertension: improved long-term effects and survival with continuous intravenous epoprostenol infusion. J Am Coll Cardiol 1997;30:343–349.
10 McLaughlin VV, Shillington A, Rich S: Survival in primary pulmonary hypertension: the impact of epoprostenol therapy. Circulation 2002;106:1477–1482.
11 Simonneau G, et al: Continuous subcutaneous infusion of treprostinil, a prostacyclin analogue, in patients with pulmonary arterial hypertension: a double-blind, randomized, placebo-controlled trial. Am J Respir Crit Care Med 2002;165:800–804.
12 Laliberte K, Arneson C, Jeffs R, Hunt T, Wade M: Pharmacokinetics and steady-state bioequivalence of treprostinil sodium (Remodulin) administered by the intravenous and subcutaneous route to normal volunteers. J Cardiovasc Pharmacol 2004;44:209–214.
13 Gomberg-Maitland M, et al: Transition from intravenous epoprostenol to intravenous treprostinil in pulmonary hypertension. Am J Respir Crit Care Med 2005;172:1586–1589.
14 Kallen AJ, et al: Bloodstream infections in patients given treatment with intravenous prostanoids. Infect Control Hosp Epidemiol 2008;29:342–349.
15 Channick RN, et al: Safety and efficacy of inhaled treprostinil as add-on therapy to bosentan in pulmonary arterial hypertension. J Am Coll Cardiol 2006;48:1433–1437.
16 McLaughlin VV, et al: Addition of inhaled treprostinil to oral therapy for pulmonary arterial hypertension: a randomized controlled clinical trial. J Am Coll Cardiol 2010;55:1915–1922.
17 Tapson V, et al: Results of the FREEDOM-C study: a pivotal study of oral treprostinil used adjunctively with an ERA and/or PDE5-inhibitor for the treatment of PAH. Am J Respir Crit Care Med 2009;179:A1040.
18 Galie N, et al: Effects of beraprost sodium, an oral prostacyclin analogue, in patients with pulmonary arterial hypertension: a randomized, double-blind, placebo-controlled trial. J Am Coll Cardiol 2002;39:1496–1502.
19 Barst RJ, et al: Beraprost therapy for pulmonary arterial hypertension. J Am Coll Cardiol 2003;41:2119–2125.
20 Olschewski H, et al: Aerosolized prostacyclin and iloprost in severe pulmonary hypertension. Ann Intern Med 1996;124:820–824.
21 Olschewski H, et al: Inhaled iloprost for severe pulmonary hypertension. N Engl J Med 2002;347:322–329.
22 Opitz CF, et al: Clinical efficacy and survival with first-line inhaled iloprost therapy in patients with idiopathic pulmonary arterial hypertension. Eur Heart J 2005;26:1895–1902.
23 Higenbottam T, Butt AY, McMahon A, Westerbeck R, Sharples L: Long-term intravenous prostaglandin (epoprostenol or iloprost) for treatment of severe pulmonary hypertension. Heart 1998;80:151–155 .
24 Olschewski H, et al: Pharmacodynamics and pharmacokinetics of inhaled iloprost, aerosolized by three different devices, in severe pulmonary hypertension. Chest 2003;124:1294–1304.
25 Giaid A, et al: Expression of endothelin-1 in the lungs of patients with pulmonary hypertension. N Engl J Med 1993;328:1732–1739.
26 Seo B, Oemar B, Siebenmann R, von Segesser L, Lüscher T: Both ET_A and ET_B receptors mediate contraction to endothelin-1 in human blood vessels. Circulation 1994;89:1203–1208.
27 Hirata Y, et al: Endothelin receptor subtype B mediates synthesis of nitric oxide by cultured bovine endothelial cells. J Clin Invest 1993;91:1367–1373.
28 Channick RN, et al: Effects of the dual endothelin-receptor antagonist bosentan in patients with pulmonary hypertension: a randomised placebo-controlled study. Lancet 2001;358:1119–1123.

29 Rubin LJ, et al: Bosentan therapy for pulmonary arterial hypertension. N Engl J Med 2002;346:896–903.
30 Humbert M, et al: Results of European post-marketing surveillance of bosentan in pulmonary hypertension. Eur Respir J 2007;30:338–344.
31 Sitbon O, et al: Effects of the dual endothelin receptor antagonist bosentan in patients with pulmonary arterial hypertension: a 1-year follow-up study. Chest 2003;124:247–254.
32 Sitbon O, et al: Survival in patients with class III idiopathic pulmonary arterial hypertension treated with first line oral bosentan compared with an historical cohort of patients started on intravenous epoprostenol. Thorax 2005;60:1025–1030.
33 McLaughlin VV, et al: Survival with first-line bosentan in patients with primary pulmonary hypertension. Eur Respir J 2005;25:244–249.
34 Galie N, et al: Treatment of patients with mildly symptomatic pulmonary arterial hypertension with bosentan (EARLY study): a double-blind, randomised controlled trial. Lancet 2008;371:2093–2100.
35 Galiè N, et al: Bosentan therapy in patients with Eisenmenger syndrome: a multicenter, double-blind, randomized, placebo-controlled study. Circulation 2006;114:48–54.
36 Rosenzweig E, et al: Effects of long-term bosentan in children with pulmonary arterial hypertension. J Am Coll Cardiol 2005;46:697–704.
37 Sitbon O, et al: Bosentan for the treatment of human immunodeficiency virus-associated pulmonary arterial hypertension. Am J Respir Crit Care Med 2004;170:1212–1217.
38 Degano B, et al: Long-term effects of bosentan in patients with HIV-associated pulmonary arterial hypertension. Eur Respir J 2009;33:92–98.
39 Hoeper M, et al: Bosentan therapy for portopulmonary hypertension. Eur Respir J 2005;25:502–508.
40 Hoeper MM, et al: Experience with inhaled iloprost and bosentan in portopulmonary hypertension. Eur Respir J 2007;30:1096–1102.
41 Opitz CF, Ewert R, Kirch W, Pittrow D: Inhibition of endothelin receptors in the treatment of pulmonary arterial hypertension: does selectivity matter? Eur Heart J 2008;29:1936–1948.
42 Wu C, et al: Discovery of TBC11251, a potent, long acting, orally active endothelin receptor-A selective antagonist. J Med Chem 1997;40:1690–1697.
43 Galie N, et al: Ambrisentan for the treatment of pulmonary arterial hypertension: results of the ambrisentan in pulmonary arterial hypertension, randomized, double-blind, placebo-controlled, multicenter, efficacy (ARIES) study 1 and 2. Circulation 2008;117:3010–3019.
44 McGoon M, et al: Ambrisentan therapy in patients with pulmonary arterial hypertension who discontinued bosentan or sitaxsentan due to liver function test abnormalities. Chest 2009;135:122–129.
45 Oudiz R, et al: Long-term ambrisentan therapy for the treatment of pulmonary arterial hypertension. J Am Coll Cardiol 2009;54:1971–1981.
46 Giaid A, Saleh D: Reduced expression of endothelial nitric oxide synthase in the lungs of patients with pulmonary hypertension. N Engl J Med 1995;333:214–221.
47 Galie N, et al: Sildenafil citrate therapy for pulmonary arterial hypertension. N Engl J Med 2005;353:2148–2157.
48 Rubin LJ, et al: Long-term treatment with sildenafil citrate in pulmonary arterial hypertension: the SUPER-2 study. Chest 2011;140:1274–1283.
49 Galie N, et al: Tadalafil therapy for pulmonary arterial hypertension. Circulation 2009;119:2894–2903.
50 Barst RJ, et al: Tadalafil monotherapy and as add-on to background bosentan in patients with pulmonary arterial hypertension. J Heart Lung Transplant 2011;30:632–643.
51 O'Callaghan DS, Gaine SP: Combination therapy and new types of agents for pulmonary arterial hypertension. Clin Chest Med 2007;28:169–185.
52 Hoeper MM, Markevych I, Spiekerkoetter E, Welte T, Niedermeyer J: Goal-oriented treatment and combination therapy for pulmonary arterial hypertension. Eur Respir J 2005;26:858–863.
53 Galiè N, Palazzini M, Manes A: Pulmonary arterial hypertension: from the kingdom of the near-dead to multiple clinical trial meta-analyses. Eur Heart J 2010;31:2080–2086.
54 Mereles D, et al: Exercise and respiratory training improve exercise capacity and quality of life in patients with severe chronic pulmonary hypertension. Circulation 2006;114:1482–1489.
55 Provencher S, et al: Deleterious effects of beta-blockers on exercise capacity and hemodynamics in patients with portopulmonary hypertension. Gastroenterology 2006;130:120–126.
56 Frank H, et al: The effect of anticoagulant therapy in primary and anorectic drug-induced pulmonary hypertension. Chest 1997;112:714–721.
57 Bonnin M, et al: Severe pulmonary hypertension during pregnancy: mode of delivery and anesthetic management of 15 consecutive cases. Anesthesiology 2005;102:1133–1137, discussion 5A–6A.
58 Sitbon O, et al: Long-term response to calcium channel blockers in idiopathic pulmonary arterial hypertension. Circulation 2005;111:3105–3111.
59 Higenbottam TW, et al: Treatment of pulmonary hypertension with the continuous infusion of a prostacyclin analogue, iloprost. Heart 1998;79:175–179.
60 O'Callaghan DS, et al: Treatment of pulmonary arterial hypertension with targeted therapies. Nat Rev Cardiol 2011;8:526–538.

Prof. Sean P. Gaine
National Pulmonary Hypertension Unit, Department of Respiratory Medicine
Mater Misericordiae University Hospital, University College Dublin
Eccles St., Dublin 7 (Ireland)
Tel. +353 1 803 2000, E-Mail sgaine@mater.ie

Chapter 25
Humbert M, Souza R, Simonneau G (eds): Pulmonary Vascular Disorders.
Prog Respir Res. Basel, Karger, 2012, vol 41, pp 246–253

Lung Transplantation and Role for Novel Extracorporeal Support in Pulmonary Hypertension

Marius M. Hoeper
Hannover Medical School, Department of Respiratory Medicine, Hannover, Germany

Abstract
Although medical therapies are now available for patients with pulmonary arterial hypertension (PAH), lung transplantation remains an important therapeutic option, especially for those patients not responding sufficiently to optimized medical therapy. Bilateral lung transplantation is the preferred procedure for most patients with PAH, while heart-lung transplantation is usually performed in patients with some forms congenital heart disease or other intractable cardiac conditions. In many cases, patients with PAH are referred for transplantation only late during the course of their disease, typically once medical therapy has been exhausted and right heart failure is imminent. These patients are difficult to treat as there are no effective drugs to treat right heart failure in this setting. Recently, there has been a renaissance of extracorporeal life support systems in the management of these patients. The use of venoarterial extracorporeal membrane oxygenation (ECMO) in awake, nonintubated patients has provided an option to stabilize patients for several weeks allowing bridging to transplantation. Positive results have also been reported with pumpless lung assist devices inserted between the pulmonary artery and the left atrium. Finally, the use of ECMO systems after transplantation appears to improve the outcome of PAH patients after lung transplantation.

Historical Perspective

Once considered the only therapeutic option for patients with end-stage pulmonary hypertension (PH), lung transplantation (LTx) and heart-lung transplantation (H/LTx) have become the last resort in an increasing therapeutic armamentarium. The era of clinical H/LTx began in the early 1980s with the publication of the first three successful H/LTx procedures by the Stanford group [1]. Interestingly, all 3 patients had suffered from pulmonary arterial hypertension (PAH), one of them from the idiopathic form and the other 2 from PAH associated with congenital heart disease. Later, the Toronto group and others reported on the first unilateral and bilateral LTx [2].

The pioneering achievements in H/LTx and LTx by the Stanford group, the Toronto group, and others raised new hopes for many patients with incurable cardiopulmonary diseases. This was particularly the case for patients with PAH for whom no effective medical therapy was available at that time. Hence, in those days PAH was one of the leading indications for H/LTx, but mortality on the waiting list was also particularly high for this patient group [3]. As a consequence, lung transplant centers began investigating medical therapies, among them various vasodilators, catecholamines, phosphodiesterase-3 inhibitors, and prostacyclin derivatives. However, only the prostacyclin derivative epoprostenol proved to be efficacious [4]. In fact, physicians were thrilled to see many patients not only stabilizing, but substantially improving with epoprostenol treatment. It turned out that some of these patients could effectively be removed from the waiting list [5, 6].

The implementation of intravenous epoprostenol therapy for PAH marked a turning point for this disease and was later followed by a rapid development of other therapies for the PH spectrum of diseases. It is a footnote in medical history that many of those centers pioneering in H/LTx were also the ones that later contributed substantially to the development of medical therapies that eventually made transplantation unnecessary in more and more patients with PAH. However, despite the remarkable achievements in medical therapy of PAH, some of these patients still have progressive disease and eventually require transplantation.

When to Consider Heart-Lung Transplantation in Patients with Pulmonary Arterial Hypertension

Current guidelines for the management of PAH list H/LTx as the last therapeutic option to be considered once other treatments have been exhausted [7–10]. The proportion of patients with PAH requiring transplantation, however, has been constantly declining over the years. In the early 1990s, more than 10% of LTx recipients had PAH [11]. Between 2002 and 2005, patients diagnosed with idiopathic PAH consisted of 6.8% of those listed for LTx in the United Network of Organ Sharing (UNOS) data base, and between 2005 and 2008 this proportion decreased to 3.7% [12]. This development reflects – at least partly – the effectiveness of modern therapy for PAH. However, some patients continue to deteriorate in spite of maximal medical therapy. Survival of patients with idiopathic PAH treated with intravenous epoprostenol has been approximately 63% at 3 years after the diagnosis [13, 14]. These numbers have somewhat improved in the meantime and some centers now report 3-year survival rates up to 80% [15], but the mortality rate of PAH remains high. This is particularly true when cohorts of newly diagnosed so-called incident cases are investigated [16, 17]. LTx therefore remains a viable and important treatment option for patients with PAH.

The pattern of PAH patients referred for LTx has changed considerably over the past years. Twenty years ago, i.e. when no effective medical therapies were available, many of these patients were immediately listed for transplantation once a diagnosis of PAH had been made. The spectrum of patients undergoing transplantation at that time ranged from patients with end-stage right heart failure to relatively stable patients with milder symptoms. The introduction of medical therapies together with new donor organ allocation systems has led to an entirely different pattern. In most circumstances, patients with PAH are now only being considered for transplantation when medical therapy is failing. In reality this means that most of these patients have been treated for several years with various combinations of endothelin receptor antagonists, phosphodiesterase-5 inhibitors, and prostacyclin derivatives. With these treatments, many patients can be stabilized for extended periods of time, but once treatment fails these patients may rapidly die from right heart failure. The same may happen if seemingly stable patients are affected by intercurrent problems such as infections, trauma, or surgery. Therefore, the timing of listing patients with PAH for transplantation has always been and remains to be a major challenge. As some PAH patients now live for many years with good quality of life, avoiding premature transplantation is as critical as avoiding missing the right time window before patients become too ill for transplantation. It is current practice in many PH referral centers to initiate PAH treatment with oral drugs, i.e. endothelin receptor antagonists and/or phosphodiesterase-5 inhibitors, and add a prostacyclin derivative once the oral treatments are not or no longer sufficiently effective. The most recent European guidelines for PH provide detailed recommendations for treatment goals and the stepwise use of combination therapy [7, 8]. Establishing contact with a transplant center should be considered once patients are not or no longer stable on oral combination therapies and require parenteral prostanoids.

Selecting Patients with Pulmonary Hypertension for Lung Transplantation

There are few circumstances that impact life more than having a deadly disease and being confronted with organ transplantation. Covering the broad implications of these topics in depth is beyond the scope of this book chapter. Eventually, the decision to move towards transplantation is always an individual one made between patients and caregivers. Factors such as survival and quality of life are among the most important aspects to be considered, but certainly not the only ones.

There are some general and disease-specific criteria that need to be taken into account when LTx is being considered. Tables 1 and 2 list absolute and relative contraindications as proposed by the International Society of Heart and Lung Transplantation (ISHLT). Tables 3 and 4 list specific criteria for patient referral and transplantation in patients with PAH [18].

Type of Transplantation

Single-lung transplantations (SLTx), bilateral sequential lung transplantations (BLTx), and combined heart-lung transplantations (H/LTx) have been performed in patients with PAH. SLTx had some appeal as this procedure has

Table 1. Absolute contraindications for LTx (modified from the 2006 guidelines of the ISHLT [18])

Malignancy within the last 2 years; in general a 5-year disease-free interval is prudent
Advanced dysfunction of another organ system (e.g. heart, liver, or kidney); in some cases of heart disease, combined H/LTx may be considered
Noncurable chronic infection, including chronic active hepatitis B, hepatitis C, and human immunodeficiency virus
Significant chest wall/spinal deformity
Documented nonadherence or inability to follow through with medical therapy
Unstable psychiatric or psychological conditions associated with the inability to cooperate or comply with medical therapy
Substance addiction (e.g. tobacco, alcohol, or narcotics) that is either active or within the last 6 months

Table 2. Relative contraindications for lung transplantation (modified from the 2006 guidelines of the ISHLT [18])

Age >65 years
Critical or unstable clinical condition despite optimized therapy
Severely limited functional status with poor rehabilitation potential
Severe cachexia (BMI <17) or severe obesity (BMI >30)
Severe or symptomatic osteoporosis
Mechanical ventilation (with exceptions in carefully selected candidates)
Colonization with highly resistant or highly virulent bacteria, fungi, or mycobacteria

Table 3. Referring patients with PAH for LTx (modified from the 2006 guidelines of the ISHLT [18])

Persistent functional class III or IV, irrespective of ongoing therapy
Rapidly progressive disease
Clinical or radiological features suggesting pulmonary venoocclusive disease

Table 4. LTx in patients with PAH (modified from the 2006 guidelines of the ISHLT [18])

Persistent functional class III or IV despite optimized medical therapy
Progressive disease with low (<350 m) or declining 6-min walking distance
Failing therapy with parenteral prostanoids
Cardiac index of less than 2.0 $l/min/m^2$
Right atrial pressure exceeding 15 mm Hg

the potential to increase the donor organ availability compared to BLTx and H/LTx. The transplantation of one lung in patients with PAH results in normalization of hemodynamics with the pulmonary blood flow being shifted almost completely away from the remaining native lung and into the graft. This concept is successful as long as ventilation is not impaired in the transplanted lung. However, complications such as infection, rejection, or the bronchiolitis obliterans syndrome result in a ventilation-perfusion mismatch with the ventilation going predominantly into the native lung and the perfusion going predominantly into the graft. As a consequence, gas exchange is profoundly impaired and these patients develop severe hypoxemia. These problems together with poor postoperative outcomes have led most centers to abandon this procedure in patients with PAH [19].

The choice between H/LTx and BLTx remains open and is mainly determined by organ shortage and center preferences. Early postoperative management tends to be more difficult after BLTx as high pulmonary artery pressure, high cardiac output, and a low compliance of the left ventricle may result in primary graft failure [20]. Those problems, however, can be successfully managed and cardiac function usually resolves within a few days after transplantation (see below for further details). Most transplantation centers currently prefer BLTx over H/LTx for patients with PAH.

In patients with congenital heart disease and PAH, BLTx also is the preferred option as long as the congenital heart defect has already been repaired or can be repaired during transplantation. A typical example is an atrial septum defect. For patients with complex congenital heart disease that cannot be corrected surgically, H/LTx may be the only therapeutic option. These patients, however, may have extensive systemic-to-pulmonary collateral vascularization which can make H/LTx very demanding, and sometimes even impossible.

Outcome

According to the 2010 ISHLT registry data, the cumulative median survival for all procedures performed was 6.6 years after BLTx and 4.6 years after SLTx [21]. Only 5% of all BLTx procedures and 1% of all SLTx procedures were performed for PAH. The short-term mortality rate after transplantation is still considerably higher for patients with idiopathic PAH than for other indications (e.g. chronic obstructive lung disease, cystic fibrosis, idiopathic pulmonary fibrosis,

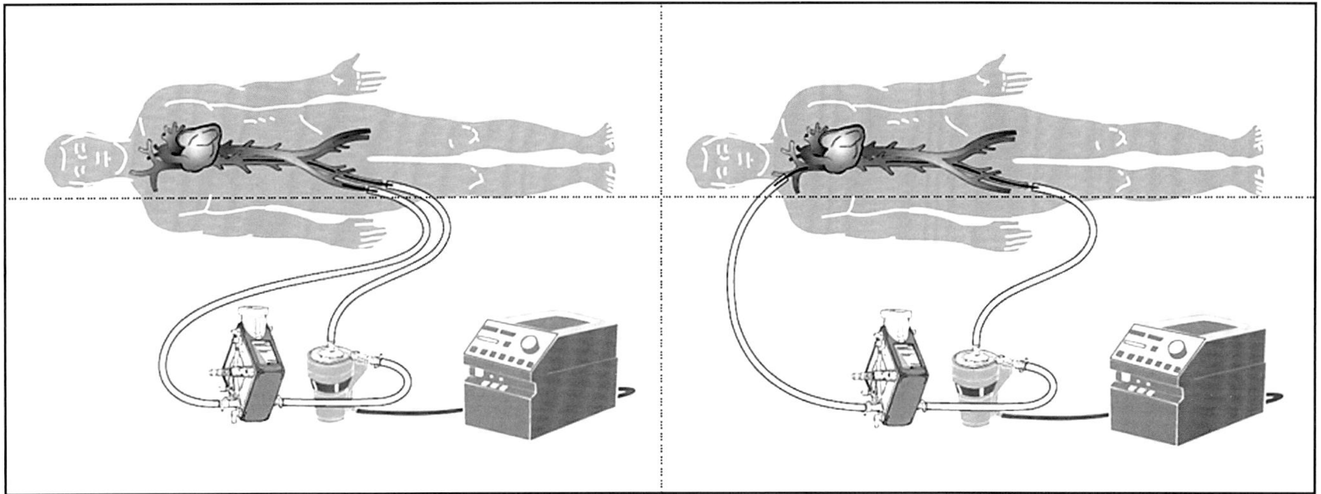

Fig. 1. Schematics of venovenous (left) and venoarterial (right) ECMO. In the venovenous system, the blood is removed from the right atrium via the femoral cannula and reinfused via the jugular cannula after oxygenation. This approach requires normal cardiac function. In contrast, the venoarterial approach (right) can fully replace cardiopulmonary function. As in the venovenous approach, the blood is removed from the right atrium but reinfused into the aortic cannula, usually inserted in a femoral artery.

etc.) but the long-term outcome is almost identical to that of patients undergoing lung transplantation for chronic obstructive pulmonary disease, with 5-year-survival rates of approximately 50% [21]. A diagnosis of PAH remains the single most important risk factor for 1-year mortality in the ISHLT registry. However, for patients who survive the first year after transplantation, the long-term outcome is significantly better for patients with PAH than for most of the other indications, most notably chronic obstructive pulmonary disease and idiopathic pulmonary fibrosis [21].

Bridging to Transplantation

It is crucial to refer patients with PAH to a transplant center if they do not respond sufficiently to medical therapy (see above for more details). In this patient population, transplantation is usually performed once medical therapy has been exhausted. This approach is in agreement with current guidelines, but creates the problem that many patients are in a terminal stage of their disease when lung transplantation is seriously considered. It is still a difficult task to bridge these patients to transplantation once they develop right heart failure while receiving optimized medical therapy. There are few other drugs that may be supportive in this scenario. Catecholamines, especially dobutamine, may help to maintain cardiac output, but efficacy is limited and often short-lasting. Levosimendan is a promising agent, but limited clinical experience suggests that it is not effective in patients with terminal right heart failure due to PAH. Today, extracorporeal life support may offer the best option to bridge these patients successfully to transplantation.

The standard modes of extracorporeal life support are venovenous and venoarterial systems (fig. 1). Venovenous systems can be used to treat lung failure, but cardiopulmonary failure as seen in patients with terminal PAH requires a venoarterial approach. Venoarterial extracorporeal membrane oxygenation (ECMO) has been used for almost 40 years to treat various conditions associated with pulmonary or cardiac failure, or both. The results, however, have been modest, mostly due to technical limitations and complications resulting from infection, bleeding, thromboembolism, hemotrauma with hemolysis, platelet activation, and the systemic inflammatory syndrome. The development of newer devices with centrifugal blood pumps and low-resistance heparin-coated biocompatible oxygenators has substantially improved the results of extracorporeal life support in various conditions. Other major steps have been the application of such devices in awake nonintubated patients [22] as well as the use of pumpless devices inserted between the pulmonary artery and the left atrium [23]. Both strategies still have to be considered experimental, but hold great promise, also in terms of future developments towards devices to be used over extended periods of time.

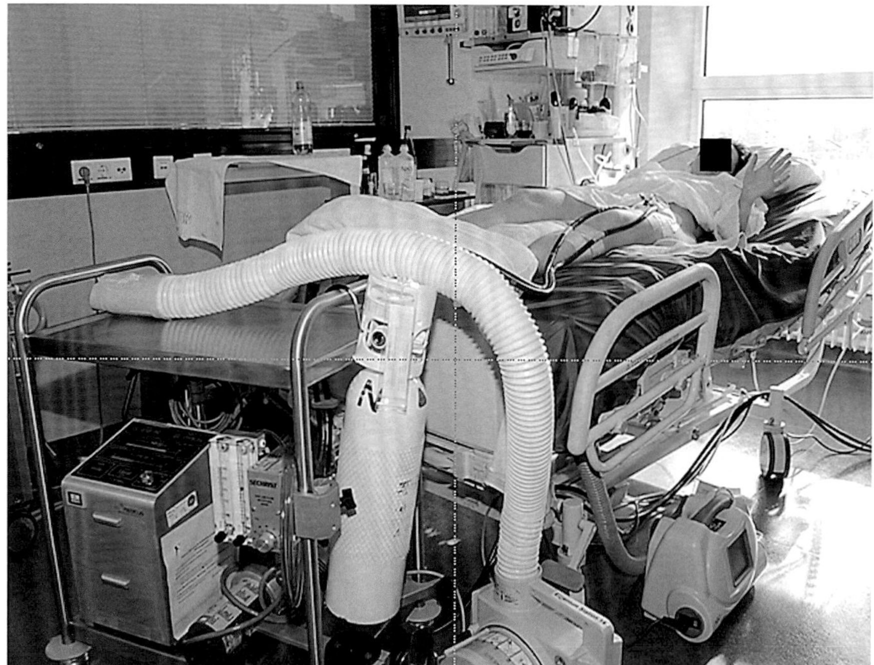

Fig. 2. Use of venoarterial ECMO in a 29-year-old nonintubated female with idiopathic PAH. The ECMO pump is standing on the table in front of the bed. The oxygenator is not visible as it is covered by the pump. Both the venous and the arterial cannulae are inserted in the left femoral vessels (note the different color of the blood before and after oxygenation). This patient received ECMO support for 42 days prior to transplantation and made a full recovery.

Venoarterial Extracorporeal Membrane Oxygenation in Nonintubated Patients with Pulmonary Arterial Hypertension as a Bridge to Transplantation

In patients with PAH and right heart failure, endotracheal intubation and mechanical ventilation is usually not a viable option as this strategy carries a high risk of right heart failure. ECMO has been used as bridge to transplantation in patients with right heart failure [24, 25], but until recently only in patients receiving mechanical ventilation. These patients are therefore exposed not only to the risks associated with ECMO, but also to the risks and complications of prolonged sedation and mechanical ventilation, especially pneumonia and septicemia [26].

In 2010, Olsson et al. [22] from Hannover Medical School (Hannover, Germany) reported on a series of 5 patients with PH and right heart failure who were treated with venoarterial ECMO while awake and breathing spontaneously (fig. 2). All patients were moribund at the time of ECMO insertion, but recovered rapidly afterwards, including an almost immediate recovery of renal function in those patients who presented with kidney failure. The patients remained on ECMO support without sedation, were breathing spontaneously, and were able to eat and drink without requiring artificial nutrition. In addition, they received passive and active physiotherapy as well as psychological support. Four patients were successfully bridged to transplantation after 18–35 days on ECMO support and 3 of them survived. None of the patients in this series had signs of limb ischemia, hemolysis, platelet activation, or systemic inflammatory response, and there were no clinically apparent systemic embolic events.

The ECMO cannulae were inserted under local anesthesia without sedation. The preferred access sites were the femoral artery and the ipsilateral femoral vein. Cannulation of both legs was avoided in order to allow the patient to move as much as possible. A 15-Fr Novalung® cannula was used for the femoral artery and a 20-Fr Heartport® cannula was placed in the femoral vein and advanced into the right atrium. Another 7-Fr introducer sheath was inserted in the femoral artery distal from the ECMO cannula and connected to the arterial branch of the ECMO circuit to ensure sufficient blood flow to the limb. Systemic oxygenation and blood pressure were measured via a line inserted in the right radial artery. The mean device flow was maintained between 3.2 and 3.5 l/min and oxygen flow was adapted to the patients' blood gases. PAH medications and catecholamines were discontinued once ECMO blood flow had been established.

This small case series showed that the use of venoarterial ECMO is feasible in patients with terminal right heart failure and that it results in immediate hemodynamic stabilization, thus offering a salvage strategy for these patients. The main disadvantages and drawbacks include the risk of

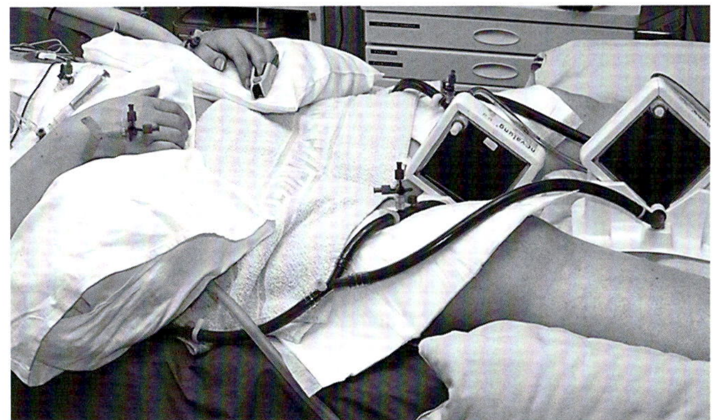

Fig. 3. Pumpless lung assist device. In this 41-year-old woman with pulmonary venoocclusive disease, a pumpless approach was applied. In this case, two Novalung oxygenators were inserted between the pulmonary artery and the left atrium. Blood flow is maintained by the elevated pulmonary artery pressure obviating the need for a pump. The cannulae were inserted after sternotomy. The patient underwent successful bilateral lung transplantation after being treated with this device for 9 days.

bleeding complications resulting from anticoagulation and the fact that the patients cannot be fully mobilized with the device in place.

Pumpless Lung Assist Devices Inserted into the Pulmonary Circulation

An alternative bridging strategy is the use of pumpless devices inserted between the pulmonary arteries and the left atrium (PA-LA). The first report on the successful application of the PA-LA approach was published in 2009 by the groups from Hannover, Germany and Toronto, Canada [27]. They used the interventional lung assist device designed by Novalung (Hechingen, Germany) a low resistance oxygenator, which was originally developed for insertion between a femoral artery and a femoral vein to allow extracorporeal CO_2 removal [23]. In order to be used in patients with PAH, the device was connected between the main pulmonary artery and the left atrium (fig. 3). Hence, this approach takes advantage of the patient's PH which is used to maintain blood flow through the device, thus obviating the need for a pump.

The insertion of this device requires general anesthesia and sternotomy. The centers that have used this technique so far prefer to insert a venoarterial ECMO prior to the procedure to avoid hemodynamic instability after intubation. The ECMO cannulae are later removed once blood flow through the Novalung device has been established. As with venoarterial ECMO, this approach also results in immediate stabilization of hemodynamics and gas exchange. Most of the patients could be rapidly extubated after the procedure.

The initial insertion of the PA-LA device is more elaborate than implanting a venoarterial ECMO device. However, the advantages of the PA-LA approach are that no pump is needed and that the patients can be fully mobilized.

Postoperative Management of Pulmonary Arterial Hypertension Patients after Lung Transplantation

It has already been mentioned above that the short-term survival after BLTx is worse for patients with PAH compared to most other indications. The reason is the particular hemodynamic situation of these patients. The right ventricle is still capable of generating high pulmonary vascular pressures. At the same time, the left ventricle of these patients, often small, stiff, and adapted to a low cardiac output, is not capable of handling a normal or elevated cardiac output as it occurs after transplantation. The consequences are PH in the graft and increased left-sided filling pressures. This is a disastrous scenario for newly transplanted lungs with a leaky alveolar-capillary membrane. Severe reperfusion injury is the consequence, which tends to develop predominantly once sedation is reduced in order to wean these patients from the ventilator. Conservative measures including a negative fluid balance, the administration of high doses of β-blockers, inhaled nitric oxide, and others, are often not successful to stabilize these patients. Some centers have tried pulmonary artery banding during the postoperative period to overcome this problem, but with limited success. Other centers have switched from BLTx to H/LTx, but the shortage of donor organs has been the main limitation for this approach.

It appears that the hemodynamic problems occurring after BLTx in patients with PAH can be successfully managed with venoarterial ECMO. This approach effectively unloads the pulmonary vasculature by reducing pulmonary artery pressures as well as left ventricular filling pressures. Many centers now routinely use this approach whenever they perform BLTx in patients with severe PH. The patients leave the operating room with ECMO support and are often weaned from the ventilator within the first 24–48 h after transplantation with the ECMO device still in place. The blood flow through the ECMO system is gradually reduced over a period of 5–10 days before the ECMO cannulae are removed. During this period, the heart usually adapts to the new hemodynamic situation and the problems described above can be avoided. Centers using this approach routinely no longer find the postoperative mortality of patients with PAH to be elevated.

Conclusion and Outlook

Despite major therapeutic advances, a proportion of patients with PAH require lung transplantation and this is not going to change in the near future. Close cooperation between PH centers and transplant teams is crucial to ensure the optimal timing of the procedure. Today, PAH patients are often referred too late for transplantation and there is still no effective therapy for end-stage right heart failure once PAH therapy has been exhausted. New strategies including the use of extracorporeal support systems in awake, nonintubated patients have been applied successfully to bridge such patients to transplantation. It is expected that new technical advancements will make these devices more convenient and more efficient, eventually allowing their long-term use, possibly even independent from a transplant perspective.

References

1 Reitz BA, Wallwork JL, Hunt SA, Pennock JL, Billingham ME, Oyer PE, Stinson EB, Shumway NE: Heart-lung transplantation: successful therapy for patients with pulmonary vascular disease. N Engl J Med 1982;306:557–564.

2 Patterson GA, Maurer JR, Williams TJ, Cardoso PG, Scavuzzo M, Todd TR: Comparison of outcomes of double and single lung transplantation for obstructive lung disease. The Toronto Lung Transplant Group. J Thorac Cardiovasc Surg 1991;101:623–631, discussion 631–622.

3 Trulock EP: Lung transplantation for primary pulmonary hypertension. Clin Chest Med 2001;22:583–593.

4 Higenbottam T, Wheeldon D, Wells F, Wallwork J: Long-term treatment of primary pulmonary hypertension with continuous intravenous epoprostenol (prostacyclin). Lancet 1984;1:1046–1047.

5 Jones DK, Higenbottam TW, Wallwork J: Treatment of primary pulmonary hypertension intravenous epoprostenol (prostacyclin). Br Heart J 1987;57:270–278.

6 Higenbottam T, Butt AY, McMahon A, Westerbeck R, Sharples L: Long-term intravenous prostaglandin (epoprostenol or iloprost) for treatment of severe pulmonary hypertension. Heart 1998;80:151–155.

7 Galie N, Hoeper MM, Humbert M, Torbicki A, Vachiery JL, Barbera JA, Beghetti M, Corris P, Gaine S, Gibbs JS, Gomez-Sanchez MA, Jondeau G, Klepetko W, Opitz C, Peacock A, Rubin L, Zellweger M, Simonneau G: Guidelines for the diagnosis and treatment of pulmonary hypertension. The task force for the diagnosis and treatment of pulmonary hypertension of the European Society of Cardiology (ESC) and the European Respiratory Society (ERS), endorsed by the International Society of Heart and Lung Transplantation (ISHLT). Eur Respir J 2009;34:1219–1263.

8 Galie N, Hoeper MM, Humbert M, Torbicki A, Vachiery JL, Barbera JA, Beghetti M, Corris P, Gaine S, Gibbs JS, Gomez-Sanchez MA, Jondeau G, Klepetko W, Opitz C, Peacock A, Rubin L, Zellweger M, Simonneau G, Vahanian A, Auricchio A, Bax J, Ceconi C, Dean V, Filippatos G, Funck-Brentano C, Hobbs R, Kearney P, McDonagh T, McGregor K, Popescu BA, Reiner Z, Sechtem U, Sirnes PA, Tendera M, Vardas P, Widimsky P, Al Attar N, Andreotti F, Aschermann M, Asteggiano R, Benza R, Berger R, Bonnet D, Delcroix M, Howard L, Kitsiou AN, Lang I, Maggioni A, Nielsen-Kudsk JE, Park M, Perrone-Filardi P, Price S, Domenech MT, Vonk-Noordegraaf A, Zamorano JL: Guidelines for the diagnosis and treatment of pulmonary hypertension: the Task Force for the Diagnosis and Treatment of Pulmonary Hypertension of the European Society of Cardiology (ESC) and the European Respiratory Society (ERS), endorsed by the International Society of Heart and Lung Transplantation (ISHLT). Eur Heart J 2009;30:2493–2537.

9 McLaughlin VV, Archer SL, Badesch DB, Barst RJ, Farber HW, Lindner JR, Mathier MA, McGoon MD, Park MH, Rosenson RS, Rubin LJ, Tapson VF, Varga J: ACCF/AHA 2009 expert consensus document on pulmonary hypertension a report of the American College of Cardiology Foundation Task Force on Expert Consensus Documents and the American Heart Association developed in collaboration with the American College of Chest Physicians; American Thoracic Society, Inc.; and the Pulmonary Hypertension Association. J Am Coll Cardiol 2009;53:1573–1619.

10 McLaughlin VV, Archer SL, Badesch DB, Barst RJ, Farber HW, Lindner JR, Mathier MA, McGoon MD, Park MH, Rosenson RS, Rubin LJ, Tapson VF, Varga J, Harrington RA, Anderson JL, Bates ER, Bridges CR, Eisenberg MJ, Ferrari VA, Grines CL, Hlatky MA, Jacobs AK, Kaul S, Lichtenberg RC, Moliterno DJ, Mukherjee D, Pohost GM, Schofield RS, Shubrooks SJ, Stein JH, Tracy CM, Weitz HH, Wesley DJ: ACCF/AHA 2009 expert consensus document on pulmonary hypertension: a report of the American College of Cardiology Foundation Task Force on Expert Consensus Documents and the American Heart Association: developed in collaboration with the American College of Chest Physicians, American Thoracic Society, Inc., and the Pulmonary Hypertension Association. Circulation 2009;119:2250–2294.

11 Taylor DO, Edwards LB, Boucek MM, Trulock EP, Keck BM, Hertz MI: The Registry of the International Society for Heart and Lung Transplantation: twenty-first official adult heart transplant report–2004. J Heart Lung Transplant 2004;23:796–803.

12 Chen H, Shiboski SC, Golden JA, Gould MK, Hays SR, Hoopes CW, De Marco T: Impact of the lung allocation score on lung transplantation for pulmonary arterial hypertension. Am J Respir Crit Care Med 2009;180:468–474.

13 McLaughlin VV, Shillington A, Rich S: Survival in primary pulmonary hypertension: the impact of epoprostenol therapy. Circulation 2002;106:1477–1482.

14 Sitbon O, Humbert M, Nunes H, Parent F, Garcia G, Herve P, Rainisio M, Simonneau G: Long-term intravenous epoprostenol infusion in primary pulmonary hypertension: prognostic factors and survival. J Am Coll Cardiol 2002;40:780–788.

15 Hoeper MM, Markevych I, Spiekerkoetter E, Welte T, Niedermeyer J: Goal-oriented treatment and combination therapy for pulmonary arterial hypertension. Eur Respir J 2005;26:858–863.

16 Humbert M, Sitbon O, Chaouat A, Bertocchi M, Habib G, Gressin V, Yaici A, Weitzenblum E, Cordier JF, Chabot F, Dromer C, Pison C, Reynaud-Gaubert M, Haloun A, Laurent M, Hachulla E, Cottin V, Degano B, Jais X, Montani D, Souza R, Simonneau G: Survival in patients with idiopathic, familial, and anorexigen-associated pulmonary arterial hypertension in the modern management era. Circulation 2010;122:156–163.
17 Humbert M, Sitbon O, Yaici A, Montani D, O'Callaghan DS, Jais X, Parent F, Savale L, Natali D, Gunther S, Chaouat A, Chabot F, Cordier JF, Habib G, Gressin V, Jing ZC, Souza R, Simonneau G: Survival in incident and prevalent cohorts of patients with pulmonary arterial hypertension. Eur Respir J 2010;36:549–555.
18 Orens JB, Estenne M, Arcasoy S, Conte JV, Corris P, Egan JJ, Egan T, Keshavjee S, Knoop C, Kotloff R, Martinez FJ, Nathan S, Palmer S, Patterson A, Singer L, Snell G, Studer S, Vachiery JL, Glanville AR: International guidelines for the selection of lung transplant candidates: 2006 update – a consensus report from the Pulmonary Scientific Council of the International Society for Heart and Lung Transplantation. J Heart Lung Transplant 2006;25:745–755.
19 Trulock EP, Christie JD, Edwards LB, Boucek MM, Aurora P, Taylor DO, Dobbels F, Rahmel AO, Keck BM, Hertz MI: Registry of the International Society for Heart and Lung Transplantation: twenty-fourth official adult lung and heart-lung transplantation report-2007. J Heart Lung Transplant 2007;26:782–795.
20 Waddell TK, Bennett L, Kennedy R, Todd TR, Keshavjee SH: Heart-lung or lung transplantation for Eisenmenger syndrome. J Heart Lung Transplant 2002;21:731–737.
21 Christie JD, Edwards LB, Kucheryavaya AY, Aurora P, Dobbels F, Kirk R, Rahmel AO, Stehlik J, Hertz MI: The Registry of the International Society for Heart and Lung Transplantation: twenty-seventh official adult lung and heart-lung transplant report – 2010. J Heart Lung Transplant 2010;29:1104–1118.
22 Olsson KM, Simon A, Strueber M, Hadem J, Wiesner O, Gottlieb J, Fuehner T, Fischer S, Warnecke G, Kuhn C, Haverich A, Welte T, Hoeper MM: Extracorporeal membrane oxygenation in nonintubated patients as bridge to lung transplantation. Am J Transplant 2010;10:2173–2178.
23 Fischer S, Simon AR, Welte T, Hoeper MM, Meyer A, Tessmann R, Gohrbandt B, Gottlieb J, Haverich A, Strueber M: Bridge to lung transplantation with the novel pumpless interventional lung assist device NovaLung. J Thorac Cardiovasc Surg 2006;131:719–723.
24 Strueber M: Extracorporeal support as a bridge to lung transplantation. Curr Opin Crit Care 2010;16:69–73.
25 Hammainen P: Re: use of extracorporeal membrane oxygenation as a bridge to primary lung transplant: 3 consecutive, successful cases and a review of the literature. J Heart Lung Transplant 2008;27:1186.
26 Chastre J, Fagon JY: Ventilator-associated pneumonia. Am J Respir Crit Care Med 2002;165:867–903.
27 Strueber M, Hoeper MM, Fischer S, Cypel M, Warnecke G, Gottlieb J, Pierre A, Welte T, Haverich A, Simon AR, Keshavjee S: Bridge to thoracic organ transplantation in patients with pulmonary arterial hypertension using a pumpless lung assist device. Am J Transplant 2009;9:853–857.

Prof. Marius M Hoeper, MD
Hannover Medical School
Department of Respiratory Medicine
DE–30623 Hannover (Germany)
Tel. +49 511 532 3530, E-Mail hoeper.marius@mh-hannover.de

Chapter 26
Humbert M, Souza R, Simonneau G (eds): Pulmonary Vascular Disorders.
Prog Respir Res. Basel, Karger, 2012, vol 41, pp 254–261

Atrial Septostomy

Jean-Luc Vachiéry

Clinique de l'Hypertension Pulmonaire et de l'Insuffisance Cardiaque, Service de Cardiologie, Cliniques Universitaires de Bruxelles, Hôpital Erasme, Brussels, Belgium

Abstract

Pulmonary arterial hypertension (PAH) is a severe and rapidly progressive condition, ultimately leading to right heart failure and death. Although medical therapy has improved over the past 15 years, PAH remains incurable and many patients will be in need of lung transplantation. However, very few will eventually be transplanted, due to contraindication precluding listing or unavailability of suitable organs. Therefore, atrial septostomy (AS) is an attractive option for selected patients either as a bridge to transplantation or as destination therapy for patients failing on medical treatment. The physiopathological reasoning in favor of AS is based on the decompression of right heart chambers together with a decrease in the neurohumoral overactivation due to right heart failure. The technique of AS has considerably improved over the years. A stepwise dilation procedure of the interatrial septum together with careful patient selection has led to a significant reduction of procedure-related death, currently as low as 2%. The procedure is indicated in patients remaining in NYHA-FC III/IV despite optimal medical therapy with appropriate oxygenation (saturation on room air ≥90%) and controlled right heart failure (right atrial pressure <18 mm Hg). Recent data suggest that AS may improve survival, especially in the era of modern therapy. Despite the success of this technique in expert centers, several issues remain to be addressed, such as long-term benefit and risk (>5–10 years). Finally, the best timing for AS should be redefined, due to the theoretical advantage of earlier intervention.

Pulmonary arterial hypertension (PAH) is a clinical syndrome of dyspnea and fatigue, characterized by the presence of precapillary hypertension in the absence of cardiac or respiratory causes [1, 2]. PAH is a severe and progressive condition, rapidly leading to right heart failure and death [2]. Over the last two decades, significant advances were made in the understanding of PAH, including pathogenesis, genetics, and diagnosis. In addition, international collaboration and improved therapies led to the establishment of specific guidelines for diagnosis and management [2], which is unique for a rare disease. Unfortunately, PAH remains incurable, quality of life is still far from ideal, and survival is limited. As an example, recent data from the French PAH network revealed that, for incident cases, the estimated survival of the most common causes of PAH (idiopathic, heritable, and anorectic drug-induced PAH) at 1, 2, and 3 years was 85.7, 69.6, and 54.9%, respectively [3]. In other words, even established aggressive medical therapy is insufficient to provide long-term benefit. Currently, lung transplantation remains the only cure for PAH [4]. However, access to transplantation is still limited due to the unavailability of suitable organs and high mortality rates for individuals on waiting lists. In addition, many patients may not be accepted for surgery because of comorbidities and/or age limitation [4]. For these patients, atrial septostomy (AS) is an acceptable option either as a destination therapy or as a bridge to transplantation. This chapter reviews the pathophysiological reasoning for AS, technical aspects, results (short- and long-term), and position in the treatment algorithm of PAH.

Physiopathology

Rationale: Role of Right Ventricular Function in Pulmonary Arterial Hypertension

In PAH, exercise tolerance, symptoms, and survival are highly dependent on right ventricular (RV) function. The RV adaptation to a chronic increase in afterload is best characterized by pulmonary vascular impedance, a combination of resistance, compliance, and reflected waves [2, 5, 6]. The consequences of pulmonary hypertension on the right ventricle are a cascade of events including increased contractility and hypertrophy, followed by dilation and failure to cope with chronically increased afterload [6]. This phenomenon is common to all

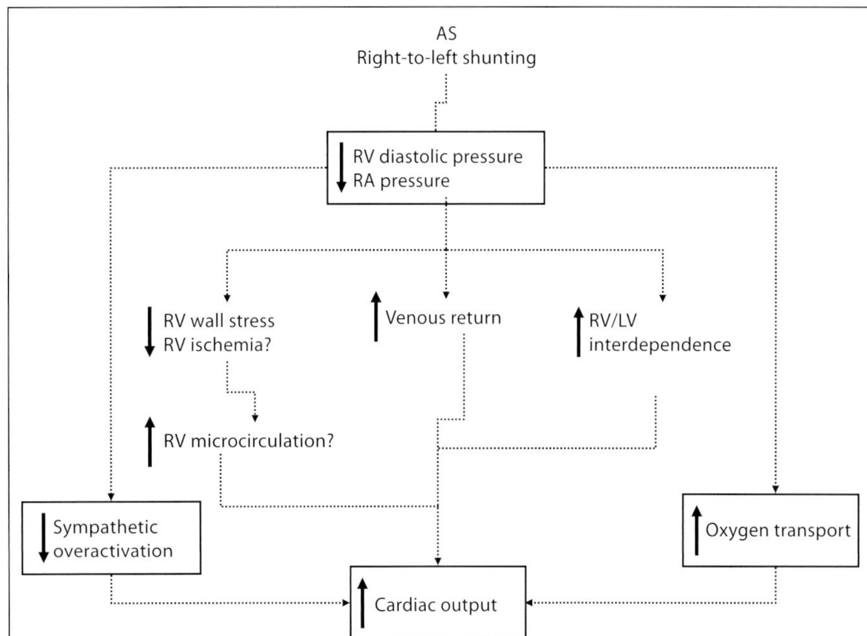

Fig. 1. Physiological effects of AS. The effects of the creation of a right-to-left shunt are mediated by a decompression of the right heart chambers, a decrease in sympathetic overactivation, and an improvement in oxygen transport, resulting in an increase in systemic cardiac output. LV = Left ventricular; RA = right atrium.

causes of pulmonary hypertension. However, compared with idiopathic PAH (IPAH), patients with PAH due to congenital heart disease appear to have a longer preservation of RV function [2, 5, 7], with only 15% of patients presenting significant RV failure [7, 8]. In addition, patients suffering from PAH in the context of Eisenmenger 's syndrome fare better awaiting transplantation, compared with patients suffering from other forms of PH [8]. The same reasoning may apply to IPAH as it has been suggested that the presence of a patent foramen ovale may be associated with a better prognosis [9].

Therefore, as the presence of 'natural' intracardiac communication is likely associated with a better outcome in PAH, the creation of shunt at the atrial level appears to be a valuable option to unload the RV under pressure.

Consequences of Atrial Septostomy: Decreased Sympathetic Overactivation

Decompression of the RV is the first event explaining the improvement observed after AS, i.e. the acute decrease in right atrial pressure (RAP) rapidly leads to an improvement in congestion, together with an improvement of systemic oxygen delivery [10, 11]. The latter occurs despite a decrease in oxygen saturation, which is compensated by an increase in cardiac output [10–15]. This can be explained by an improvement in venous return, decreased wall stress, and improvement in ventricular interdependence through the interventricular septum (fig. 1).

Decreased sympathetic overactivation is one of the key mechanisms by which AS improves hemodynamics, clinical manifestations of RV function, and exercise capacity (fig. 1) [14]. Our group hypothesized that septostomy would decrease sympathetic nervous system overactivity if the beneficial effects of the improved cardiac hemodynamics could compensate for the shunt-induced, hypoxemia-associated chemoreflex activation. In this study, 10 matched healthy controls were compared to 11 patients studied immediately before and the day after AS. Sympathetic activity was assessed by means of muscle nerve sympathetic nerve activity (MSNA) by microneurography and measurement of circulating neurohormones. Compared to the control subjects, the PAH patients had lower mean blood pressure (75 ± 2 vs. 96 ± 3 mm Hg, respectively; $p < 0.001$) and arterial oxygen saturation (SaO_2; 92 ± 1 vs. 97 ± 0%, respectively; $p < 0.001$), higher heart rate (HR); (84 ± 4 vs. 68 ± 3 beats/min, respectively; $p < 0.01$), and MSNA (76 ± 5 vs. 29 ± 2 bursts/min, respectively; $p < 0.001$). As expected, AS significantly decreased RAP (from 11 ± 1 to 8 ± 1, $p < 0.01$) and SaO_2 (from 91 ± 1 to 84 ± 1%; $p < 0.001$) while increasing left atrial pressure (4 ± 1 to 6 ± 1, $p < 0.01$) and cardiac output (3.0 ± 0.3 to 3.8 ± 0.3; $p < 0.01$; all values are expressed as means ± SD). MSNA significantly decreased after septostomy, despite a drop in SaO_2, while plasma levels of norepinephrine, aldosterone, and plasma renin activity remained unaffected. This improvement was directly correlated with the drop in RAP (fig. 2) [14].

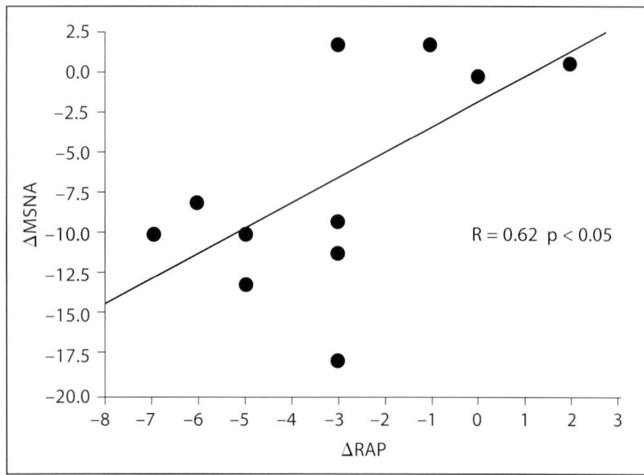

Fig. 2. Decrease in sympathetic overactivity following AS [14]. Changes in sympathetic overactivity, measured by MSNA at baseline and 24 h after AS (Y-axis, in burst/min), correlate with the observed decrease in RAP (mm Hg).

Improvement in oxygen delivery is another important mechanism explaining the benefit of right-to-left shunting. Diller et al. [16] used mathematical and computer modeling to study the physiological effects of shunting under fixed pulmonary blood flow. In their model, increasing right-to-left shunting improved systemic cardiac output, arterial blood pressure, and arterial delivery of oxygen. This contrasted with an unchanged mixed venous content of oxygen, suggesting that increasing the volume of right-to-left shunting cannot compensate for RV failure and that the benefit of AS may represent the result of improved flow of blood rather than augmented tissue oxygenation [16]. Finally, right atrial mechanics and systemic perfusion may be improved by low-flow interatrial shunting, as observed in an animal model of pulmonary hypertension [17].

In summary, the key physiological effects of AS include the following: RV decompression, decreased sympathetic overactivation, and improved oxygen transport despite arterial oxygen desaturation without directly affecting the pulmonary circulation (fig. 1).

Technique of Atrial Septostomy

The idea to create a shunt at the atrial level to alleviate an overloaded RV was put forward in the early 1960s. Blade septostomy was a surgical technique consisting of a single blade opening of the interatrial septum (IAS) through a thoracotomy. It has been initially performed in children presenting severe forms of congenital heart disease [18, 19]. With the development of interventional cardiology, the technique was modified in the late 1980s. The blade opening was performed percutaneously under general anesthesia for patients awaiting transplantation before medical treatments for PAH were made available [20, 21]. The procedure-related mortality of blade septostomy was as high as 50%, very likely because it was performed as a 'last resort' option in patients with end-stage RV failure [19–21].

The technique has considerably improved over the years, with most of the procedures performed worldwide using the same protocol, termed 'balloon-dilation atrial septostomy', as described by Sandoval et al. [12]. This technique combines the creation of a septostomy by perforation of the IAS, followed by progressive dilation using balloons of increasing size (fig. 3). The procedure is performed in the setting of the cardiac catheterization laboratory. Although a light sedation may be used in some cases, most patients are awake and the intervention is performed under local anesthesia with continuous monitoring of transcutaneous oxygen saturation, HR, and systemic blood pressure. A Swan-Ganz (or Cournand) catheter, for right heart pressure measurements, is inserted into a femoral vein, while a conventional pigtail catheter is positioned in the ascending aorta for systemic pressure monitoring, blood gas analysis, and measurement of left ventricular end diastolic pressure. A long (>100 cm) sheath is then introduced into the other femoral vein and positioned at the level of the foramen ovale, using the pigtail as a landmark in the profile plane. A Brockenbrough needle is then introduced in the long sheath to puncture the IAS. The sheath is then advanced in the left atrium (LA). Some centers use transesophageal echocardiography to guide the puncture of the IAS, although this has the major disadvantage of requiring general anesthesia. A pigtail Inoue guide wire positioned in the LA then replaces the needle. Once the Inoue guide is in place, the sheath is withdrawn and the first balloon (4–8 mm diameter) is progressively mounted across the IAS and inflated to stretch the orifice of the AS. After thorough monitoring of SaO_2, RAP, and left ventricular diastolic or LA pressure, a larger balloon (8–20 mm) is used until one of the following targets is reached: (1) decrease in SaO_2 by >10% compared to baseline, with SaO_2 maintained at >84%; or (2) doubling of the LA pressure, which must be maintained <15–18 mm Hg [10, 12, 22, 23]. An important elastic recoil may be observed, leading to a functional orifice around 1 mm and secondary closure of the defect from 8 to 29% [10, 12, 13, 22, 23].

To avoid this, a modified technique of stent fenestration of the IAS has been performed [24]. However the risk/benefit ratio and the long-term effects of this procedure remain unknown.

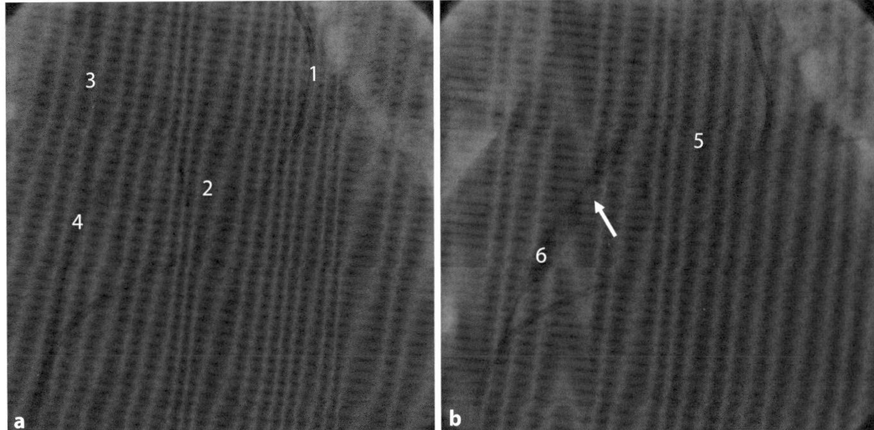

Fig. 3. Technical aspects of balloon-dilation AS. **a** The first step consists of a puncture of the IAS with a Brockenbrough needle (AS), followed by the positioning of an introducer in the LA across the IAS (4). The following can be seen on the picture: a catheter in the pulmonary artery for monitoring of right heart pressures (1), a pigtail in the descending aorta just above the aortic valve as a landmark to identify the IAS (2), and a permanent catheter for prostacyclin infusion (3). **b** A pigtail Inoue guide wire (5) is positioned in the LA through the introducer (4, in **a**). A balloon (size 8 mm) filled with contrast (6) is then inserted over the guide wire and progressively inflated across the IAS, with a clearly visible imprint (white arrow).

Patient Characteristics and Short-Term Effects of Atrial Septostomy

Clinical Outcome

More than 250 procedures have been reported worldwide, both in the adult and the pediatric population of PAH [10–13, 15, 20–26]. Patient characteristics are described in table 1. While recently published data have not been included [23], they match almost identically with the overall population described in the table. In most cases, AS has been performed in patients with IPAH (82%) in a context of RV failure (43%), syncope (38%), or both (19%). In about half of the cases, AS was performed after failure of medical therapy, with 61% of the patients receiving parenteral prostanoids [22].

Postprocedure hemodynamics have been reported in 52.5% of the published cases [22], showing expected immediate effects such as a 26% decrease in RAP and a 38% increase in cardiac index despite a 10% in SaO_2 [13, 14, 22]. These results also suggest that a greater benefit is expected in patients with a RAP >11 mm Hg before intervention [22].

Procedure-Related Mortality

The procedure-related mortality rate has been reported to be as high as 16% in patients with overt RV failure [10, 12, 22]. Interestingly enough, the experience reported after 2001 suggests that AS is performed earlier both in the adult [11, 13, 15] and the pediatric population [25, 26]. Importantly, most patients are now under PAH-targeted therapies presenting with less severe RV failure. As a result, the procedure-related mortality rate has decreased to 7.1% after 24 h and 14.8% after a month [22]. In the most experienced center who pioneered AS, only 1 death has been reported out of 50 procedures performed in 34 patients, a 2% mortality rate [23]. Advanced symptoms (NYHA IV) and a higher RAP level prior to the procedure, together with an exaggerated drop in SaO_2 during AS are amongst the key factors associated with the worst outcome [10, 22, 23]. Refractory hypoxemia, hypoxia-induced shock, progressive RV failure, and multiple organ dysfunctions are the main causes of procedure-related deaths [22, 23].

Long-Term Benefits of Atrial Septostomy

Clinical Outcome

After AS, most patients report an improvement in symptoms, reflected by a decrease in NYHA functional class (3.49 + 0.6 to 2.1 + 0.7), together with a decrease in episodes of syncope and RV failure in 88% of the cases [22, 23]. In addition, exercise tolerance is improved with a benefit in 6-min walk distance up to 150 m [10, 11, 13, 15, 22], despite a significant reduction in SaO_2 at the end of exercise

Table 1. Clinical and functional characteristics of a population receiving an AS from 223 reported cases [22]

Characteristics	
Age, years	28 ± 17
Etiology	
IPAH	82%
PAH due to corrected L-R shunt	8%
PAH due to connective tissue disease	5%
CTEPH	3%
Other cause	3%
NYHA functional class	3.6±0.4
Main indication for intervention	
Right heart failure	43%
Syncope	38%
Association of both previous indication	19%
Bridge to transplantation	14%
Medical therapy at time of intervention	n = 93 (43%)
Intravenous prostanoids	61%
Inhaled or subcutaneous prostacyclin	8%
Single oral therapy	34%
Combined therapy (any combination)	11%

All values are expressed as means ± SD, unless otherwise indicated. CTEPH = Chronic thromboembolic pulmonary hypertension; L-R = left-to-right.

that is typically decreased below 75% on room air [11, 13]. Secondary closure of the defect is higher when dilation is performed with small-sized balloons: 29 and 21% with balloon sizes of 8.5 + 2.5 mm [23] and up to 14 mm [15], respectively, compared with only 8% for sizes between 12 and 20 mm [13]. Patency of the AS orifice and right-to-left shunting can be monitored by transthoracic echocardiography (fig. 4) and measurement of SaO_2 at peak exercise. If in doubt, contrast echocardiography and cardiopulmonary exercise testing may be useful prior to considering another procedure.

Survival

Long-term outcome has been reported in 128 of the cases published, allowing the calculation of a median survival of 60 months for the whole cohort and 63.1 months after procedure-related deaths have been excluded [22]. Risk factors for mortality include older age (HR 1.04), PAH due to systemic sclerosis (HR 8.32), and severe symptoms with higher NYHA-FC (HR 4.71) [22, 23], whereas a better baseline 6-min walk time and a higher resting SaO_2 were associated with a better prognosis [23]. An elevated baseline RAP no longer appears to be associated with a worse outcome, which is likely explained by the consistent use of a risk-minimizing strategy excluding patients with overt RV failure [22]. Whether or not AS improves survival is difficult to establish in the absence of a randomized clinical trial. On the other hand, some investigators [23, 26, 27] have used the equation derived from the NIH registry, based on hemodynamic variables [28]. Although less than ideal, it is an acceptable way to identify a signal for improved survival in the IPAH population. Compared to the NIH equation, 1-year, 2-year, and 3-year survival rates following AS were reported to be as high as 90 vs. 65, 81 vs. 52, and 77 vs. 43%, respectively (table 2) [23, 26, 27]. In a recent study, Sandoval et al. [23] reported the longest experience with AS in severe PAH. In this retrospective analysis, the authors performed 50 procedures in 34 patients. Only 1 death was observed during the procedure. The patients were followed for close to 5 years (58.5 ± 38 months). Interestingly enough, the median survival of 60 months (95% CI: 43–77) matched the previously published data, with an improvement in survival compared with the NIH equation (table 2 and fig. 5a) One of the important lessons of this single-center experience was that of a subgroup of 11 patients (32.6%) who received PAH-targeted pharmacologic treatment at different time intervals after AS (mean: 18 ± 13 months), most of them (82%) within the first 2 years. In this subgroup of 'treated' patients, the median survival for patients on pharmacotherapy additional to AS was 83 months (95% CI: 57–109), which was better than that for patients with AS alone (53 months, 95% CI: 39–67; log-rank: 6.52; p = 0.010; fig. 5b). Although retrospective, this analysis confirms that AS is a safe and effective intervention that may exert a beneficial impact on long-term survival in selected patients. In addition, survival appears to be improved when AS is combined with PAH-specific pharmacotherapy.

Atrial Septostomy in the Current Treatment Algorithm for Pulmonary Arterial Hypertension

Risk-Minimizing Strategy

Despite a significant decrease in procedure-related mortality, AS remains a high-risk intervention as it is performed in compromised patients; however, the risk may be controlled and minimized (table 3). A higher mortality rate has been reported when patients are in overt uncontrolled RV failure, advanced NYHA-FC, and have elevated RAP >20 mm Hg [10, 12, 22]. On the other hand, the

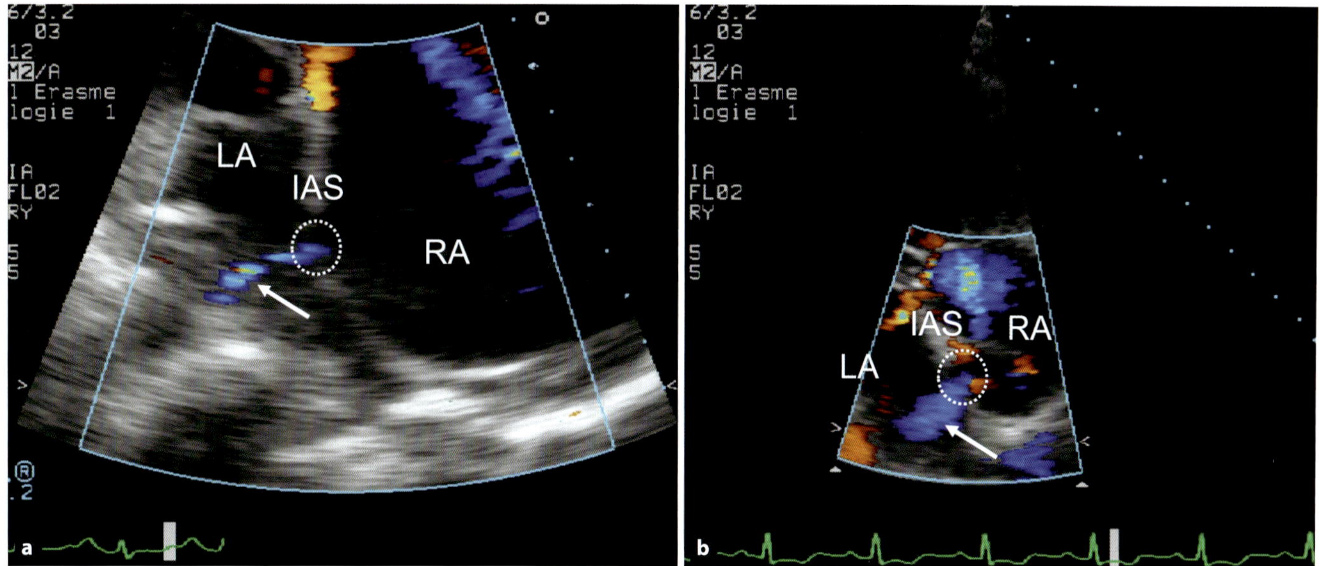

Fig. 4. Visualization of a functional AS by transthoracic echocardiography. **a** Presence of a functional septostomy orifice (dotted circle) 24 h postintervention. The right-to-left shunt is visible in color Doppler (arrow). **b** Persistence and increase in shunt in the same patient, 2 years postintervention. RA = Right atrium.

Table 2. Survival after AS

Study	Number (procedures)	1-year		2-year		3-year	
		predicted	observed	predicted	observed	predicted	observed
Kerstein et al. [28]	13 (13)	62	86	48	73	39	65
Law et al. [26]	43 (46)	68	84	55	77	46	69
Sandoval et al. [23]	34 (50)	65	90	52	81	43	77

Survival values are percentages.

benefit of AS is better in patients with a higher transatrial gradient 10, SaO_2, and 6-min walk time at baseline [23], and in patients receiving PAH-targeted therapies following AS [23].

Timing of Atrial Septostomy

It has to be emphasized that AS should not be offered to patients with end-stage disease or presenting with end-organ damage, such as liver or renal failure. In fact, recent data suggest that the benefit of the procedure may be superior when performed at an earlier stage of disease [13, 15, 23]. As with other high-risk procedures, AS should only be performed in specialized PAH centers with a team of interventional cardiologists experienced in the transseptal approach. A greater clinical benefit is expected in patients with persistent signs of RV failure and/or syncope despite background therapy [22]. In the pediatric population, centers are reporting a remarkable effect on syncope [25]. At our center, it is also considered for all patients who are potential candidates for lung transplantation at time of listing. Table 4 reports the recommendations to minimize the risk of AS [22].

Conclusions

The creation of a right-to-left shunt by AS is an important component of the current treatment strategy for PAH. It is indicated in patients with uncontrolled or rapidly progressive symptoms despite appropriate management. It is also a

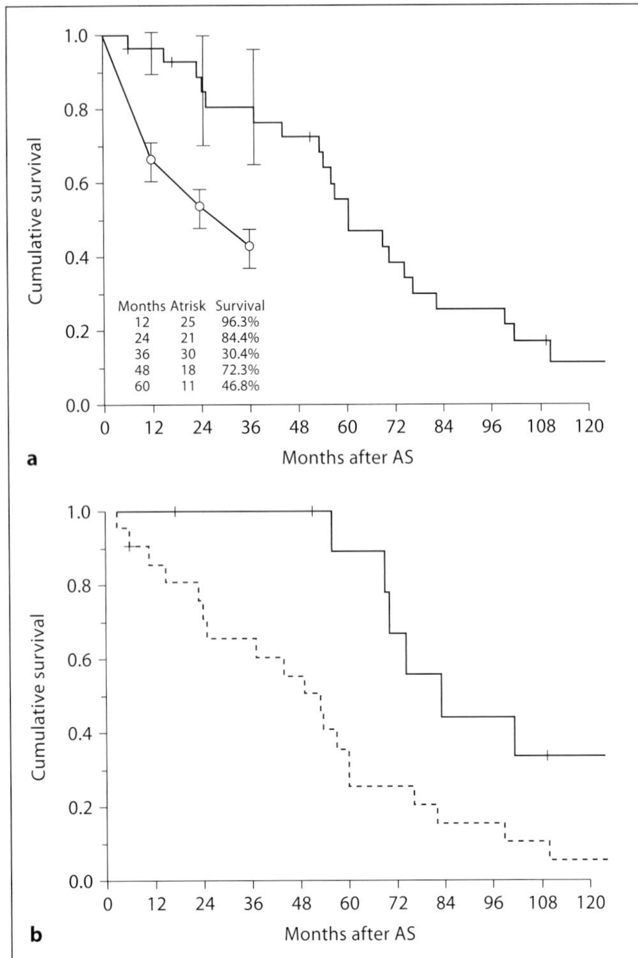

Fig. 5. Survival following AS [23]. **a**: Kaplan-Meier survival estimates after AS in patients with PAH (upper line), compared with predicted survival (open circles, calculated from D'Alonso et al. [28]). Vertical bars represent the 95% CI. **b** Improved survival in patients with AS plus PAH-specific pharmacologic treatment (continuous line) vs. patients with (p = 0.01).

Table 3. Recommendations for a risk-minimizing strategy to decrease mortality [22]

Setting	Strategy
Environment	only in specialized centers for PAH with expertise in transseptal puncture
Preconditioning	in case of severe right heart failure, improve RV function and filling pressures with intravenous diuretics and inotropic support (dobutamine); correction of metabolic and hematological disturbances (hyponatremia, hypokalemia, anemia, thrombocytopenia)
During the procedure	oxygen supplement to achieve an SaO_2 >85–90% anxiolytics and light sedation continuous monitoring of systemic pressure, RAP, and SaO_2 maintain SaO_2 <10% vs. baseline values and >85% stepwise dilatation of the IAS by balloons of increased size (4–16 mm on average), under thorough monitoring of the above-mentioned variables
After the procedure	oxygen therapy to maintain SaO_2 >90% consider blood transfusion in case of fall in hemoglobin level

Table 4. Indications and contraindications for AS

Indications	failure of medical therapy with persisting signs of right heart failure and/or syncope clinical deterioration despite rapid and timely treatment escalation absence of alternative or denial of medical therapy bridge-to-transplantation
Contraindications	RAP >20 mm Hg and/or LA pressure ≥18 mm Hg SaO_2 <90% on room air severely decompensated and/or unstable right heart failure patients under permanent inotropic and/or ventilatory support end-stage disease with short life expectancy (<6 months)

valuable treatment option in countries where medical therapies are too expensive or not available. Although it remains a high-risk procedure, careful patient selection, preconditioning the patients, and thorough stepwise intervention can considerably reduce the risk of serious adverse events. When performed in expert hands, AS not only is able to alleviate symptoms, but may also confer a survival benefit. Many questions remain unanswered, including the benefit of earlier intervention (in less severe patients in whom the benefit of AS may only be present during exercise) and the long-term deleterious effects of chronic hypoxemia in adult patients. Although desirable, a randomized-controlled trial addressing these issues is unlikely to happen, mainly due to cost issues and selection biases, as it cannot be performed in a large number of centers. A more realistic goal may be to establish an international registry with the hope of further exploring the place of this procedure in the management of PAH.

References

1 Simonneau G, Robbins IM, Beghetti M, et al: Updated clinical classification of pulmonary hypertension. J Am Coll Cardiol 2009;54(suppl 1):S43–S54.
2 Galie N, Hoeper MM, Humbert M, et al: Guidelines for the diagnosis and treatment of pulmonary hypertension: the Task Force for the Diagnosis and Treatment of Pulmonary Hypertension of the European Society of Cardiology (ESC) and the European Respiratory Society (ERS), endorsed by the International Society of Heart and Lung Transplantation (ISHLT). Eur Heart J 2009;30:2493–2537.
3 Humbert M, Sitbon O, Chaouat A, et al: Survival in patients with idiopathic, familial, and anorexigen-associated pulmonary arterial hypertension in the modern management era. Circulation 2010;122:156–163.
4 Lordan JL, Corris PA: Pulmonary arterial hypertension and lung transplantation. Expert Rev Respir Med 2011;5:441–454.
5 Bristow MR, Zisman LS, Lowes BD, et al: The pressure-overloaded right ventricle in pulmonary hypertension. Chest 1998;114:101S–106S.
6 Champion HC, Michelakis ED, Hassoun PM: Comprehensive invasive and noninvasive approach to the right ventricle-pulmonary circulation unit: state of the art and clinical and research implications. Circulation 2009;120: 992–1007.
7 Hopkins WE: The remarkable right ventricle of patients with Eisenmenger syndrome. Coron Artery Dis 2005;16:19–25.
8 Hopkins WE, Ochoa LL, Richardson GW, Trulock EP: Comparison of the hemodynamics and survival of adults with severe primary pulmonary hypertension or Eisenmenger syndrome. J Heart Lung Transplant 1996;15:100–105.
9 Rozkovec A, Montanes P, Oakley CM: Factors that influence the outcome of primary pulmonary hypertension. Br Heart J 1986;55:449–458.
10 Sandoval J, Rothman A, Pulido T: Atrial septostomy for pulmonary hypertension. Clin Chest Med 2001;22:547–60.
11 Reichenberger F, Pepke-Zaba J, McNeil K, Parameshwar J, Shapiro LM: Atrial septostomy in the treatment of severe pulmonary arterial hypertension. Thorax 2003;58:797–800.
12 Sandoval J, Gaspar J, Pulido T, et al: Graded balloon dilation atrial septostomy in severe primary pulmonary hypertension: a therapeutic alternative for patients nonresponsive to vasodilator treatment. J Am Coll Cardiol 1998;32:297–304.
13 Vachiéry JL, Stoupel E, Boonstra A, Naeije R. Balloon atrial septostomy for pulmonary hypertension in the prostacyclin era (abstract). Am J Respir Crit Care Med 2003;167:A692.
14 Ciarka A, Vachiéry JL, Houssière A, et al: Atrial septostomy decreases sympathetic overactivity in pulmonary arterial hypertension. Chest 2007;131:1831–1837.
15 Kurzyna M, Dabrowski M, Bielecki D, et al: Atrial septostomy in treatment of end-stage right heart failure in patients with pulmonary hypertension. Chest 2007;131:977–983.
16 Diller GP, Lammers AE, Haworth SG, et al: A modelling study of atrial septostomy for pulmonary arterial hypertension, and its effect on the state of tissue oxygenation and systemic blood flow. Cardiol Young 2010;20:25–32.
17 Zierer A, Melby SJ, Voeller RK, Moon MR: Interatrial shunt for chronic pulmonary hypertension: differential impact of low-flow vs high-flow shunting. Am J Physiol Heart Circ Physiol 2009;296:H639–H644.
18 Austen WG, Morrow AG, Berry WB: Experimental studies of the surgical treatment of primary pulmonary hypertension. J Thorac Cardiovasc Surg 1964;48:448–455.
19 Rashkind WJ: Atrial septostomy in congenital heart disease. Adv Pediatr 1969;16:211–232.
20 Rich S, Lam W: Atrial septostomy as palliative therapy for refractory primary pulmonary hypertension. Am J Cardiol 1983;51:1560–1561.
21 Nihill MR, O'Laughlin MP, Mullins CE: Effects of atrial septostomy in patients with terminal cor pulmonale due to pulmonary vascular disease. Cathet Cardiovasc Diagn 1991;24:166–172.
22 Keogh AM, Mayer E, Benza RL, et al: Interventional and surgical modalities of treatment in pulmonary hypertension. J Am Coll Cardiol 2009;54:S67–S77.
23 Sandoval J, Gaspar J, Peña H, et al: Effect of atrial septostomy on the survival of patients with severe pulmonary arterial hypertension. Eur Respir J 2011;38:1343–1348.
24 Troost E, Delcroix M, Gewillig M, Van Deyk K, Budts W: A modified technique of stent fenestration of the interatrial septum improves patients with pulmonary hypertension. Catheter Cardiovasc Interv 2009;73:173–179.
25 Micheletti A, Hislop AA, Lammers A, et al: Role of atrial septostomy in the treatment of children with pulmonary arterial hypertension. Heart 2006;92:969–972.
26 Law MA, Grifka RG, Mullins CE, Nihill MR: Atrial septostomy improves survival in select patients with pulmonary hypertension. Am Heart J 2007;153:779–784.
27 Kerstein D, Levy PS, Hsu DT, Hordof AJ, Gersony WM, Barst RJ: Blade balloon atrial septostomy in patients with severe primary pulmonary hypertension. Circulation 1995;91:2028–2035.
28 D'Alonso GE, Barst RJ, Ayres SM, et al: Survival in patients with primary pulmonary hypertension. Results of a national prospective study. Ann Intern Med 1991;115:343–349.

Prof. Jean-Luc Vachiéry
Clinique de l'Hypertension Pulmonaire et de l'Insuffisance Cardiaque, Service de Cardiologie
Cliniques Universitaires de Bruxelles, Hôpital Erasme
808 Route de Lennik
BE–1070 Brussels (Belgium)
Tel. +32 25555602, E-Mail Jean-Luc.Vachiery@ulb.ac.be

Humbert M, Souza R, Simonneau G (eds): Pulmonary Vascular Disorders.
Prog Respir Res. Basel, Karger, 2012, vol 41, pp 262–275

Pulmonary Vascular Disorders in Hereditary Hemorrhagic Telangiectasia

Vincent Cottin[a,c] · Chahéra Khouatra[a,c] · Sophie Dupuis-Girod[b,c] · Jean-François Cordier[a,c]

[a]Hospices Civils de Lyon, Hôpital Louis Pradel, Service de Pneumologie, Centre de référence national des maladies pulmonaires rares, Université de Lyon, Université Lyon I, INRA, UMR754 INRA-Vetagrosup EPHE IFR 128, [b]Hospices Civils de Lyon, Hôpital Louis Pradel, Service de génétique, and [c]Centre de référence national de la maladie de Rendu-Osler; Research Network on Rendu-Osler Disease, Lyon, France

Abstract

Hereditary hemorrhagic telangiectasia (HHT) is a genetic disorder with autosomal dominance and variable penetrance, characterized by epistaxis, telangiectasia, and visceral manifestations, with an estimated prevalence of 1 in 6,000. Causative mutations have been identified in either the *ENG* or the *ACVRL1* genes coding for endoglin and ALK1, respectively. Pulmonary vascular manifestations of HHT include especially pulmonary arteriovenous malformations (PAVMs; mainly in patients with mutations of *ENG*) and less frequently pulmonary hypertension (PH; mainly in patients with mutations of *ACVRL1*). PAVMs are present in 10–25% of patients with *ACVRL1* mutations and up to 50% of patients with *ENG* mutations. Although PAVMs may remain asymptomatic, they may cause a variety of manifestations, which are often severe and include hypoxemia due to right-to-left shunting, dyspnea on exertion, transient ischemic attacks or cerebral strokes, systemic severe infections (especially cerebral abscesses), and rarely massive hemoptysis or hemothorax. Treatment of PAVMs is based on transcatheter coil vaso-occlusion, which dramatically reduces the risk of complications. However, long-term follow-up is warranted after treatment due to possible recanalization of treated PAVMs and development or growth of untreated PAVMs. Systematic screening for PAVM is recommended in all adult HHT patients and symptomatic children. Contrast echocardiography (preceded by chest radiograph) is the method of choice for noninvasive screening, with the alternative of chest CT. Patients with HHT and their relatives should be informed of the risk of serious complications from PAVMs frequently occurring in asymptomatic individuals. PH is rare in HHT. Detected by echocardiography, PH is confirmed by right heart catheterization showing elevated mean pulmonary arterial pressure. Distinguishing between PH associated with liver AVMs causing high cardiac output and left heart failure, or genuine pulmonary arterial hypertension (PAH), is critical for management. In PH with high-output heart failure, the cardiac output is elevated, pulmonary vascular resistance is normal or decreased, and pulmonary capillary wedge pressure is often elevated; management includes diuretics, correction of anemia, consideration for liver transplantation, and possibly bevacizumab. In PAH, cardiac output is normal or decreased, pulmonary capillary wedge pressure is normal, and pulmonary vascular resistance is elevated; whether medical therapy specific for pulmonary arterial pressure may be beneficial in these patients is unknown.

Overview and Diagnosis of Hereditary Hemorrhagic Telangiectasia

Clinical Diagnosis of Hereditary Hemorrhagic Telangiectasia

Hereditary hemorrhagic telangiectasia (HHT), or Rendu-Osler-Weber disease, is a genetic disease, with autosomal dominant inheritance. Common symptoms are dominated by frequent (several times a week in some patients) and possibly abundant epistaxis (which may alter the quality of life), telangiectases on the lips and fingertips, and anemia often requiring iron supplementation due to recurrent nasal and gastrointestinal bleeding. However, the severity of the disease is mostly related to lung (and occasionally liver or brain) involvement by arteriovenous malformations (AVMs) [1].

HHT affects approximately 1 in 6,000 individuals, with important geographic disparities. In particular, there are areas of higher prevalence such as the French department of Ain, Vermont in the USA, and the Netherlands Antilles.

Table 1. Diagnostic criteria ('Curaçao criteria') for the diagnosis of HHT [2]

Epistaxis	spontaneous, recurrent nose bleeds
Telangiectases	multiple, at characteristic sites: lips, oral cavity, fingers, nose
Visceral lesions	gastrointestinal telangiectasia (with or without bleeding) PAVM hepatic AVM cerebral AVM spinal AVM
Family history	a first-degree relative with HHT according to these criteria

The diagnosis is definite if 3 criteria are present, possible or suspected if 2 criteria are present, and unlikely if fewer than 2 criteria are present.

HHT is therefore one of the most common monogenic diseases, although nonsevere cases without visceral involvement or uncomplicated AVMs are likely underdiagnosed.

Clinical manifestations may gradually appear or worsen over time, with penetrance generally complete by the fifth decade. Epistaxes, usually the first symptom, often begin by the age of 10 years, are present by the age of 20 years in half the patients, and later increase in severity. Telangiectases similarly develop with age, generally between the second and fifth decades of life, and are present in half the patients by the age of 30 years. Telangiectases in HHT typically affect the lips, tongue, palate, fingers, and face, and may resemble those found in systemic sclerosis. Telangiectases of conjunctiva, trunk, arms, and nail beds are less characteristic of HHT.

The diagnosis of HHT is based on the clinical so-called 'Curaçao criteria' [2] (table 1). The clinical diagnosis of HHT may, however, be challenging especially in young subjects with epistaxis yet no or few telangiectases, in patients with limited or no epistaxis and telangiectasia, and in subjects who have little medical information about their relatives [3].

Molecular Diagnostic Testing and Genetic Counseling

Molecular diagnostic testing for HHT can confirm the diagnosis in a given individual and his/her family. However, molecular testing is not necessary in every patient with HHT, especially if clinically established. Direct sequencing of the *ENG* and *ACVRL1* genes may be useful in subjects with possible HHT according to the Curaçao criteria [4] and for early diagnosis. As no mutation is found in 15–20% of HHT families, absence of mutation does not rule out the diagnosis.

Molecular testing is mostly useful for genetic counseling, i.e. evaluation of risk of transmission of disease in apparently unaffected individuals. However, genetic counseling is complex in HHT due to late onset penetrance, variable expressivity, partially understood phenotype-genotype correlations, and molecular diversity of the disease. In children of patients with HHT (who have a theoretical risk at birth of having HHT of 50%, but with progressive onset of clinical manifestations with age), the diagnosis cannot be ruled out on the basis of absence of symptoms and signs; however, molecular diagnosis can be proposed if the causative mutation has been identified in the family. The potential impact of genetic testing on psychological issues and insurance should not be underestimated and should be balanced with the anticipated medical benefit after informed discussion with the individual.

Overview of Hereditary Hemorrhagic Telangiectasia Complications

The potential severity of HHT emanates from visceral manifestations (table 2), and especially from pulmonary vascular manifestations, with frequent pulmonary AVMs (PAVMs) that may cause right-to-left shunting with hypoxemia and increased risk of cerebral abscess and ischemic cerebral stroke, and rarely pulmonary hypertension (PH) of varied mechanisms. Nosebleeds may manifest as massive hemorrhaging requiring blood perfusion. Gastrointestinal telangiectasia may be responsible for acute hemorrhages, which may require multiple blood perfusion and endoscopic treatment in a minority of patients. Liver AVMs may cause left-to-right shunting and hyperdynamic PH. Cerebral AVMs rarely cause intracerebral and subarachnoidal hemorrhaging; however, central nervous symptoms in HHT patients are more often related to infections complicating PAVMs. Complications may arise from associated juvenile polyposis, but rarely. Overall, HHT can shorten the life expectancy by a mean of 7 years, especially when left untreated.

Other complications of visceral involvement by HHT include chronic bleeding from gastrointestinal telangiectasia, with iron deficiency and anemia, and bleeding from telangiectasia of the skin or oral mucosa (rarely severe). Cerebral AVMs may cause headaches. The prevalence of migraine is higher than in the general population, especially in patients with PAVMs. More recently, a potential immune dysfunction and a prothrombotic state associated

Table 2. Visceral manifestations of HHT and management principles

Manifestation/lesion	Prevalence	Presentation	Treatment principles
Epistaxis/telangiectasia of nasal mucosa	>90%	epistaxis beginning in childhood, often inaugural of HHT; mild epistaxis, recurrent epistaxis causing anemia, or massive acute hemorrhage	acute bleeding: local treatment with packing; recurrent bleeding: humidification, lubricants, septal dermatoplasty, KTP laser, iron supplementation, tranexamic acid, bevacizumab (?)
Mucocutaneous telangiectasia (face, lips, oral cavity, tongue, ears, fingertips)	80%	cosmetic consequences; bleeding usually mild	usually none indicated
Telangiectasia (and rarely aneurysms, or AVMs) of the gastrointestinal tract	15–30%	asymptomatic anemia detected by annual screen over 35 years, or iron deficiency from chronic bleeding, occasionally acute gastrointestinal hemorrhage	iron supplementation, blood transfusion, one or two endoscopic laser therapy, consider medical therapy (hormonal, antifibrolytic)
Pulmonary AVMs	5–10% in HHT2, 50% in HHT1	asymptomatic in most; hypoxemia, exercise dyspnea, systemic abscess especially cerebral abscess, ischemic cerebral stroke; increased risk of migraine; rarely hemoptysis or hemothorax	transcatheter vaso-occlusion; surgical resection in life-threatening bleeding; antibiotic prophylaxis for any procedure at risk of bacteremia; avoid scuba diving and particular caution to avoid injection of air through intravenous access
PAH	<1%	dyspnea on exertion; screening and detection by echocardiography; diagnosis by right heart catheterization	medical therapies of PAH
Hepatic vascular malformations	>30%	asymptomatic in most; dyspnea on exertion if high cardiac output and passive PH (hepatic AVMs); portal hypertension (hepatoportal malformations); biliary ischemia (portohepatic venous malformations)	treatment of liver AVMs (consider liver transplantation), avoid liver biopsy and hepatic artery embolization
Cerebral AVMs	15%	asymptomatic, headache, epilepsy, ischemia due a vascular steal effect, hemorrhage	follow-up, microsurgical excision, stereotactic radiotherapy, embolization, according to individual risk assessment
Conjunctival telangiectasia	up to 45%	asymptomatic, 'bloody tears'	usually none indicated

with increased plasma levels of factor VIII have been reported in HHT, the clinical relevance of which is still unclear.

HHT must be differentiated from other disorders with epistaxis, telangiectasia, and/or visceral AVMs that may falsely fulfill the Curaçao criteria, including the syndrome of cutaneous capillary malformation and visceral AVM, the Adams-Oliver syndrome (with cutaneous telangiectasia, PAVMs, and scalp and limb congenital defects), the Wyburn-Mason syndrome with retinocephalic vascular malformation, and von Willebrand disease with frequent epistaxis and possible telangiectasia.

Pathogenesis of Hereditary Hemorrhagic Telangiectasia: From Genes to Vessel Malformations

Genotypes of Hereditary Hemorrhagic Telangiectasia

HHT clinically segregates as an autosomal dominant inherited disease, with variable inter- and intrafamilial expressivity and late onset penetrance. Most patients with HHT carry mutations in the genes *ENG* coding for endoglin or *ACVRL1* coding for the activin receptor-like kinase (ALK1) [5] (table 3). The respective frequency of *ENG* or *ACVRL1* mutations in HHT patients varies between series and according to potential bias in patient selection (e.g. predominance of

Table 3. Locus and genes identified in HHT

Locus	Gene (location)	Protein	OMIM No.	Clinical specificities
HHT1	*ENG* (9q33-34)	endoglin	187300	increased risk of pulmonary and cerebral AVMs; symptomatic liver involvement rare
HHT2	*AVCRL1* (12q11-14)	ALK-1 (activin receptor-like kinase)	600376	increased risk of hepatic AVMs and postcapillary PH, and of PAH; increased risk of pancreatic AVMs (?); earlier cutaneous telangiectasia, later onset of epistaxis
HHT3	? (5q)	?	N/A	
HHT4	? (7p)	?	N/A	
?	*MADH4* (18q21.1)	SMAD4	175050	associated with juvenile polyposis; this genotype represents no more than 1–2% of cases of HHT

Additional loci have been reported on chromosome 5 and 7p14 with unidentified genes. N/A = Not applicable.

ENG mutations in families with high prevalence of PAVM). In addition, germinal mutations have been described in the gene *madh4 (mothers against decapentaplegic homologue 4)* coding for the protein Smad4 in patients with a syndrome of combined familial juvenile polyposis (otherwise caused by mutations of *BMPRIA*) and HHT. At least two further loci (and unidentified genes) seem to be involved in patients with HHT. In addition, some cases of HHT with no detectable mutation may be caused by a mosaic *ENG* or *ACVRL1* mutation below the current limit of detection of molecular screening methods. The involvement of several genes in HHT may contribute to the clinical heterogeneity of the disease. Whether the disease phenotype may be influenced by modifier genes or environmental factors is unknown.

More than 600 mutations (deletions, duplications, splice site mutations, missense mutations) have been described throughout the *ENG* and *ACVRL1* genes [5], with most mutations causing haploinsufficiency, and some causing a dominant-negative effect. Confirmation of the responsibility of these genes in the pathogenesis of the disease has been obtained from experimental animal models, with vascular abnormalities (including telangiectases and epistaxis) reproduced by gene inactivation [5]. Founder effects were demonstrated especially for mutations of *ACVRL1*.

Genotype-Phenotype Correlations

Genotype-phenotype correlations in HHT have identified different prevalence rates of visceral involvement according to the genotype (table 3). Mutations of the *ENG* gene (HHT1) are associated with an increased risk of PAVMs (approx. 50%), as compared to those of the *ACVRL1* gene (approx. 10–25%) [6, 7]. No correlation has been consistently found between specific mutations and the risk of PAVM. The risk of developing PAVM may vary considerably among family members. Interestingly, PAVMs may be clustered in families with mutations of *ENG* [6], suggesting that screening for PAVM may be of particular importance in patients with a family history of PAVM, symptomatic or not. Both postcapillary PH and pulmonary arterial hypertension (PAH) are more frequently found in patients carrying mutations of *ACVRL1* (HHT2).

Molecular Signaling

All three genes implicated in HHT code for members of the transforming growth factor-β (TGF-β) superfamily of proteins and play a role in signal transduction in endothelial cells [5]. TGF-β signaling is involved in a variety of cellular physiologic processes, including cell proliferation, apoptosis, and cell homeostasis of endothelial cells and smooth muscle cells. Defects in TGF-β signaling may explain abnormalities in vasculogenesis and angiogenesis in HHT.

ALK1 and endoglin function as type I and type III membrane receptors, respectively, and Smad4 is an intracellular signaling second messenger (activated following ligand binding to a cell surface heteromeric complex of type I and type II receptors). Endoglin associates with multiple receptor complexes including ALK1. ALK1 mostly interacts with bone morphogenetic protein receptor type 2 (BMPR2) and TβRII. Ligands for ALK1 are BMP9 and BMP10. It is currently considered that endoglin, ALK1, and Smad4 may be components of a common signal transduction pathway that is perturbed in HHT [5], with cooperative effects of type I and type II receptors. In the future, better understanding of the fine regulation of this signaling pathway by members of the TGF-β superfamily of proteins may clarify the pathogenesis of HHT.

Further progress in disease pathogenesis has come from the identification of mutations in *BMPR2* in up to 58–74% of patients with familial (or heritable) PAH and in 3–40% of patients with idiopathic PAH [8]. Mutations of the *ACVRL1* and *Smad8* genes have also been described in a few patients with idiopathic PAH in the absence of clinical HHT. Such mutations may schematically contribute to proliferation of smooth muscle cells and apoptosis of endothelial cells, and predispose to PAH. Individuals carrying mutations of *BMPR2* or *ACVRL1* develop more severe PAH, with earlier onset, as compared to their counterparts without identified mutation [9, 10]. In HHT, both postcapillary PH resulting from increased cardiac output due to liver AVMs, and much more rarely isolated PAH indistinguishable from idiopathic PAH, mostly occur in patients who have mutations of the *ACVRL1* gene. Another case of PAH has been described in an HHT patient with a mutation in the *ENG* gene and who had taken dexfenfluramine. These findings support the notion that endothelium cell dysfunction related to mutations within the TGF-β signaling pathway may both cause HHT and predispose to PAH, with other environmental and possibly genetic factors involved. How mutations within the *ACVRL1* gene can give rise to HHT, PAH, or both, remains to be elucidated.

Development of Abnormal Vessels

How mutations of *ENG*, *ACVRL1*, or *Smad4* can give rise to vascular malformations in HHT has been reviewed [5]. Recent work has shown that AVMs represent enlargement and stabilization of normally transient arteriovenous connections. Based on mouse models of HHT which develop HHT-like AVMs, haploinsufficiency of the endoglin or ALK1 proteins (caused by mutations within one of two gene alleles) may result in the inability of blood vessels to mature appropriately, with ensuing aberrant response to vessel injury and angiogenesis. According to this model, AVMs would therefore develop in HHT preferentially in the local setting of angiogenesis, with proliferation of endothelial cells driven by vascular endothelial growth factor-A, but impaired recruitment of surrounding mural cells (pericytes or smooth muscle cells) to angiogenic sprouts due to the mutations of *ENG* or *ACVRL1* [5]. This process may be amplified by reactive oxygen species. ALK1 has further been shown to play a role in transducing hemodynamic forces into a biochemical signal required to limit nascent vessel caliber; altered blood flow in pathologically enlarged arteries may precipitate a flow-dependent adaptive response with further development of arteriovenous connections that are normally transient.

Pulmonary Arteriovenous Malformations

Definition and Prevalence

PAVMs are abnormal communications between pulmonary arteries and pulmonary veins, i.e. direct communication of arteries and veins without the intermediary of a normal capillary network, and PAVMs cause right-to-left shunting and potentially hypoxemia. In less than 5% of cases, the PAVM may involve a systemic artery rather than pulmonary artery, with no consequences on hematosis [11]. PAVMs vascularized by more than one branch of pulmonary artery or drained by multiple segmental pulmonary veins are labeled complex PAVMs.

PAVMs predominate in the lower lobes (60–95%) and are multiple in about half the cases [3] (fig. 1). They are more frequent in women, with a sex ratio varying between 1:1.5 and 1:1.9 [11]. No side predominance has been reported. The median age at the diagnosis of a PAVM was 42 years in a large series, with extreme values of 10–79 years, and equal distribution between the ages of 20 and 75 years [3]. PAVMs have also been reported in children and infants.

Similar to other manifestations of HHT, the prevalence of PAVMs has been reported to increase with age, with a prevalence of up to 50% during the fifth decade in patients with *ENG* mutations, and an estimated prevalence of 23% of PAVM in HHT patients undergoing systematic screening [6]. A higher frequency (41–65%) has been reported when considering the presence of intrapulmonary right-to-left shunting as evidenced by contrast echocardiography rather than definite PAVMs on chest CT.

Up to 15% of patients with PAVM do not have other manifestations of HHT and do not carry mutations of HHT genes. So-called idiopathic PAVMs are anatomically similar to HHT-related PAVMs except for a greater number of solitary PAVMs (80%) and a lack of lower lobe predominance [12]. The clinical manifestations and complications of idiopathic PAVMs are similar to those associated with HHT.

Occasionally, HHT patients present with countless 'diffuse' PAVMs of various size and are responsible for massive right-to-left shunting [13] (fig. 2). More common in women, diffuse PAVMs (defined as at least one segment of the lungs diffusely involved by PAVMs) are associated with an increased risk of death from various causes including hemoptysis of bronchial artery origin. Management is particularly difficult and should be conducted in experimented centers;

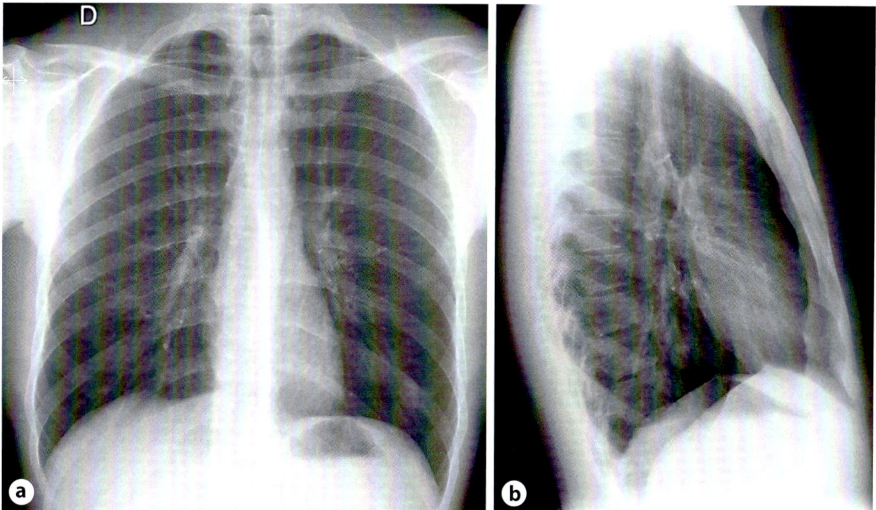

Fig. 1. Chest radiograph of a PAVM of the left lower lobe: anteroposterior view (**a**) and lateral view (**b**).

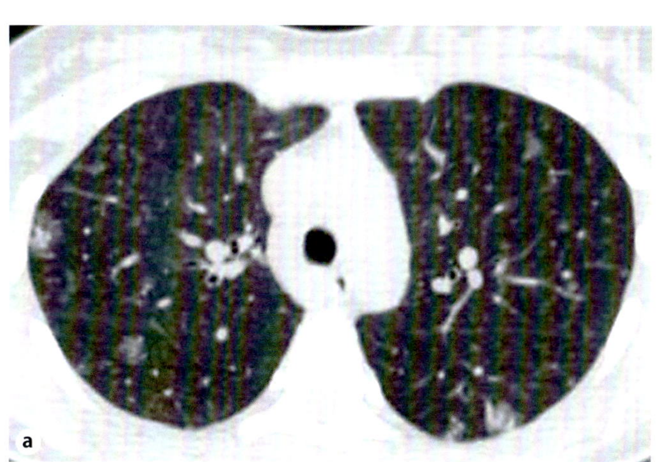

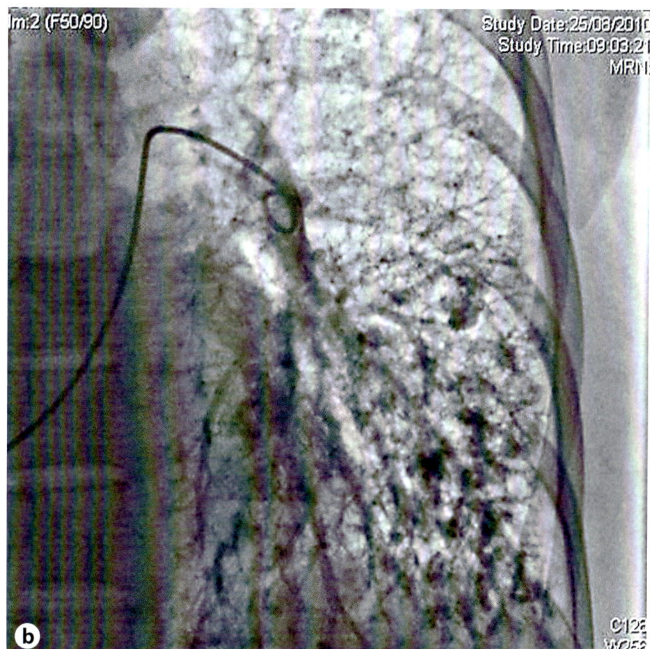

Fig. 2. Diffuse PAVMs: CT of the chest (**a**) and pulmonary angiography (**b**).

however, transcatheter percutaneous vaso-occlusion of diffuse PAVMs can be performed in a majority of cases [14]. Lung transplantation may be indicated in selected cases.

Clinical Manifestations and Complications
Most PAVMs are currently diagnosed by systematic screening or incidental imaging findings, or revealed by neurological complications, while dyspnea reveals the presence of PAVMs in only 22% of cases [3]. Dyspnea on exertion, present in about half of the patients with PAVM, is the most frequent respiratory symptom of PAVM and is related to the severity of right-to-left shunting. However, a large number of patients with PAVM may tolerate severe hypoxemia with only little dyspnea. Therefore, screening for PAVMs cannot rely simply on clinical symptoms.

Other respiratory symptoms may include hemoptysis (about 10% of patients), chest pain (6%), finger clubbing (about 20%), cyanosis (18%), and thoracic murmur (3%)

at clinical examination [3]. Cyanosis may be absent in anemic patients with recurrent nose or gastrointestinal bleeding and iron deficiency, or rarely may be prominent in case of hypoxemia-related erythrocytosis. Hemoptysis in patients with HHT may be due to either bronchial telangiectasia or PAVM (with risk of massive hemoptysis in case of bleeding PAVM).

Severe and possibly lethal hemorrhagic complications of PAVM have been described in fewer than 10% patients with HHT and PAVM, related to the intrabronchial or intrapleural rupture of PAVM with ensuing hemoptysis or hemothorax [1]. The risk of severe bleeding from PAVMs may be decreased by vaso-occlusion, but this has not been prospectively evaluated.

PAVMs may cause potentially severe complications, especially severe infections and central nervous system manifestations such as transient ischemic attack, cerebral stroke, and cerebral abscess. Such complications frequently reveal the diagnosis of PAVM and even of HHT itself. Infectious and embolic manifestations are attributed to the right-to-left shunting that bypasses the capillary bed and facilitates the passage of thrombotic emboli and bacteria into the systemic and especially cerebral circulation, similarly to what is observed in congenital cyanotic heart disease. Other severe infections may occur [15], including abscesses of the kidney, knee, spinal cord, liver, and soft tissue, as well as meningitis, septicemia, endocarditis, and bacterial spondylodiscitis. Moderate abnormalities of the immune system, especially phagocytic cells in HHT, might contribute to infections independently of right-to-left shunting and PAVM.

Brain abscess, which may be (not exceptionally) the presenting manifestation leading to the diagnosis of HHT, occurs in 5–9% of patients with HHT and 5–19% of patients with HHT and PAVM [3, 11] (9.1% in the largest series to date [7]) (fig. 3). Brain abscess occurs at a younger age than in the general population. The risk of brain abscess is mostly influenced by the severity of the right-to-left shunting, and may be increased in patients with multiple PAVMs, especially when the feeding artery of the PAVM exceeds 3 mm in diameter. Cerebral abscesses in HHT are frequently due to multiple anaerobic organisms, and may follow dental or parondontal procedures, but septic foci are seldom identified.

PAVMs are also associated with an increased risk of ischemic cerebral events, including ischemic strokes in 10–19% of patients with PAVMs, and transient cerebral ischemic attack in 6–37% of patients [3]. Clinical consequences of ischemic cerebral complications are particularly devastating considering their young age of onset in HHT patients (41 years of age in HHT compared to 63 years in the general population). Neurologic manifestations are much more frequently related to the PAVM than to hemorrhagic cerebral AVM.

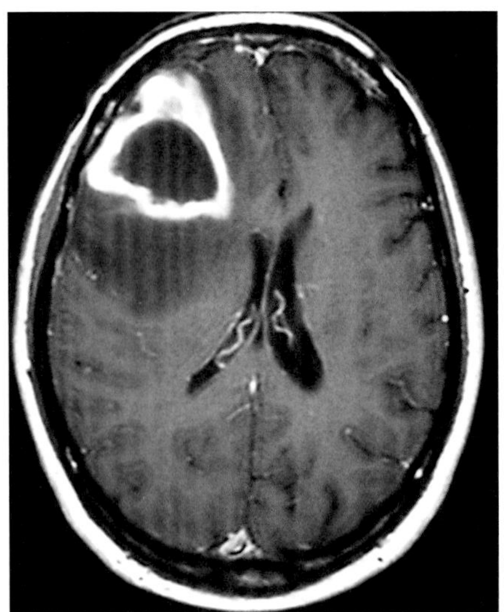

Fig. 3. CT of the brain showing cerebral abscess revealing PAVMs in a patient with HHT.

The presence of PAVMs is also associated with a significant increase in the prevalence of migraine (particularly with aura), as also reported in non-HHT patients with patent foramen ovale. Similarly, the prevalence of PAVM is higher in patients with migraine among the HHT population (50 vs. 36%). The risk of migraine in patients with PAVMs may be increased by the lack of trapping of vasoactive substances by bypassing the pulmonary capillary circulation.

Imaging

Helical multidetector CT scan of the chest is now the gold standard for the diagnosis of PAVM, based on the presence of a nodular or rounded opacity of variable size, with both afferent and efferent vessels (the latter with larger size) (fig. 4, 5). Unenhanced multidetector thoracic CT with thin cut (1–2 mm) reconstructions is the recommended method for PAVM screening and diagnosis [4]. Intravenous injection of contrast medium shows considerable enhancement of the PAVM, allowing differential diagnosis from other nodules, and assessment of perfusion [16]. Posttreatment CT images and 3-dimensional reconstruction may contribute to the definitive diagnosis of PAVM. In addition, chest CT may show nonspecific micronodules potentially corresponding to small (and not treatable) PAVMs [17]. Other vascular

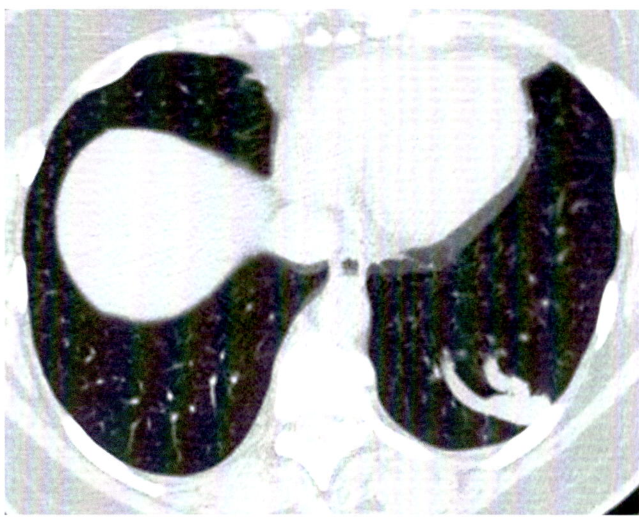

Fig. 4. CT of the chest showing a PAVM of the left lower lobe. Note the visibility of both the afferent and efferent vessels.

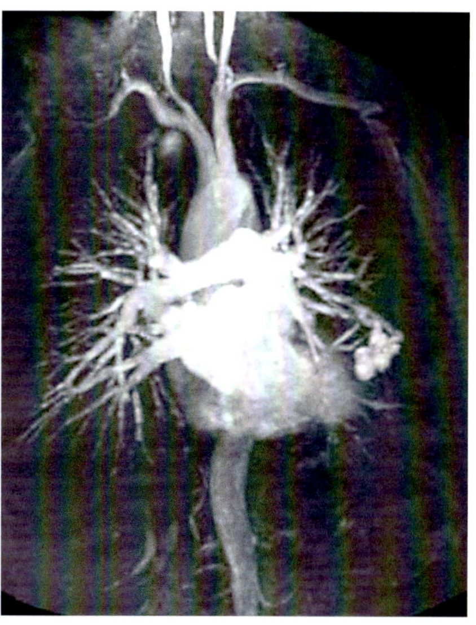

Fig. 6. MRI of the chest showing PAVM. Note the visibility of both the afferent and efferent vessels.

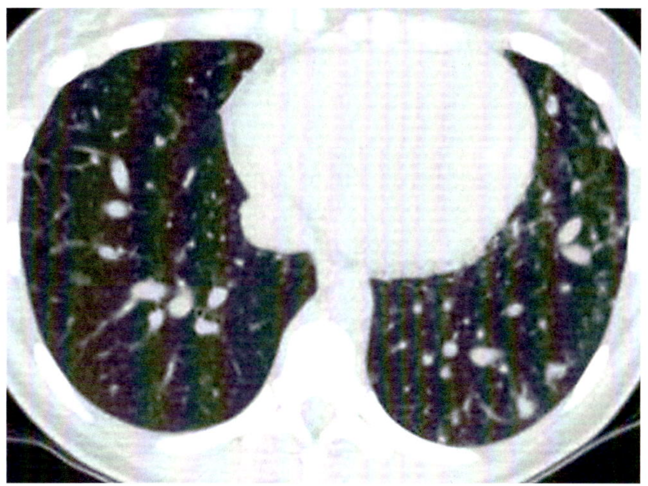

Fig. 5. CT of the chest showing multiple PAVMs in a patient with HHT.

malformations such as pulmonary varices (not reported in HHT) may be occasionally mistaken for PAVM, although the diagnosis may be corrected when checking for the presence of both the afferent and efferent vessels of the putative PAVM.

The sensitivity of chest CT has been demonstrated to be higher (97%) than that of pulmonary angiography [16]. The main limitation to the use of chest CT is related to irradiation. The use of pulmonary angiography is now restricted to transcatheter treatment of PAVMs. Angiographic MRI is not as efficient as helical CT for the diagnosis of PAVM; however, 4-dimensional time-resolved magnetic resonance angiography (fig. 6) is a promising tool for the noninvasive and radiation-free evaluation of PAVM patency [18]. PAVM may be also visible on a plain chest radiograph as a rounded or oblong opacity, 1–5 cm in diameter, and with branching vessels, but smaller PAVM may not be visible.

Assessment of Right-to-Left Shunting

Transthoracic contrast echocardiography is the method of choice for the assessment of right-to-left shunting in HHT [17]. Transthoracic contrast echocardiography is performed by injecting 4–5 ml of agitated modified fluid gelatin or isotonic saline solution with 0.5 ml room air into a peripheral vein while simultaneously imaging the atria with 2-dimensional echocardiography. It allows to directly visualize the right-to-left shunt and to differentiate intracardiac shunting (that may be due to coincidental patent foramen ovale) from intrapulmonary shunting (due to PAVMs in HHT, hepatopulmonary syndrome in patients with liver cirrhosis, etc.). Semiquantification of the shunt by echocardiography improves the prediction of PAVM [19]. One pitfall of contrast echocardiography is that it is positive in a proportion of patients with no visible PAVM on chest CT [17]. It also remains positive after endovascular treatment of PAVM in up to 90% of patients, even when no residual PAVM is seen on pulmonary angiography [20], likely corresponding to microscopic PAVMs not amenable to vaso-

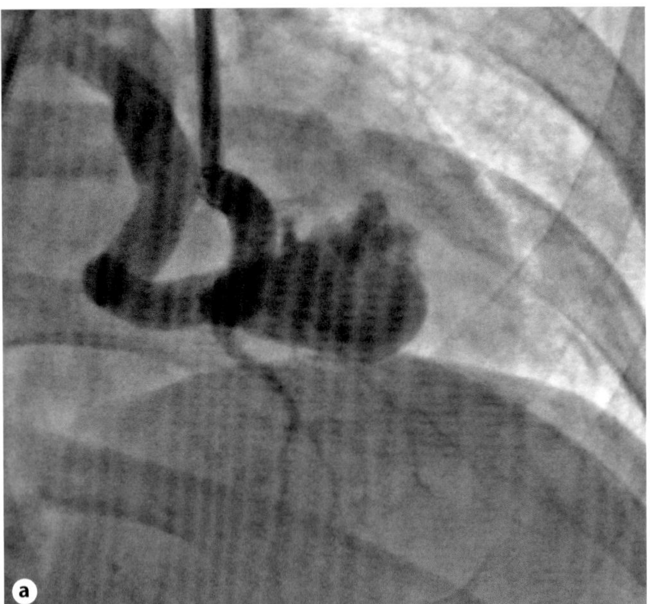

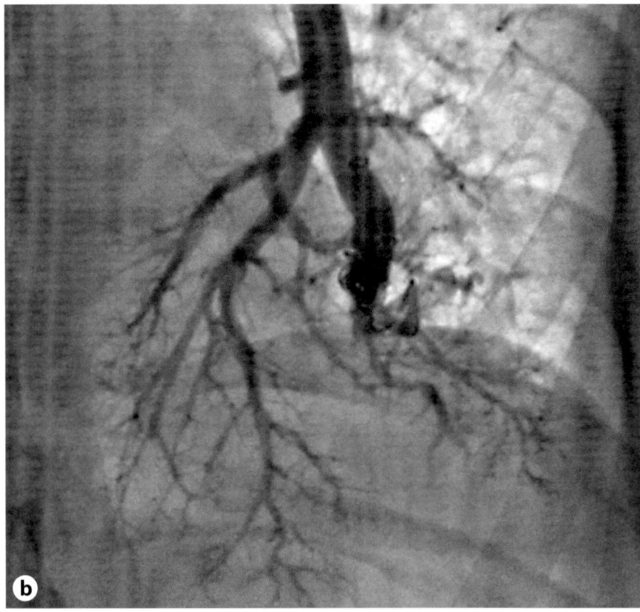

Fig. 7. Pulmonary angiography of a PAVM before (**a**) and after (**b**) transcatheter vaso-occlusion using coils.

occlusion therapy. It is not known whether such microscopic PAVMs can evolve over the years to treatable PAVMs with a risk of complications; long-term follow-up may be appropriate in these patients, with repeated diagnostic investigations for PAVM after several years.

Hypoxemia due to right-to-left shunting may be severe in patients with PAVMs. Classical orthodeoxia present in only a minority of patients with large PAVMs has low diagnostic value [17]. Increased alveolar-arterial oxygen difference of partial pressure of oxygen under 100% oxygen indicates with excellent specificity that hypoxemia is related to PAVMs causing right-to-left shunting; however, this test has insufficient sensitivity for screening and suffers from suboptimal reproducibility. It may be used for quantification of right-to-left shunting rather than for screening purposes. Of note, alveolar-arterial oxygen difference of partial pressure of oxygen under 100% oxygen is usually normal in patients with hepatopulmonary syndrome, another cause of intrapulmonary right-to-left shunting with positive contrast echocardiography. Partial pressure of carbon dioxide is normal or low. Radionuclide lung scanning, which has been largely used in the past to assess for right-to-left shunting, is expensive, not widely available, and no longer recommended in HHT. Spirometry is normal in a majority of HHT patients. A mild decrease in transfer coefficient for carbon monoxide has been reported in patients with HHT.

Treatment of Pulmonary Arteriovenous Malformations

Treatment of PAVMs in HHT aims at preventing severe complications, especially brain abscesses, ischemic strokes, and hemorrhage; therefore, treatment is warranted even in asymptomatic patients [4]. Occlusion of PAVM will also correct hypoxemia and dyspnea on exertion when present. Antibiotic prophylaxis is recommended in patients with PAVM prior to potentially bacteremic procedures [4]. We also advocate prophylactic treatment in all HHT patients with positive contrast echocardiography, including those with no visible PAVM on chest CT. Antibiotic prophylaxis in HHT patients should follow recommendations for the prevention of infectious endocarditis [4]. Scuba diving is contraindicated due to the risk of air embolism [4]. The use of air filters is recommended for intravenous infusion to prevent air embolism and transient ischemic attacks.

Transcatheter vaso-occlusion of PAVMs using detachable steel coils ('embolization therapy') is the recommended therapy [4, 21] (fig. 7). Other devices are occasionally used, especially Amplatzer occluders for PAVMs with very large feeding vessels [21]. Treatment of PAVMs is particularly indicated when the feeding vessel(s) of the PAVM is (are) 3 mm or more, but treatment of smaller PAVMs with right-to-left shunting is also justified when technically feasible [4]. Five to 10 PAVMs can be occluded within one procedure, but several procedures can be required to occlude all visible PAVMs. The vaso-occlusion must be performed by radiologists experienced in the management and treatment of HHT-related PAVMs to decrease the risk of complications and improve efficacy [4].

Major complications of the vaso-occlusion of PAVMs are rare. These include symptomatic lung infarction, systemic migration of the coils, as well as air embolism and exceptionally transient angina, cardiac arrhythmia, deep venous thrombosis, or pneumothorax. Infections related to the procedure are prevented by prophylactic antibiotherapy. More frequent benign complications such as pleural pain and transient pleural effusion improve with symptomatic treatment.

Vaso-occlusion of PAVMs immediately decrease right-to-left shunting, improves arterial blood gases, and corrects dyspnea [4], whereas residual hypoxemia and positive cardiac contrast echocardiography are frequent. Indirect evidence has demonstrated that the risk of infection and cerebral ischemic events is greatly reduced (yet not totally suppressed) by transcatheter embolization. Reduction in the frequency and severity of migraines is also obtained. Vaso-occlusion may decrease the risk of bleeding from PAVMs.

The overall long-term success rate of vaso-occlusion is greater than 75–80%; however, a proportion of patients will need further therapy. Long-term follow-up is therefore mandatory in all HHT patients diagnosed with PAVMs, treated or not. PAVMs may repermeabilize over time, or initially small PAVMs not requiring vaso-occlusion may grow. Vaso-occlusion of large PAVMs may unmask or facilitate the development of new PAVMs. Detection of reperfused PAVMs is recommended, as they may be successfully treated by repeated vaso-occlusion in a majority of cases.

The best monitoring modalities following vaso-occlusion have not been established. Chest CT is currently the best investigation to evaluate potential perfusion of previously treated PAVMs and the need to repeat the procedure, especially evaluation of efferent vessels (that should be collapsed if vaso-occlusion is efficient). Chest CT may be performed 3–12 months after the vaso-occlusion, then repeated every 3 years thereafter; small untreated PAVMs may be followed every 1–5 years. MRI may also be useful for follow-up [18], obviating the frequent artefacts of chest CT in patients with metallic coils.

Although high-flow PAVMs contribute to low pulmonary vascular resistance and may, therefore, protect from PH, they may coexist with PH in a small proportion of HHT patients, with significant challenge for management. PH and (or) increased cardiac output may increase the risk of rupture of the PAVMs [22]. When present, severe PH is usually considered a contra-indication for vaso-occlusion of pulmonary AVMs because of potential worsening of PH and possible increased risk associated with the procedure. However, vaso-occlusion of PAVMs does not consistently increase the mean pulmonary artery pressure in HHT patients without severe PH, although it may increase in selected individuals.

Surgical treatment of PAVMs consisting of conservative resection of lung lobes or segments is now restricted to complex or multiple PAVMs not amenable to transcatheter therapy, or is used as an emergency procedure for hemothorax (occasionally in combination with endovascular treatment). Lung transplantation has been done in rare HHT patients with severe and diffuse PAVMs.

Screening for Pulmonary Arteriovenous Malformations

Screening for PAVMs is justified in all patients with HHT due to the high risk of severe complications that are largely prevented by treatment of PAVM. Patients and their relatives (and especially – but not exclusively – HHT families with identified cases of PAVMs, cerebral abscess, and/or a mutation of the *ENG* gene) should be informed of the potential consequences of asymptomatic PAVMs when left untreated, and should be offered screening in HHT reference centers. Screening may be repeated after 5–10 years in adult HHT patients with negative screening tests.

Noninvasive methods are preferred for screening. Contrast echocardiography is the most sensitive test to detect right-to-left shunting, with a sensitivity and negative predictive value of 93% [17], and is most appropriate for screening for PAVM. Graded contrast echocardiography may be useful in selecting HHT patients in whom thoracic CT scan is indicated. An anteroposterior chest radiograph is useful to detect large PAVMs, and may be performed prior to contrast echocardiography (thus rendered no longer necessary if PAVM is visible on the chest radiograph). This simple screening algorithm (fig. 8) obviates the need of chest CT in the majority of HHT patients without PAVM; furthermore, it has the advantage of very large availability, lower cost, and especially much lower radiation exposure than chest CT. Screening based on chest CT is an alternative to this algorithm frequently used in the community, especially in centers without expertise in contrast transthoracic echocardiography; however, it causes significant radiation exposure.

Pulmonary Arteriovenous Malformations in Pregnancy and in Children

PAVMs often increase in size and number during pregnancy, which is likely due to increased blood volume and cardiac output, and may occasionally give rise to potentially lethal complications, such as hemorrhage, requiring emergency surgical treatment or embolization therapy. Systematic screening and treatment of PAVM are therefore recommended prior to pregnancy when possible. Pregnant HHT patients

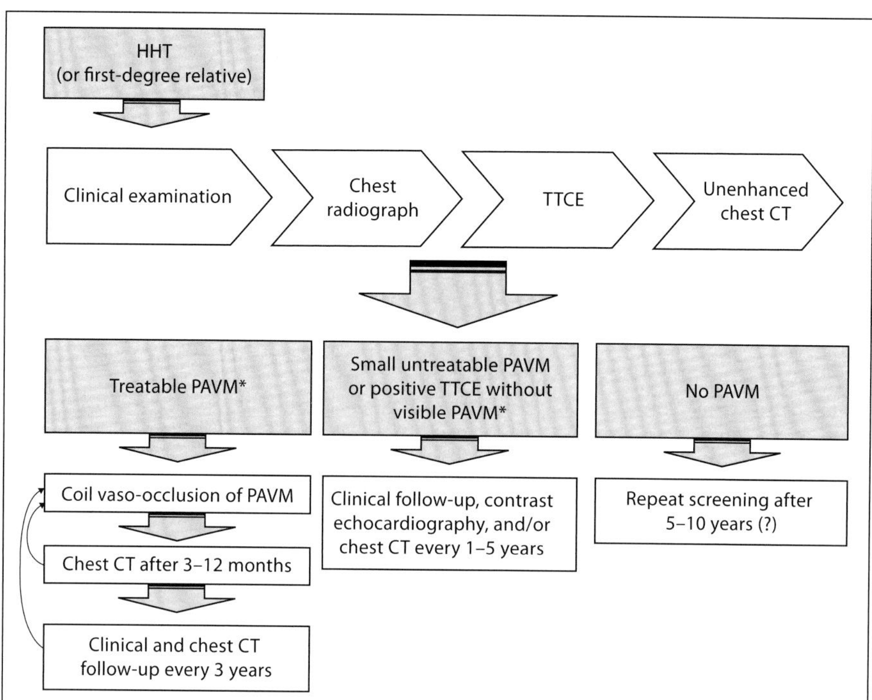

Fig. 8. Proposed algorithm for the screening and follow-up of PAVMs in adult patients with HHT. * Antibiotic prophylaxis is recommended in patients with PAVM prior to potentially bacteremic procedures. TTCE = Transthoracic contrast echocardiography.

with PAVM should be offered close follow-up throughout pregnancy, and the risk of fetal irradiation should be weighed against that of serious PAVM-related complications; transcatheter vaso-occlusion has been performed effectively and safely after 16 weeks of gestational age.

HHT is increasingly diagnosed in children, especially since genetic testing has been made available. PAVM may already be present in children, or even at birth, with potentially the same complications as in adults. As in adults, transcatheter vaso-occlusion is the treatment of choice for PAVMs. Screening in asymptomatic children with HHT is debated; however, a minimal evaluation with clinical examination (cyanosis) and pulse oximetry are routinely performed, and screening contrast echocardiography may be performed when technically feasible.

Pulmonary Hypertension in Hereditary Hemorrhagic Telangiectasia

Clinical Context and Detection

PH is the other severe pulmonary vascular complication of HHT, which is only rarely observed. PH in HHT may result from increased cardiac output and hyperdynamic state, or may be isolated and similar to idiopathic PAH in the absence of liver AVM. Other factors may be present in patients with HHT and may contribute to the pathogenesis of PH. Venous thromboembolism must be ruled out. Pulmonary capillary hemangiomatosis has been described in a patient with HHT. Portal hypertension and liver cirrhosis also have to be excluded in the context of HHT with liver involvement.

Systematic screening for PH is not recommended in asymptomatic HHT patients. However, echocardiography should be systematically performed in any patient with unexplained shortness of breath. Echocardiography is therefore an important investigation in patients with HHT, contributing to both screening for PAVM and right-to-left shunting using the contrast method, and further evaluating possible PH whatever its mechanism (high cardiac output, or high pulmonary vascular resistance). The presence of dilated right cavities and/or increased velocity of the tricuspid regurgitation at echocardiography should prompt right heart catheterization, which is required to confirm PH and characterize its mechanism. Conversely, undiagnosed HHT may be detected in patients presenting with PAH. PH specialists should look for telangiectasia, recurrent epistaxis, and family history of HHT.

Increased Cardiac Output and Hyperdynamic State

Increased cardiac output and heart failure result from systemic AVMs, mostly in the liver (hepatic artery to hepatic vein). Only the most significant liver AVMs with high cardiac output may be symptomatic in about 5% of patients, with dyspnea on exertion, palpitations, and peripheral edema [1]. Left ventricular failure is often precipitated by associated severe anemia or onset of atrial fibrillation (facilitated by left atrial enlargement). A liver bruit and hepatic pulsatility may be found. Patients may also present with other manifestations associated with liver vascular malformations independently of PH, including abdominal pain from biliary or mesenteric ischemia, ascites or hematemesis from portal hypertension, or hepatic encephalopathy [1].

Echocardiography demonstrates dilated right ventricle and atrium, with tricuspid valvular regurgitation, and normal left ventricle ejection fraction. The left atrium is often dilated. Pleural effusion may be present. Inferior vena cava may be enlarged. Right heart catheterization, the gold standard for the diagnosis of PH and its mechanism, demonstrates elevated mean pulmonary artery pressure, with above normal cardiac index (>3.0 and often up to 5–10 l/min/m^2), normal or decreased pulmonary vascular resistance, normal transpulmonary gradient (difference greater than 12 mm Hg between mean pulmonary arterial pressure and pulmonary capillary wedge pressure), and frequently increased left atrial pressure and pulmonary capillary wedge pressure. Despite left ventricular failure, no overt left ventricular systolic dysfunction is found. Doppler sonography is the method of choice for diagnosing liver AVMs (associated with enlarged hepatic arteries) [23], which are also well visualized by CT scan of the abdomen. Mutations in the *ACVRL1* gene are typically present; however, *ENG* mutations have also been reported in this context.

Management of such patients with PH related to liver AVM is difficult. Liver transplantation is considered in patients with life-threatening intractable cardiac failure. It resolves the hyperdynamic circulation state and provides long-term efficacy, although liver AVMs may reoccur on the transplant [24].

Medical therapy includes correction of atrial fibrillation, salt restriction, and diuretics, as clinically indicated. Chronic anemia due to iron deficiency, as well as other causes of increased cardiac output not related to HHT (Paget's disease, hyperthyroidism, thiamine deficiency, polycythemia vera, and arteriovenous access for hemodialysis) must be ruled out. The antiangiogenic vascular endothelial growth factor-antagonist bevacizumab has led to dramatic improvement of liver AVMs in some HHT patients [25, 26], and is currently being evaluated in several clinical trials; however, the routine use of bevacizumab is not recommended until further long-term evaluation of the risks and benefits of this approach is available. Pulmonary vasodilators are not indicated. Banding of the hepatic artery has been used successfully as a palliative therapy to reduce the hepatic artery flow. Transjugular intrahepatic portosystemic shunt may worsen the hyperdynamic circulatory state and is thus contraindicated. Transarterial subselective embolization of liver AVMs in patients with high-output cardiac failure may be followed by significant complications especially biliary ischemia or necrosis and should be generally avoided [23].

Pulmonary Arterial Hypertension

PAH is caused by remodeling of small pulmonary arteries with lumen narrowing, subsequent right heart failure, and death. PAH in the absence of liver AVM is very rare in HHT, although the prevalence has not been studied; moderate PH may be found more frequently. PAH in HHT is clinically indistinguishable from idiopathic PAH, with dyspnea on exertion and progressive right heart failure. Furthermore, it is histologically similar to idiopathic PAH, with intimal hyperplasia, medial thickening and remodeling, in situ thrombosis, and plexiform lesions. PAH mostly occurs in HHT patients with mutations of the *ACVRL1* gene (ALK1); however, it is currently unknown how mutations of *ACVRL1* may give rise to either HHT (potentially with PAVM, or liver AVM and hyperdynamic PH), or to idiopathic PAH. Modifier genes and (or) environmental factors are likely to contribute to pathogenesis.

PAH is defined at right heart catheterization by an increase in mean pulmonary artery pressure (≥25 mm Hg at rest), with normal pulmonary capillary wedge pressure (≤15 mm Hg). Cardiac output may be decreased. Pulmonary vascular resistance and transpulmonary gradient are increased.

PAH and PAVMs are only rarely associated, as high-flow and low-resistance PAVMs may contribute to decrease the pulmonary artery pressure and pulmonary vascular resistance [27], thereby masking nonsevere PAH. However, a minority of patients may present with both PH and PAVMs. In this situation, vaso-occlusion of PAVM may theoretically increase the pulmonary arterial pressure and unmask a genuine PAH, as observed in individual patients. In one series, however, vaso-occlusion of PAVMs was not followed by either increase in normal or mildly elevated pulmonary arterial pressure or right heart failure [28]. Vaso-occlusion of small PAVM responsible for hemoptysis has been performed effectively in a patient with severe PAH. Overall, vaso-occlusion of PAVMs in patients with known PH should be considered with extreme caution, balancing the risk of PAVMs (and especially hemorrhage due to increased pressure) and of vaso-occlusion (i.e. worsening in right ventricular function due to PH) [22, 29]. When necessary, the hemodynamic consequences of PAVM vaso-occlusion may be tested by transient occlusion of the feeding vessel by an inflatable balloon.

The natural history and long-term outcome of HHT-associated PAH is unknown, but is likely similar to that of PAH with a dim prognosis. Whether patients with HHT and PAH may benefit from specific PAH therapy remains to be determined, although sparse case reports have suggested some hemodynamic improvement.

Financial Support

Hospices Civils de Lyon, Université Lyon I.

References

1 Faughnan ME, Granton JT, Young LH: The pulmonary vascular complications of hereditary haemorrhagic telangiectasia. Eur Respir J 2009; 33:1186–1194.

2 Shovlin CL, Guttmacher AE, Buscarini E, Faughnan ME, Hyland RH, Westermann CJ, Kjeldsen AD, Plauchu H: Diagnostic criteria for hereditary hemorrhagic telangiectasia (Rendu-Osler-Weber syndrome). Am J Med Genet 2000;91:66–67.

3 Cottin V, Chinet T, Lavole A, Corre R, Marchand E, Reynaud-Gaubert M, Plauchu H, Cordier JF, Groupe d'etudes et de recherche sur les maladies 'orphelines' pulmonaires (GERM'O'P): Pulmonary arteriovenous malformations in hereditary hemorrhagic telangiectasia: a series of 126 patients. Medicine (Baltimore) 2007;86:1–17.

4 Faughnan ME, Palda VA, Garcia-Tsao G, Geisthoff UW, McDonald J, Proctor DD, Spears J, Brown DH, Buscarini E, Chesnutt MS, Cottin V, Ganguly A, Gossage JR, Guttmacher AE, Hyland RH, Kennedy SJ, Korzenik J, Mager JJ, Ozanne AP, Piccirillo JF, Picus D, Plauchu H, Porteous ME, Pyeritz RE, Ross DA, Sabba C, Swanson K, Terry P, Wallace MC, Westermann CJ, White RI, Young LH, Zarrabeitia R: International guidelines for the diagnosis and management of hereditary haemorrhagic telangiectasia. J Med Genet 2011;48:73–87.

5 Shovlin CL: Hereditary haemorrhagic telangiectasia: Pathophysiology, diagnosis and treatment. Blood Rev 2010;24:203–219.

6 Lesca G, Olivieri C, Burnichon N, Pagella F, Carette MF, Gilbert-Dussardier B, Goizet C, Roume J, Rabilloud M, Saurin JC, Cottin V, Honnorat J, Coulet F, Giraud S, Calender A, Danesino C, Buscarini E, Plauchu H: Genotype-phenotype correlations in hereditary hemorrhagic telangiectasia: Data from the French-Italian HHT network. Genet Med 2007;9:14–22.

7 Post MC, Letteboer TG, Mager JJ, Plokker TH, Kelder JC, Westermann CJ: A pulmonary right-to-left shunt in patients with hereditary hemorrhagic telangiectasia is associated with an increased prevalence of migraine. Chest 2005;128:2485–2489.

8 Machado RD, Eickelberg O, Elliott CG, Geraci MW, Hanaoka M, Loyd JE, Newman JH, Phillips JA, 3rd, Soubrier F, Trembath RC, Chung WK: Genetics and genomics of pulmonary arterial hypertension. J Am Coll Cardiol 2009;54:S32–S42.

9 Sztrymf B, Coulet F, Girerd B, Yaici A, Jais X, Sitbon O, Montani D, Souza R, Simonneau G, Soubrier F, Humbert M: Clinical outcomes of pulmonary arterial hypertension in carriers of BMPR2 mutation. Am J Respir Crit Care Med 2008;177:1377–1383.

10 Girerd B, Montani D, Coulet F, Sztrymf B, Yaici A, Jais X, Tregouet D, Reis A, Drouin-Garraud V, Fraisse A, Sitbon O, O'Callaghan DS, Simonneau G, Soubrier F, Humbert M: Clinical outcomes of pulmonary arterial hypertension in patients carrying an ACVRL1 (ALK1) mutation. Am J Respir Crit Care Med 2010;181:851–861.

11 Cottin V, Dupuis-Girod S, Lesca G, Cordier JF: Pulmonary vascular manifestations of hereditary hemorrhagic telangiectasia (Rendu-Osler disease). Respiration 2007;74:361–378.

12 Wong HH, Chan RP, Klatt R, Faughnan ME: Idiopathic pulmonary arteriovenous malformations: clinical and imaging characteristics. Eur Respir J 2011;38:368–375.

13 Pierucci P, Murphy J, Henderson KJ, Chyun DA, White RI Jr: New definition and natural history of patients with diffuse pulmonary arteriovenous malformations: twenty-seven-year experience. Chest 2008;133:653–661.

14 Lacombe P, Lagrange C, Beauchet A, El Hajjam M, Chinet T, Pelage JP: Diffuse pulmonary arteriovenous malformations in hereditary hemorrhagic telangiectasia: long-term results of embolization according to the extent of lung involvement. Chest 2009;135:1031–1037.

15 Dupuis-Girod S, Giraud S, Decullier E, Lesca G, Cottin V, Faure F, Merrot O, Saurin JC, Cordier JF, Plauchu H: Hemorrhagic hereditary telangiectasia (Rendu-Osler disease) and infectious diseases: an underestimated association. Clin Infect Dis 2007;44:841–845.

16 Remy J, Remy-Jardin M, Wattinne L, Deffontaines C: Pulmonary arteriovenous malformations: evaluation with CT of the chest before and after treatment. Radiology 1992;182:809–816.

17 Cottin V, Plauchu H, Bayle JY, Barthelet M, Revel D, Cordier JF: Pulmonary arteriovenous malformations in patients with hereditary hemorrhagic telangiectasia. Am J Respir Crit Care Med 2004;169:994–1000.

18 Boussel L, Cernicanu A, Geerts L, Gamondes D, Khouatra C, Cottin V, Revel D, Douek P: 4D time-resolved magnetic resonance angiography for noninvasive assessment of pulmonary arteriovenous malformations patency. J Magn Reson Imaging 2010;32:1110–1116.

19 Zukotynski K, Chan RP, Chow CM, Cohen JH, Faughnan ME: Contrast echocardiography grading predicts pulmonary arteriovenous malformations on CT. Chest 2007;132:18–23.

20 Lee WL, Graham AF, Pugash RA, Hutchison SJ, Grande P, Hyland RH, Faughnan ME: Contrast echocardiography remains positive after treatment of pulmonary arteriovenous malformations. Chest 2003;123:351–358.

21 Trerotola SO, Pyeritz RE: PAVM embolization: an update. AJR Am J Roentgenol 2010;195:837–845.

22 Cottin V, Gamondes D, Schuller A, Coudurier M, Dupuis-Girod S, Tronc F, Cordier JF: Near-fatal haemorrhage from pulmonary arteriovenous malformation in HHT with increased cardiac output. Eur Respir Rev 2009;18:190–192.

23 Buscarini E, Plauchu H, Garcia Tsao G, White RI Jr, Sabba C, Miller F, Saurin JC, Pelage JP, Lesca G, Marion MJ, Perna A, Faughnan ME: Liver involvement in hereditary hemorrhagic telangiectasia: consensus recommendations. Liver Int 2006;26:1040–1046.

24 Dupuis-Girod S, Chesnais AL, Ginon I, Dumortier J, Saurin JC, Finet G, Decullier E, Marion D, Plauchu H, Boillot O: Long-term outcome of patients with hereditary hemorrhagic telangiectasia and severe hepatic involvement after orthotopic liver transplantation: a single-center study. Liver Transpl 2010;16:340–347.

25 Flieger D, Hainke S, Fischbach W: Dramatic improvement in hereditary hemorrhagic telangiectasia after treatment with the vascular endothelial growth factor (VEGF) antagonist bevacizumab. Ann Hematol 2006;85:631–632.

26 Mitchell A, Adams LA, MacQuillan G, Tibballs J, van den Driesen R, Delriviere L: Bevacizumab reverses need for liver transplantation in hereditary hemorrhagic telangiectasia. Liver Transpl 2008;14:210–213.

27 Trembath RC, Thomson JR, Machado RD, Morgan NV, Atkinson C, Winship I, Simonneau G, Galie N, Loyd JE, Humbert M, Nichols WC, Morrell NW, Berg J, Manes A, McGaughran J, Pauciulo M, Wheeler L: Clinical and molecular genetic features of pulmonary hypertension in patients with hereditary hemorrhagic telangiectasia. N Engl J Med 2001;345:325–334.

28 Shovlin CL, Tighe HC, Davies RJ, Gibbs JS, Jackson JE: Embolisation of pulmonary arteriovenous malformations: no consistent effect on pulmonary artery pressure. Eur Respir J 2008;32: 162–169.

29 Montani D, Price LC, Girerd B, Chinet T, Lacombe P, Simonneau G, Humbert M: Fatal rupture of pulmonary arteriovenous malformation in hereditary haemorrhagic telangiectasis and severe PAH. Eur Respir Rev 2009;18:42–46.

Vincent Cottin
Hôpital Louis Pradel, Service de pneumologie
FR–69677 Lyon (Bron) Cedex, (France)
Tel. +33 472 357 072, E-Mail vincent.cottin@chu-lyon.fr

Chapter 28
Humbert M, Souza R, Simonneau G (eds): Pulmonary Vascular Disorders.
Prog Respir Res. Basel, Karger, 2012, vol 41, pp 276–279

Future Perspectives in Pulmonary Arterial Hypertension

Lewis J. Rubin

Division of Pulmonary and Critical Care Medicine, School of Medicine, University of California at San Diego, La Jolla, Calif., USA

Abstract

In a remarkably short interval of time, pulmonary artery hypertension (PAH) has evolved from a disease of unknown pathogenesis devoid of effective therapy to a condition whose cellular and molecular underpinnings are unfolding, and for which three treatment classes have been developed. Nevertheless, PAH remains incurable and is often refractory to medical therapy, underscoring the need for further research. This chapter will highlight some of the anticipated approaches to research in pathogenesis, diagnosis and monitoring, and novel therapies that are anticipated to yield clinical applications in the future.

The remarkable progress achieved in elucidating the pathogenesis of pulmonary arterial hypertension (PAH) over the past two decades has led to the development of disease-targeted therapies for this condition. Despite these achievements, however, the diagnosis is often established late in the course of the disease, the response to therapy is often incomplete in many patients, and survival remains poor. Accordingly, new diagnostic and treatment strategies must be developed for PAH that identify patients with early disease, optimize the treatments currently available, and capitalize on the identification of novel pathogenic pathways. This article will provide a glimpse into the future, based on recent developments in the field that hold promise for enhancing the management of PAH.

Identification of mutations in the bone morphogenetic protein receptor 2 (BMPR2) in the majority of cases of familial PAH was a major advance in the elucidation of the pathogenic sequence in PAH [1, 2]. However, fewer than 20% of individuals with a BMPR2 mutation develop familial PAH, and most individuals with PAH do not have an identifiable mutation [3]; accordingly, it is likely that other factors, including genes and external stimuli (a 'second hit'), are needed to initiate the sequence that leads to vascular injury and the pulmonary hypertensive state. Both the role of these other factors in initiating the vascular injury and the mechanisms through which they interface with genetic abnormalities are unknown [4].

A variety of cellular abnormalities have been described that may play important roles in the development and progression of PAH [5–9]. These include altered cellular metabolism, impaired synthesis of nitric oxide, prostacyclin and endothelin, impaired potassium channel and growth factor receptor function, altered serotonin transporter regulation, increased oxidant stress, and enhanced matrix production. However, the relative importance of each of these processes is unknown, and the interactions between these various pathways need to be explored. Additionally, the intermediate steps involved in the transduction of signals related to BMPR2 are unknown; clarification of these pathways will lead to a more complete understanding of how impaired BMPR2 signaling, both inherited and acquired, leads to hypertensive pulmonary vascular disease [10–12].

Pulmonary Arterial Hypertension Therapy

Less than a decade ago, therapy for PAH was based on a limited understanding of the disease pathogenesis, largely empiric, and usually ineffective. The treatment of PAH has advanced dramatically since then, with a number well-designed and executed clinical trials demonstrating sustained efficacy of several therapies that target specific abnormalities present in PAH [13–16]. Furthermore, the complexity of these treatments has devolved from continuous intravenous delivery to oral and inhaled modes of drug delivery. Future studies targeting newly identified alterations in endothelial and smooth muscle cell function may provide novel treatments. Several of the most promising targets are discussed below.

Serotonin Receptor and Transporter Function

Serotonin [5-hydroxytryptamine (5-HT)] is a potent vasoconstrictor and smooth muscle mitogen that has long been suspected to play a pathogenic role in PAH [17]. Recent work suggests that the $5\text{-HT}2_B$ receptor may be upregulated in PAH, providing a novel therapeutic target since antagonists to this receptor have been developed. Others have shown that the serotonin transporter, a molecule that facilitates transmembrane transport of serotonin into the cell, is upregulated in PAH [9]. Interestingly, the fenfluramine anorexigens, which are known to increase the risk of developing PAH, stimulate an upregulation of the serotonin transporter in vitro, supporting a pathogenic mechanism for this system in PAH. Drugs that downregulate the serotonin transporter, such as selective serotonin reuptake inhibitors, may be worthy of study as treatment options in the future.

Vasoactive Intestinal Polypeptide

Vasoactive intestinal polypeptide (VIP) is a substance produced by cells from a variety of organs that exerts cellular antiproliferative effects. VIP is also a neuropeptide with potent vasodilating properties. VIP deficiency has been described in lung tissues from patients with idiopathic PAH (IPAH). In a preliminary case series, 8 patients with IPAH who were treated with inhaled VIP at daily doses of 200 μg in four single inhalations showed marked clinical and hemodynamic improvement [18]. However, a recent double-blinded trial with inhaled VIP was negative. The reasons for these discrepant findings are unclear, and may be due to dosing or delivery systems.

Rho Kinase Inhibitors

Rho kinase is part of a family of enzymes that is involved in the processes of cellular growth and, in particular, smooth muscle tone. Studies in animal models of pulmonary hypertension suggest that fasudil, an inhibitor of Rho kinase, may ameliorate the hemodynamic and pathologic severity of pulmonary vascular injury, as well as provide a rationale for clinical development of this agent in PAH [19, 20].

Inhibitors of Growth Factor Synthesis and Promoters of Apoptosis

PAH is characterized pathologically by uncontrolled angiogenesis and impaired apoptosis, processes that are reminiscent of malignant transformation. In support of this concept, monoclonal expansion has been demonstrated in the plexiform lesions of IPAH. Additionally, unique cellular metabolic abnormalities that result in resistance to apoptosis have been reported in cells from patients with IPAH [21]. Recently published reports in which imatinib, a tyrosine kinase inhibitor that is approved for the treatment of hematopoietic malignancies, produced improvement in an animal model of pulmonary hypertension [22] and a handful of PAH patients refractory of other available treatments [23] suggests that this novel approach may be of benefit in PAH and warrants further study. Large-scale clinical trials are now underway.

Adrenomedullin is a peptide that causes vasodilation and inhibits proliferation of pulmonary vascular smooth muscle cells [24, 25]. Both intravenous and inhaled adrenomedullin lower pulmonary vascular resistance in patients with IPAH [26, 27]. Long-term data are not available, but the substance has the potential of becoming a promising future treatment for PAH [25].

Cell-Based Therapy

Several recent publications have demonstrated that infusions of endothelial progenitor cells in animal models of pulmonary hypertension attenuate the injury, particularly when these cells are transfected with nitric oxide synthase, the enzyme responsible for the generation of nitric oxide from the precursor L-arginine [28]. Thus, while cell-based therapies have yet to fulfill their promise in clinical studies, particularly in cardiovascular diseases, pilot safety and efficacy trials are now underway with progenitor cell infusions in patients with severe PAH refractory to medical therapy [29].

Drugs currently marketed to treat other conditions may have effects that are beneficial in PAH as well. For example, the hydroxymethylglutaryl-coenzyme-A reductase inhibitors (statins) manifest pleiotropic effects that have been suggested to be responsible for a component of their benefit in arteriosclerotic disease [30], and these agents attenuate the pulmonary arteriopathy induced by the administration of monocrotaline to experimental animals [31, 32]. Formal clinical studies with statins may, therefore, be appropriate. Similarly, currently available platelet inhibitors (i.e. aspirin) and newer antithrombotic agents may have a role in the treatment of PAH, in light of the beneficial effects (and inherent risks) of anticoagulation with warfarin in IPAH.

As with other diseases with a complex pathogenesis, targeting a single pathway in PAH is unlikely to be uniformly successful. With the development of several pathway-specific therapies, the opportunity exists for evaluating multidrug therapy in PAH. Uncontrolled small trials have suggested that the addition of bosentan to patients failing oral or inhaled prostanoid therapy with beraprost or iloprost, respectively, resulted in improved exercise capacity. Similarly, the addition of sildenafil to inhaled iloprost therapy resulted in potentiation of the clinical effects. Recently, randomized clinical trials have demonstrated that the addition of inhaled iloprost to background therapy with bosentan [33], or oral sildenafil to background intravenous epoprostenol therapy, resulted in further improvement in hemodynamics, exercise capacity, and time to clinical worsening [34]. The role of initial combination therapy compared with monotherapy followed by escalation to combination therapy is currently being investigated in a multicenter trial.

Unresolved questions exist regarding combination therapy for PAH include:

- Which combinations are the most potent, i.e. which pathways are the most pivotal targets for treatment, and how many should be targeted?
- What is the optimal timing for combination therapy? Should combination therapy be initiated early in the course of the disease in order to maximize the response, or should it be considered only if monotherapy fails to achieve the desired clinical response?
- What are the appropriate criteria for assessing response to therapy?

Measuring Outcomes and Monitoring the Course of Therapy

The development of treatments for PAH has prompted the challenge of how to best assess and monitor the efficacy of long-term therapy. Because it is believed that randomized placebo-controlled trials using survival as an end point would be unethical to perform in PAH, alternative strategies are required to measure and compare the relative effects of the available treatments. Similarly, noninvasive markers of disease severity, i.e. biomarkers, imaging studies, or physiological tests, are needed that can be widely applied to reliably monitor clinical course. Studies that assess the value of these outcome measures, alone or in combination, will enable physicians to time and select therapy in a more structured fashion. Furthermore, more attention needs to be focused on the state of right ventricular function in PAH since this is arguably the single most important determinant of outcome [35]. MRI may be particularly useful in this regard since both structure and function of the right ventricle may be assessed noninvasively and sequentially over the course of treatment [36]. Additionally, MRI may prove useful in noninvasive assessment of the pulmonary vasculature, for example in determination of operability for patients with chronic thromboembolic pulmonary hypertension.

Conclusions

Although major advances in our understanding of the mechanism of disease development and in the treatment of PAH have been achieved over the past decade, substantial gaps in our knowledge remain. Bringing together physicians and scientists representing multiple disciplines and expertise, all sharing an interest in PAH, affords the opportunity to develop collaborations that will narrow these gaps of knowledge in the future.

References

1 Deng Z, Morse JH, Slager SL, et al: Familial primary pulmonary hypertension (gene PPH1) is caused by mutations in the bone morphogenetic protein receptor-II gene. Am J Hum Gen 2000;67:737–744.

2 Lane KB, Machado RD, Pauciulo MW, et al: Heterozygous germline mutations in BMPR2, encoding a TGF-beta receptor, cause familial primary pulmonary hypertension. The International PPH Consortium. Nat Genet 2000;26: 81–84.

3 Thomson JR, Machado RD, Pauciulo MW, et al: Sporadic primary pulmonary hypertension is associated with germline mutations of the gene encoding BMPR2, a receptor member of the TGF-beta family. J Med Genet 2000;37:741–745.

4 Derynck R, Zhang YE: TGF-beta-induced signalling pathways. Nature 2003;425:581–583.

5 Christman BW, McPherson CD, Newman JH, et al: An imbalance between the excretion of thromboxane and prostacyclin metabolites in pulmonary hypertension. N Engl J Med 1992;327:70–75.
6 Tuder RM, Cool CD, Geraci MW, et al: Prostacyclin synthase expression is decreased in lungs from patients with severe pulmonary hypertension. Am J Respir Crit Care Med 1999;159:1925–1932.
7 Yuan JX, Aldinger AM, Juhaszova M, et al: Dysfunctional voltage gated K^+ channels in pulmonary artery smooth muscle cells of patients with primary pulmonary hypertension. Circulation 1998;98:400–406.
8 Mandegar M, Remillard CV, Yuan JX: Ion channels in pulmonary arterial hypertension. Prog Cardiovasc Dis 2002;45:81–114.
9 Eddhaibi S, Humbert M, Fadel E, et al: Serotonin transporter overexpression is responsible for pulmonary artery smooth muscle hyperplasia in primary pulmonary hypertension. J Clin Invest 2001;108:1141–1150.
10 Du L, Sullivan CC, Chu D, et al: Signaling molecules in nonfamilial pulmonary hypertension. N Engl J Med 2003;348:500–509.
11 Krick S, Platoshyn O, McDaniel SS, et al: Augmented K^+ currents and mitochondrial membrane depolarization in pulmonary artery myocyte apoptosis. Am J Physiol Lung Cell Mol Physiol 2001;281:L887–L894.
12 Yuan JXJ, Rubin LJ: Pathogenesis of pulmonary artery hypertension: need for multiple hits. Circulation 2005;111:534–538.
13 Barst RJ, Rubin LJ, Long WA, et al: A comparison of continuous intravenous epoprostenol (prostacyclin) with conventional therapy for primary pulmonary hypertension. The Primary Pulmonary Hypertension Study Group. N Engl J Med 1996;334:296–302.
14 Rubin LJ, Badesch DB, Barst RJ, et al: Bosentan therapy for pulmonary arterial hypertension. N Engl J Med 2002;346:896–903.
15 Galie N, Humbert M, Vachiery JL, et al: Effects of beraprost sodium, an oral prostacyclin analogue, in patients with pulmonary arterial hypertension: a randomized, double-blind, placebo-controlled trial. J Am Coll Cardiol 2002;39:1496–1502.
16 Olschewski H, Simonneau G, Galie N, et al: Inhaled iloprost for severe pulmonary hypertension. N Engl J Med 2002;347:322–329.
17 Fanburg BL, Lee SL: A new role for an old molecule: serotonin as a mitogen. Am J Physiol 1997;272:L795–L806.
18 Petkov V, Mosgeoller W, Ziesche R, et al: Vasoactive intestinal polypeptide as a new drug for treatment of primary pulmonary hypertension. J Clin Invest 2003;111:1339–1346.
19 Oka M, Homma N, Taraseviciene-Stewart L, Morris KG, Kraskauskas D, Burns N, Voelkel NF, McMurtry IF: Rho kinase-mediated vasoconstriction is important in severe occlusive pulmonary arterial hypertension in rats. Circ Res 2007;100:923–929.
20 Abe K, Shimokawa H, Morikawa K, Uwatoku T, Oi K, Matsumoto Y, Hattori T, Nakashima Y, Kaibuchi K, Sueishi K, Takeshit A: Long-term treatment with a Rho-kinase inhibitor improves monocrotaline-induced fatal pulmonary hypertension in rats. Circ Res 2004;94:385–393.
21 Sutendra G, Bonnet S, Rochefort G, Haromy A, Folmes KD, Lopaschuk GD, Dyck JRB, Michelakis ED: Fatty acid oxidation and malonyl-CoA decarboxylase in the vascular remodeling of pulmonary hypertension. Science Transl Med 2010;44:1–13.
22 Schermuly RT, Dony E, Ghofrani HA, et al: Reversal of experimental pulmonary hypertension by PDGF inhibition. J Clin Invest 2005;115:2811–2821.
23 Ghofrani HA, Seeger W, Grimminger F: Imatinib for the treatment of pulmonary arterial hypertension. N Engl J Med 2005;353:1412–1413.
24 Nagaya N, Kangawa K: Adrenomedullin in the treatment of pulmonary hypertension. Peptides 2004;25:2013–2018.
25 Said SI: Mediators and modulators of pulmonary arterial hypertension. Am J Physiol Lung Cell Mol Physiol 2006;291:547–558.
26 von der Hardt K, Kandler MA, Chada M, Cubra A, Schoof E, Amann K, Rascher W, Dotsch J: Brief adrenomedullin inhalation leads to sustained reduction of pulmonary artery pressure. Eur Respir J 2004;24:615–623.
27 Nagaya N, Nishikimib T, Uematsua M, Satoha T, Oyaa H, Kyotania S, Sakamakia F, Uenoa K, Nakanishia N, Miyatakea K, Kangawab K: Haemodynamic and hormonal effects of adrenomedullin in patients with pulmonary hypertension. Heart 2000;84:653–658.
28 Zhao YD, Courtman DW, Deng Y, Kugathasan L, Zhang Q, Stewart DJ: Rescue of monocrotaline-induced pulmonary arterial hypertension using bone marrow-derived endothelial-like progenitor cells: efficacy of combined cell and eNOS gene therapy in established disease. Circ Res 2005;96:442–450.
29 Wang XX, Zhang FR, Shang YP, Zhu JH, Xie XD, Tao QM, Zhu JH, Chen JZ: Transplantation of autologous endothelial progenitor cells may be beneficial in patients with idiopathic pulmonary arterial hypertension: a pilot randomized controlled trial. J Am Coll Cardiol 2007;49:1566–1571.
30 Indolfi C, Cioppa A, Stabile E, et al: Effects of hydroxymethylglutaryl coenzyme-A reductase inhibitor simvastatin on smooth muscle cell proliferation in vitro and neointimal formation in vivo after vascular injury. J Am Coll Cardiol 2000;35:214–221.
31 Nishimura T, Faul JL, Berry GJ, et al: Simvastatin attenuates smooth muscle neointimal proliferation and pulmonary hypertension in rats. Am J Respir Crit Care Med 2002;166:1403–1408.
32 Nishimura T, Vaszar LT, Faul JL, et al: Simvastatin rescues rats from fatal pulmonary hypertension by inducing apoptosis in neointimal smooth muscle. Circulation 2003;108:1640–1645.
33 McLaughlin VV, Oudiz RJ, Frost A, Tapson VF, Murali S, Channick RN, Badesch DB, Barst RJ, Hsu H, Rubin LJ: A randomized, double-blind, placebo-controlled study of iloprost inhalation as add-on therapy to bosentan in pulmonary arterial hypertension. Am J Resp Crit Care Med 2006;174:1257–1263.
34 Simonneau G, Rubin LJ, Galie N, Barst RJ, Fleming T, Burgess G, Collings L, Cossons N, Badesch DB: safety and efficacy of sildenafil-epoprostenol combination therapy in patients with pulmonary arterial hypertension (abstract). Am J Resp Crit Care Med 2007;175:A300.
35 Voelkel NF, Quaife RA, Leinwand LA, Barst RJ, McGoon MD, Meldrum DR, Dupuis J, Long CS, Rubin LJ, Smart FW, Suzuki YJ, Gladwin M, Denholm EM, Gail DB: Right ventricular function and failure: report of a National Heart, Lung, and Blood Institute working group on cellular and molecular mechanisms of right heart failure. Circulation 2006;114:1883–1891.
36 Merten LL, Friedberg MK: Imaging the right ventricle-current state of the art. Nature Reviews Cardiology 2010;7:551–563.

Lewis J. Rubin, MD
Division of Pulmonary and Critical Care Medicine
University of California at San Diego
La Jolla, CA 92037-1330 (USA)
E-Mail ljrubin@ucsd.edu

Author Index

Adir, Y. 161

Beghetti, M. 122
Bolliger, C.T. VII
Bouillon, K. 76
Brauner, M. 178

Canuet, M. 169
Chaouat, A. 169
Chemla, D. 23
Cordier, J.-F. 262
Cottin, V. 262
Coulet, F. 65

Dauriat, G. 178
Degano, B. 105
Di, R.-M. 199
Dias, B. 59
Dorfmüller, P. 14, 149
Ducoloné, A. 169
Dupuis-Girod, S. 262

Eyries, M. 65

Fernandes, C.J.C. 143

Gaine, S.P. 237
Galiè, N. 161
Gille, T. 178
Girerd, B. 65

Hassoun, P.M. 94
Hervé, P. 23, 113
Hoeper, M.M. 246
Hoette, S. 23, 59, 143
Hovnanian, A. 143
Huertas, A. 149
Humbert, M. VIII, 65, 76, 85, 105, 149

Jais, X. 226
Jardim, C. 59, 143
Jiang, X. 85
Jing, Z.-C. 85, 199

Kambouchner, M. 178
Kessler, R. 169
Khouatra, C. 262

Lang, I.M. 226
Le Gal, G. 218
Le Pavec, J. 94
Leroyer, C. 218

Mainguy, V. 37
Maitre, B. 137
Meyer, G. 207
Montani, D. 1, 65, 149
Morinaga, L.K. 143
Mottier, D. 218

Naeije, R. 48
Nunes, H. 178

O'Callaghan, D.S. 237

Parent, F. 137
Peacock, A. 48
Price, L. 76
Provencher, S. 37

Rubin, L.J. 276

Sanchez, O. 207
Savale, L. 113, 137
Simonneau, G. VIII, 1, 137
Sitbon, O. 105, 113
Soubrier, F. 65
Souza, R. VIII, 59, 143

Tissot, C. 122

Uzunhan, Y. 178

Vachiéry, J.-L. 254
Valeyre, D. 178
Valmary, S. 105
Vonk Noordegraaf, A. 48

Weitzenblum, E. 169
Whyte, K.F. 23
Wort, S.J. 76

Yaici, A. 65

Subject Index

ACVRL1
hereditary hemorrhagic telangiectasia mutation 264, 265
pulmonary arterial hypertension mutation 66, 69, 72
Aging, pulmonary hemodynamics studies
exercise pulmonary hemodynamics 28
resting pulmonary hemodynamics 28
Ambrisentan
congenital heart disease-associated pulmonary arterial hypertension management 132
efficacy in pulmonary arterial hypertension 242
Aminorex fumarate, pulmonary arterial hypertension induction 78
Angiography, pulmonary
chronic thromboembolic pulmonary hypertension diagnosis 229, 230
hepatopulmonary syndrome diagnosis 119
Anticoagulants, *see specific anticoagulants*
Aortic valve disease, pulmonary hypertension association 166–168
Apixaban, venous thromboembolism management 222, 223
Apoptosis, therapeutic targeting in pulmonary arterial hypertension 277
Arteriovenous malformation, *see* Pulmonary arteriovenous malformation
Asymmetric dimethylarginine (ADMA), pulmonary arterial hypertension marker 60, 61
Atrial septostomy
congenital heart disease-associated pulmonary arterial hypertension management 133
long-term effects
clinical outcome 257, 258
survival 257, 258, 260
right ventricle dysfunction in pulmonary arterial hypertension 254, 255
risk minimization 258–260
short-term effects
clinical outcome 257
mortality 257
surgical technique 256, 257
sympathetic overactivation decrease 255, 256
timing 259

Balloon pulmonary angioplasty, chronic thromboembolic pulmonary hypertension management 231
Benfluorex, pulmonary arterial hypertension induction 80
Beraprost
chronic thromboembolic pulmonary hypertension management 231, 232
efficacy in pulmonary arterial hypertension 240, 241
Bevacizumab, pulmomary arterial hypertension induction 80, 81
Biomarkers, pulmonary arterial hypertension
asymmetric dimethylarginine 60, 61
brain natriuretic peptide 61, 62
D-dimer 61
endothelin 61
ideal properties 59
prospects for study 62, 63
troponin 60
uric acid 59
von Willebrand factor 61
Bone morphogenetic protein receptor type 2 (BMPR2)
cellular function 68
gene mutation in pulmonary arterial hypertension
clinical features 72
effects on receptor 67
frequency 67
genetic counseling and testing 70–72
overview 1–3
penetrance 68, 69
types 67, 68
signaling 67
structure 67

Bosentan, *see also* Endothelial receptor antagonists
chronic thromboembolic pulmonary hypertension management 232, 233
congenital heart disease-associated pulmonary arterial hypertension management 132
connective tissue disease-associated pulmonary arterial hypertension management 99
efficacy in pulmonary arterial hypertension 241, 242
human immunodeficiency virus pulmonary arterial hypertension management 109
sickle cell disease pulmonary hypertension management 141
Brain natriuretic peptide (BNP)
congenital heart disease-associated pulmonary arterial hypertension findings 127, 128
interstitial lung disease-associated pulmonary hypertension diagnosis 181, 182
pulmonary arterial hypertension biomarker studies 61, 62
venous thromboembolism risk stratification 213
Bronchoalveolar lavage (BAL), pulmonary veno-occlusive disease findings 155

Calcium channel blockers (CCBs)
congenital heart disease-associated pulmonary arterial hypertension management 131
HIV-associated pulmonary arterial hypertension management 109
Cardiac catheterization, *see* Hemodynamics
Cardiopulmonary exercise testing, *see* Hemodynamics
Carmustine (BCNU), pulmonary arterial hypertension induction 82
Chest X-ray
congenital heart disease-associated pulmonary arterial hypertension 126, 127
high-altitude pulmonary hypertension 204
schistosomiasis-associated pulmonary arterial hypertension 146
Chronic hemolytic anemia, pulmonary arterial hypertension association 5
Chronic mountain syndrome (CMS)
clinical features 200
epidemiology 199
Chronic obstructive pulmonary disease (COPD), pulmonary hypertension
classification 169
clinical features 172, 173
course 174
definition 169, 170
diagnosis 171, 172
pathology 170
pathophysiology 170, 171
prevalence 170
prognosis 174, 175
severe pulmonary hypertension 173, 174
treatment
oxygen therapy 175
vasodilators 175
Chronic thromboembolic pulmonary hypertension (CTEPH)
angiography 229, 230
classification 7, 8
clinical presentation 229
course 228, 229
definition 226, 227
diagnosis 229, 230
epidemiology 227, 228
etiology 228
hemodynamics 230
overview 226
pathophysiology 228, 229
prognosis 233
treatment
balloon pulmonary angioplasty 231
endothelin receptor antagonists 232, 233
prospects 233, 234
prostacyclin and analogs 231, 232
pulmonary endarterectomy 230, 231
sildenafil 233
ventilation-perfusion scanning 229
Classification, pulmonary hypertension
Group 1 1–5
Group 1' 5, 6
Group 2 6, 7
Group 3 7
Group 4 7
Group 5 7–9
Cocaine
human immunodeficiency virus and pulmonary arterial hypertension association 107
pulmonary arterial hypertension induction 81
Combined pulmonary fibrosis and emphysema (CPFE) syndrome, features and management 186, 187
Computed tomography (CT)
interstitial lung disease-associated pulmonary hypertension diagnosis 181
pulmonary arteriovenous malformation 268, 269
pulmonary hemodynamics studies 51
pulmonary veno-occlusive disease 154
venous thromboembolism diagnosis 210, 211
Congenital heart disease-associated pulmonary arterial hypertension, *see also specific diseases*
assessment
brain natriuretic peptide 127, 128
cardiac catheterization 127
chest X-ray 126, 127
echocardiography 126–129
electrocardiography 126
exercise capacity 127
physical examination and history 125
classification 4, 124

definition 124
epidemiology 125
genetics 125
management
atrial septostomy 133
bosentan 132
calcium channel blockers 131
combination therapy 132, 133
nitric oxide 131, 133
organ transplantation 134
outcomes 134, 135
postoperative care 130
prostacyclin 131
pulmonary artery banding 130
sildenafil 132
special conditions 133
surgery 128–130, 133, 134
overview 122
pathophysiology 122, 123
postoperative hypertension 125
pulmonary vascular resistance elevation secondary to large volume left-to-right shunt 125
secondary to small volume left-to-right shunt 125
Connective tissue disease-associated pulmonary arterial hypertension, *see also specific diseases*
overview 3, 4, 94
rheumatoid arthritis 98
Sjögren's syndrome 98
systemic lupus erythematosus 97, 98
systemic sclerosis 95–97
treatment
anti-inflammatory drugs 98
anticoagulation 100
combination therapy 100
endothelin receptor antagonists 99
general measures 98
lung transplantation 101
phosphodiesterase inhibitors 99, 100
prostaglandins 98, 99
tyrosine kinase inhibitors 100, 101
venous lesions 20, 21
Connective tissue disease-related interstitial lung disease, *see also specific diseases*
clinical impact 188
diagnosis 188
epidemiology 187
overview 187
pathogenesis 187, 188
prognosis 188
treatment 188
Cyclophosphamide 80

Dabigatran, venous thromboembolism management 221, 222
Dasatinib, pulmonary arterial hypertension induction 81
D-dimer
pulmonary arterial hypertension marker 61
venous thromboembolism diagnosis 209
Dexfenfluramine, pulmonary arterial hypertension induction 78–80
Diethylpropion, pulmonary arterial hypertension induction 80
Drug- and toxin-induced pulmonary arterial hypertension
classification 3
drugs and toxins in induction
aminorex fumarate 78
benfluorex 80
bevacizumab 80, 81
carmustine 82
cocaine 81
cyclophosphamide 80
dasatinib 81
dexfenfluramine 78–80
diethylpropion 80
fenfluramine 78–80
interferon-α_2 80
mazindol 80
methamphetamine 81
mitomycin-C 82
overview 76, 78
pergolide 80
phendimetrazine 80
phenformin 80
phenylpropanolamine 80
propylhexedrine 80
pyrrolizidine alkaloids 81, 82
Saint John's wort 81
structures 79
thalidomide 80
3,4-methylenedioxymethamphetamine 81
toxic rapeseed oil 82
tryptophan 82
pathophysiology 77, 78

Echocardiography
congenital heart disease-associated pulmonary arterial hypertension 126–129
hepatopulmonary syndrome diagnosis 119
high-altitude pulmonary hypertension 204
interstitial lung disease-associated pulmonary hypertension diagnosis 180
pulmonary hemodynamics studies 49
pulmonary veno-occlusive disease 154
right ventricular function 51–53
sickle cell disease pulmonary hypertension 137–140
Ecstasy (MDMA), pulmonary arterial hypertension induction 81
Edoxaban, venous thromboembolism management 222, 223
Eisenmenger syndrome
features 125
management 130, 132, 133

prognosis 134, 135
Electrocardiography
congenital heart disease-associated pulmonary arterial hypertension 126
high-altitude pulmonary hypertension 203
End-stage renal disease, pulmonary hypertension association 9
Endothelin-1 (ET-1)
pulmonary arterial hypertension marker 61
virus induction 110
Endothelin receptor antagonists, *see also* Bosentan
chronic thromboembolic pulmonary hypertension management 232, 233
congenital heart disease-associated pulmonary arterial hypertension management 132
connective tissue disease-associated pulmonary arterial hypertension management 99
efficacy in pulmonary arterial hypertension 241, 242
HIV-associated pulmonary arterial hypertension management 109
portopulmonary hypertension management 115, 116
ENG
hereditary hemorrhagic telangiectasia mutation 264, 265
pulmonary arterial hypertension mutation 66, 69
Epoprostenol, efficacy in pulmonary arterial hypertension 237, 238
Exercise hemodynamics, *see* Hemodynamics
Exercise-induced pulmonary hypertension
cardiac abnormalities 37, 38
exercise hemodynamics, *see* Hemodynamics
hemodynamics 25
Extracorporeal membrane oxygenation (ECMO), lung transplantation bridge therapy 250, 251

Fenfluramine, pulmonary arterial hypertension induction 78–80
Fondaparinux, venous thromboembolism management 219
Fractionated heparin, venous thromboembolism management 218, 219

Gaucher's disease, pulmonary hypertension association 8
Genetic counseling
hereditary hemorrhagic telangiectasia 263
heritable pulmonary arterial hypertension 70–72
Growth differentiation factor-15 (GDF-15), venous thromboembolism risk stratification 213

Heart-type fatty acid-binding protein (H-FABP), venous thromboembolism risk stratification 213
Hemodynamics
aging effects on resting pulmonary hemodynamics 28
chronic thromboembolic pulmonary hypertension 230
congenital heart disease-associated pulmonary arterial hypertension findings 127
end-expiratory pressure measurements 29
exercise hemodynamics
aging effects 28
exercise limitations in pulmonary artery hypertension 37, 38
incremental test characteristics in pulmonary artery hypertension 38, 39
left heart disease-associated pulmonary hypertension diagnosis 31–33
methodology 30, 31
normal adults 28, 37
pulmonary vascular disease effects 28, 29
role in catheter laboratory 31
high-altitude pulmonary hypertension 204
idiopathic pulmonary arterial hypertension 88
interstitial lung disease-associated pulmonary hypertension diagnosis 180, 181
invasive hemodynamics indications and utility 23, 24
noninvasive testing, *see also* Right ventricle
computed tomography 51
echocardiography 49
magnetic resonance imaging 50, 51
overview 48
prognostic study prospects 33, 34
pulmonary capillary wedge pressure
exercise capacity
diagnosis of pulmonary artery hypertension findings 43, 44
health-related quality of life 43
therapy of pulmonary artery hypertension findings 44
nonidiopathic pulmonary arterial hypertension testing 44, 45
normal values 30
screening for pulmonary artery hypertension 43
utility 30
pulmonary circulation physiology 24, 25, 48
pulmonary hypertension definition 25
pulmonary vascular reactivity testing 33
pulmonary vascular resistance equation 48
pulmonary veno-occlusive disease 152, 153
right heart catheterization
discriminative properties of tests 42
evaluative properties of tests 42, 43
rationale and relevance for testing in pulmonary artery hypertension 40, 42
safety 29
technique 29
walking test responses in pulmonary artery hypertension 39, 40
right ventricle adaptation to increased load 27
right ventricular afterload
impedance 26, 27
resistive load 25, 26
sickle cell disease pulmonary hypertension 139, 140
Heparin, venous thromboembolism management
low-molecular-weight heparins 219

unfractionated heparin 218, 219
Hepatopulmonary syndrome (HPS)
clinical presentation 118, 119
diagnosis
angiography 119
echocardiography 119
perfusion lung scanning 119
pulmonary function testing 119
epidemiology 117
hypoxemia mechanisms 118
management
liver transplantation 119
medical therapy 119
overview 113, 117
pathophysiology 117, 118
portopulmonary hypertension comparison 114
signaling pathway dysregulation 118
Hereditary hemorrhagic telangiectasia (HHT)
BMPR2 mutations, *see* Bone morphogenetic protein receptor type 2
classification 1–3, 67
clinical features
ACVRL1 mutation 72
BMPR2 mutation 72
overview 262
complications 263, 264
diagnosis 262, 263
gene mutations 1–3, 65, 66, 69
genetic counseling and testing 70–72
genetic testing and counseling 263
Heritable pulmonary arterial hypertension
linkage analysis 65, 66
pathogenesis
gene mutations 264, 265
genotype-phenotype correlation 265
signaling 265, 266
vessel abnormality development 266
prospects for study 72, 73
pulmonary hypertension
cardiac output and hyperdynamic state 272, 273
detection 272
pulmonary arterial hypertension 273, 274
High-altitude pulmonary hypertension (HAPH)
chest X-ray 204
definition 199–201
distribution 199
echocardiography 204
electrocardiography 203
epidemiology 201
genetics 203
hemodynamics 204
pathogenesis 202
pathology 201, 202
pathophysiology 202
physical examination 203
prospects for study 205
pulmonary function testing 203, 204
symptoms 203
treatment 204, 205
Human herpesvirus-8 (HHV-8), pulmonary arterial hypertension role 109, 110
Human immunodeficiency virus (HIV), pulmonary arterial hypertension association
cocaine synergy 107
diagnosis 107
epidemiology 105, 106
genetic predisposition 106
infection pathophysiology 106, 107
overview 4, 105
pathology 106
portal hypertension 107
prognostic factors 108
pulmonary veno-occlusive disease 107, 108
treatment
antiretroviral therapy 108
bosentan 109
calcium channel blockers 109
prostacyclin 109
sildenafil 109
supportive therapy 108
Hypoxia, pulmonary hypertension association 7

Idiopathic pulmonary arterial hypertension (IPAH)
China
diagnosis
acute pulmonary vasodilator testing 86
catheterization 86
differential diagnosis 86
registries 85, 86
treatment 86
classification 1
comparison between developed and developing countries
comorbidity 88, 90
demographics 87, 88
early detection 88
epidemiology 87
hemodynamics 88, 89
initial medications 89, 90
prognosis 90, 91
pulmonary veno-occlusive disease comparison 150, 157
Idiopathic pulmonary fibrosis (IPF), pulmonary hypertension
clinical impact 185, 186
diagnosis 185
epidemiology 183
pathogenesis 183–185
prognosis 186
treatment 186

Idrabiotaparinux, venous thromboembolism management 222
Idraparinux, venous thromboembolism management 222
Iloprost
  chronic thromboembolic pulmonary hypertension management 232
  efficacy in pulmonary arterial hypertension 241
Imatinib, connective tissue disease-associated pulmonary arterial hypertension management 100
Inferior vena cava filter, venous thromboembolism management 215
Interferon-α_2, pulmonary arterial hypertension induction 80
Interstitial lung disease (ILD), *see also specific diseases*
  classification 178, 179
  pulmonary hypertension
    classification 179
    diagnosis
      brain natriuretic peptide 181, 182
      computed tomography 181
      echocardiography 180
      hemodynamics 180, 181
      pulmonary function testing 182
    out of proportion pulmonary hypertension 179, 180
    treatment 182, 183
  connective tissue disease-related interstitial lung disease
    clinical impact 188
    diagnosis 188
    epidemiology 187
    overview 187
    pathogenesis 187, 188
    prognosis 188
    treatment 188
Invasive hemodynamics, *see* Hemodynamics

Left heart disease (LHD), pulmonary hypertension association
  heart failure
    diastolic heart failure 164, 165
    reduced left ventricular ejection fraction 162–164
  overview 6, 7, 161, 162
  pulmonary capillary wedge pressure studies 31–33
  valvular disease 166–168
Liver transplantation
  hepatopulmonary syndrome management 119
  portopulmonary hypertension management 116, 117, 120
Low-molecular-weight heparin (LMWH), venous thromboembolism management 219
Lung assist device, lung transplantation bridge therapy 251
Lung transplantation
  bridge therapy
    extracorporeal membrane oxygenation 250, 251
    lung assist device 251
    overview 249
  congenital heart disease-associated pulmonary arterial hypertension management 134
  connective tissue disease-associated pulmonary arterial hypertension management 101
  historical perspective 246, 247
  idiopathic pulmonary fibrosis-associated pulmonary hypertension 186
  indications in pulmonary arterial hypertension 247
  outcomes 248, 249
  patient selection 247
  postoperative management 251, 252
  pulmonary veno-occlusive disease 157
  types 247, 248
Lymphangioleiomyomatosis, pulmonary hypertension association 8

Magnetic resonance imaging (MRI)
  pulmonary hemodynamics studies 50, 51
  right ventricular function 53–56
Mazindol, pulmonary arterial hypertension induction 80
Mean pulmonary arterial pressure (mPAP)
  echocardiography 49
  exercise testing, *see* Hemodynamics
  magnetic resonance imaging 50
  pulmonary hypertension definition 25
Mediastinitis, pulmonary hypertension association 9
Methamphetamine, pulmonary arterial hypertension induction 81
Mitomycin-C, pulmonary arterial hypertension induction 82
Mitral valve disease, pulmonary hypertension association 166–168

Neurofibromatosis type 1, pulmonary hypertension association 8, 69, 70
Nitric oxide (NO)
  chronic obstructive pulmonary disease pulmonary hypertension management 175
  congenital heart disease-associated pulmonary arterial hypertension management 131, 133

Out of proportion pulmonary hypertension
  chronic obstructive pulmonary disease 173, 174
  interstitial lung disease 179, 180

Perfusion lung scanning
  chronic thromboembolic pulmonary hypertension 229
  hepatopulmonary syndrome diagnosis 119
Pergolide, pulmonary arterial hypertension induction 80
Phendimetrazine, pulmonary arterial hypertension induction 80
Phenformin, pulmonary arterial hypertension induction 80
Phenylpropanolamine, pulmonary arterial hypertension induction 80
Portopulmonary hypertension (PoPH)
  diagnostic criteria 113, 114
  epidemiology 114

hepatopulmonary syndrome comparison 114
management
endothelin receptor antagonists 115, 116
liver transplantation 116, 117, 120
overview 115
prostacyclin 116
sildenafil 116
overview 4
pathophysiology 114, 115
survival 117
Positron emission tomography (PET), right ventricular function 55, 56
Primary pulmonary arterial hypertension, *see* Idiopathic pulmonary arterial hypertension
Propylhexedrine, pulmonary arterial hypertension induction 80
Prostacyclin
analogs, *see specific analogs*
chronic thromboembolic pulmonary hypertension management 231, 232
congenital heart disease-associated pulmonary arterial hypertension management 131
connective tissue disease-associated pulmonary arterial hypertension management 98, 99
HIV-associated pulmonary arterial hypertension management 109
portopulmonary hypertension management 116
sickle cell disease pulmonary hypertension management 141
Pulmonary arterial hypertension (PAH)
arterial lesions
complex lesions 16–18
concentric laminar intimal fibrosis 16
inflammation 18, 19
intimal fibrosis 15, 16
medial hypertrophy 15
biomarkers, *see* Biomarkers, pulmonary arterial hypertension
classification 1–5
hemodynamics, *see* Hemodynamics
histology 14
medical treatment, *see also specific therapies*
combination therapy 243
endothelin receptor antagonists 241, 242
phosphodiesterase inhibitors 242, 243
prospects 276–278
prostanoids 237–241
supportive therapy 243, 244
venous lesions 19–21
Pulmonary arterial pressure, *see* Mean pulmonary arterial pressure
Pulmonary arteriovenous malformation (PAVM)
children 272
clinical manifestations and complications 267, 268
definition 266
imaging 268, 269
pregnancy 271, 272
prevalence 266
right-to-left shunting assessment 269, 270
treatment 270, 271
Pulmonary artery banding, congenital heart disease-associated pulmonary arterial hypertension management 130
Pulmonary artery sarcoma, pulmonary hypertension association 9
Pulmonary capillary hemangiomatosis (PCH)
classification 5, 6
vascular lesions
arterial 15
venous 20
Pulmonary capillary wedge pressure (PCWP), *see also* Hemodynamics
left heart disease-associated pulmonary hypertension diagnosis 31–33
normal values 30
pulmonary hypertension definition 25
pulmonary veno-occlusive disease 152, 153
utility 30
Pulmonary endarterectomy (PEA)
chronic thromboembolic pulmonary hypertension management 230
surgical technique 230, 231
Pulmonary hemodynamics, *see* Hemodynamics
Pulmonary hypertension, *see specific conditions*
Pulmonary Langerhans cell histiocytosis (PLCH), pulmonary hypertension association
clinical impact 194
diagnosis 194
epidemiology 192
overview 8, 192
pathogenesis 192, 194
prognosis 194
treatment 194, 195
Pulmonary vascular resistance, *see* Hemodynamics
Pulmonary veno-occlusive disease (PVOD)
classification 5, 6
clinical presentation 151
diagnosis
acute vasodilator testing 153, 154
bronchoalveolar lavage 155
computed tomography 154
echocardiography 154
hemodynamics 152, 153
histopathology 151, 152
pulmonary function testing 154, 155
epidemiology 149–151
five-year review 157, 158
idiopathic pulmonary arterial hypertension comparison 150, 157
overview 149
prognosis 155

treatment
conventional therapy 155, 156
immunomodulation 156, 157
lung transplantation 157
pulmonary arterial hypertension therapies 156
vascular lesions
arterial 15
venous 20
Pyrrolizidine alkaloids, pulmonary arterial hypertension induction 81, 82

Rheumatoid arthritis (RA), pulmonary arterial hypertension association 98
Rho kinase, therapeutic targeting in pulmonary arterial hypertension 277
Right ventricle
adaptation to increased load 27
afterload
impedance 26, 27
resistive load 25, 26
catheterization, *see also* Hemodynamics
safety 29
technique 29
noninvasive imaging of function
echocardiography 51–53
magnetic resonance imaging 53
prognostic relevance and therapeutic sensitivity 53, 54
structure and function 55, 56
pulmonary arterial hypertension pathophysiology 254, 255
venous thromboembolism risk stratification and dysfunction 212, 213
Rivaroxaban, venous thromboembolism management 222, 223

Saint John's wort, pulmonary arterial hypertension induction 81
Sarcoidosis, pulmonary hypertension association
clinical impact 191
diagnosis 191
epidemiology 188, 189
overview 8, 188
pathogenesis 188–191
prognosis 191
treatment 191–193
Schistosomiasis, pulmonary arterial hypertension association
clinical features 146, 147
diagnosis 146, 147
epidemiology 143, 144
life cycle of parasite 144
overview 4
pathophysiology 144–146
treatment 147
Serotonin system, therapeutic targeting in pulmonary arterial hypertension 277
Sickle cell disease (SCD), pulmonary hypertension
clinical presentation 138, 140
crisis and pulmonary pressures 140
epidemiology 138
hemodynamics 139, 140
overview 137
pathophysiology
hemolysis 140
thrombosis 141
screening 140
treatment 141
Sildenafil
chronic thromboembolic pulmonary hypertension management 233
congenital heart disease-associated pulmonary arterial hypertension management 132
connective tissue disease-associated pulmonary arterial hypertension management 99, 100
efficacy in pulmonary arterial hypertension 242, 243
HIV-associated pulmonary arterial hypertension management 109
portopulmonary hypertension management 116
sickle cell disease pulmonary hypertension management 141
Sitaxsentan, congenital heart disease-associated pulmonary arterial hypertension management 132
Sjögren's syndrome, pulmonary arterial hypertension association 98
Smad8, mutation in pulmonary arterial hypertension 69
Statins, therapeutic prospects in pulmonary arterial hypertension 277
Systemic lupus erythematosus (SLE), pulmonary arterial hypertension association 97, 98
Systemic sclerosis, pulmonary arterial hypertension association
clinical features 96
early diagnosis 97
epidemiology 95
pathophysiology 95, 96
prognosis 97
risk factors 96
treatment 98–101

Tadlafil, efficacy in pulmonary arterial hypertension 243
Thalidomide, pulmonary arterial hypertension induction 80
Thyroid disease, pulmonary hypertension association 8
Toxic rapeseed oil, pulmonary arterial hypertension induction 82
Treprostinil
chronic thromboembolic pulmonary hypertension management 232
efficacy in pulmonary arterial hypertension 238–240
Tricuspid annular plane systolic excursion (TAPSE), right ventricular function 51, 56
Tricuspid regurgitation (TRV)
mean pulmonary arterial pressure estimation 49
sickle cell disease pulmonary hypertension 137–140

Troponins
  pulmonary arterial hypertension marker 60
  venous thromboembolism risk stratification 213
Tryptophan, pulmonary arterial hypertension induction 8

Ultrasonography
  echocardiography, *see* Echocardiography
  venous thromboembolism diagnosis with compression ultrasonography 210
Uric acid (UA), pulmonary arterial hypertension marker 59

Vasoactive intestinal polypeptide (VIP), therapeutic prospects in pulmonary arterial hypertension 277
Venous thromboembolism (VTE)
  biomarkers for risk stratification
    brain natriuretic peptide 213
    growth differentiation factor-15 213
    heart-type fatty acid-binding protein 213
    right ventricular dysfunction 212, 213
    troponins 213
  diagnosis
    algorithms 211, 212
    clinical probability 208, 209
    compression ultrasonography 210
    computed tomography 210, 211
    D-dimer testing 209
  frequency 207
  long-term outcomes
    mortality 215
    persistent perfusion defects 216
    recurrence 215, 216
  risk factors
    cancer 207, 208
    genetics 208
    hormone replacement therapy and oral contraceptives 208
    pregnancy 207
  risk prediction for recurrence and bleeding 224
  treatment
    anticoagulant development
      apixaban 222, 223
      challenges 223
      dabigatran 221, 222
      edoxaban 222, 223
      idrabiotaparinux 222
      idraparinux 222
      rivaroxaban 222, 223
    cancer patients 220
    duration of anticoagulant therapy 220
    fondaparinux 219
    heparin
      low-molecular-weight heparins 219
      unfractionated heparin 218, 219
    home treatment 214, 215
    inferior vena cava filter 215
    initiation 219, 220
    personalized care 223, 224
    pregnant patients 220, 221
    prospects and study design 221
    thrombolytic therapy overview 214
    vitamin K antagonists 219
Vitamin K antagonists, venous thromboembolism management 219
Von Willebrand factor, pulmonary arterial hypertension marker 61

Warfarin, *see* Vitamin K antagonists